▼▼▼▼

CURRENT
VETERINARY
DERMATOLOGY

The Science and Art of Therapy

▼ ▼ ▼ ▼

CURRENT
VETERINARY
DERMATOLOGY

The Science and Art of Therapy

CRAIG E. GRIFFIN, D.V.M.
Diplomate, American College of
Veterinary Dermatology
Animal Dermatology Clinic
San Diego, California

KENNETH W. KWOCHKA, D.V.M.
Diplomate, American College of
Veterinary Dermatology
Associate Professor of Dermatology
Chief, Dermatology Service
Department of Veterinary Clinical Sciences
College of Veterinary Medicine
The Ohio State University
Columbus, Ohio

JOHN M. MACDONALD, D.V.M.
Diplomate, American College of
Veterinary Dermatology
Associate Professor
Department of Small Animal Surgery and Medicine
College of Veterinary Medicine
Auburn University
Auburn, Alabama

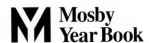

St. Louis Baltimore Boston Chicago London Philadelphia Sydney Toronto

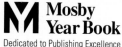

Mosby Year Book
Dedicated to Publishing Excellence

Publisher: George Stamathis
Editor: Robert W. Reinhardt
Assistant Editor: Susie H. Baxter
Production Editor: George B. Stericker, Jr.
Designer: Julie Taugner

Printed in the United States of America

Mosby–Year Book, Inc.
11830 Westline Industrial Drive
St. Louis, Missouri 63146

Library of Congress Cataloging in Publication Data

Current veterinary dermatology / [compiled by] Craig E. Griffin,
  Kenneth W. Kwochka, John M. MacDonald.
     p.   cm.
   ISBN 0-8016-3384-2
   1. Dogs—Diseases.   2. Cats—Diseases.   3. Veterinary dermatology.
 I. Griffin, Craig E.   II. Kwochka, Kenneth W.   III. MacDonald, John M.
 SF992.S55C87   1992
 636.7089′65—dc20
                                                               92-7164
                                                                 CIP

92 93 94 95 96 GW/WA/WA 9 8 7 6 5 4 3 2 1

Contributors

DONNA WALTON ANGARANO, D.V.M.
Diplomate, American College of Veterinary
  Dermatology
Associate Professor
Department of Small Animal Surgery and
  Medicine
College of Veterinary Medicine
Auburn University
Auburn, Alabama

HAZEL C. CARNEY, D.V.M., M.S.
Feline Medical Clinic
Baton Rouge, Louisiana

CAROL S. FOIL, D.V.M., M.S.
Diplomate, American College of Veterinary
  Dermatology
Associate Professor
Department of Veterinary Clinical Sciences
School of Veterinary Medicine
Louisiana State University
Baton Rouge, Louisiana

CRAIG E. GRIFFIN, D.V.M.
Diplomate, American College of Veterinary
  Dermatology
Animal Dermatology Clinic
San Diego, California

ROBERT J. KEMPPAINEN, D.V.M., Ph.D.
Director, Endocrine Diagnostic Laboratory
Associate Professor
Department of Physiology and Pharmacology
College of Veterinary Medicine
Auburn University
Auburn, Alabama

KENNETH W. KWOCHKA, D.V.M.
Diplomate, American College of Veterinary
  Dermatology
Associate Professor of Dermatology
Chief, Dermatology Service
Department of Veterinary Clinical Sciences
College of Veterinary Medicine
The Ohio State University
Columbus, Ohio

JOHN M. MACDONALD, D.V.M.
Diplomate, American College of Veterinary
  Dermatology
Associate Professor
Department of Small Animal Surgery and
  Medicine
College of Veterinary Medicine
Auburn University
Auburn, Alabama

KENNETH V. MASON, M.VSc.
Fellow, Australian College of Veterinary
  Scientists (Dermatology)
Albert Animal Hospital
Springwood, Queensland
Australia

KAREN A. MORIELLO, D.V.M.
Diplomate, American College of Veterinary
  Dermatology
Clinical Associate Professor of Dermatology
Department of Medical Sciences
School of Veterinary Medicine
University of Wisconsin
Madison, Wisconsin

WAYNE S. ROSENKRANTZ, D.V.M.
Diplomate, American College of Veterinary
  Dermatology
Animal Dermatology Clinic
Garden Grove, California

EDMUND J. ROSSER JR, D.V.M.
Diplomate, American College of Veterinary
    Dermatology
Associate Professor of Dermatology
Department of Small Animal Clinical Sciences
College of Veterinary Medicine
Michigan State University
East Lansing, Michigan

CAROLE A. ZERBE, D.V.M.
Assistant Professor of Medicine
Department of Clinical Studies
School of Veterinary Medicine
University of Pennsylvania
Philadelphia, Pennsylvania

For **Tricia**
(CEG)

For **Joshua**
(KWK)

For **April, Kristin, Julia,** *and* **Claire**
and
To **Marni Lazear,**
who is a source of inspiration to all,
through the dedicated treatment by her owners,
Bob *and* **Marylyn**
(JMM)

Preface

This book evolved from our recognition of a need for a reference text for practicing veterinarians that would serve as a comprehensive yet practical resource in diagnosing and treating dermatologic diseases of small animals. The path we followed from conception to the final text was truly an educational experience. We made a concerted effort to present information based on the actual mental and physical processes of diagnosis, treatment, and total case management that we utilize in our practices.

Early in the development of the book we decided to work closely with our contributors to achieve a comprehensive viewpoint for each chapter that would represent a collection of the experiences of all authors and editors rather than one individual's viewpoint. Although this was more time-consuming, we think the effort has been well worth it.

As the body of knowledge in dermatology has expanded, an ever-increasing challenge has arisen to select the most clinically relevant information. Our intention was to write not a "textbook" but a clinical guide on selected topics. These topics were chosen because they are common in routine practice or represent areas where new and important information has become available.

There are three basic types of chapters in the book. The first (1, 2, 4 to 15, 20, 21, and 25 to 30) focuses on a specific disease. The second (16, 17, 22 to 24, 31, and 32) provides an overview of clinical examination findings or problems (with emphasis on the differential diagnosis). The third (3, 18, and 19) concentrates on a treatment or therapeutic modality used in handling common clinical problems.

Most chapters are organized into introductory, clinical disease, diagnosis, and treatment sections. The **introductory** material covers such features as the importance of the disease to the practitioner and discusses relevant or new information regarding its pathogenesis. The **clinical disease** section provides a comprehensive account of historical and physical examination findings pertinent to the disease. Emphasis is placed on the features most valuable in suggesting a differential for the patient's clinical problem. In the **diagnosis** section tests and procedures are covered. In the **treatment** section the preferred regimen is presented and, where appropriate, a variety of options. Many treatments suggested are actually plans for management rather than mere discussions of a single drug.

We recognize that in practice a definitive diagnosis cannot always be established due to client restraints or poor access to the required tests and procedures. To assist the reader in developing as strong a diagnosis as possible, boxes have been positioned on the first page of each chapter listing findings that are suggestive of the disease, compatible with its diagnosis, and finally (in the editors' and authors' opinion) necessary for a tentative or definitive diagnosis. Chapters that review specific clinical problems or findings contain a list of differential diagnoses (instead of the diagnostic criteria) to provide a basis for logical diagnostic pursuit. Chapters that focus on specific therapeutic agents contain a list of those drugs with indications for their use. Finally, a formulary of dermatologic drugs, diagnostic procedures, and recommended techniques appears in Appendixes A and B. Drugs are listed in alphabetical order (for easy location), along with the name(s) of their manufacturer(s) and their dosages, indications, and common side effects. Manufacturers' addresses are provided in Appendix C.

We hope that this text proves useful in the diagnosis and treatment of dermatologic diseases for the practicing veterinarian and that it is useful as a practical introduction to clinical veterinary dermatology for veterinary students. We could not have accomplished the project without the knowledge and help of many veterinary dermatologists and practicing veterinarians around the world. To them we are grateful. We are especially indebted to all the contributors, who unselfishly provided

their expertise in respective areas. We wish to
thank, in particular, our mentors and friends Richard Anderson, Richard Halliwell, Peter Ihrke, Robert Kirk, Gail Kunkle, Danny Scott, and Tony Stannard, who have been a source of inspiration and
motivation in our pursuit of the science of veterinary dermatology. The culmination of their inspiration is this book.

Craig Griffin
Kenneth Kwochka
John MacDonald

Contents

Notice

Every effort has been made to ensure that the drug dosage schedules and current therapy contained herein are accurate and in accord with the standards accepted at the time of publication. However, as new research and experience broaden our knowledge, changes in treatment and drug therapy occur. Therefore, the reader is advised **to check the product information sheet included in the package of each drug or vaccine he/she plans to administer** to be certain that changes have not been made in the recommended dose or in the contraindications. This is of particular importance in regard to new or infrequently used drugs.

Infectious Diseases

1

Recurrent Pyoderma

Kenneth W. Kwochka

Differential Diagnosis of Pyoderma and Major Causes of Recurrent Pyoderma in Dogs

DIFFERENTIAL FOR SUPERFICIAL PYODERMA LESIONS

Demodicosis, dermatophytosis, drug eruptions, chronic allergic dermatoses, pemphigus foliaceus, pemphigus erythematosus, subcorneal pustular dermatosis, sterile eosinophilic pustulosis, linear IgA dermatosis

DIFFERENTIAL FOR DEEP PYODERMA LESIONS

Foreign body granulomas, mycotic granulomas, sterile granulomas, panniculitis, vasculitis, cutaneous neoplastic disorders

PRURITIC CAUSES OF RECURRENT PYODERMA

Flea allergy dermatitis, atopy, food allergy dermatitis, canine scabies, cheyletiellosis

NONPRURITIC CAUSES OF RECURRENT PYODERMA

Hypothyroidism, hyperadrenocorticism, reproductive hormone imbalances, idiopathic keratinization defects, canine demodicosis, severe metabolic diseases, immune system abnormalities, chronic steroid administration, environmental factors, poor nutritional status, idiopathic chronic recurrent pyoderma

---

Importance

Pyoderma is commonly defined as a pyogenic or pus-producing bacterial infection of the skin. The classic primary lesion is a pustule or draining tract with purulent exudate. Unfortunately, this information can be confusing and misleading in a clinical setting because the pustular or purulent lesion may be visible only by histologic examination. There is a great degree of variation in the cutaneous lesions seen at the time of presentation in dogs. It is important to be familiar with the multitude of clinical presentations of the disease. Additionally, there are nonbacterial causes of pustular lesions, which may add further complexity to establishing the diagnosis.

Recurrent pyoderma is a chronic relapsing bacterial infection of the skin usually associated with an underlying predisposing disease. The bacterial infection can be cleared with a proper antibiotic and topical antibacterial therapy but recurs, usually rapidly, after discontinuation of treatment. Recurrent pyoderma is associated with such a long list of underlying diseases that the diagnostic approach is complex. Adding to this complexity is the fact that many dogs with pyoderma are pruritic. It must be determined whether the pruritus is due to the pyoderma itself or associated with the underlying predisposing disease. **Any plan for controlling the pyoderma without serious consideration of the predisposing diseases will fail.** However, there are cases in which a diligent search does not reveal a cause for the recurrent pyoderma. The practitioner at this point still has treatment options for long-term successful management of the patient.

Pyoderma is one of the most common and frustrating dermatoses seen by veterinarians in small animal practice. One study (Sischo et al., 1989) revealed it to be the second most common inflammatory skin disorder diagnosed in dogs in the United States, behind only flea allergy dermatitis. In fact, many flea allergy cases will also be complicated by secondary pyoderma.

Successful management of recurrent pyoderma requires (1) recognition of its various clinical manifestations, (2) formulation of a logical differential diagnosis and diagnostic plan for potential predisposing diseases, and (3) development of a rational therapeutic plan that will control the pyoderma and the predisposing disease.

Pathogenesis

Coagulase-positive *Staphylococcus intermedius* is the infective organism most frequently associated with canine pyoderma. *Staphylococcus aureus*, the most common pathogen in human cutaneous infections, is implicated in a low number of cases. *S. intermedius* is not considered of public health significance for humans. Although there are biochemical differences between the two species, antibiotic susceptibility test patterns are similar; thus the same antibiotics can be used on an empirical basis. Gram-negative bacteria such as *Proteus* spp, *Pseudomonas* spp, and *Escherichia coli* may be found as secondary invaders with pyoderma.

Identification of a specific carriage site of the pathogenic bacteria on dogs would be helpful in therapeutic management of recurrent pyoderma, but such a site has not been definitively determined for *S. intermedius*. Reports have suggested that coagulase-positive staphylococci are normally carried on the hair coat, providing a source of infectious organisms for the skin under appropriate conditions (White et al., 1983; Cox et al., 1988). However, long-term quantitative studies have not been conducted to differentiate between persistent colonization and contamination from external sources, particularly in exposed areas such as the hair coat.

Normal skin has a number of primary physical and immunologic defense mechanisms against pathogenic bacterial invasion. These include the hair coat, epidermal turnover with exfoliation, the stratum corneum, epidermal lipids, sebum, immunoglobulins, interferon, and normal nonpathogenic skin flora. Very little information is available about the microclimate at the skin surface of dogs and how changes in this climate might affect the development of cutaneous infections. No doubt, some dogs develop seasonal pyoderma associated with environmental factors, especially increases in temperature and humidity. Recent work (Chesney,

1990) has shown that deep in the hair coat near the skin surface the temperature is high (37° C) but in the sun this temperature rises even further to 43° C. The pH of the skin surface in the dorsal lumbosacral area of 40 kennel dogs was found to range from 6 to 10 (Chesney, 1990). The skin surface appears to be a very moist area with high ambient relative humidity affected by many factors including rain, sun, wind, saliva, glandular secretions, and foreign material. At least 11 species of coagulase-negative staphylococci that likely contribute to normal defense mechanisms have been isolated on the skin surface of normal dogs (Kwochka, 1986).

Pathophysiologic mechanisms important in the establishment of skin infection at the cellular and biochemical level are largely unknown. There may be anatomic and physiologic factors in the epidermis of dogs versus other species that predispose to bacterial infections (Mason and Lloyd, 1990). The stratum corneum is thinner and more compact than that of other species and may contain less intercellular material. There is also no obvious lipid seal at the hair follicle infundibula.

Microorganisms must become attached to the epithelial cell surface before an infection can occur. After attachment the bacteria multiply to large numbers, colonize the skin, penetrate to the deeper layers, and release various toxins that cause tissue damage and clinical disease. A canine corneocyte bacterial adherence assay has been developed (McEwan, 1990). Dogs with atopic disease and dogs with pyoderma were shown to have a significantly higher adherence of *S. intermedius* to corneocytes than were seborrheic or normal dogs. This may partially explain the predisposition of atopic dogs to development of secondary pyoderma.

Local cutaneous hypersensitivity reactions may promote the penetration of bacterial antigens from the stratum corneum into the dermis, leading to cutaneous damage. A quantitative study of penetration of staphylococcal protein A, an important bacterial toxin, through canine skin under experimentally induced inflammation (intradermal histamine injections) was conducted by Mason and Lloyd (1990). These workers found that the absorption of protein A was enhanced by prior injection of histamine, supporting the hypothesis that release of inflammatory mediators from mast cells during hypersensitivity reactions may facilitate percutaneous absorption of staphylococcal products and lead to the development of pyoderma. This again may explain the high incidence of secondary pyoderma in allergic diseases.

Pyoderma should always be considered a secondary clinical manifestation of an underlying primary problem. In most cases the pathophysiologic cause of the secondary pyoderma has not been established. Some common predisposing causes include environmental factors (high temperature and humidity), allergic dermatitides (including flea allergy, atopy, and food allergy), endocrinopathies (hypothyroidism, hyperadrenocorticism, sex hormone abnormalities), poor nutritional status, immunologic incompetency (sometimes related to neoplasia), idiopathic keratinization defects, ectoparasites (demodicosis, scabies, cheyletiellosis), and inappropriate prior therapy such as the excessive use of glucocorticoids. The major predisposing factors in most parts of the United States are allergic dermatitis and long-term administration of glucocorticoids.

"Bacterial hypersensitivity" has been implicated in the pathogenesis of recurrent superficial pyoderma in humans and dogs. Elevated antistaphylococcal IgE has been detected in human patients with recurrent superficial skin infections. Dogs with circular, expanding, severely erythematous lesions with extreme pruritus have often been thought to have "bacterial hypersensitivity." Animals with recurrent pyoderma and such lesions were shown to have elevations in antistaphylococcal IgG and IgE (Halliwell and Gorman, 1989). This syndrome needs further study as regards pathophysiology and treatment.

CLINICAL DISEASE

There are two general causes for poor response to therapy and the development of a chronic recurrent pyoderma. First is the failure to recognize the presence and severity of the bacterial infection and to treat it correctly on initial presentation. Second is the failure to recognize predisposing factors and primary diseases that precipitated the relapsing infection.

Lesions of Recurrent Pyoderma

A number of clinical classification systems have been used for cutaneous bacterial infections. The most useful is based on depth of the infection within the skin. This system directly influences selection of the type and duration of appropriate therapy. Surface pyodermas are not true infections but superficial erosions of the skin with associated increased colonization of pathogenic staphylococci. Superficial pyodermas are true infections in which the epidermis (impetigo) or hair follicles (folliculitis) are involved without extension into the dermis. Deep pyodermas extend into the dermis and in some cases to the subcutaneous tissue. This classification is discussed more extensively in another review paper (White and Ihrke, 1987).

Recurrent Superficial Pyoderma

There are certain types of lesions that increase the suspicion that a pyoderma is present. Folliculitis is the most common clinical type of recurrent pyoderma. In its active erupting stage the lesions consist of papules and pustules associated with hair follicles. Papules are more common, since the pustules are fragile and transient and quickly become crusted when traumatized (Fig. 1-1). On close inspection it is not unusual to see a hair protruding from the middle of the lesion, indicating active inflammation and infection of the follicle. Nonfollicular papules may also be present, since many cases of recurrent superficial pyoderma are associated with allergy. If the lesions are diffuse, there may also be generalized erythroderma (Fig. 1-2). Active folliculitis lesions usually have mild to severe pruritus.

In many cases, especially if antiinflammatory medication has been used, it is more common to see advanced resolving lesions or what have been referred to as "footprint" lesions of folliculitis. These include mutifocal areas of postinflammatory (postinfection) hyperpigmentation, a "moth-eaten" alopecia (Fig. 1-3), and bull's-eye-type lesions (characterized by focal alopecia, central hyperpigmentation, epidermal collarettes, and a halo of erythema) (Fig. 1-4). Very chronic lesions with associated pruritus and self-trauma will appear as crusted, hyperpigmented, lichenified plaques that may involve large areas of the skin surface.

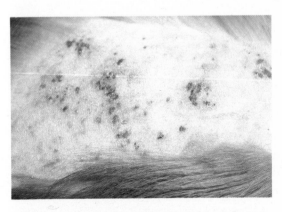

Figure 1-1. Papules, pustules, erythema, and crusts on the trunk of a Golden Retriever with superficial staphylococcal folliculitis. Prior to clipping, these type of lesions can usually be palpated more easily than they can be visualized.

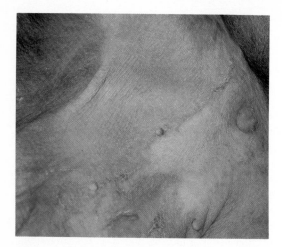

Figure 1-2. Diffuse erythroderma, alopecia, and scaling on the ventrum of a Shetland Sheepdog with superficial staphylococcal folliculitis secondary to hypothyroidism.

The clinical lesions seen on presentation may be related to the coat type. Short-coated breeds, such as Dalmatians and English Bulldogs, generally have papules, multifocal alopecia, and a moth-eaten appearance of the hair coat. In dogs on steroids and in Chinese Shar-Peis there may be no active lesions present but simply the "footprints" of the pyoderma. In long-coated breeds it is more common to part the hair and see pustules along with papules, hyperpigmented macules, and bull's-eye-type lesions.

Recurrent superficial pyoderma may have any distribution from focal to generalized, but it is most common for lesions to be regionalized and related to the underlying primary disease. Most dogs have an allergic skin condition as the primary cause. Flea-allergic animals usually have secondary folliculitis of the dorsal lumbosacral area, ventral abdomen, and medial thighs. Atopic dogs commonly have lesions involving the ventral abdomen, axillae, and extremities. The face may also be involved in some atopic dogs, especially the short-coated breeds. Animals with food allergy will have a more varied distribution of lesions. Dogs that have a secondary folliculitis associated with endocrinopathies, metabolic diseases, immune system dysfunction, and idiopathy tend to have a more generalized distribution of lesions involving the trunk.

Recurrent Deep Pyoderma

Chronic recurrent deep pyoderma is less commonly encountered in practice than is recurrent superficial pyoderma. However, the disease is more debilitating and harder to control, and it can be life-threatening if septicemia develops, especially

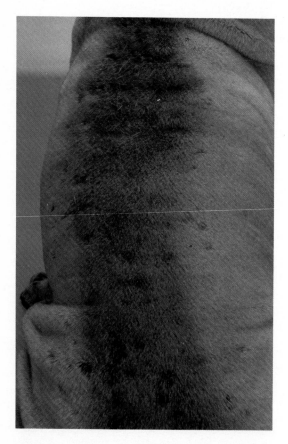

Figure 1-3. "Moth-eaten" pattern of alopecia on the dorsum of a Chinese Shar Pei with superficial staphylococcal folliculitis.

(Courtesy Dr. Patricia White, Columbus, Ohio.)

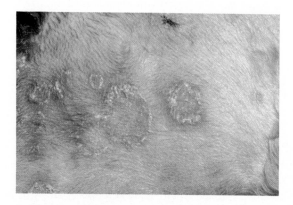

Figure 1-4. Multiple "bull's-eye-type" lesions characterized by alopecia, central hyperpigmentation, epidermal collarettes, and a "halo" of erythema on the trunk of a mixed breed dog with superficial staphylococcal folliculitis.

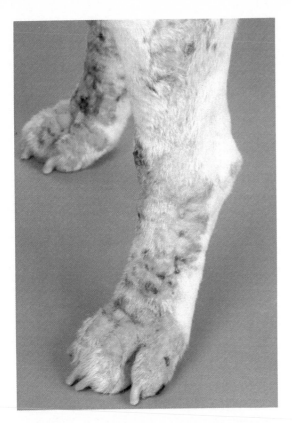

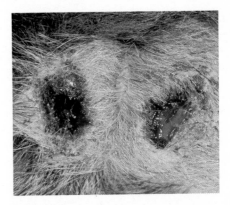

Figure 1-6. Crusted lesion (left) and ulcerated, necrotic lesion with a purulent exudate after crust removed (right) on the trunk of a German Shepherd Dog with deep pyoderma due to *Pseudomonas aeruginosa*.

(Courtesy Dr. Patricia White, Columbus, Ohio.)

Figure 1-5. Multiple alopecic nodular lesions draining a hemorrhagic and purulent exudate on the leg and foot of a Bull Terrier with deep staphylococcal pyoderma.

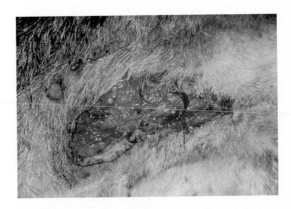

Figure 1-7. Large ulcerated cellulitis lesion with extensive tissue necrosis down to muscle on the lateral thigh of a German Shepherd Dog with deep pyoderma due to *Pseudomonas aeruginosa*.

(Courtesy Dr. Patricia White, Columbus, Ohio.)

if secondarily complicated by gram-negative bacteria.

Chronic relapsing deep pyoderma is more common in short-coated breeds probably due to an intense foreign body reaction to keratin from ruptured infected follicles pushed into the dermis by the short stubby hair shafts. Deep pyoderma lesions are characterized by red or purple, raised, nodules from which blood and purulent exudate can be expressed (Fig. 1-5). Fistulous tracts may form, and the tissue may become necrotic and extremely friable. Older "footprint" lesions consist of multifocal, tightly adherent crusts that when removed reveal ulcerated, necrotic skin (Fig. 1-6). Such lesions are usually not pruritic but are painful for the dog. Cellulitis may also develop in which the infection and inflammation dissect through tissue planes resulting in diffuse massive swelling, edema, erythema, ulceration, tissue necrosis, multiple draining tracks, and high fever (Fig. 1-7).

It is most common to see recurrent deep pyoderma in large short-coated breeds and in a generalized distribution. However, more localized areas of the body may be affected in different breeds. Recurrent deep pyoderma of the chin and lips is seen primarily in Doberman Pinschers, Great Danes, and English Bulldogs. Other short-coated breeds such as Dalmatians, Bull Terriers, and American Staffordshire Terriers develop a pressure point deep pyoderma. The lesions are most common over the hock and elbow joints. Interdigital pyoderma is also most often seen in short-coated breeds. Lesions consist of erythema, nodules (interdigital abscesses, interdigital "cysts"), fistulas, ulcers, severe swelling, moist dermatitis, pain, and peripheral lymphadenopathy. German Shepherd

Dogs develop a severe deep pyoderma of the hind limbs and dorsal lumbosacral area.

Pruritus and Recurrent Pyoderma

Most cases of chronic recurrent superficial pyoderma have a history of pruritus. In fact, the primary presenting complaint is usually pruritus. A complete history may help determine if the pruritus is due only to the pyoderma or whether a concurrent underlying pruritic skin disease is present. It is important to establish exactly when the pruritus developed in the course of the disease so a logical diagnostic plan can be formulated. If pruritus was the initial clinical sign before skin lesions were noticed, or if significant pruritus remains when existing pyoderma has cleared with antibiotics and topical therapy, then pruritic causes of pyoderma (e.g., allergic diseases and ectoparasites) should be considered. If, however, pruritus developed after skin lesions were present, if it clears *completely* when the pyoderma has been treated, or if the pyoderma is nonpruritic, then nonpruritic causes of recurrent pyoderma such as the endocrinopathies and metabolic diseases should be eliminated from the list of differentials.

Another important aspect of the history in helping to make a diagnosis of pyoderma and determine the role of pruritus is the response to previous medications, especially antibiotics and steroids. If proper antibiotic therapy has been used without steroids and the owner reports full recovery (skin lesions and pruritus completely resolve) while on treatment but recurrence shortly after discontinuation of therapy, then nonpruritic causes of recurrent pyoderma should be considered. If, however, the owner reports only partial improvement, with pruritus remaining, then pruritic causes of recurrent pyoderma should be considered.

Initial use of corticosteroids as sole therapy or use of corticosteroids in addition to antibiotics to control inflammation and pruritus associated with pyoderma makes assessment of clinical response difficult. Steroids will not allow the veterinarian to judge the pruritic component of the pyoderma in order to establish a logical list of differentials. The pyoderma will quickly improve because of the antiinflammatory effects of steroids, but relapses with combined therapy are more common and will be more severe. In fact, a simple first-occurrence pyoderma may be made into a chronic relapsing pyoderma due to chronic steroid usage.

Differential Diagnosis

The diagnosis of pyoderma is usually made by a combination of history, clinical lesions, cytology, and response to antibiotics. Culture and susceptibility testing and biopsies may also be needed in some cases. Although the vast majority of papular, pustular, and bull's-eye-type lesions are associated with superficial pyoderma, important differentials include demodicosis, dermatophytosis, drug eruptions, chronic allergic dermatoses, pemphigus foliaceus, pemphigus erythematosus, subcorneal pustular dermatosis, sterile eosinophilic pustulosis, and linear IgA dermatosis. Primary differentials for deep pyoderma lesions include foreign body, mycotic and sterile granulomas, panniculitis, vasculitis, and cutaneous neoplastic disorders.

The more important lists of differentials are diseases and factors that may contribute to the development of chronic recurrent pyoderma.

Pruritic Causes of Recurrent Pyoderma

These are the primary diseases that most commonly cause chronic recurrent superficial pyoderma. They include allergic and parasitic dermatoses. Flea allergy, atopy, and food allergy are all associated with recurrent pyoderma. Canine scabies and cheyletiellosis are less commonly complicated by secondary infection.

Nonpruritic Causes of Recurrent Pyoderma

Nonpruritic diseases may lead to recurrent superficial pyoderma and are the most common causes of chronic recurrent deep pyoderma. They include endocrinopathies such as hypothyroidism, hyperadrenocorticism, and reproductive hormone imbalances. Most of the idiopathic keratinization defects and canine demodicosis are also nonpruritic until complicated by a secondary pyoderma. This is also the category for pyoderma associated with severe metabolic diseases, pyoderma associated with immune system abnormalities, and idiopathic recurrent pyoderma.

Additional Factors

Although not diseases per se, other factors to consider as possibly contributing to chronic recurrent pyoderma include inappropriate previous usage of antibiotics, environmental factors such as high temperature and humidity, poor grooming practices, poor nutritional status, and excessive use of glucocorticoids.

DIAGNOSIS

A diagnosis of pyoderma is usually made in practice by observing the response to antibiotics and topical antibacterial therapy without any diagnostic techniques employed. No tests are needed for a "simple," first-occurrence, superficial pyoderma. However, there are techniques that will be helpful in certain clinical situations.

Diagnostic Techniques

It is usually easy to make a diagnosis of superficial or deep pyoderma when pustules are present or when there is a productive purulent lesion. However, classical lesions are not always present and all pustules are not always due to pyoderma.

Cytology

If classical-type lesions are present, then smears should be made of purulent exudate and stained with a modified Wright's stain (Diff-Quik) or Gram stain. A supportive finding for pyoderma is cellular exudate consisting primarily of healthy and degenerative neutrophils with intracellular and extracellular cocci. In older superficial lesions and in deep lesions it may at times be difficult to actually find cocci. Eosinophils are occasionally seen in the exudate from deep lesions. Large numbers of acantholytic keratinocytes from pustular contents should arouse suspicion that an autoimmune disease may be present, especially if there has been poor response to previous antibiotics. Cytologic findings compatible with pyoderma are enough information to start antibiotic therapy on an empirical basis.

Culture and Susceptibility

Bacterial culture and susceptibility tests are not necessary on the first visit with a mild, previously untreated pyoderma. If an antibiotic has been chosen empirically and response has been excellent, culture is also not needed. In fact, most cases even of recurrent pyoderma can be successfully diagnosed and managed without ever performing a culture. When cost is a consideration, it is probably more valuable to spend the client's money on diagnostics for the underlying disease than on routine culture and susceptibility testing.

Culture and susceptibility testing is useful in suspected pyodermas that fail to respond to empirical antibiotics, when there is a question about the presence of pyoderma because of atypical or unusual clinical lesions, when chronic antibiotic therapy is being used and there is concern about development of resistance, when large numbers of rods are found on cytology, and when a deep pyoderma is present. Cytology performed along with the culture and susceptibility is valuable to document that the organisms grown are actually causing the pyoderma.

The proper method for obtaining a specimen to culture depends on the clinical lesion. A pustular lesion should not be prepared with alcohol or other topical antiseptics prior to culture. Pustular contents can be obtained by vigorously rubbing a sterile swab over several lesions. If difficulty is encountered, the pustules may first be pricked open with a sterile needle. Small numbers of nonpathogenic organisms may contaminate the culture, but an experienced laboratory technician should be able to select the pathogenic staphylococci for susceptibility testing based on gross morphology and hemolytic pattern. Swabs should be sent to the laboratory in a suitable transport medium (e.g., Modified Amies). When crusts are present, the specimen should be obtained with a swab, collecting the exudate from under the crust.

Swabs are also used to collect purulent exudate from deep, draining lesions. Nondraining abscesses will need to be lanced with a needle to express purulent exudate to the surface. The surface of deep lesions may be disinfected prior to culture with alcohol or an antiseptic.

Tissue collected by skin biopsy is utilized when classical lesions are not present. These include papules, focal alopecia, bull's-eye-type lesions, focal hyperpigmentation, and nonexudative nodules. Hair is clipped, the surface disinfected, a 4 or 6 mm sterile punch (Acu-Punch) used with sterile technique, and the biopsy submitted to the laboratory in transport medium or wrapped in sterile gauze soaked with sodium chloride. The microbiology laboratory should mince the tissue with a tissue grinder, scissors, or mortar and pestle prior to culture.

Skin Biopsy

A skin biopsy submitted for routine histopathologic examination may be helpful in cases of chronic recurrent pyoderma. Not only will a biopsy confirm the presence of a folliculitis or deep pyoderma, other pathologic changes may help in diagnosis of the precipitating disease.

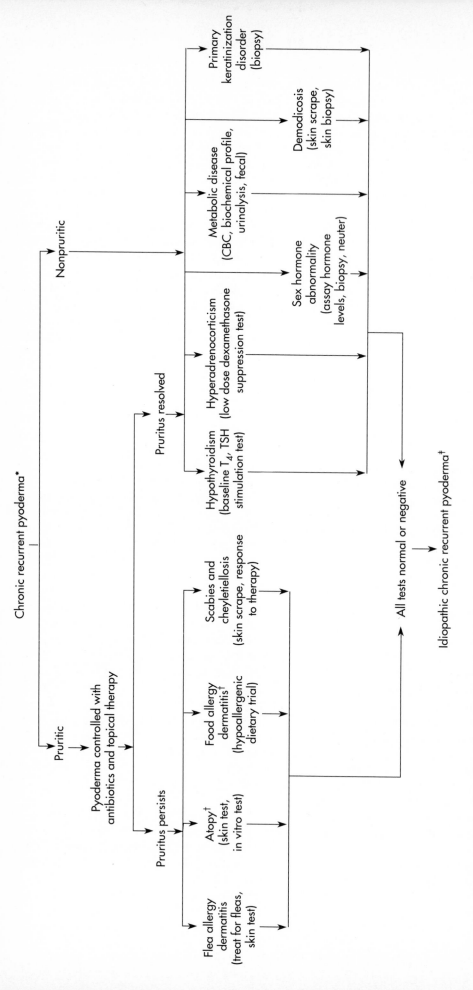

Figure 1-8. Flow chart for diagnostic evaluation of chronic recurrent pyoderma in dogs.

* All cases should be controlled with antibiotics, groomed and bathed with an antibacterial shampoo, and placed on a balanced commercial diet during the course of the diagnostic work.

† A very small number of dogs may have recurrent pyoderma due to atopy or food allergy with minimal or no pruritus.

‡ Some of these dogs may have immune system dysfunction.

The pathologist may be able to report a folliculitis with a pattern of inflammation consistent with allergic dermatitis. This would encourage diagnostics such as intradermal allergy testing and a food-elimination diet. Conversely, the pathologist may report pyoderma devoid of severe inflammation, with epidermal and dermal atrophy suggestive more of an endocrine dermatosis such as endogenous or iatrogenic hyperadrenocorticism. A good dermatopathologist will be familiar with the various primary keratinization disorders that may predispose to pyoderma. Finally, a biopsy also allows for a complete examination for cutaneous parasites, such as *Demodex canis* mites, to complement skin scraping findings.

Plan to Investigate the Precipitating Dermatoses

In many cases what has been termed a chronic recurrent pyoderma is really a skin infection that has been treated wrong. Before an extensive diagnostic evaluation of underlying diseases is recommended, it must be determined that the pyoderma is truly recurrent. A chronic recurrent pyoderma will respond completely to antibiotic therapy but relapse within several days to several weeks after discontinuation of treatment. To determine that the pyoderma has been treated correctly, there are several important considerations:

1. Has the correct antibiotic been selected?
2. Has the right dose been used for the proper duration?
3. Has a clinical reevaluation been performed prior to discontinuation of therapy?
4. Has the owner been giving the drug as prescribed?
5. Have antibiotics been used without steroids or other immunosuppressive drugs?

If the answers to all these questions are "yes" but the pyoderma recurs whenever therapy is discontinued, a complete diagnostic evaluation (Fig. 1-8) is warranted. The diagnostic plan should be organized to take into account the degree of pruritus associated with the pyoderma. Since many of the tests may be adversely affected by a concurrent pyoderma, it is best to keep the infection controlled with antibiotics and topical therapy during the course of the diagnostic evaluation.

TREATMENT

The best form of therapy for chronic recurrent pyoderma is control of the infection with systemic antibiotics and topical antibacterial therapy *and* specific therapy for the underlying precipitating disease. Complete information on the treatment of these diseases is found in the appropriate chapters.

Antibiotics and topical therapy may be needed on a continual or intermittent basis for long periods until the primary disease is controlled. For example, it may take several weeks or even months before atopic dermatitis is controlled with hyposensitization. One course of antibiotics may resolve the pyoderma but it may quickly return until the allergy is controlled. Several courses of antibiotics and continual antibacterial shampoos may be needed during this time. If a client calls to report that his atopic dog has relapsed with pruritus while on a program of hyposensitization and medical treatment, then that animal should be reevaluated for evidence of pyoderma. It may need antibiotics rather than glucocorticoids or a higher dosage of glucocorticoids. The same may be true of recurrent pyoderma associated with hypothyroidism or hyperadrenocorticism. Several months of antibiotics may be needed to control pyoderma until all the cutaneous changes associated with the endocrinopathy have resolved.

A special situation exists in immature dogs that develop a superficial impetigo or folliculitis. They will usually have some degree of pruritus associated with the infection. This condition may recur at frequent intervals until full sexual maturity and cause no problems thereafter. Several courses of systemic antibiotics and antibacterial shampoos are required until that time. If these dogs are treated with antibiotics and corticosteroids in combination (many are, because of the pruritus), the likelihood that this juvenile problem will develop into a chronic recurrent pyoderma into adulthood increases. It may then take months for reversal of the cutaneous effects of the steroids to adequately control the skin infection.

True idiopathic chronic recurrent pyoderma is diagnosed when an underlying precipitating disease cannot be found after an extensive diagnostic evaluation. Some dogs may fall into this category by default when owners cannot afford, or for some other reason will not allow, such an evaluation. The most successful therapy for long-term maintenance of these cases is still antibiotics and topical antibacterials. Immunostimulating drugs may also be helpful in a low percentage of cases but seldom afford total control of the problem.

Specific therapy for idiopathic chronic recurrent pyoderma depends on the frequency of relapse. In some cases a mild superficial pyoderma may occur only two to four times per year. It is most practical and economical to manage these with antibiotics and antibacterial shampoos during the episodes without extensive diagnostics and adjunctive therapy. This may also be true of some cases of recurrent pyoderma due to allergies or keratinization defects. However, the owner should be warned that the frequency of relapse may increase with time.

In cases of idiopathic recurrent pyoderma with frequent relapses, I prefer to start by using a bactericidal antibiotic selected by culture and susceptibility testing, an antibacterial shampoo selected by the condition of the hair coat and skin, and no corticosteroids for a period of 12 to 16 weeks. If the condition is cleared and there is still a relapse after this time, antibiotics and topical antibacterials are again used but this time with an immunostimulant. If there is still an unsatisfactory response, maintenance antibiotic administration is discussed with the owner.

If the client has decided not to pursue a full diagnostic evaluation or if no cause can be found and a diagnosis of idiopathic chronic recurrent pyoderma is made, the owner must be informed that the disease is controllable but noncurable and will require some form of topical/systemic therapy for the rest of the dog's life. Treatment options should be discussed, including differences in efficacy, labor intensiveness, and cost. Most cases of chronic recurrent pyoderma can be controlled, but the amount of work and expense of the drugs, especially in large breeds, may result in an owner's electing euthanasia.

Antibiotics (Table 1-1)

When large areas of the skin are affected, systemic antibiotic therapy is required for successful management of first-occurrence and chronic recurrent superficial and deep pyodermas. There are general principles of antibiotic usage that apply in all cases. Antibiotics are divided for clinical use into one group for "simple" first-occurrence pyodermas, a second group for refractory cases, and

Table 1-1. Systemic antibiotics for dogs with staphylococcal pyoderma

ANTIBIOTIC	TRADE NAME (MANUFACTURER)	DOSE	COMMENTS	MAJOR SIDE EFFECTS
Amoxicillin trihydrate–clavulanate potassium	Clavamox (SmithKline Beecham)	22 mg/kg q12h PO, higher than manufacturer's recommended dose	Resistance rare, moisture sensitive	Vomiting, diarrhea
Cefadroxil	Cefa-Tabs, Cefa-Drops (Fort Dodge)	22 mg/kg q12h PO, severe deep pyoderma may require q8h administration	Resistance very rare	Vomiting, diarrhea
Cephalexin	Generics (various)	22 mg/kg q12h PO, severe deep pyoderma may require q8h administration	Resistance very rare	Vomiting, diarrhea
Cephradine	Generics (various)	22 mg/kg q12h PO, severe deep pyoderma may require q8h administration	Resistance very rare	Vomiting, diarrhea
Chloramphenicol hydrochloride	Generics (various)	50 mg/kg q8h PO	In humans life-threatening blood dyscrasias may occur; therefore concern for accidental ingestion	—

Table 1-1. Systemic antibiotics for dogs with staphylococcal pyoderma—cont'd

ANTIBIOTIC	TRADE NAME (MANUFACTURER)	DOSE	COMMENTS	MAJOR SIDE EFFECTS
Clindamycin hydrochloride	Antirobe (Upjohn)	5.5-11 mg/kg q12h PO, depends on depth of infection	Good for deep fibrosing pyoderma, but rapid development of resistance	—
Erythromycin	Stearate and estolate generics (various)	10-15 mg/kg q8h PO, stearate on empty stomach	Rapid development of resistance	Vomiting in 50% of dogs
Lincomycin hydrochloride	Lincocin (Upjohn)	22 mg/kg q12h PO, on empty stomach	Rapid development of resistance	—
Ormetoprim-sulfadi-methoxine	Primor (Roche)	55 mg/kg q24h PO, on day 1, then 27.5 mg/kg q24h PO	Advantage of once-a-day dosage	Concern for sulfonamide hypersensitivity reactions, although incidence may be lower
Oxacillin	Oxacillin Capsules ℞ (Biocraft), Prostaphlin (Squibb)	22 mg/kg q8h PO, on empty stomach	Resistance very rare	Vomiting, diarrhea
Rifampin	Rifadin (Marion Merrell Dow), Rimactane (Ciba)	5-10 mg/kg q24h PO	Excellent penetration of chronic deep granulomatous scarred lesions; rapid development of resistance, so give with a beta-lactamase–resistant antibiotic; toxicity limits usage in recurrent pyoderma	Hepatitis, thrombocytopenia, hemolytic anemia, anorexia, vomiting, diarrhea, death
Trimethoprim-sulfadiazine	Tribrissen (Coopers), Di-Trim (Syntex)	20-30 mg/kg q12h PO	Potential for side effects limits usage in recurrent pyoderma	Keratoconjunctivitis sicca, multisystemic drug-induced hypersensitivity
Trimethoprim-sulfamethoxazole	Generics (various)	20-30 mg/kg q12h PO	Potential for side effects limits usage in recurrent pyoderma	Keratoconjunctivitis sicca, multisystemic drug-induced hypersensitivity

a third for resistant infections and long-term maintenance of chronic recurrent pyodermas.

General Principles

There are several general principles of antibiotic therapy that must be considered. The antibiotic should have known spectrum of activity against *S. intermedius* and be resistant to beta-lactamase, which is produced in a large percentage of isolates. If possible, a narrow-spectrum agent should be used since the long-term therapy required for most pyodermas has the potential to alter gastrointestinal flora. Actual clinical problems reported with continued use of broad-spectrum antibiotics are rare in dogs. However, a recent report (Plant, 1991) has suggested that such chronic usage may predispose to cutaneous *Malassezia pachydermatis* infection.

Another common question is whether it is more beneficial to use bactericidal over bacteriostatic antibiotics. In general, if the host has a normal immune system, bacteriostatic drugs are just as effective. Bactericidal antibiotics should be used with confirmed or suspected immunodeficiencies, when indicated by susceptibility testing, and in severe cases of deep pyoderma and mixed infections (gram-positive and gram-negative bacteria). Since resistance to most bacteriostatic antibiotics used in dogs is quick to develop, bactericidal agents are usually needed for cases of chronic recurrent pyoderma.

When interpreting results of a bacterial susceptibility test prior to selecting an antibiotic, it is important to remember that the in vitro and in vivo sensitivities may not always directly correlate. Only about 40% of blood flow reaches the dermal/epidermal junction, so pharmacokinetic studies done with blood levels may not match levels in the skin. It may be difficult to achieve adequate tissue levels in the presence of dermal abscesses, purulent exudate, and keratin foreign bodies. A client may call to report a poor clinical response when the susceptibility test indicated that an effective antibiotic was utilized. Conversely, the practitioner may call a client to change an antibiotic only to find that it has been working although the susceptibility indicated to the contrary. I have seen this discrepancy most often with the macrolides, potentiated sulfonamide combinations, and chloramphenicol. Antibiotic responsiveness may also change during therapy, so repeat bacterial culture and susceptibilities may be needed. This is especially true of erythromycin and lincomycin, to which resistance can develop quickly.

A bacterial culture may indicate mixed infection with gram-negative organisms as well as gram-positive staphylococci, even in superficial pyodermas. Generally, treating the staphylococci alone will also control the opportunistic gram-negatives. The exception would be severe deep infection with pure *Pseudomonas* spp in the immunocompromised host such as a dog with generalized demodicosis or on chemotherapy.

Other considerations in selecting an antibiotic include cost (since cutaneous infections require long-term administration), ease of administration (oral vs parenteral), frequency of administration (q24h, q12h, q8h), and potential side effects.

Initially, the choice of an antibiotic may be based on empirical considerations of known spectrum of activity against *S. intermedius* and resistance to inactivation by beta-lactamase. Narrow-spectrum antibiotics fulfilling these criteria include erythromycin, lincomycin, clindamycin, and beta-lactamase–resistant penicillins. Lack of response to empirical therapy warrants culture and susceptibility testing and reassessment of the diagnosis.

It should be stressed to the owner that full dosage of the antibiotic (based on an accurate body weight), for the entire prescribed duration, must be used for cure or control. For superficial pyoderma the antibiotic should be used for a minimum of 21 consecutive days or for 7 to 14 days after clinical cure. Deep pyodermas should be treated for a minimum of 4 to 6 weeks, and 8 to 12 weeks is not unusual. Treatment should continue for 2 weeks after a complete clinical cure. In all cases the veterinarian should reevaluate the animal after 3 weeks of therapy and before discontinuation of antibiotics. The client does not have the ability to do a complete examination and determine if any papules, pustules, crusts, or nodules remain, especially under a thick hair coat. Detection of remaining lesions may even be difficult for the veterinarian. Clipping a small area of hair to better visualize the skin surface is helpful. Extensive palpation of the skin and subcutis will confirm that all deep pyoderma lesions have resolved.

Poor Antibiotic Choices for the Skin

Because of inadequate skin levels or rapid development of resistance, the following antibiotics should not be used for pyoderma: penicillin, ampicillin, amoxicillin, hetacillin, streptomycin, tetracycline, and nonpotentiated sulfas.

Antibiotic Choices for First-Occurrence Pyoderma

The agents under this heading are usually effective against first-occurrence superficial pyodermas that have not been previously treated. (Clindamycin is also effective in deep pyodermas caused by susceptible staphylococci.) They are less effective with the prolonged usage needed for chronic recurrent pyoderma due to development of resistance. The narrow-spectrum, beta-lactamase–resistant antibiotics in this category include erythromycin, lincomycin, and clindamycin.

Erythromycin (generics, 10 to 15 mg/kg q8h PO) is a bacteriostatic macrolide antibiotic that inhibits ribosomal protein synthesis. It is inexpensive and of low toxicity but must be given three times per day, which may limit usage.

Erythromycin is an efficient inducer of plasmid-mediated resistance, and cross-resistance with lincomycin is almost universal. It is effective in 80% to 90% of cutaneous staphylococcal isolates, but resistance develops readily, lowering this figure to 40% or 50% with previous usage (Kunkle, 1990). Thus, although it is a good initial antibiotic in superficial pyoderma, efficacy is reduced, especially after multiple usage. This antibiotic has been used so heavily in many parts of the country that geographical resistance has developed, limiting its use.

Generally erythromycin is used in larger dogs because of easier dosing and lower cost whereas lincomycin is easier to dose in small dogs. Enteric coated formulations are most often utilized. Vomiting is a common side effect of erythromycin, occurring in up to 50% of dogs. Most will tolerate the drug after 48 hours, but in a few the antibiotic will need to be changed. Some guidelines should be followed to try to decrease the incidence and severity of vomiting:

1. The estolate rather than the stearate form may be used; however, unfortunately, the estolate form is almost twice as expensive.
2. Careful adherence to the recommended dosage, especially staying at the low end of the wide dosage range, may also decrease incidence of gastrointestinal upset.
3. Giving medication with a small amount of food will help, but the stearate should be given on an empty stomach for maximum absorption. The estolate may be given with food.
4. In large dogs requiring high dosages, starting with half the dose and then increasing to the full dose after 2 to 3 days enables the antibiotic to be better tolerated.
5. An antiemetic given for the first 2 to 3 days may control gastrointestinal upset. If mild gastrointestinal symptoms result, the drug will usually be tolerated within 48 hours and can be continued without further adverse effects.

Lincomycin hydrochloride (Lincocin, 22 mg/kg q12h PO) is a macrolide-like antibiotic with a mode of action similar to that of erythromycin. If resistance is recognized to one, the other should not be utilized. It is more expensive than erythromycin, especially in large dogs, but is easier to dose in small dogs. It has the advantages of being a twice-a-day drug without the side effect of vomiting. Lincomycin is best administered on an empty stomach. Geographic resistance has also been seen.

Clindamycin hydrochloride (Antirobe) is closely related to lincomycin and shows cross-resistance. It is better absorbed and more potent, attaches to white blood cells, and attains good levels in bone. It therefore has demonstrated activity in superficial and deep infections, including osteomyelitis, and is used in dermatology for deep pyoderma, especially fibrosed lesions, caused by susceptible staphylococci. Unfortunately, resistance develops readily and it is very expensive used at the higher dosage. Clindamycin is available in capsules and an oral liquid. Two dosages are suggested, one for superficial (5.5 mg/kg q12h PO) and one for deep (11 mg/kg q12h PO) infections.

Antibiotic Choices for Refractory Pyoderma

The drugs discussed next are usually chosen either empirically or on the basis of culture and susceptibility when erythromycin, lincomycin, and clindamycin are no longer effective. They may continue to be effective for long periods in cases of recurrent pyoderma, but potential side effects are a concern with the long-term use of some of them.

Potentiated sulfonamides are among the most common antibiotics now used to treat staphylococcal pyodermas. They work by inhibiting sequential steps in bacterial metabolism and are effective against many strains of staphylococci and some gram-negative rods. Potentiated sulfonamides are effective against 80% to 90% of cutaneous staphylococcal isolates, but resistance may develop with chronic usage, lowering this figure to 60% to 65% (Kunkle, 1990). These drugs may not work as well in vivo as in vitro. They are inexpensive compared to other broad-spectrum bactericidal agents.

Trimethoprim-sulfadiazine (Tribrissen, Di-Trim) has been the potentiated sulfa most commonly used in veterinary medicine. Doses range from 20 to 30 mg/kg q12h PO. One investigator (Zertuche, 1990) showed trimethoprim-sulfadiazine to have a longer half-life in the skin of dogs than in serum and suggested that 30 mg/kg q24h PO is adequate for the treatment of superficial canine pyoderma. However, clinical response is not as impressive in many dogs with once-a-day dosing. Trimethoprim-sulfamethoxizole (20 to 30 mg/kg q12h PO) has also been used extensively because the generics are inexpensive and efficacy appears comparable to that of trimethoprim-sulfadiazine.

Ormetoprim and sulfadimethoxine (Primor), a new potentiated sulfonamide, has been licensed for veterinary usage. It is given at 55 mg/kg q24 PO the first day and then at 27.5 mg/kg q24h PO. It has a claim for increased clinical efficacy and true once-a-day dosage, since sulfadimethoxine has a blood half-life of 13 hours versus 6 hours for sulfadiazine. Although this work has not been conducted in the skin, clinical use of ormetoprim-sulfadimethoxine over the last 12 months has shown excellent results with once-a-day dosing.

Another possible advantage is that sulfadimethoxine has less reported potential for inducing keratoconjunctivitis sicca and other (more serious) drug reactions associated with sulfadiazine. The combination has not been used long enough, however, to determine whether this claim is true in dogs, although there are anecdotal reports of reactions similar to those seen with other sulfonamides. The cost is comparable to that of other potentiated sulfonamides.

Side effects associated with potentiated sulfonamides include keratoconjunctivitis sicca and a multisystemic drug-induced hypersensitivity, like a type III Arthus reaction (Werner and Bright, 1983; Giger et al., 1985). The latter has been recognized most often in Doberman Pinschers, but similar reactions have also been seen in multiple breeds. In Doberman Pinschers the reaction has been linked to the sulfonamide component of the drug combination. Multisystemic reactions include fever, nonseptic polyarthritis, lymphadenopathy, polymyositis, retinitis, glomerulonephritis, hepatitis, erythema multiforme, toxic epidermal necrolysis, anemia, leukopenia, and thrombocytopenia. Concern about the development of such a hypersensitivity reaction warrants extreme caution in long-term usage of sulfonamides in any breed.

Chloramphenicol (generics, 50 mg/kg q8h PO) is a broad-spectrum, bacteriostatic antibiotic that inhibits bacterial ribosomal protein synthesis. It is relatively inexpensive and in dogs has few side effects. As with potentiated sulfonamides, there may be discrepancies between its in vivo responsiveness and in vitro susceptibility. It has 80% to 90% sensitivity against cutaneous staphylococci, and this value remains high even after previous use.

The drug is inactivated by the liver and causes reversible depression of liver microsomal enzymes. Chloramphenicol is utilized heavily in some parts of the country though hardly at all in others. There is concern about human exposure to it because of potential life-threatening blood dyscrasias and the development of resistant enterics that may affect humans. Therefore caution should be exercised when dispensing chloramphenicol for any pyoderma in dogs.

Antibiotic Choices for Resistant Infections and for Long-Term Maintenance of Chronic Recurrent Pyoderma

As a group, the antibiotics discussed under this heading are most often utilized in cases of chronic recurrent superficial and deep pyoderma because of the low incidence of resistance, even with prolonged use, and minimal side effects. Unfortunately, they are among the most expensive antibiotics for pyoderma in dogs.

Beta-lactamase–resistant penicillins are excellent bactericidal antibiotics that work by inhibiting bacterial cell wall synthesis. They have the desirable characteristic of being narrow spectrum against gram-positive cocci. However, they are often reserved as one of the last antibiotics chosen because of expense. Cloxacillin, dicloxacillin, nafcillin, and oxacillin are all members of this group. Oxacillin (Oxacillin Capsules ℞, Prostaphlin) at 22 mg/kg q8h PO is reportedly the most effective (95% to 100%), with staphylococcal resistance extremely rare. Food interferes with absorption, so this group of antibiotics must be administered at least 1 hour before or after feeding. Adverse reactions are rare but may be seen as with other penicillins.

Amoxicillin trihydrate with clavulanate potassium (Clavamox) is another effective broad-spectrum, bactericidal antibiotic combination. It works by inhibiting cell wall biosynthesis and is effective in 95% to 100% of staphylococcal isolates; resistance to it is rare. However, amoxicillin is not an effective antibiotic for most pyodermas when used alone because it is not beta-lactamase–resistant. The combination is moisture-sensitive so should be dispensed in the manufacturer's foil packaging. There has been some concern about cases relapsing while on this antibiotic in spite of favorable susceptibility results. It works better in the skin at 22 mg/kg q12h PO rather than at the recommended 13.75 mg/kg q12h PO.

Cephalosporins are broad-spectrum, bactericidal antibiotics that attack bacterial cell walls by interfering with polypeptide cross-linkages. They are 95% to 100% active against *S. intermedius* as well as many of the secondary invaders, such as *Proteus mirabilis* and some species of *Pseudomonas*. Resistance develops rarely, and this antibiotic is especially effective in controlling recurrent deep pyoderma. Commonly used cephalosporins include cefadroxil (Cefa-Tabs), cephalexin (generics), and cephradine (generics). The usual dosage is 22 mg/kg q12h PO, although some cases of deep pyoderma will require q8h administration. Cephalosporins are extremely effective and should be reserved for severe infections or when indicated based on susceptibility testing.

Rifampin (Rifadin, Rimactane, 5 to 10 mg/kg q24h PO) is a bactericidal antibiotic that inactivates DNA-dependent RNA polymerases of the bacteria. It is extremely active against susceptible species of staphylococci and is included in this discussion because it is usually reserved for deep staphylococcal pyodermas with chronic, granulomatous, scarring lesions (interdigital pyoderma, pressure point pyoderma, infected acral pruritic nodules), which other antibiotics have failed to penetrate. Rifampin penetrates such lesions because of its high lipid solubility and concentrating ability in neutrophils and macrophages.

Problems with rapid development of resistance and potential for toxicity may limit use of rifampin in chronic recurrent deep pyodermas. A beta-lactamase–resistant antibiotic should be given with rifampin to minimize resistance. Side effects, especially at the high end of the dosage range, are common and include elevated liver enzymes, hepatitis, thrombocytopenia, hemolytic anemia, anorexia, vomiting, diarrhea, and death. Rifampin should not be used in dogs with preexisting liver disease, and liver enzymes should be monitored every 2 weeks.

Antibiotic Choices for Mixed Infections

It is rare for chronic recurrent pyodermas to be complicated by significant gram-negative organisms. Therefore, the antibiotics discussed next are rarely utilized except in cases of gram-negative infections in an immunocompromised animal.

Fluoroquinolones are derivatives of nalidixic acid. They are broad-spectrum bactericidal antibiotics that work by inhibiting DNA replication. They are especially effective against *E. coli* and *Salmonella* and moderately effective against staphylococci and *Pseudomonas*. Resistance is rare but may develop by mutation over many generations. The recommended dosage for enrofloxacin (Bay-

tril) is 2.5 to 5 mg/kg q12h PO on an empty stomach. Gastrointestinal signs may be seen, and the drug should not be used in growing dogs since articular cartilage may be damaged. This antibiotic is being overused for superficial and deep pyodermas due to staphylococci. It penetrates granulomatous tissue reactions well and should be reserved for severe deep pyoderma with resistant staphylococci or mixed infections based on culture and susceptibility testing.

Aminoglycosides are not commonly utilized in pyodermas because of parenteral administration, nephrotoxicity, ototoxicity, and cost. The one exception is severe mixed gram-positive and gram-negative deep infections, especially in immunocompromised hosts, in which the aminoglycoside is often combined with a beta-lactamase–resistant penicillin or cephalosporin. Gentamicin (Gentocin, 2 mg/kg q8h SQ or IM) is most commonly utilized, but amikacin (Amiglyde-V, 10 mg/kg q12h SQ or IM) is also effective and has less potential for nephrotoxicity than gentamicin.

Antibiotic Failure

There are a number of factors to consider when antibiotic therapy has failed to adequately clear a pyoderma. The antibiotic chosen may have been inappropriate for the type of infection or susceptibility pattern of the bacteria. At this point an alternate antibiotic should be chosen or, better, a bacterial culture and susceptibility performed. It must also be established that the correct dose, administration frequency, and duration of therapy were used without concurrent glucocorticoids. Steroids may contribute to recurrent pyoderma for several months after discontinuation, especially if large doses or repositol forms were used over long periods.

If there is no response after these factors have been investigated and corrected, the proper diagnosis may not have been made or other conditions may be adversely affecting response. Further diagnostics, such as cutaneous biopsies, would be indicated in this situation. In nonresponsive or recurrent deep infections such as pressure point pyodermas, interdigital pyodermas, and infected acral pruritic nodules, the biopsy may reveal deep microabscesses, hair shafts embedded in the dermis, or severe scar tissue, all of which limit antibiotic penetration and clinical response even when the bacteria are susceptible to the drug.

For cases that respond but quickly relapse within days upon discontinuation of therapy, one should still question whether the duration of antibiotics was long enough. If so, concomitant diseases should then be investigated as described above.

A superficial or deep pyoderma may become a chronic recurrent problem even after all proper diagnostic and therapeutic programs have been followed. These cases are completely antibiotic-responsive but relapse quickly when medication is discontinued. They have no demonstrable underlying cause for the recurrent pyoderma but may have some type of abnormality in the immune system. They have what is termed "idiopathic chronic recurrent pyoderma."

Maintenance Antibiotics

The practitioner is often faced with giving the client an economically feasible alternative for long-term control of idiopathic chronic recurrent pyoderma or euthanizing the animal. I prefer to try better control of recurrence by use of an immunostimulating agent, topical antibacterial therapy, and antibiotics administered only as needed. However, this plan does not always work and many cases will be controlled only with antibiotics administered on a continual basis.

Maintenance antibiotics should be considered as long as both the practitioner and the client are aware of possible risks for the development of resistant organisms. Although usually considered a last resort, they are the most efficacious form of therapy in dogs with true idiopathic chronic recurrent pyoderma.

Maintenance antibiotic therapy entails using the agent on a continual basis at a subminimal dosage or pulsed periodically at full dosage to prevent recurrent infections. In vitro studies have shown that subminimal doses may work by structural alterations in the bacteria, enhanced phagocytosis, increased bactericidal activity of serum, decreased ability to adhere to corneocytes, and alterations in enzyme systems. There is no solid evidence to indicate that either subminimal dosing or pulse dosing is more effective or less likely to induce resistance than the other. Both have been used successfully in dogs with chronic recurrent pyoderma, with little problem concerning resistance as long as appropriate antibiotics were used. Maintenance antibiotic therapy will save clients money over the life of their animal and keep the pet comfortable and relatively free of pyoderma.

A bactericidal drug with low potential for development of resistance and minimal side effects (e.g., a cephalosporin, amoxicillin–clavulanate potassium, or beta-lactamase–resistant penicillin) should be used. When subminimal dosing, a single daily or alternate-day dose is given. For example, the dog that requires a full dosage of 500 mg of cephalexin q8-12h should be weaned slowly to 250 mg q24h or q48h for long-term management. When pulse dosing, a full dose is used for 1 week followed by no drug the following week. This may gradually be decreased to 1 week on and 2 to 3 weeks off. Some dermatologists prefer to use subminimal dosing if relapses occur within 1 week of stopping antibiotics and will use pulse therapy if it normally takes longer than a week for the pyoderma to recur.

For relapses a culture and susceptibility test should be performed to ensure that resistance has not developed. If it has not, then full-dose antibiotic therapy may bring the pyoderma under control, followed again by slowly decreasing the dosage to maintenance. An alternate antibiotic should also be considered. Dogs on maintenance antibiotics should be monitored regularly for side effects.

Topical Therapy

Rarely a dog with chronic recurrent pyoderma may be completely controlled with topical therapy alone, without systemic antibiotics. However, this is extremely labor-intensive and not practical for most clients. Antibacterial shampoos are usually needed two to three times a week to have any chance of achieving this goal. However, topical therapy is an important adjunct in the management of recurrent superficial and deep pyodermas. It is most helpful when used prophylactically to decrease the severity and frequency of recurrence of the infection.

In deep pyodermas clipping the hair coat followed by warm water soaks, whirlpool baths, and shampoos are very helpful. Povidone-iodine solution (generics) and chlorhexidine solution (Nolvasan Solution) are excellent antimicrobial agents when added to the soaking or whirlpool solutions. Local soakings or hot compresses are helpful in localized deep pyodermas, especially when there is a foreign body reaction to keratin in the dermis (e.g., with pressure point pyodermas and callus pyodermas).

Antibacterial shampoos are the most commonly employed method of topical therapy for superficial and deep pyodermas. In most cases of chronic recurrent pyoderma they must be used at least weekly to have efficacy. Benzoyl peroxide products (OxyDex Shampoo, Sulf OxyDex Shampoo, Pyoben Shampoo) are especially effective, not only because of their excellent antimicrobial activity but because they possess a follicular flushing activity. Benzoyl peroxide was shown in a controlled quantitative study (Kwochka and Kowalski, 1991) to have superior prophylactic activity against *S. intermedius* when compared to chlorhexidine, complexed iodine, and triclosan. Benzoyl peroxide shampoos lather quite well and are aesthetically pleasing. Human formulations should not be used, unless the benzoyl peroxide concentration is under 5%, since the higher-percentage products are irritating to dog skin. Benzoyl peroxide is also keratolytic and degreasing. Whereas these actions will be beneficial in many cases, they can inhibit long-term usage in others because of excessive drying of the skin. Then a bath oil or humectant rinse (HyLyt*efa Bath Oil Coat Conditioner, Humilac Dry Skin Spray and Rinse, Alpha-Sesame Oil Dry Skin Rinse) should be used after each bathing to rehydrate the skin and hair coat.

Benzoyl peroxide is also found in gel formulations (OxyDex Gel, Pyoben Gel) for use on localized pyodermas such as furunculosis of the chin and pressure point pyoderma.

Chlorhexidine is another excellent antimicrobial agent found in shampoo formulations (Chlorhexi-Derm Shampoo, Nolvasan Shampoo). Although it does not have the follicular flushing activity of benzoyl peroxide, it has the advantage of being in an emollient formulation for long-term use on dry skin and coat. Iodine is also found in scrub and shampoo (Weladol) formulations but is more irritating than benzoyl peroxide or chlorhexidine and has the disadvantage of staining light colored hair coats.

Mupirocin (Bactoderm) is a topical antibiotic in a polyethylene glycol base for localized pyoderma. It has excellent activity against gram-positive cocci, is bactericidal, works well at an acid pH, is not systemically absorbed, and is not chemically related to other antibiotics. Mupirocin penetrates very well into granulomatous deep pyoderma lesions such as interdigital abscesses. Owners are able to significantly decrease severity and relapse rate of superficial and deep pyodermas if they immediately apply mupirocin q12h when they first notice early lesions developing. This is especially true of localized conditions such as chin pyoderma, pressure point pyoderma, and interdigital abscesses.

Immunostimulants

Other therapy for chronic recurrent pyoderma usually falls into the category of nonspecific im-munostimulation or immunomodulation. It should be reserved for cases in which the pyoderma responds completely to antibiotics but recurs very quickly after discontinuation of therapy and all other potential causes of recurrent pyoderma have been eliminated by proper diagnostic testing. Even in these well-screened cases, response to immunostimulation is seldom complete and there is no practical way to predict which dogs might respond without a therapeutic trial. This is probably accounted for by the fact that most of these dogs are not immunosuppressed or, if they are, the immunostimulant does not affect the portion of the immune system that is defective. Results of immunostimulation will be exceedingly poor if immunomodulation is used routinely for all cases of pyoderma without the proper screening. This probably accounts for the lack of faith in this therapy by many practitioners.

Staphage Lysate is the most commonly utilized immunostimulating agent and is licensed for use in the dog. This product contains lysed cultures of serologic type I and III *S. aureus* with a polyvalent *Staphylococcus* bacteriophage. The major benefit is thought to be associated with stimulation of antibacterial antibody formation or a nonspecific stimulation of T cell reactivity and macrophage killing of staphylococci. Some investigators feel that the best response is seen in cases with pruritic superficial pyodermas. I have seen less response using this drug for recurrent deep pyoderma in comparison to superficial pyoderma.

There have been many different dosages reported for Staphage Lysate. Currently, most dermatologists use 0.5 ml twice per week SQ, or 1 ml once a week, with apparently equal success. Therapy continues for 12 to 14 weeks before a final assessment of efficacy. It is mandatory that the existing pyoderma be controlled with antibiotics while initiating therapy. Response is determined by observing for relapse in the pyoderma when antibiotics are discontinued 6 to 8 weeks into therapy. Complete response would be a case which needs no further antibiotics but is controlled with immunomodulation alone. Partial response would include the ability to use antibiotics with less frequency, such as three to four times a year rather than continually.

In my experience, 30% to 40% of properly screened cases of idiopathic chronic recurrent pyoderma will show some response. A double-blind, placebo-controlled study (DeBoer et al., 1990) showed 40% efficacy. Occasionally, the dosage can be decreased to 1 ml every 2 to 3 weeks for maintenance, but this is rare. Cases that show partial response will sometimes benefit from 1 ml twice per week or 2 ml once a week. Side effects are rare and reversible. They include vomiting, diarrhea, quivering, fever, malaise, nonseptic polyarthritis, and injection site reactions. There are at least two anecdotal reports of signs of anaphylaxis after administration of the drug.

Other injectable immunomodulators include autogenous bacterins, Immunoregulin, and Staphoid AB. All of these agents have reported efficacy for recurrent pyoderma either in the literature or in anecdotal reports. However, none have been evaluated in well-designed, clinical trials. Additionally, Immunoregulin is impractical for long-term use because of IV administration. Autogenous bacterins require proper microbiological facilities and personnel to be made properly. Autogenous bacterins and Staphoid AB are also associated with more local injection site reactions than Staphage Lysate.

Levamisole (Levasole) has immunomodulatory properties including normalization of T cell and phagocyte function in immunocompromised hosts. The empirical dosage is 2.2 mg/kg q48h PO. It should be adhered to strictly since larger or smaller doses may result in immunosuppression. Efficacy has been reported to be no better than 10% to 15%. Toxicity includes gastrointestinal disturbance, neurotoxicity, lethargy, granulocytopenia, erythema multiforme, and toxic epidermal necrolysis. The author has occasionally had positive results with a Staphage Lysate and levamisole combination when the individual drugs did not work well by themselves.

Other products currently under investigation for their immunomodulatory properties include cimetidine, ketoconazole, hydroxyzine, fish oil, and evening primrose oil. Cimetidine (Tagamet) may act as an immunostimulator by reversing T-suppressor–mediated immune suppression in patients with chronic infectious diseases. It has shown efficacy in dogs with recurrent superficial pruritic pyoderma. However, the dosage of 3 to 4 mg/kg q12h PO is cost prohibitive for chronic administration.

Miscellaneous Treatments

Low-dose alternate-day glucocorticoids may be helpful in controlling chronic recurrent pyoderma in two types of cases. First, dogs with severe inhalant or food allergies that cannot be managed with avoidance, nonsteroidal antipruritic agents, topical therapy, or hyposensitization may benefit

from prednisone or prednisolone given at 0.2 to 0.5 mg/kg q48h PO. Second, dogs with severe, pruritic, idiopathic seborrheic dermatitis may also be helped by glucocorticoids. This should be the *last alternative* in these cases since, more often than not, the glucocortiocids will contribute to rather than help control the pyoderma.

Some cases of chronic fibrosing interdigital pyoderma may become so severe that the infection will no longer respond to any form of medical therapy (including continual antibiotics) or medical therapy becomes too expensive and euthanasia contemplated. A viable alternative if infection is localized to the interdigital spaces is complete surgical removal of the diseased tissue. Excellent results have been obtained (Swaim et al., 1991) using a fusion podoplasty technique in seven dogs with bacterial and demodectic fibrosing interdigital pyoderma. Although this is an expensive, major surgical procedure, long-term prognosis is better than continuation of medical therapy.

REFERENCES

Chesney C: Shampoos and other topical therapy (Workshop report 13). In von Tscharner C, Halliwell REW (eds): Advances in veterinary dermatology, vol 1, London, 1990, Baillière Tindall, p 434.

Cox HU, et al: Temporal study of staphylococcal species on healthy dogs, Am J Vet Res 49:747, 1988.

DeBoer DJ, et al: Evaluation of a commercial staphylococcal bacterin for management of idiopathic recurrent superficial pyoderma in dogs, Am J Vet Res 51:636, 1990.

Giger U, et al: Sulfadiazine-induced allergy in six Doberman Pinschers, J Am Vet Med Assoc 186:479, 1985.

Halliwell REW, Gorman NT: Nonatopic allergic skin diseases. In Halliwell REW, Gorman NT (eds): Veterinary clinical immunology, Philadelphia, 1989, WB Saunders, p 253.

Kunkle GA: Update on antimicrobial therapy. In Proceedings, Dermatologics For Veterinary Medicine, fall skin seminar, 1990, p 66.

Kwochka KW: Qualitative and quantitative incidence of staphylococci on normal canine skin and hair coat: an investigation into the possibility of two different microbial populations (abstr). In Proceedings, Annual members' meeting AAVD & ACVD, 1986, p 31.

Kwochka KW, Kowalski JJ: Prophylactic efficacy of four antibacterial shampoos against *Staphylococcus intermedius* in dogs, Am J Vet Res 52:115, 1991.

Mason IS, Lloyd DH: Factors influencing the penetration of bacterial antigens through canine skin. In von Tscharner C, Halliwell REW (eds): Advances in veterinary dermatology, vol 1, London, 1990, Baillière Tindall, p 370.

McEwan NA: Bacterial adherence to canine corneocytes. In von Tscharner C, Halliwell REW (eds): Advances in veterinary dermatology, vol 1, London, 1990, Baillière Tindall, p 454.

Plant JD: Factors associated with and prevalence of increased *Malassezia pachydermatis* numbers on dog skin (abstr): In Proceedings, Annual members' meeting AAVD & ACVD, 1991, p 22.

Sischo WM, et al: Regional distribution of ten common skin diseases in dogs, J Am Vet Med Assoc 195:752, 1989.

Swaim SF, et al: Fusion podoplasty for the treatment of chronic fibrosing interdigital pyoderma in the dog, J Am Anim Hosp Assoc 27:264, 1991.

Werner LL, Bright JM: Drug-induced immune hypersensitivity disorders in two dogs treated with trimethoprim sulfadiazine: case reports and drug challenge studies, J Am Anim Hosp Assoc 19:783, 1983.

White SD, Ihrke PJ: Pyoderma. In Nesbitt GH (ed): Contemporary issues in small animal practice: dermatology, New York, 1987, Churchill Livingstone, p 95.

White SD, et al: Occurrence of *Staphylococcus aureus* on the clinically normal hair coat, Am J Vet Res 44:332, 1983.

Zertuche HOP: Trimethoprim and sulfadiazine in the dog: Plasma and skin concentrations after oral administration (abstr). In Proceedings, Annual members' meeting AAVD & ACVD, 1990, p 39.

2

Dermatophytosis

Carol S. Foil

Diagnostic Criteria for Dermatophytosis in Dogs and Cats

SUGGESTIVE
Clinical signs

COMPATIBLE
Suggestive plus a positive Wood's lamp examination of hair and scale

TENTATIVE
Positive direct examination of hair and scale for arthrospores and hyphae

DEFINITIVE
Positive DTM culture
Biopsy identification of fungal elements

Importance

When clinicians rely on clinical signs alone, dermatophytosis is overdiagnosed, especially in dogs. In all studies of skin diseases of dogs and cats the incidence of dermatophyte infection is low. In one study of dermatology cases presented to a university practice (Blakemore, 1974) ringworm constituted only 2% of the diagnoses. Analysis of cultures submitted from suspect ringworm cases generally reveals that between 11% and 22% are positive. Nevertheless, the veterinary practitioner must maintain a high index of suspicion because of the protean clinical manifestations of dermatophytosis in pet animals, and because these infections are transmissible to humans.

Normal Microflora

A wide variety of molds and yeasts may be cultured from normal dogs and cats, both those with dermatitis and those suspected of having dermatophytosis. An important point is that it is possible to isolate dermatophytes from the hair coats of normal dogs and cats. The extent to which these are resident flora (inapparent carriers) or transient organisms is not entirely clear. Most of the saprophyte isolates probably represent transient contamination of the pelage by air-borne or soil-acquired spores. Undeniably, *Microsporum canis* is present as a persistent infection of asymptomatic long-haired cats. The presence of other potentially pathogenic fungi on the hair and skin of normal animals is of unknown significance.

Pathogenic Dermatophytes

The term "dermatophytosis" implies cutaneous infection with one of a number of keratinophilic species of fungi. Over 20 species have been reported to infect domestic dogs and cats (Foil, 1990). The great majority of these are one of three species: *Microsporum canis*, *Trichophyton mentagrophytes*, or the geophilic *Microsporum gypseum*. In cats 98% of cases are reportedly caused by *M. canis*. However, among the isolates in our caseload at Louisiana State University from 1980 to 1989, 6% (4/61) of feline infections were caused by *M. gypseum*. In dogs the importance of the three common etiologic agents varies geographically (Table 2-1).

Several reports have documented the simultaneous infection with more than one dermatophyte species in dogs. *Microsporum gypseum* and *Trichophyton mentagrophytes* have been the most common.

Etiologic identification of dermatophytosis has more value than just academic curiosity. Each species of dermatophyte that infects humans and domestic animals exhibits unique epidemiologic features. The source in cases of *M. canis* infections is usually an infected cat. *Trichophyton* sp infections are generally acquired directly or indirectly by exposure to the typical host animal. To determine the probable source of *T. mentagrophytes*, subspecific identification is required. In most instances dogs and cats are suspected of being exposed by contact with rodents or their burrows. *Microsporum gypseum* is a geophilic organism that inhabits rich soil. Dogs and cats are exposed by digging in contaminated areas. Infections with the anthropophilic species are acquired as reverse zoonoses by direct contact with infected persons.

Zoonotic Ringworm

Symptomatic or asymptomatic carriage of any dermatophyte, especially *Microsporum canis*, represents a great threat to exposed persons. In this regard it is important to note that asymptomatic carriage in long-haired cattery cats may be especially common. (See Chapter 3.) One study (Quaife and Womar, 1982) has identified a 35% incidence of asymptomatic carriage of *M. canis* in long-haired show cats. In another (Pepin and Oxenham, 1986) the magnitude of risk was demonstrated when it was found that 50% of persons exposed to symptomatic or asymptomatic infected cats acquired the infection; in 69.6% of all households with infected cats, at least one person became infected.

Zoophilic infections were identified in 15% of all cases of ringworm in children in another survey (Svejgaard, 1986). Worldwide, the rate of infection among humans with *M. canis* is reportedly rising. The role of the veterinarian in controlling this important zoonosis will be concomitantly emphasized in the ensuing discussion.

The veterinarian and employees are at great risk of acquiring dermatophytosis as an occupational hazard (Fig. 2-1). In a study of government veterinarians and animal health workers conducted in Great Britain (Constable and Harrington, 1982) animal ringworm was the most commonly reported zoonosis; the overall prevalence was 24%.

Table 2-1. Relative distribution (%) of dermatophyte species causing infection in dogs in the United States and New Zealand

SPECIES	NATIONAL[a]	PURDUE[b]	LSU[c]	FLA[d]	NZ[e]
M. canis	70	63	42.8	2	75
M. gypseum	20	5	44.3	28	8
T. mentagrophytes	10	32	11.4	69	11

a, Kaplan W. In Kirk RW (ed): Current veterinary therapy III, Philadelphia, 1968, WB Saunders.
b, Blakemore JC. In Kirk RW (ed): Current veterinary therapy V, Philadelphia, 1974, WB Saunders.
c, Lewis DT, et al: Vet Dermatol (in press, 1992).
d, Bone WJ, Jackson WF: Vet Med Small Anim Clin 66:140, 1971.
e, Carman MG, et al: NZ Vet J 27:136, 143, 1979.

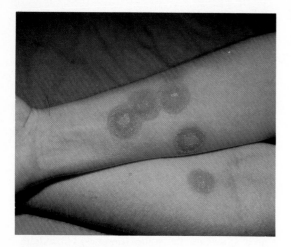

Figure 2-1. Highly inflamed dermatophytosis on the arms of a veterinarian.

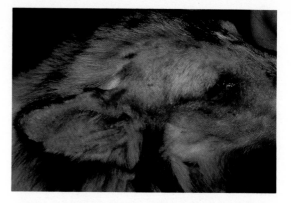

Figure 2-2. Periocular alopecia and erythema, mimicking demodicosis, on a young adult Collie.

Pathogenesis

Dermatophyte infections of dogs and cats are infections of the hair shafts and follicles. Infected hair shafts are fragile, and hair fragments containing infectious arthrospores are the most efficient means of transmission to other hosts. Such material may remain infectious in the environment for many months. Transmission is by direct contact or by contact with infected hair and scale in the environment or on fomites.

Host factors are poorly documented, but the host's ability to mount an inflammatory response plays a crucial role in terminating an infection. Dermatophyte infections in healthy dogs are often self-limiting. On the other hand, corticosteroid therapy is likely to make these infections more widespread and prolonged by inhibiting local inflammation. Other, more subtle, aberrations in the host's immune or inflammatory response may influence the likelihood of acquiring and retaining a dermatophyte infection. For example, atopic persons are at increased risk of dermatophytosis due to local inhibition of T cell function.

As is the case with many other infectious diseases, young animals are at increased risk of acquiring symptomatic dermatophyte infections. This increased risk is caused partly by the delayed development of inflammation due to a lack of specific immunity. The relatively poor inflammatory response of most typical feline ringworm lesions attests to the cat's relative tolerance of *M. canis*. This may account for the high rate of asymptomatic carriage of this species among cats. The nature and intensity of a host's immune and inflammatory response determine the nature of the dermatophyte lesion.

CLINICAL DISEASE
History

History taking may be of limited benefit with dermatophytosis unless a known exposure has occurred, because the clinical disease is so variable and the incubation period poorly defined. The disease may or may not be pruritic. In cases affecting the face or feet, infection may be associated with digging habits or with exposure to rodents.

Whenever confronted with a dermatophyte suspect, the clinician should ask about lesions on exposed persons. The source of kittens presented for examination should be ascertained, because cats from some breeding establishments may have a high incidence of infection. Dogs may be exposed and become symptomatic from an asymptomatic cat, so the number, types, and sources of contact animals should be determined.

Physical Examination

Dermatophytosis should not be diagnosed on the basis of clinical signs alone. High variability in dermatologic findings exists in true cases of ringworm, and there are several other common skin diseases that mimic the classical ringworm lesion. The most important feature of dermatophytosis in dogs and cats is the follicular location of the infection. Therefore, the most consistent clinical sign is one or more patches of alopecia (Fig. 2-2). Another fairly consistent feature is that most lesions are scaly (Fig. 2-3). Some patients may develop

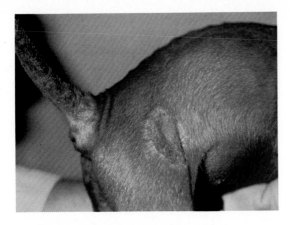

Figure 2-3. Classical patchy alopecia with associated scale in a dog with dermatophytosis.
(Courtesy Dr. Craig Griffin, San Diego, Calif.)

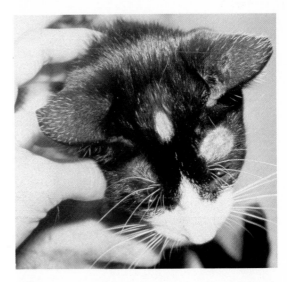

Figure 2-4. Circular alopecia with scale in a kitten with *Microsporum canis* infection.

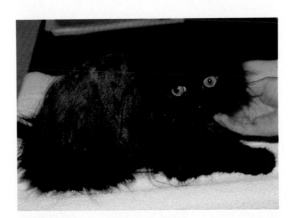

Figure 2-5. Generalized *Microsporum canis* infection in a young Persian that had been treated with repositol corticosteroids and megestrol acetate for pruritic dermatitis.

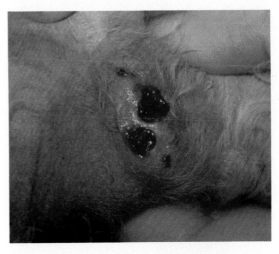

Figure 2-6. Granulomatous ulcerated nodule caused by *Microsporum canis* in a Persian with generalized dermatophytosis.

the "classical" circular ringworm, with central healing and fine follicular papules on the periphery; but signs and symptoms, in general, are highly varied and depend on the host-fungus interaction.

Feline dermatophytosis most often appears as irregular or circular alopecia with or without scale (Fig. 2-4). The alopecia may be severe and widespread with minimal evidence of inflammatory response (Fig. 2-5). Other presenting syndromes in feline dermatophytosis include miliary dermatitis, focal or multifocal pruritic dermatitis (especially in cats on corticosteroid or megestrol acetate therapy), onychomycosis, and granulomatous dermatitis. Granulomatous dermatitis, an uncommon syndrome recognized most often in cats, takes the form of a well-circumscribed, ulcerated, or fistulated dermal nodule (Fig. 2-6). The lesions usually occur on cats that are afflicted with generalized *M. canis* infection. Nodular forms have been called mycetomas, pseudomycetomas, and Majocci's granulomas. The asymptomatic carrier is important in feline dermatophytosis.

Dogs more often exhibit the classical foci of alopecia, with follicular papules and scale admixed with crust (Fig. 2-7). However, less common syndromes are frequent enough that dermatophytosis should be considered with any papular or pustular eruption. Facial folliculitis and furunculosis, mimicking an autoimmune skin disease, may be caused by a dermatophyte, often a *Trichophyton* species (Fig. 2-8). *Trichophyton* infections may also pre-

sent as folliculitis and furunculosis affecting only one leg. A seborrhea-like syndrome with greasy scale may develop in generalized cases. A nodular form of ringworm seen in dogs is the dermatophyte kerion. The kerion is a boggy, exudative, variably circumscribed type of furunculosis (Fig. 2-9) that is a common presenting sign of *M. gypseum* infection. Onychomycosis may be manifested as chronic ungual fold inflammation, with or without footpad involvement (Fig. 2-10), or the claw alone may be infected, causing claw deformity and fragility.

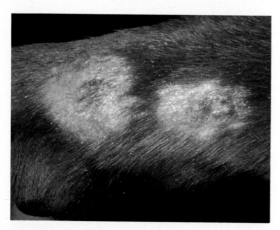

Figure 2-7. Classical circular ringworm with folliculitis on the forelimb of a Doberman Pinscher puppy. Note that the lesion has been scraped to rule out demodicosis.

(Courtesy Dr. Valerie Fadok, Denver, Colo.)

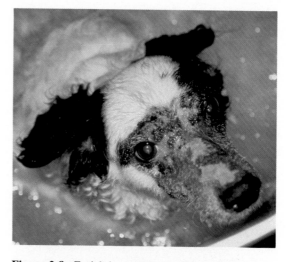

Figure 2-8. Facial dermatitis caused by *Trichophyton* infection.

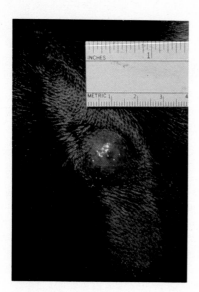

Figure 2-9. Dermatophyte kerion caused by *Microsporum gypseum* on the shoulder of a young Rottweiler.

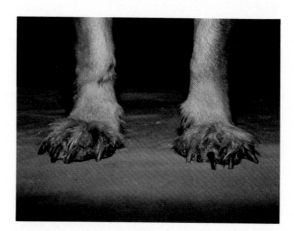

Figure 2-10. Onychomycosis caused by *Trichophyton* infection.

(Courtesy Dr. Valerie Fadok, Denver, Colo.)

Differential Diagnoses

The most important skin diseases to be differentiated from ringworm in dogs are demodicosis and staphylococcal folliculitis. Most practitioners are familiar enough with the signs and symptoms of demodicosis that it is seldom overlooked when there are circular patches of hair loss and foci of folliculitis in a young dog. Nonetheless, the clinical features of the diseases are indistinguishable. This is not surprising given the similarity of their pathogeneses—each being a follicular infection. Superficial staphylococcal folliculitis, especially when accompanied by spreading rings of erythema and exfoliation, is more often mistaken for dermatophytosis (Fig. 2-11). Also a hyperkeratotic staphylococcal lesion in a seborrheic spaniel is quite often misdiagnosed as ringworm (Fig. 2-12). Moreover, the greasy scale that accumulates on seborrheic lesions can give a false-positive Wood's lamp examination. Staphylococcal skin diseases are so much more common in dogs than dermatophyte infections are that it can truly be said of dog skin disease: "If it looks like ringworm, it's probably Staph."

The differential diagnosis in cats varies with the presentation. Alopecic lesions should be scraped to rule out feline demodicosis. Self-inflicted alopecia in the pruritic or psychogenic alopecic patient may mimic ringworm lesions. Dermatophytosis is an important rule-out in feline miliary dermatitis, although allergic skin disease is the most common cause of this syndrome.

In both dogs and cats, nodules are more often caused by other infectious agents or neoplasms. However, dermatophytes should still be considered in the differential diagnosis.

Misshapen, brittle, and sloughing nails, with or without accompanying paronychia, may be caused by bacterial infection, autoimmune skin disease, or drug eruption or may be the result of a developmental defect or rarely a nutritional disease. Dermatophytosis is a rather uncommon cause of this presentation in either dogs or cats.

DIAGNOSIS
Fungal Culture

Definitive diagnosis of dermatophytosis is made by positive culture or biopsy. Dermatophytosis is such a variable skin disease in cats that many veterinary dermatologists consider culturing for fungi a part of the minimum data base in the workup of virtually every feline skin disease. It should also be included in the workup of any case of folliculitis or patchy alopecia in dogs. This is readily performed by the clinician in private practice through the use of the dermatophyte test medium (DTM). The medium consists of Sabouraud's dextrose agar with phenol red as pH indicator and antimicrobials to inhibit bacterial and saprophytic mold growth.

There are several important principles for the accurate use of the culture medium so that both false-negative and false-positive culture results will be avoided.

Obtaining specimens. Lesions to be cultured should be clipped and cleaned. This will reduce contaminant growth on the DTM, which might lead to false-positive readings, and if performed properly will not reduce the likelihood of fungus iso-

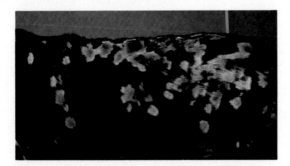

Figure 2-11. This patient had multiple patches of alopecia and erythema with epidermal collarettes. The disease superficially resembles generalized dermatophytosis; however, it was caused by staphylococcal folliculitis and responded rapidly to antibiotics.

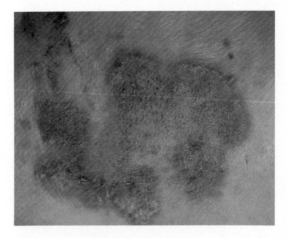

Figure 2-12. Superficial folliculitis lesions on a seborrheic Cocker Spaniel. Such lesions are often mistaken for dermatophytosis. They respond well to standard antibiotic therapy.

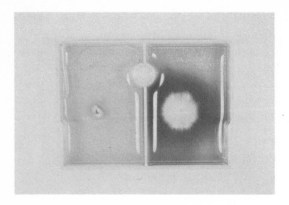

Figure 2-13. Seven-day old *Microsporum canis* colony on dermatophyte test medium *(right)* and rapid sporulation medium *(left)*. Color change has occurred simultaneously with mycelial growth.

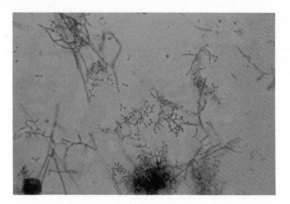

Figure 2-14. Microscopic appearance of *Trichophyton mentagrophytes* stained with lactophenol cotton blue. (×120.) Note the numerous microconidia. These features may be confused with the features of saprophytic species of fungi, so all such colonies should be submitted to a microbiology laboratory for identification.

lation. Using only the short stubble of clipped hair also will allow a larger number of individual hairs to be placed on the medium. The hair should be clipped to 0.5 cm, and the area patted (not rubbed) clean with a 70% alcohol-moistened gauze and then allowed to dry. Samples are chosen thoughtfully and should include hairs that are already broken or associated with inflammatory lesions or scale. Several lesions are sampled. Hair is collected with hemostats by grasping the hair shafts close to the skin and rolling the hairs from the follicles. This allows collection of intrafollicular portions of the hairs and increases the likelihood of obtaining infected material. If possible, hair that is Wood's lamp–positive is used. Some scale is included in the sample to be cultured, but avoid putting exudate or antiseptics on the medium.

Using the DTM. An appropriate storage site for inoculated DTM is chosen. Bottles are left loosely capped, at room temperature, and are protected from UV light and desiccation. Samples are stored where they may be easily observed and inspected daily. For proper interpretation, one must observe the medium color changing to red simultaneously with growth of a cottony mycelium (Fig. 2-13). A false-positive reading may result from saprophytic growth if the color change is observed later.

Fungal growth should be examined microscopically. After 7 to 10 days most colonies begin to produce macrospores, which will allow specific identification (Figs. 2-14 to 2-16). If a suspect colony fails to produce spores or is difficult to identify (as is often the case with *Trichophyton* spp), refer the culture to a diagnostic laboratory for identifi-

cation. This information can be important in case management and for public health decisions.

Some information can be gleaned from the color of fungal growth. Zoophilic dermatophyte colonies are always white to buff-colored. Anthropophilic species may be pinkish to yellow. Blue, green, dark brown, or black fungi are contaminants (although one geophilic species, *Trichophyton ajelloi*, does produce a black pigment in the medium). If such fungi have overgrown a colony suspected of being a dermatophyte, subculturing will be necessary and the specimens should be referred to a diagnostic laboratory.

Culturing asymptomatic animals. It may be necessary to attempt dermatophyte cultures from asymptomatic patients when human infection from an animal source is suspected or a dermatophytosis in a cattery or other multiple-cat household is being investigated.

It is also good practice to follow treatment with cultural investigations. Brush culturing (MacKenzie brush technique) is the preferred method of obtaining such specimens. (See Chapter 3.) A newly purchased toothbrush or a sterile scrub brush is satisfactory for this. The hair coat is brushed thoroughly on many parts of the body. The bristles are then impressed directly onto the culture medium in several sites. Any animal producing enough infective elements to be a source of infection to others will be identified by this technique.

Culturing onychomycosis. Special culture techniques may be needed with suspected onychomycosis. In some cases the hair surrounding the

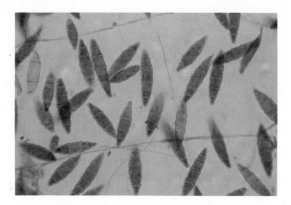

Figure 2-15. Microscopic appearance of *Microsporum gypseum* macroconidia. (×120.) The macroconidia are relatively thin-walled and have six or fewer septations.

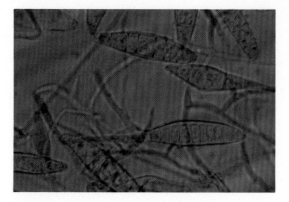

Figure 2-16. Microscopic appearance of *Microsporum canis* macroconidia. (×400.) The macroconidia are thick-walled, have a knobby "beak" on the end, and often present more than six septations.

ungual fold will be infected and may be cultured as for more common types of dermatophytosis. In obtaining samples from the feet, special care is needed to reduce contaminant growth by clipping and cleaning as described under "Obtaining specimens" p. 27. The transient carriage of fungi on the feet of dogs is common enough to warrant correlating cultural findings with histopathologic demonstration of fungi in hair or claw. Otherwise, repeated isolation of the fungus from the lesions may be regarded as evidence of causation. If the claws alone are affected, a scalpel blade may be used to shave fine pieces from the proximal end of trimmed or surgically excised claws for culture. Untreated Sabouraud's dextrose agar as well as DTM should be used, because nondermatophyte species of fungi may cause onychomycosis.

Biopsy

Biopsy is not as sensitive as culture and should not normally be relied on as the method for definitively diagnosing most superficial ringworm infections. On the other hand, when the true significance of a cultural isolation is questioned, demonstration of the organism in biopsy specimens is definitive proof of true infection. Histopathologic examination is most useful in the nodular forms of dermatophytosis—the kerion and granulomatous ringworm. It may be impossible to culture the organisms in such cases by collecting hair and scale. If surgical biopsy is performed, aseptically collected and transported tissue should be submitted for cultural as well as histopathologic study. Care must be taken to collect material with tissue grains,

for grains are what contain the infective material. Cytologic examination of the grains will help determine if bacterial (including actinomycetes) or fungal culturing is necessary. With onychomycosis, shaved or clipped or surgically excised samples of claws may be submitted for histopathologic examination. Some pathologists prefer to have claws soaked in water or detergent prior to processing, so it is appropriate to submit these specimens in a dry container. If fungal organisms are present, they will be readily visible to the pathologist within the substance of the claw, after processing and staining.

Direct Examination

Some veterinarians become skilled in the microscopic inspection of hair and scale from suspicious lesions. Such specimens may be mounted in 10% potassium hydroxide (KOH) overnight for clearing. More rapid processing may be accomplished by gently warming the specimens. Even in experienced hands, however, this technique is diagnostic in relatively few cases of dog and cat ringworm. It is time-consuming and may lead to misinterpretation when saprophytic fungal spores are present in the specimen. It is important to remember when interpreting such specimens that dermatophytes never form macrospores in tissue. Elements that superficially resemble macrospores microscopically include pollen grains and saprophyte spores. Dermatophyte elements expected to be present in hair and scale are hyphae and arthrospores (Fig. 2-17). Oily sebaceous debris or med-

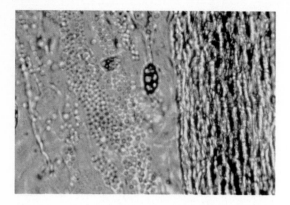

Figure 2-17. Microscopic examination of an infected hair which is surrounded by small refractile round arthrospores. (×400, KOH with Parker's blue ink.) Note that the macroconidium is a saprophyte spore. Dermatophytes never form macroconidia in tissue.

ications may be mistaken for arthrospores by persons who have little experience.

Wood's Lamp Examination

Microsporum canis infections may be positive on a Wood's lamp examination. This technique can be very valuable in the hands of an experienced diagnostician; but it should not be used to rule out dermatophytosis, since not all infections fluoresce. However, recent reports have shown that probably more than 80% of true infections with *M. canis* will be positive with careful examination (Pepin and Oxenham, 1987). On the other hand, it is easy for the less experienced clinician to overinterpret this examination, as scale and medication can have a greenish hue. True fluorescence is quite bright, apple green, and should be only *within* the shafts of the infected hairs.

The Wood's lamp should be turned on for 5 minutes prior to use and should be applied to suspect lesions for 3 to 5 minutes, since some *M. canis* strains require time before fluorescence becomes obvious.

The Physical Examination

Although clinical signs can be suggestive, as discussed above, it is dangerous to make a diagnosis on the basis of clinical signs alone. Furthermore, it is unwise to reject the possibility of dermatophytosis based on the clinical signs, the direct examination of hairs and scale, or the Wood's lamp examination. Because of the expense of specific therapy, the possible toxicity of systemic therapy,

and the public health implications of this disease, it is advisable to seek a confirmed diagnosis whenever dermatophytosis is suspected.

TREATMENT
Treatment Goals

Treatment should be aimed at eliminating the infection from the host. It should be remembered, however, that healthy dogs and short-haired cats in single-cat households may undergo spontaneous remission. Other goals of therapy include reducing contagion and satisfying the client's desires to hasten resolution.

Topical Therapy

Every confirmed case of dermatophytosis should receive topical therapy. Hair is clipped from a wide margin surrounding all lesions. Long-haired animals should be clipped entirely.

Antiseptic baths and rinses will remove the scale, crusts, exudate, and infected hairs, reducing the potential for spread of the infection. For this type of therapy, benzoyl peroxide, captan, or chlorhexidine shampoos or enilconazole, povidone-iodine, or chlorhexidine rinses may be employed. Sulfurated lime rinses are also effective antifungal topicals (Table 2-2). When sparsely haired sites are infected and the infection is localized, topical antifungal therapy alone may be sufficient to hasten resolution. Creams and lotions are available for use on focal lesions. For highly inflamed lesions, topical corticosteroids in combination with antifungal agents may hasten resolution of clinical disease. As long as one of the newer imidazole, triazole, or allylamine topicals is chosen for the treatment of lesions, there is no particular advantage of one product over another. There is a wide variety of topical antifungals available for use in human medicine, but only miconazole, clotrimazole, and (in Europe) enilconazole and ketoconazole have received veterinary labeling to date. The compounds labeled for use on persons are significantly more expensive than these.

Kerions do not require specific antifungal therapy unless widespread disease is present, in which case systemic therapy should be given. The kerion should be cleaned gently to remove exudate and avoid potentiation of scarring. Granulomatous ringworm in cats is usually associated with generalized dermatophytosis, which should be treated systemically.

Table 2-2. Products recommended for topical therapy in dermatophytosis of dogs and cats

PRODUCT	ADMINISTRATION	COMMENTS
Povidone-iodine[a]	1:4 in water qd	Irritating, sensitizing
Chlorhexidine solution[b]	2% rinse qd	
Chlorhexidine shampoo[c]	Bathe q5d	Good option
Lime-sulfur[d]	2% rinse q5-7d	Odorous, not for white animals
Na hypochlorite (bleach)	1:20 (0.5%) rinse q5-7d	Not for black animals
Captan[e]	2% (2 Tbsp/gal) rinse or spray shampoo q5d	
Enilconazole[f]	0.2% rinse q3d × 4	Not in U.S.
Miconazole cream or lotion[g]	Apply q12h	For localized lesions, can be irritating
Clotrimazole cream[h]	Apply q12h	For localized lesions, can be irritating
Ketoconazole cream[i]	Apply q12h	Prescription for use in people, several other azole topicals available[j]
Lotrisone cream[k]	Apply q12h	For highly inflamed lesions, short-term
Naftin cream[l]	Apply q12-24h	An allylamine

Modified from Foil CS. In Kirk RW (ed): Current veterinary therapy IX, Philadelphia, 1986, WB Saunders.
a, Betadine Solution; b, Nolvasan Solution; c, Nolvasan Shampoo and ChlorhexiDerm Shampoo; d, Lym Dyp; e, Orthocide Spray and Antifungal/Antibacterial (2% Captan) Shampoo; f, Imaveral (available in Europe, not the U.S.); g, Conofite Cream and Conofite Lotion; h, Veltrim and Lotrimin; i, Nizoral 2% Cream; j, sulconazole (Exelderm 1% Solution or Exelderm Cream); oxiconazole (Oxistat 1% cream); k, Lotrisone Cream (contains clotrimazole and betamethasone dipropionate); l, Naftin 1% Cream.

Systemic Therapy

Griseofulvin (Grifulvin V, Fulvicin, Grisactin, Gris-PEG). Griseofulvin is poorly water soluble, and thus gastrointestinal absorption is variable and incomplete. Absorption is enhanced by administration with a fat-containing meal or by formulations using polyethylene glycol (PEG). Particle size (micronization) also greatly affects oral absorption. Divided dosage regimens provide higher absorption levels.

Dosages recommended for dogs and cats are not based on modern pharmacologic studies. Those that have proved effective in the largest numbers of cases (Table 2-3) are high, and significant toxicities may be encountered. The most common side effects are vomiting, diarrhea, and anorexia. These can often be managed by dividing the doses more frequently or lowering the dose slightly. Bone marrow suppression, manifested as neutropenia, ane-

mia, or pancytopenia, may follow prolonged use at higher doses or may be seen as non–dose dependent idiosyncratic reactions in some cats. Of these, neutropenia is most often severe and may be fatal despite withdrawal of the drug. It is recommended to follow a CBC weekly or biweekly during the course of griseofulvin therapy in cats. Severe neutropenic reactions may be associated with feline immunodeficiency virus infection (Shelton et al., 1990), so this drug should probably be avoided in cats with such infections. Neurologic side effects have also been recorded in cats. Griseofulvin is a teratogen and must never be given during the first two thirds of pregnancy.

Ketoconazole (Nizoral, Ketofungol). Ketoconazole has moderately effective fungistatic action against *Microsporum canis* and *Trichophyton mentagrophytes*. The treatment regimen should be carried out for at least 3 weeks. Some animals will

Table 2-3. Drugs for systemic therapy of dermatophytosis in dogs and cats

DRUG	DOSE[a]	ROUTE	INTERVAL (HR)	DURATION[b] (WK)
Griseofulvin				
Microsized[c]	25-60	PO	12	4-6
Ultramicrosized[d]	2.5-5	PO	12-24	4-6
Ketoconazole[e]	10	PO	24	3-4

a, Dose per administration at specified interval, expressed in mg/kg.
b, Follow-up brush culture should be negative before discontinuing therapy.
c, Trade names: Grifulvin V, Fulvicin U/F, Grisactin.
d, Trade names: Fulvicin PG, Grisactin Ultra, Gris-PEG.
e, Trade name in U.S.: Nizoral; in Europe: Ketofungol.

remain culture-positive after this treatment period, but few relapse clinically. As with griseofulvin, ketoconazole may be less successful in the treatment of long-haired cats than other types of patients. Specifically, there is concern about its less than favorable fungicidal activity against *Microsporum canis*. Also it is not labeled for use in dogs and cats in the United States. Since griseofulvin is a fairly safe and effective approved drug for the treatment of dermatophytosis, most veterinary dermatologists in the United States reserve ketoconazole for use in selected cases in which resistance to griseofulvin is strongly suspected or the patient cannot tolerate griseofulvin. Among European veterinary dermatologists, however, ketoconazole has supplanted griseofulvin as the standard approach to systemic therapy. Along with topical enilconazole, it has proved particulary helpful in treating cattery infestations (Carlotti and Couprie, 1988).

Side effects of ketoconazole include anorexia (common), hepatotoxicity and/or icterus problems (uncommon), and inhibition of steroidal hormone synthesis. Testosterone production is particularly sensitive to this drug.

Newer antifungal drugs. New triazole compounds such as itraconazole (Sporonox) and saperconazole may soon be available in human medicine and in oral formulations. These drugs have been shown to be highly efficacious against human dermatophytosis and to produce less systemic toxicity. Unfortunately, as was the case with ketoconazole, some clinical studies (Saul and Bonifaz, 1990) have also shown that their efficacy against *M. canis* may not be as great as against anthropophilic *Trichophyton* species. In a study of *M. canis* scalp dermatophytosis, however, which, like animal ringworm, is follicular, itraconazole was very successful (93% culture-negative in 4 to 8 weeks) (Legendre and Esola-Macre, 1990). Pre-

liminary work with itraconazole in dogs and cats with systemic fungal disease would also indicate a lower potential for toxicity in these species compared to ketoconazole. Unfortunately, the triazole that has received labeling for human use in the United States, fluconazole (Diflucan), is probably not highly efficacious against dermatophytes.

The allylamine drug terbinafine (Lamisil) may be available for human use in the United States as an oral agent in the near future. It is presently available in some European countries and has shown great promise against chronic dermatophytosis, especially onychomycosis, with virtually no serious systemic toxicity. It remains to be seen whether terbinafine will prove useful in veterinary mycology.

Specific Treatment Recommendations

Dermatophytosis should always be treated topically, but not every infected animal will require systemic therapy. Long-haired cats and any dog or cat with generalized dermatophytosis should be totally clipped and receive systemic therapy. Since *Trichophyton* infections often spread, become generalized, and cannot be expected to resolve spontaneously, they should be treated systemically.

Monitoring Treatment

A mycologic as well as clinical cure should be the goal in treating dermatophytosis. Most affected animals are treated for a minimum of 1 month. Asymptomatic animals should be tested culture-negative with the brush technique (described earlier) prior to cessation of therapy. Patients receiving griseofulvin are monitored with a CBC once every 2 weeks, if doses are moderate, or more frequently, if doses have been chosen from the high end of the recommended range. Griseofulvin- and ketoconazole-treated patients should have liver enzyme activities evaluated once a month.

Environmental Cleanup

Some environmental cleanup should be performed in cases of generalized *Microsporum canis* infection. For specific recommendations see Chapter 3.

REFERENCES

Blakemore JC: Dermatomycosis. In Kirk RW (ed): Current veterinary therapy V, Philadelphia, 1974, WB Saunders, p 422.

Carlotti D, Couprie B: Dermatophyties du chien et du chat, Actual Pratique Medicale Chirurgicale Anim Compagnie, September-October, p 449, 1988.

Constable PJ, Harrington JM: Risks of zoonoses in a veterinary service, Br Med J 284:246, 1982.

Foil CS: Dermatophytosis. In Greene CE (ed): Infectious diseases of the dog and cat, Philadelphia, 1990, WB Saunders, p 659.

Legendre R, Esola-Macre J: Itraconazole in the treatment of tinea capitis, J Am Acad Dermatol 23:559, 1990.

Pepin G, Oxenham M: Zoonotic dermatophytosis (ringworm), Vet Rec 118:110, 1986.

Pepin GA, Oxenham M: Feline dermatophytosis: the diagnosis of subclinical infection and its relevance to control, Vet Dermatol Newslett 11:21, 1987.

Quaife RA, Womar SM: *Microsporum canis* isolations from show cats, Vet Rec 110:333, 1982.

Saul AS, Bonifaz A: Itraconazole in common dermatophyte infections of the skin: fixed treatment schedules, J Am Acad Dermatol 23:554, 1990.

Shelton GH, et al: Severe neutropenia associated with griseofulvin therapy in cats with feline immunodeficiency virus infection, J Vet Intern Med 4:317, 1990.

Svejgaard E: Epidemiology and clinical features of dermatomycoses and dermatophytoses, Acta Derm Venereol (Stockh) Suppl 121:19, 1986.

3

Dermatophytosis: Cattery Management Plan

Hazel C. Carney   Karen A. Moriello

Treatment Plan for Elimination of Dermatophytosis From a Cattery

Identification of affected cats
Isolation of affected cats
Environmental decontamination
Topical treatment
Systemic treatment if necessary
Reevaluation with serial fungal cultures
Integration of cured cats back into the normal population

Importance

The exact incidence of dermatophytosis in cats or catteries is unknown. Ringworm is not a reportable disease. It has a stigma associated with it in the breeding and showing cattery. Cattery owners are reluctant to admit the presence of the disease in any of their cats, often ignoring the problem until the entire facility is contaminated. Even cats that appear healthy may, in fact, be infected. Many times breeders admit the magnitude of the infection only after they have been confronted by someone who contracted the disease from contact with an infected kitten. Most breeders realize that treatment is expensive. Practitioners must be aware of the exhaustive methods needed to fully diagnose the extent of the dermatophyte infection and then develop a treatment eradication program that a breeder will utilize.

Pathogenesis

Causative Organisms

Microsporum canis is the cause of 96% or more of the dermatophytosis seen in cattery source animals (Menges and George, 1955; Quaife and Womar, 1982). *M. canis* is a keratinophilic organism that invades superficial layers of the skin, hair, and nails. It is so well-adapted to the cat that long-term asymptomatic carrier states are routinely encountered. Previously from 5.9% to 91% of the cats in a given cattery could be considered clinically normal yet culture positive for the organism (Woodard, 1983). Recent research, however (Moriello and DeBoer, 1991), has demonstrated that if only one cat in the cattery is infected with *M. canis* all cats will culture positive.

Microsporum gypseum is a soil saprophyte that occasionally causes dermatophyte lesions in cattery animals, especially when cats are housed in outdoor facilities that accumulate in-blown dust and debris. One author (Moriello, unpublished data, 1989) finds *M. canis* to be the cause of all cases of dermatophytosis in purebred long-haired cats. Another, however (Carney, unpublished data, 1989), has cultured *M. gypseum* from two Himalayan catteries in which animals were housed in screened porch buildings on farms in the South. Although rare asymptomatic carrier states have been documented for *M. gypseum,* the existence of a long-term carrier state has not been demonstrated (Fuentes et al., 1954).

Trichophyton mentagrophytes also should be considered as a potential cause of ringworm in cattery cats that are housed in outdoor facilities to which rodents have access (Blank, 1957). Both catteries from which one author (Carney, unpublished data, 1989) has cultured this organism have housed short-haired breeds, one Abyssinian and the other Russian Blue. In both catteries animals were housed in outdoor runs. *Trichophyton mentagrophytes* was cultured from another Abyssinian at a show in England (Quaife and Womar, 1982). The organism also has been recovered from clinically normal cats. Whether these cats are short-term transporters or long-term carriers is unknown (Fuentes et al., 1954).

Predisposing Factors

No sex or breed predispositions have been documented for feline dermatophytosis. Age, nutrition, poor management, and concurrent disease have been shown to influence whether a cat becomes infected. Ringworm lesions are seen most commonly in kittens, which are more susceptible to diseases. Nutrition is not adequate in many catteries because breeders usually insist on feeding any number of dietary concoctions. Diseases are common in catteries when owners fail to vaccinate at optimal frequency. Some cattery owners do not maintain FeLV-, FIV-, and FIP-negative status. This decreases the effectiveness of cell-mediated immune responses in the cats. Many catteries have poor ventilation and no sunshine or fresh air. The cats are crowded into small areas. Ectoparasites irritate the cats, causing them to scratch and produce skin defects. Grooming potions used to develop show-coats may also damage skin and increase the likelihood of infection.

Exposure to *Microsporum canis* or another dermatophyte may or may not result in an infection. (Readers should refer to the preceding chapter to review how an infection can become established in a cat.)

Transmission of Dermatophytosis

Dermatophytes are spread by direct contact with an infected cat or fomite. In a cattery, in-house transmission can occur rapidly from clinically affected animals or from asymptomatic carriers. The meticulous grooming habits of the cat probably account for this rapid dissemination. Communal grooming transfers organisms between cats, and scratching cats aerosolize hairs infected with ectothrix spores. Cats returning from shows or breeding loans are always potential sources of infection.

Microsporum canis has been reported anecdotally to persist in the environment for 13 to 52 months (Muller et al., 1989). Any building or room where infected cats have been housed could potentially be a source of infections. Organisms have been cultured from dust, heating vents, and furnace filters (Moriello, unpublished data, 1989). Visitors to a cattery may introduce the organism into a clean colony. Brushes, bedding, transport cages, and other grooming and show paraphernalia are all potential sources of infection or reinfection.

CLINICAL DISEASE
History

Consider dermatophytes as a possible cause of any dermatosis seen in a cattery-source animal. To help a cattery owner eliminate a dermatophyte from a cattery, the veterinarian must have a thorough understanding of the type of cattery, its physical plant, and the management protocols. To determine this information, we ask the following questions of all catteries with which we work:

1. How many cats are in the cattery? (This should include breeding queens, toms, kittens that are nursing, kittens that are in show competition, premiers [spays or castrates] on the show circuit, and pet cats that interact with cattery residents.)
2. What vaccination protocol is followed?
3. What is the FeLV, FIV, and FIP status of each cat?
4. What is the floorplan of the cattery? (Owners are asked to draw a sketch of the cattery and label the kitten room, grooming area,

feeding area, stud quarters, and connections to human living premises.)

5. What type ventilation systems and heating and cooling units are used?
6. What type cages are used? How are they cleaned? Are they submersible in cleaning solutions?
7. What has been the breeding schedule for the past 2 years? What outside cats were brought into this cattery, and which cats have been loaned for breeding purposes?
8. Who feeds, cleans, plays with, grooms, or in any way interacts with the cats?
9. What topical products currently are in use on any of the cats? (Include in the list show shampoos, rinses, etc.)
10. What systemic medications are being given to any of the cats, whether veterinarian or owner-prescribed?
11. How long has the cattery owned each cat?
12. Which cats have had any form of skin disease?

Presenting Signs and Physical Examination Findings

Unfortunately, cats with dermatophytosis may be clinically normal; they may also present with a myriad of hair coat abnormalities. Suggestive lesions are most commonly observed in kittens, less frequently in queens and toms, and least often in castrates or spayed females.

In kittens initial lesions usually appear as well-circumscribed scaly patches of hair loss on ear tips, chin, bridge of the nose, upper lips, and the supraoptic/preauricular area. The lesions may progress to thin, dry, grayish crusts. If secondary bacteria invade the lesions, thicker moister crusts will develop. From the face, lesions progress via grooming to the digits, paws, and legs and eventually over the entire body. The areas gradually heal, being replaced with short, soft, almost downy new fur that may be darker than the cat's normal coat. Disseminated ringworm in kittens may cause a moth-eaten appearance (Holzworth, 1987).

Adult queens may have patchy hair loss, recurrent chin acne, miliary scabs, a nonluxurious hair coat, or folliculitis. Rarely a cat may present with only blepharitis; fungi are cultured from periocular hair follicles or corneal scrapings. Often queens appear normal and are found to be infected only after their kittens develop lesions at 3 to 6 weeks of age (Holzworth, 1987).

Toms usually present with a single scratch that becomes infected after a mating tussle with an asymptomatic queen. Rarely they may have lesions similar to what has been described in queens (Holzworth, 1987).

Premieres usually show cyclic thin scruffy coats with or without miliary crusts. Others have paronychia.

Any cat with dermatophytosis may scratch, but pruritus is not a common symptom of the disease.

Sentinel lesions for a particular cattery may appear in a first litter from a recently acquired queen, in new cattery workers, or in a kitten new to the show circuit.

Remember, asymptomatic carrier cats are just that: they look great but are infection "time bombs" that continuously spread fungal organisms.

DIAGNOSIS

Tests Needed to Confirm a Dermatophyte Infection

Physical examination. Basic physical examination with drawings of lesion distribution and a written description of the type lesions found on each cat will help determine the extent of disease and will aid in the assessment of response to therapy.

Wood's lamp evaluation. A Wood's lamp will detect the presence of fluorescing strains of *Microsporum canis*. Wood's lamps must be used correctly if they are to give reliable information. (Refer to the preceding chapter for a full explanation of the physiologic basis of fluorescence and the proper technique in using the lamp.)

Direct examination "clearing" technique. The "clearing" technique will detect ectothrix spores and hyphae. It is more fully described in the preceding chapter.

Fungal culture. The most reliable means for detecting a dermatophyte on the haircoat of cats is the MacKenzie brush technique. This protocol minimizes the chance of false-negative culture from lesions, maximizes the opportunity to identify carrier cats, and seems reliable even when the owner has treated the cat topically.

A new toothbrush in its original cellophane package is sterile for fungi. For either lesional or asymptomatic cats the toothbrush is aggressively brushed over the cat's **entire** body for 2 to 3 minutes. Hairs **must** be visible in the bristles of the brush. The bristles are then gently embedded in the fungal culture medium. If screw-type media bottles are used, a child's toothbrush will more readily fit into the bottle; Sab-Duet plates can be inoculated with any-size toothbrush. The culture should be kept at room temperature. The cap of the screw-type jar must be slightly loosened. A cup of water placed in a container with the vials will increase the relative humidity and improve the likelihood that a pathogenic fungus when present is not overgrown by contaminants. *Microsporum canis* usually grows within 7 to 10 days and sometimes in as little as 3 days. Cultures from asymptomatic carrier cats may require 14 to 21 days for identifiable growth to occur. Positive identification of organisms should be made using lactophenol cotton blue stain on samples taken from the colony with cellophane tape.

When sterile toothbrushes are not available, individual hairs may be cultured. If only a few lesions fluoresce, the hairs for culture should be taken from these areas. Any lesion to be cultured is first patted with 70% isopropyl alcohol and allowed to dry. Hairs are plucked from the periphery of the lesion, gently in the direction of growth so as to obtain the hair bulb root. This end of the hair most frequently is culture-positive. Random selection of hairs is **not** recommended in any clinically normal cat.

Colony identification. Some generalities are important to remember. Gross colonies of pathogenic fungi are **never** colored or heavily pigmented. Color change in the culture medium alone is **not** diagnostic of a pathogenic fungus. The most suspicious growth is white, fluffy colonies with concomitant agar color changes, from which pathogenic spores can be identified. Spores must be examined microscopically for confirmation. Media color change is suggestive but not diagnostic of *Microsporum canis*. (See the preceding chapter for further explanation of colony identification.)

Biopsy testing. Rarely all the above tests are negative but one or more cats have skin lesions. In this case biopsies of the lesions should be obtained and submitted for fungal, bacterial, and histologic evaluation as recommended in the previous chapter. The history submitted with the biopsies should indicate that the patient lives in a ringworm-suspect cattery.

TREATMENT
Available Treatment Options

Treatment regimens for use in a cattery should be designed to completely eliminate the dermatophyte organisms from the cats and the environment. This is a monumental undertaking that, in optimum form, requires aggressive topical and systemic therapy for the cats, interruption of the breeding program and show campaigns, isolation of the colony, environmental decontamination, and testing and isolation of future cattery members. (See flowchart, next page.) Cattery owners must be willing to invest time, money, and effort in the treatment program. Successful elimination of the disease also requires much communication between the veterinarian and the cattery owner. Treatment plans, the potential side effects of some treatments, and the treatment timetable must be well understood by both. Modifications of an ideal eradication program thus are made on the basis of the cattery owner's commitment, the extent of the problem, and economics.

The therapeutic options include three general approaches. The first requires total depopulation of the cattery, decontamination of the facility, and repopulation with only cats that are negative on three consecutive MacKenzie brush cultures performed at 2-week intervals. Most breeders reject this approach because of the loss of their gene pool. The second technique requires treatment of the entire colony and facilities with appropriate topical medications, systemic therapy, and environmental cleanup. The colony is isolated, and breeding and showing are interrupted. Costs escalate as the size of the colony increases. The third option is to treat just the kittens. This is practical only for catteries that produce kittens for the pet cat market. Only one feline practitioner (Stein, 1986) reports using a modification of this approach with any regularity, because in general "kitten mills" and pet shops are the least likely to treat their problems.

Ideal Treatment Plan for Elimination of Dermatophytosis From a Cattery
Identification of Affected Cats

As soon as even one cat is suspected of having ringworm, all cats in the cattery should be examined. If *Microsporum canis* is identified as the causative fungus in the index case, all cats should be considered infected. If another organism is identified the infection rate may not reach 100%. Ideally all cats, whether lesional or normal appearing, should be cultured by the MacKenzie brush technique. In large catteries this may be cost prohibitive; an alternative would be to screen first by Wood's lamp examination and microscopic examination of hairs with culture of only those cats that are negative by both tests. Another alternative is to assume that if one cat is infected all will be.

MOVEMENT OF CATS ACCORDING TO MACKENZIE BRUSH CULTURE (MKBC) RESULTS

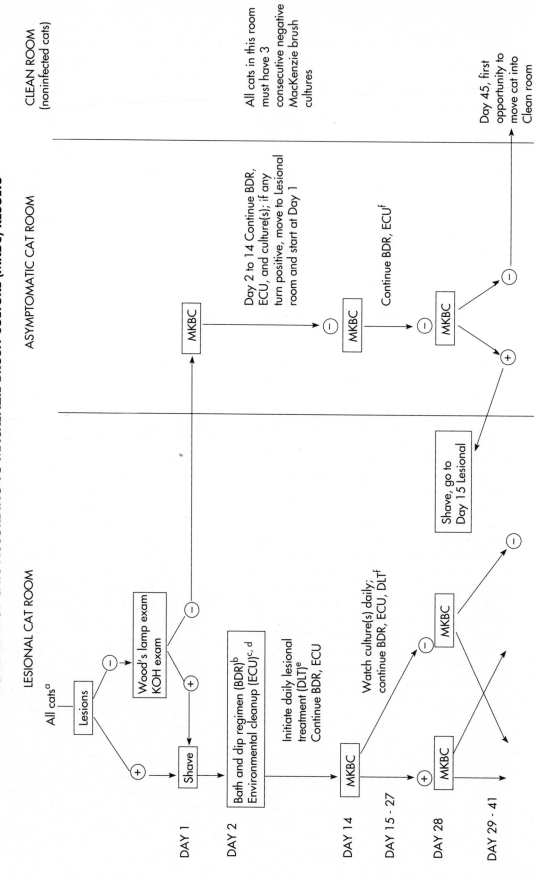

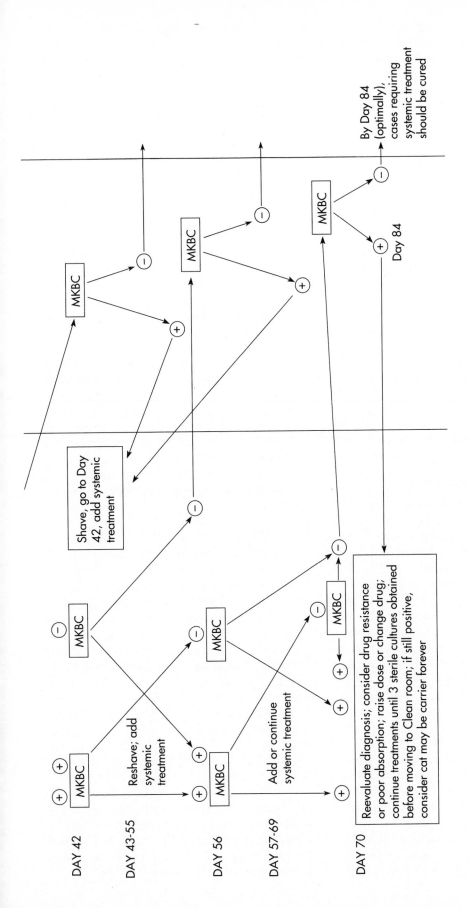

DAY 42

DAY 43-55   Reshave; add systemic treatment

DAY 56

DAY 57-69   Add or continue systemic treatment

DAY 70   Reevaluate diagnosis; consider drug resistance or poor absorption; raise dose or change drug; continue treatments until 3 sterile cultures obtained before moving to Clean room; if still positive, consider cat may be carrier forever

Shave, go to Day 42, add systemic treatment

By Day 84 (optimally), cases requiring systemic treatment should be cured

Day 84

a, Identify cats. Separate them into two groups, lesional and asymptomatic. Check all asymptomatics with a Wood's lamp and KOH exam of hairs. If a cat is positive on either test, move to the lesional group. Separate the two groups into two rooms and identify a third room that has never been occupied by cats or can be stripped and locked up.

b, Bathe and dip every cat once every fifth day using the techniques described in the text; if a cat is to have a new MKBC inoculation on the day of a bath and dip, inoculate the culture before the bath.

c, Massive cleanup of the environment is to be done every fifth day; see protocol in the text. Always clean the dermatophyte-free room first each day and clean it routinely before it is occupied on day 42. Clean the asymptomatic cat room next and then the lesional cat room.

d, Daily cleanup of the environment includes washing of litter pans and water bowls, spraying air-conditioner and heater vents, mopping floors, and doing laundry with the addition of sodium hypochlorite. Always clean the dermatophyte-free room first, then the asymptomatic cat room, and then the lesional cat room.

e, Lesional treatment of affected cats is described in the text.

f, Continue these for the entire program.

Additional cats in the environment are then not cultured until after treatment has been started. Whenever possible, samples should be taken at the cattery location so as to minimize the risk of contamination of the veterinary hospital.

Separation of Affected Cats

Cleanup of both the cats and the environment is greatly facilitated if each cat can be housed separately in a submersible, scrubable cage; either the polystyrene or the welded wire metal cage withstands the necessary heavy cleaning.

If possible, all cats that were identified as infected by Wood's lamp or microscopic examination of hairs should be moved to a separate room or building from cats that are pending results of DTM culture. When quarantine buildings or separate rooms are not available, all cats should be caged individually and the entire cattery should be closed to visitors and new cats. Whenever possible, the person who handles suspects should differ from the person who handles infected cats. Alternatively, a single caretaker must handle all the suspects first and then the known infected patients. At the end of the feeding and medication session each day, the person's clothes should be changed and laundered with the addition of 0.5% sodium hypochlorite (Chlorox) to make a 1:30 dilution in the washer.

Environmental Decontamination

All contaminated equipment, toys, feed containers, transport cages, scratching posts, grooming supplies, bedding etc., **must be removed** from the environment. Any item that cannot be washed in a bathtub or washing machine should be destroyed. Washable items should be placed in a washing machine, bathtub, or laundry wash sink as appropriate to the item. The items must then be washed in hot water using an antifungal soap (Nolvasan Scrub), rinsed, and then soaked in a 1:30 dilution of 0.5% sodium hypochlorite for 10 minutes. This should be repeated a minimum of three times.

All rooms in which the cats have lived or played may contain fungal spores. A Wood's lamp should be used at night to view the entire cattery, walls, ceilings, furnace vents, air conditioner filters, under owner's beds, behind the refrigerator where many kittens play, and all other crevices where hair and dander could collect; this will help to identify areas of high hair concentration that may otherwise be overlooked.

Next, all surfaces, whether they fluoresced earlier or not, are vacuumed, scrubbed, rinsed, and wiped down with a 1:30 dilution of 0.5% sodium hypochlorite. Vacuum bags should be burned or saturated with a 1:30 dilution of 0.5% sodium hypochlorite. One room at a time is decontaminated and allowed to dry thoroughly before a person or a cat reenters: sodium hypochlorite is very irritating to the eyes, skin, and mucous membranes. Furnace and air conditioner filters will need to be changed and discarded once a week. Initially all heating or cooling vents and furnaces should be vacuumed and cleaned by a commercial company with high-powered suction equipment (Moriello, unpublished data, 1989). Daily spraying of the filters with 2% chlorhexidine (Nolvasan Solution) will help decrease the number of spores that are recirculated. Fans should not be used in the cattery. When the cattery is a private house, books, lamps, bric-a-brac, bed linens, and furniture must also be vacuumed and wiped at least once a week with an antifungal liquid such as a 1:30 dilution of 0.5% sodium hypochlorite or a 1:4 dilution of 2% chlorhexidine solution. Rugs that cannot be destroyed or removed should be washed with an antifungal disinfectant. Steam cleaning fails to maintain water temperatures of above 43° C at the carpet level and may not be a reliable method of killing fungal spores unless an antifungal disinfectant such as chlorhexidine is added to the water (Moriello, unpublished data, 1989). All vehicles used to transport cats must likewise be decontaminated.

This massive cleanup is mandatory if a breeder wishes to remove fungi from the premises.

Topical Treatment of Cats and Cages

Asymptomatic cats should be bathed every 5 days in an antifungal shampoo (ChlorhexiDerm, Nolvasan Skin and Wound) followed by an antifungal dip (1:4 of 2% Nolvasan Solution), which is allowed to dry on the cat. On the day that the cat is bathed and dipped, the cat's cage should be washed in the bathtub or sink with hot soapy water and then soaked for 10 minutes in a 1:30 dilution of 0.5% sodium hypochlorite and rinsed. Bedding should also be washed with sodium hypochlorite and soap in the washing machine, rinsed, dried, and replaced. Daily cleaning of cages is best accomplished using a 1:4 dilution of 2% chlorhexidine in a spray bottle and wiping down the cage walls. The use of disposable 6-inch paper plates for each feeding is very inexpensive and decreases the incidence of "chin acne" ringworm as well as bacterial folliculitis of the mentum. Litter pans and water bowls should be washed daily in hot soapy water, soaked for 10 minutes in 1:30 dilution of 0.5% sodium hypochlorite, and then rinsed and dried.

Symptomatic cats should be shaved all over; **never anticipate a cure for dermatophytosis if the owner is unwilling to shave the cat.** Even whiskers must be sacrificed. General anesthesia may be required, especially to clip hair between toes and on the face. A vacuum cleaner may be used to vacuum the hairs as they are clipped from the anesthetized cat. Cats should be clipped in a draft free environment. Hair is put into a cardboard box and burned, as is the vacuum cleaner bag if one was used. Alternatively, the hair is placed in a widemouthed gallon-size jar, covered with a 1:30 dilution of 0.5% sodium hypochlorite, and discarded. Clipper blades should be sterilized by autoclave or ethylene oxide after use. A cat may be "embarrassed" and upset by the shaving, but this response can be lessened if it is anesthetized for the clipping. The cat should be allowed to fully recover from the anesthesia before any bathing and dipping are begun. General anesthesia costs may be unrealistic for a large group of cats. Many cattery owners are amazingly good with electric clippers, so you may elect to have the owner do the close clipping. This offers the advantage that the fungal spores are removed away from the veterinary hospital. In any case, the person doing the clipping should wear washable or burnable attire and immediately upon finishing the procedure dispose of the clothing or put it directly into the washing machine with soap and sodium hypochlorite. Owners should disinfect or discard their clipper blades. For disinfecting, a 1:30 dilution of 0.5% sodium hypochlorite is suitable.

After the initial shaving, bathing, and dipping as well as the environmental cleanup, **all** cats should be bathed and dipped once every week (once every 5 days being preferred). Whenever the fungal culture becomes positive on one of the asymptomatic cats, that cat should be clipped and moved into the infected cat quarters. If cultures remain negative at 2 weeks on any asymptomatic cat, that cat should be recultured; only after three consecutive cultures inoculated at 2-week intervals are negative can a specific cat be considered free of *M. canis* and not a subclinical carrier.

Topical Agents Available for Dermatophyte Control

The use of topical antifungal agents is essential in the therapy of dermatophytosis. Many products are fungicidal. Certain information helps decide which chemical is used on cats and which should be restricted to use on inanimates.

Povidone-iodine and 0.5% sodium hypochlorite are not recommended for use directly on cats because they are skin irritants and the iodines stain light-colored coats and cause gastric irritation when ingested. Sodium hypochlorite 0.5% diluted to a 1:30 concentration is the most cost-effective antifungal agent for use on inanimate surfaces; it is not recommended for use directly on cats.

Technical captan rinse irritates human skin and because it has been identified as a potential human carcinogen should no longer be recommended for routine use. We both prefer to use chlorhexidine gluconate–containing products. They are the least irritating topically to both cats and humans and may be used either full strength or diluted with up to 4 parts water. The 2% solution (Nolvasan Solution) may be kept in spray bottles to clean any surfaces or mist ventilation ducts and filters. If diluted 1:4, the chlorhexidine can be sponged directly onto any lesions on the cats once daily and used as a whole body dip as well. All chlorhexidine compounds should be kept out of the eyes because they may cause severe corneal ulceration. Chlorhexidine is available prepackaged in ointment (Nolvasan Ointment) and suspension forms (Nolvasan Suspension) for use on lesions. The surgical scrub (Nolvasan Scrub) is excellent as a dish soap and laundry detergent.

Lime sulfur (LymDyp) at a 1:32 dilution may be used as an effective, inexpensive dip but is poorly tolerated by both cats and owners because of the horrible smell it produces. The dip may also stain light-colored cats and surfaces.

Thiabendazole has reportedly been effective as a topical antifungal agent (Heymann, 1986); a commercial otic preparation (Tresaderm) does contain thiabendazole and is effective as a lesional medication; plus it has the benefit of containing a steroid to decrease the irritation occasionally seen with a dermatophyte lesion. However, the steroid can be absorbed systemically so it is not recommended in very young kittens or pregnant queens; its only practical use is in the treatment of toms or premiers with single lesions.

Other topical agents that are effective for focal lesions only are miconazole (Conofite) and clotrimazole (Lotrimin). Irritant contact reactions have been reported in some cases.

Topical agents must be used long-term: a minimum duration is for 2 weeks after **every** cat in the cattery has tested negative for dermatophytes **by fungal culture** of a MacKenzie brush on three separate tests inoculated 2 weeks apart. This means at least 12 to 20 weeks of bathing and dipping every fifth day. **Do not compromise.**

Systemic Medications

Two systemic antifungal medications currently are available. Their use may be reserved for when 3 to 4 weeks of intensive topical and environmental treatment has failed to significantly reduce the number of culture positive animals. Usage from the beginning in any lesional animal, however, seems to facilitate a cure.

Griseofulvin. Griseofulvin has long been available for treatment of dermatophytosis. It is fungistatic. **It must be given daily to be effective.** Our recommended dosages are 25 mg/kg of the microsize liquid (Grifulvin V) divided q12h PO for kittens or cats weighing less than 2 kg and 10 mg/kg of the ultramicrosize tablet (Gris-PEG or Fulvicin U/F) divided q12h PO for cats weighing 2 kg or more. Both products are given after a meal; kittens are given ½ teaspoon cream cheese as a fatty supplement after the liquid, and adult cats are given the pills in a small ball of the cream cheese, which disguises the taste of the pill and provides the fatty supplement.

Because the recognition of griseofulvin toxicity is increasing (Helton et al., 1986; Kunkle and Meyer, 1987), we recommend that cats receiving this medication be given a physical examination every 2 weeks. Ideally, a complete blood count and serum chemistry profile should be drawn on each cat before it is started on griseofulvin and CBCs should be repeated every 2 weeks while the cats are on systemic therapy. This laboratory testing can become cost-prohibitive in a large cattery; most cattery owners prefer to watch the cats closely and test only those that show signs of toxicity. Thus the veterinarian must spend time to educate the cattery owner and ensure that the owner knows to contact the veterinarian if a cat shows any signs of depression, fever, icterus, ataxia, or angioedema. In practice the milder clinical signs such as anorexia, vomiting, and diarrhea can be limited if the cat is fed just prior to medicating so food is present in the stomach with the medication.

The cattery owner should be told that griseofulvin is teratogenic and therefore contraindicated in pregnant animals prior to day 57 of gestation.

Resistance to griseofulvin is extremely rare with only one case having been documented (Scott, 1980).

Ketoconazole. Ketoconazole (Nizoral) is a broad-spectrum antifungal antibiotic that has been used successfully to treat dermatophyte infections. However, resistant strains of *Microsporum canis* have been identified (Woodard, 1983). The dosage recommended is 10 mg/kg q24h PO (Foil, 1986). Anorexia is a common side effect. Anecdotally one of us (Carney, unpublished data, 1990) has seen markedly less appetite depression if the cat's dosage is repackaged into a no. 2 gelatin capsule, which is then filled with vitamin B1 powder. Again the drug is always given when the cat is known to have food in its stomach. Because hepatic toxicity is possible, a pretreatment chemistry panel is advised; follow-up chemistry panels are recommended at 2-week intervals. Again, excessive costs usually prohibit multiple chemistry screens in large catteries so owners elect to observe for signs of vomiting, icterus, or severe depression. If these signs appear, the medication is stopped and the cat is evaluated by the veterinarian.

Treatment of Kittens Only

In some situations a cattery owner may be unable or unwilling to treat the entire cattery. If the owner wishes only to produce kittens that are not infected with *Microsporum canis,* an alternative strategy is available:

1. Isolate breeding and pregnant queens from the remainder of the cattery.
2. Clip the haircoat of the queens.
3. Treat the queens topically with chlorhexidine shampoos and dips twice weekly.
4. After the kittens are born, begin oral griseofulvin therapy in the queens. Although griseofulvin is contraindicated in pregnant queens, one feline practitioner (Stein, personal communication, 1986) routinely begins administration of griseofulvin in the last week of pregnancy and has not observed any ill effects.
5. Wean the kittens as soon as possible, preferably by 4 weeks of age. Isolate the kittens from all other cats. Some cattery owners choose to separate kittens from queens at birth and hand-raise them in isolation.
6. At 4 weeks of age, culture all kittens with a sterile toothbrush. Pending fungal culture results, begin topical therapy. Chlorhexidine or lime sulfur is safe in young kittens. If the fungal culture indicates that the kittens are infected, begin oral griseofulvin or ketoconazole therapy. Fully explain the potential for toxicity.
7. Kittens should not be sold until at least one, preferably two, negative fungal cultures are obtained.

Monitoring Responses to Therapy

Response to therapy in both cats and kittens is best monitored by fungal culture. The MacKenzie brush technique should be used. The brushing must be very aggressive so as not to obtain false-negatives.

Preventive Measures

Preventing the introduction or reintroduction of dermatophytes into a cattery requires isolation of new cats, isolation of cats returning from shows or breeding loans, and periodic culturing of the entire colony. Cats must be culture-negative before they enter or reenter a colony, and separate isolated cages must be maintained for them pending culture results. While the cultures are pending, the isolated cats should be bathed and dipped once weekly with chlorhexidine shampoos and dips. Items used with these cats must not be used elsewhere in the cattery.

Cat shows pose a tremendous threat to a ringworm-free cattery. Preventing exposure to spores while at a show is difficult. Cats should be groomed away from other cats if at all possible. Grooming tools should never be borrowed or loaned. Carriers should be covered whenever the cats are not being examined by the judges. The day the cat returns home it should be brushed with a sterile brush and a culture inoculated. Then it should be bathed and dipped for the first time and isolated. Bathing and dipping should be continued every 5 days until the culture results are available.

Fungal vaccines are successful in Europe for the management of endemic dermatophytosis in cattle. Although one report (Mosher et al., 1977) described the use of a fungal vaccine in the treatment of dermatophytosis in a cat, no controlled studies on the use of fungal vaccines to treat or prevent fungal infection have been published. Several small companies are selling "*M. canis* vaccines." Efficacy has not been shown and none of the vaccines has FDA approval. We recommend avoiding these vaccines until safety and efficacy have been shown.

REFERENCES

Blank F: Favus of mice, Can J Microbiol 3:885, 1957.

Foil CS: Antifungal agents in dermatology. In Kirk RW (ed): Current veterinary therapy IX, Philadelphia, 1986, WB Saunders.

Fuentes CA, et al: Occurrence of Trichophyton mentagrophytes and Microsporum gypseum on hairs of healthy cats, J Invest Dermatol 23:311, 1954.

Helton KA, et al: Griseofulvin toxicity in cats: literature review and report of seven cases, J Am Anim Hosp Assoc 22:453, 1986.

Heymann LD: Thiabendazole treatment of ringworm in a cat, Mod Vet Pract 6:545, 1986.

Holzworth J: Diseases of the cat: medicine and surgery, vol 1, Philadelphia, 1987, WB Saunders.

Kunkle GA, Meyer DJ: Toxicity of high doses of griseofulvin in cats, J Am Vet Med Assoc 191:322, 1987.

Menges RW, George LK: Observations on feline ringworm caused by Microsporum canis and its public health significance, Proc Am Vet Med Assoc:471, 1955.

Moriello KA, DeBoer DJ: Fungal flora of the coat of pet cats, Am J Vet Res 52:602, 1991.

Mosher CL, et al: Treatment of ringworm (Microsporum canis) with inactivated fungal vaccine, Vet Med Small Anim Clin 72:1343, 1977.

Muller GH, et al: Small animal dermatology, ed 4, Philadelphia, 1989, WB Saunders.

Quaife RA, Womar SM: Microsporum canis isolations from show cats, Vet Rec 110:333, 1982.

Scott DW: Feline dermatology 1900-1978: a monograph, J Am Anim Hosp Assoc 16:331, 1980.

Stein B: Personal communication, 1986.

Woodard DC: Ketoconazole treatment for Microsporum species, Feline Pract 13:28, 1983.

4

Cutaneous *Malassezia*

Kenneth V. Mason

Diagnostic Criteria for *Malassezia* Dermatitis

SUGGESTIVE

Greasy, yellow/gray scale, erythema, lichenification, hyperpigmentation, pruritus, and rancid seborrheic odor

COMPATIBLE

Characteristic clinical findings and observation of budding yeasts on cytologic examination

TENTATIVE

Budding yeasts on cytologic or histologic examination

Poor response to antibiotics and nonspecific topical therapy

DEFINITIVE

Budding yeasts demonstrated on diseased skin

Response to systemic ketoconazole or imidazole shampoo therapy

Malassezia pachydermatis (syn. *Pityrosporum pachydermatis* and *P. canis*) is a lipophilic nonmycelial yeast with a characteristic slightly elongated oval shape, a thick wall, and unipolar budding (Fig. 4-1). It is commonly found on normal and abnormal canine skin and within the ear canal, anal sacs, vagina, and rectum. There is an increase in incidence and organism numbers in some cases of otitis and dermatitis.

Importance

Malassezia and *Staphylococcus* play a significant role in seborrheic (oily and scaly) dermatitis and otitis. *Malassezia* dermatitis is common and should be considered a factor in any scaly, erythematous, oily, pruritic dermatitis in which other differentials have been eliminated by diagnostic tests and lack of response to treatment.

The role of *Malassezia* as a cause of disease has been controversial. The *Pityrosporum* (now *Malassezia*) was first described by Rivolta in 1873, and in 1874 Malassez suggested that it was causally related to seborrheic dermatitis and dandruff in humans. Sabouraud in 1904 made the same observation. Subsequently many authors reported on the relationship, and some even fulfilled all of Koch's postulates regarding the various species of yeast in human and animal skin diseases.

Pathogenesis

It is now apparent that alterations in skin surface microclimate or host defense may allow this normally commensal organism to become a significant

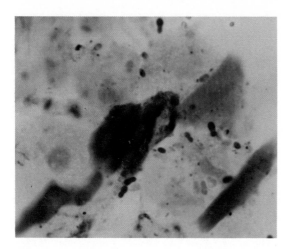

Figure 4-1. Typical peanut-shaped budding yeast of *Malassezia*.

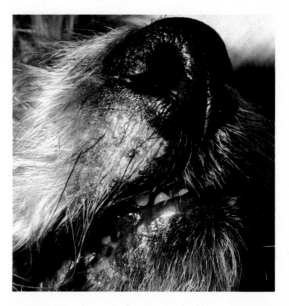

Figure 4-2. Focal area of alopecia and scale caused by *Malassezia* infection. The presenting complaint in this 6-year-old Australian Terrier was for "fits of pawing" at the nose and lip.

pathogen. Surface microclimate factors leading to *Malassezia* proliferation are excessive sebum production, accumulation of moisture and subsequent disruption of epidermal barrier. The yeast produces lipases that further alter the sebum balance. Zymogen in the yeast cell wall activates mammalian complement further damaging the host's epidermal integrity and is believed to cause epidermal spongiosis, inflammation and pruritus.

Allergic and bacterial skin disease may also be predisposing factors. *Malassezia pachydermatis* is unusual in that it can proliferate in proximity to many skin bacteria and its growth has been shown to be enhanced in the presence of *Staphylococcus*. *Malassezia* from humans is lipid dependent, but *M. pachydermatis* from animals has its growth enhanced only by sebum lipids.

A T cell–mediated hypersensitivity is responsible for recovery from acute yeast infections and the prevention of disease by normal yeast flora. In animals with *Malassezia* dermatitis the T cell response either is (presumably) overwhelmed or fails.

CLINICAL DISEASE
Dogs

Malassezia dermatitis occurs in adults of any age and any breed. Those predisposed are the Silky, Australian, Maltese, and West Highland White Terriers, Chihuahuas, Poodles, Shetland Sheepdogs, and German Shepherd Dogs. The dermatitis often starts in the summer or high-humidity months (also the allergy season) and then persists into winter. There is a second spike of cases in early spring. Clients complain of only partial relief in response to corticosteroids or a shortened relief period after increasing doses of injectable forms of the drug. Pruritus is a major sign and constant feature. Animals with generalized dermatitis have an offensive malodorous, greasy seborrheic smell that is also noticed in *Malassezia* otitis.

Regional (ear, muzzle, interdigital, and perianal) dermatitis or generalized disease occurs. The presenting complaint can be chronic face rubbing (Fig. 4-2). This may be mild or severe, with a "frenzied fit" of nose and lip scratching with the front paws. Some animals that exhibit this type of nose scratching are misdiagnosed as having central nervous system disease and are placed on anticonvulsants. Head shaking, scratching at the ears, and aural hematoma are signs of ear disease. Pododermatitis is manifested as foot licking, with discoloration of paw fur and alopecia. Perianal and ventral tail dermatitis is manifested as flank and dorsal tail self-trauma by rubbing, chewing, and scooting along the ground. Skin lesions consist of diffuse erythema, with variable scale (yellow and/or slate gray), hyperpigmentation, and traumatic alopecia. The skin and hair are greasy to waxy. Focal scaly plaques, erythematous macules, and patches that may coalesce into serpiginous tracts are occasionally recorded (Fig. 4-3).

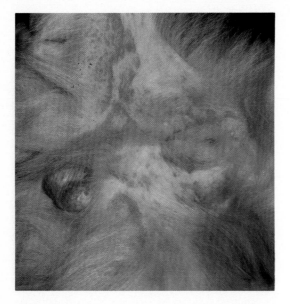

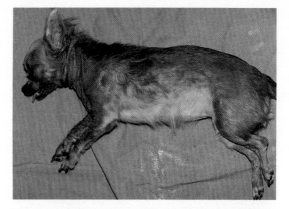

Figure 4-4. A Chihuahua with hyperpigmented, lichenified, scaly dermatitis caused by *Malassezia*. Note the anterior limb and ventral neck distribution often associated with the generalized cutaneous infection.

Figure 4-3. *Malassezia* dermatitis in a Shetland Sheepdog, manifesting as erythematous macules, papules, and plaques with scale and often joining to appear serpiginous.

Severe generalized disease presents as an exfoliative erythroderma and alopecic, hyperpigmented, lichenified areas with gray to white scale (Figs. 4-4 and 4-5).

Cats

Malassezia causes a black and waxy otitis, chin acne, and generalized erythematous scaly dermatitis in cats.

Differential Diagnosis

The clinical signs in dogs and cats are pruritic, erythematous, scaly, hyperpigmented, lichenified dermatitis and otitis; therefore, the differential diagnosis is extensive. It is even more perplexing for the clinician since *Malassezia* dermatitis is often associated with or triggered by most of the potential differential diagnoses. The prime differential features and associated predisposing diseases are atopy, flea allergy, food allergy, superficial pyoderma, and all the etiologic factors considered in an oily and scaly seborrhea complex with exfoliative erythroderma.

DIAGNOSIS
Cytology

The most useful and readily available tool to a clinician presented with a suspect case of *Malas-*

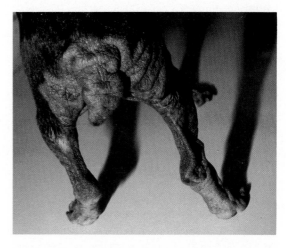

Figure 4-5. A Chihuahua with hock, perianal, and tail dermatitis caused by *Malassezia*. The skin is alopecic, hyperpigmented, and lichenified.

sezia dermatitis and/or otitis is cytology. A cotton swab vigorously rubbed on the surface of affected skin or in the ear canal and then pressed and rolled onto a glass slide is the preferred collection technique from oily skin. A superficial scrape with a blunt spatula or blunt scalpel blade will also provide an adequate sample. Scaly and erythematous lesions devoid of hair or after clipping will often reveal diagnostic samples with cellophane tape stripping. Clear cellophane tape is repeatedly pressed onto lesional skin and then stained and mounted without a coverslip. The slide is fixed with heat (skip this step if using cellophane tape) and stained with a routine cytologic stain (Diff Quik). It is then examined under high power or with an oil immersion lens on a light microscope (Fig. 4-1).

Histopathology

Biopsy of affected skin for histopathology is also useful. However, the dermatopathologist must be knowledgeable about the significance of *Malassezia* organisms in the skin and the type of cutaneous reaction pattern elicited. Until recently *Malassezia* organisms on skin biopsy were dismissed as an incidental finding, with no role in the development of dermatitis.

Culture

A swab of the skin surface processed routinely on bacteria or dermatophyte medium may produce *Malassezia* but more often will fail to isolate the yeast. Better results are obtained if the laboratory is alerted to look for yeasts and to use dextrose Sabouraud agar with chloramphenicol and gentamicin added. Yeast colonies will develop in 48 to 72 hours at 37° C. They appear as small, white, round, glistening colonies (Fig. 4-6). Oil- or sebum-enriched medium is described as helpful but is not necessary.

Trial Therapy

The only way to resolve the issue of whether a commensal-turned-pathogen has played a contributory role in the dermatitis is to remove that organism. Trial therapy with an antibiotic effective against *Staphylococcus intermedius* is a well-established diagnostic protocol to determine the role of the bacterium in a dermatosis. When *Malassezia* is demonstrated and inadequate resolution of the dermatitis occurs with removal of other identified factors, then a trial therapy for 2 weeks with ketoconazole (Nizoral) or other imidazoles helps support the yeast's role in the dermatitis. Other beneficial properties of ketoconazole (e.g., antiproliferative effects) should also be considered.

The diagnosis of a *Malassezia* dermatitis depends on identification of the yeast via cytology, culture, or histopathology, rule-out of other erythematous, scaly, pruritic dermatoses, and ultimately the response to antiyeast treatment.

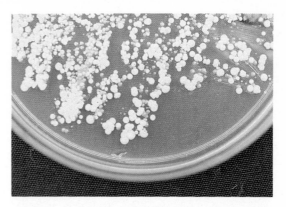

Figure 4-6. A 72-hour culture of *Malassezia pachydermatis* on dextrose Sabouraud agar.

TREATMENT
Systemic Therapy

The treatment of *Malassezia* dermatitis is best accomplished with 30 days of ketoconazole at 10 mg/kg q12h PO. Pruritis is noticeably decreased in the first week and cutaneous lesions are resolving by the second week on ketoconazole. Ketoconazole is actively secreted by sebaceous glands, which explains how this imidazole is effective against surface fungi. Vomiting and vague signs of malaise are occasionally encountered and can often be overcome by giving food with the tablets. Rarely liver damage is associated with ketoconazole in humans and cats. Ketoconazole treatment has the added disadvantage of being an expensive drug, which is compounded if monitoring of liver enzymes is recommended.

Topical Therapy

Selenium sulfide shampoo (Seleen) followed by rinses with enilconazole (Imaverol) is quite effective and cheaper than ketoconazole; however, enilconazole has an offensive odor and may not be universally available. Selenium sulfide shampoo is useful with an imidazole to remove scale and sebum, on which the yeast survive, and it has a direct but weak antimicrobial effect on the organism. Twice weekly treatments are recommended during the first 2 weeks, and weekly thereafter.

Three shampoo preparations have the potential to be effective as the sole treatment. Ketoconazole shampoo (Nizoral Shampoo) is approved in many countries for the treatment of seborrheic dermatitis in humans. Chlorhexidine shampoos (Nolvasan Surgical Scrub) containing more than 1% active ingredient are effective in some circumstances. Two to four percent chlorhexidine preparations are more reliably effective. A selenium sulfide, chlorhexidine, and miconazole shampoo (Sebolyse Foam) is available in Australia and has been evaluated on *Malassezia* dermatitis in animals and found to be effective. Since *Malassezia* dermatitis can be recurrent, with frequent relapses, an effective shampoo may be valuable for maintaining control without resorting to frequent courses of ketoconazole.

Local treatment with miconazole cream (Conofite) is valuable in pododermatitis and cheilitis, as well as for the most severely affected areas in generalized dermatitis.

Mycotic (yeast) otitis should be vigorously treated at the same time, preferably with a miconazole or nystatin and antibiotic combination otic preparation. Corticosteroids in the otic preparation help settle the inflammation, speeding resolution.

Griseofulvin is not effective against this yeast. The use of concurrent systemic antistaphylococcal antibiotics is not always indicated, but some cases have required combination antiyeast and antibacterial therapy. The cases requiring combination therapy often have a history of initially fair to good response to antistaphylococcal antibiotics and then relapse while still on a prolonged course of antibiotics or relapse soon after completing the antibiotic therapy and fail to respond again.

SUPPLEMENTAL READINGS

Dufait R: *Pityrosporum canis* as the cause of canine chronic dermatitis, Vet Med Small Anim Clin 78:1055, 1983.

Mason KV, Evans EG: Dermatitis associated with *Malassezia pachydermatis* in eleven dogs, J Am Anim Hosp Assoc 27:13, 1991.

Rosenberg EW, et al: Effect of topical application of heavy suspension of killed *Malassezia ovalis* on rabbit skin, Mycopathologia 72:147, 1980.

Shuster S: Introduction: a history. In Shuster S, Blatchford N (eds): Seborrhoeic dermatitis and dandruff, a fungal disease. International congress and symposium series, no. 132, London, 1988, Royal Society of Medicine Services, p 3.

5

Sporotrichosis

Edmund J. Rosser Jr.

Diagnostic Criteria for Sporotrichosis

SUGGESTIVE
Nonhealing intact or draining nodules

COMPATIBLE
History of a wound preceding the formation of lesions
Granulomatous or pyogranulomatous inflammation on cytologic and histologic examination of tissue and exudates

TENTATIVE
Pleomorphic population of organisms on cytologic or histologic examination of tissue and exudates

DEFINITIVE*
Positive identification of organisms on culture, cytology, histopathology, or fluorescent antibody test

*A negative outcome on any of these tests does not preclude the diagnosis.

Sporotrichosis is a mycotic disease caused by the dimorphic fungus *Sporothrix schenckii*. It is found in the yeast form in body tissues (37° C) and the mycelial form in the environment (25° to 30° C). The organism has been isolated in most regions of the world and prefers soil that is rich in decaying organic matter. *S. schenckii* has also been isolated from tree bark and sphagnum moss (Barsanti, 1984). Sphagnum moss has been an intermittent source of the organism associated with sporadic outbreaks of the infection. A multistate outbreak of sporotrichosis recently occurred in forestry workers and seedling handlers (England et al., 1989). It was associated with sphagnum moss harvested in Wisconsin and used as a packing for conifer seedlings.

Sporotrichosis infection is usually acquired via direct inoculation of the infectious organism into tissue (Rippon, 1985; Chandler and Watts, 1987). The disease in dogs is often related to an incident in which a puncture wound results from a thorn or wood splinter. For this reason the disease is more commonly observed in hunting dogs. In cats the infection is believed to be acquired by inoculation of the organism from a puncture wound by the contaminated claw of another cat (Dunstan et al., 1986a). This may partially explain why the infection is usually identified in intact male cats that roam outdoors. In humans the environmental contamination of a puncture wound is also considered an important mechanism in acquiring the disease. However, the exposure of humans to cats infected with *Sporothrix schenckii* has recently been examined (Rosser, 1989) and is now thought to be a significant means of acquiring the infection.

The zoonotic potential of this disease must be considered and respected. There have been several reports documenting the transmission of sporotrichosis to people by contact with an ulcerated wound or the exudate from an infected cat (Dunstan et al., 1986b). Human infections have also occurred, even though no known injury or penetrating wound had occurred prior to the development of disease. Transmission from animals to humans has been limited to cases of feline sporotrichosis and is presumably related to the large numbers of organisms found in contaminated tissues, exudates, and feces. The infectious organism is often difficult to demonstrate from dogs and humans with sporotrichosis. Thus dogs and humans are an unlikely source of infection. However, a case of canine sporotrichosis was recently reported (Moriello et al., 1988) in which organisms were easily observed and isolated from various tissue exudates. Therefore veterinarians, technicians, owners of infected cats, and anyone in contact with infected cats have a higher risk of infection.

CLINICAL DISEASE

Sporotrichosis of dogs and cats may appear in any one or a combination of three forms: cutaneous, cutaneolymphatic, and disseminated. The clinical presentations of this disease are different in dogs and cats.

Dogs

Sporotrichosis of dogs usually presents in the cutaneous and/or cutaneolymphatic form. The disseminated form is rare (Iwasaki et al., 1988). The disease usually begins with nodular lesions that may ulcerate and develop draining tracts. The owner should be questioned whether any injury or puncture wound may have occurred in the affected area before the nodule or draining tract was noticed. If the patient has been previously treated with soaks and systemic antibiotics for a suspected bacterial infection, there is usually a poor or partial response.

The cutaneous form of the disease is a multinodular condition most frequently affecting the trunk or head (Fig. 5-1). The nodules are in the dermis and subcutis and may ulcerate and drain a purulent exudate, with subsequent crust formation. The cutaneolymphatic form presents with a history of nodules on the distal aspect of one of the limbs. The infection ascends proximally following lymphatic vessels, and secondary nodules are formed. These may ulcerate and drain a purulent exudate

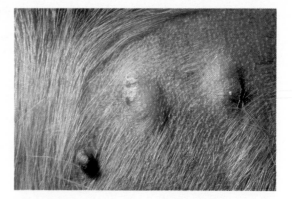

Figure 5-1. Cutaneous form of sporotrichosis in a dog with multiple nodules in the abdominal region.
(From Rosser EJ Jr, Dunstan RW. In Greene CE (ed): Infectious diseases of the dog and cat, Philadelphia, 1990, WB Saunders.)

(Fig. 5-2). The cutaneolymphatic form is usually associated with a regional lymphadenopathy.

Cats

Lesions of cats frequently occur on the distal aspects of the limbs, the head, or the tail base region. Cats initially present with fight wound abscesses, draining puncture wounds, or cellulitis. Previous treatment with soaks and systemic antibiotics for a bacterial infection results in poor or partial improvement. Affected areas become ulcerated, drain a purulent exudate, and form crusted nodules (Fig. 5-3). Extensive areas of necrosis may develop, with exposure of muscle and bone. The disease may be spread to other areas of the body by autoinoculation. This occurs when the cat licks and scratches the lesions and transfers organisms by normal grooming behavior. Lesions may then develop on the remaining extremities, face, and ears. Evidence of lymphatic system involvement (e.g., palpable lymphadenopathy or "corded" lymphatics) may not be apparent during the physical examination of an affected cat. However, when cats with sporotrichosis have been necropsied, most revealed evidence of lymph node and lymphatic vessel involvement. In addition, *Sporothrix* organisms are commonly present in many internal organs and the feces, indicating presence of the disseminated form of the disease.

Affected dogs and cats may also present with a history of lethargy, anorexia, depression, and pyrexia. These signs suggest the potential for disseminated sporotrichosis and should alert the clinician to the possibility of an immunocompromised patient.

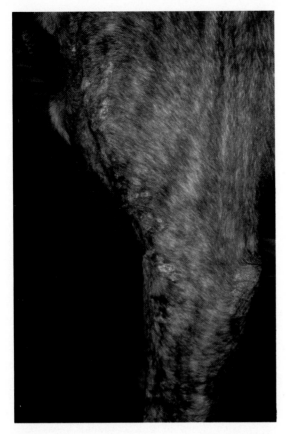

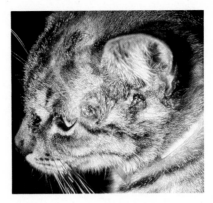

Figure 5-3. Feline sporotrichosis with multiple nodules, ulcerations, and draining tracts.
(Courtesy Dr. Nita Gulbas, Phoenix, Ariz.)

Figure 5-2. Cutaneolymphatic form of sporotrichosis in a dog with nodules and ulcers that follow the lymphatics.

Differential Diagnosis

The differential diagnosis for sporotrichosis includes the numerous causes of deep granulomatous and pyogranulomatous diseases as well as causes of folliculitis and furunculosis. Parasitic diseases to consider are demodicosis and *Pelodera* dermatitis, which are easily diagnosed by the examination of deep skin scrapings. Deep bacterial infections or pyodermas can be ruled out by submitting samples of exudate for bacterial culture (using both aerobic and anaerobic culture methods). Bacterial organisms to consider include coagulase positive staphylococci, *Pseudomonas* spp, *Proteus* spp, and anaerobic bacteria. In cats *Pasteurella multocida* and *Mycobacterium* spp should also be considered. Several other fungal diseases can demonstrate lesions similar to those of sporotrichosis and include histoplasmosis, blastomycosis, coccidioidomycosis, cryptococcosis, pheohyphomycosis, mycetoma, pseudomycetoma, and dermatophytosis. The suspected organism can usually be demonstrated

by submitting samples of exudate for fungal culture. Other conditions to consider in the differential diagnosis of sporotrichosis include neoplastic skin diseases, panniculitis, vasculitis, and idiopathic sterile granulomatous and pyogranulomatous skin diseases. These can all be confirmed by histologic examination of skin biopsies.

DIAGNOSIS

Because of the zoonotic potential of sporotrichosis, certain precautions need to be taken. All people handling cats **suspected** of having sporotrichosis should wear gloves. Gloves should also be worn when taking samples of exudates or tissues (i.e., a biopsy sample). The gloves should then be carefully removed and disposed of as biologic waste. Forearms, wrists, and hands are washed with either a chlorhexidine or a povidone-iodine scrub.

Cytologic Examination

An attempt to establish the diagnosis of sporotrichosis should begin with cytologic examination of tissue exudates. *Sporothrix schenckii* is identified as a pleomorphic yeast that is round, oval, or cigar shaped and may either be present within macrophages and inflammatory cells or located extracellularly (Fig. 5-4). Specimens should be stained with a routine cytologic stain (Diff-Quik) and examined for bacteria and fungi. Because this organism is often difficult to see with routine stains, an additional slide may be stained for the presence of fungi with either the periodic acid–Schiff (PAS) or the Gomori methenamine silver (GMS) stain.

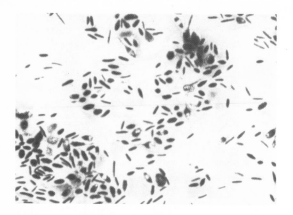

Figure 5-4. Photomicrograph of the exudate obtained from a cat with sporotrichosis (Gram stain). Note the abundance of *Sporothrix schenckii* organisms, showing the typical yeastlike cell morphology, which varies from oval and round shapes to the characteristic elongated "cigar bodies."

(Courtesy Joyce Stringfellow, Auburn, Ala.)

Even with these, the organism can be difficult to find in the exudates from dogs but is easily identified in the exudates from cats.

Cultures

When sporotrichosis is suspected, samples should be submitted for both bacterial and fungal culture. Patients with this disease may have an opportunistic bacterial infection. Therefore it is important to isolate that organism as well since it requires its own specific treatment. The samples submitted for fungal culture should include both a sample of the exudate (from deep within a draining tract) and a piece of tissue (removed surgically) for a macerated tissue culture. This is most important in dogs, in which there may be only a few organisms present. Sporotrichosis should be listed as a differential diagnosis when specimens are submitted to the laboratory.

Histopathology

The best specimens to submit for histopathologic examination are biopsy samples of early-forming, intact nodules. The histologic pattern observed in sporotrichosis of dogs and cats is nodular to diffuse pyogranulomatous inflammation (Rosser and Dunstan, 1990). The reaction is present in the dermal and subcutaneous tissues and may extend to the adjacent skeletal muscle. In cats the fungal organisms are numerous and readily demonstrated within the pyogranulomatous reaction, even on hematoxylin and eosin (H&E)–stained sections. In

dogs there are usually only a few organisms demonstrable, even when the slides are stained with a fungal stain such as PAS or GMS. Therefore each section of tissue should be carefully examined. Organisms are often found sequestered in clear spaces within the pyogranulomatous reaction.

Fluorescent Antibody Test

The fluorescent antibody test is most useful for establishing a diagnosis of sporotrichosis in dogs when the above procedures have been negative (Kaplan and Ochoa, 1963). It is quite sensitive and may be positive when attempts to culture the organism have failed. The procedure can be performed by the Centers for Disease Control, Atlanta, Ga. A sample of either the exudate or preferably a portion of affected tissue should be submitted.

TREATMENT

Glucocorticoids or any other immunosuppressive drugs are contraindicated in dogs or cats with sporotrichosis. They should be avoided both during and after treatment of the disease, since immunosuppressive doses of glucocorticoids have been shown (Raimer et al., 1983) to cause a recurrence of the clinical disease after apparent resolution. Concurrent bacterial infection should be treated with an appropriate antibiotic based on culture and sensitivity testing. Most cases will require a 4-to-8-week treatment regimen with an appropriate systemic antibiotic.

Dogs

The treatment of choice for dogs is the oral administration of a supersaturated solution of potassium iodide (SSKI), 40 mg/kg q8h PO with food (Rosser and Dunstan, 1990). Treatment must be continued for 30 days beyond complete clinical remission since recurrence is common when the duration has been inadequate. The owner should be advised to observe the dog for any signs of iodism during the treatment period. The signs of iodism include ocular and nasal discharge, a dry hair coat with excessive scaling, vomiting, depression, and collapse. If iodism is observed, the medication should be discontinued for 1 week. The drug may be reinstituted at the same dosage when side effects are mild. If iodism becomes a recurrent problem or the side effects are severe, alternative drug therapy should be considered.

The imidazole and triazole classes of drugs may be considered for dogs that do not tolerate iodides, are refractory to iodide therapy, or relapse after an apparent clinical cure. Ketoconazole (Nizoral) has been used successfully for many different types of fungal infections at dosages ranging from 5 to 30 mg/kg q12-24h PO. Administration is recommended with food, preferably in an acid environment (tomato juice). I have successfully treated one case of canine sporotrichosis using ketoconazole at 15 mg/kg q12h PO for 3½ months (1 month beyond the apparent clinical cure). Ketoconazole is well-tolerated by dogs. Side effects are mild and include anorexia, pruritus, alopecia, and lightening of the hair coat color. Itraconazole, a recently introduced triazole, is currently undergoing investigative treatment trials for various fungal diseases (including sporotrichosis) and has shown efficacy in these early studies (Restrepo et al., 1986; Kan and Bennett, 1988; Burke, 1989).

Cats

Increased sensitivity to the toxic side effects of iodides and ketoconazole in cats poses a greater challenge for the treatment of sporotrichosis. The treatment of choice for cats is the oral administration of SSKI at 20 mg/kg q12h with food. This should continue for 30 days beyond complete clinical remission. The owner should observe the cat for signs of iodism during the treatment period. Signs of iodism include vomiting, anorexia, depression, twitching, hypothermia, and cardiovascular failure (Macy and Small, 1983). The treatment should be discontinued if signs of iodism are observed and treatment with an imidazole drug considered. Ketoconazole (Nizoral) may be given at a dosage of 5 to 10 mg/kg q12-24h PO with food, preferably in an acid environment (tomato juice). This should be continued for 30 days beyond the apparent clinical cure. The owner should closely observe the cat since toxic side effects are a greater problem with this drug in cats when compared to dogs. Side effects include anorexia, depression, vomiting, diarrhea, fever, neurologic signs, and jaundice. If any of these signs are observed, the drug should be discontinued. It may become necessary to alternate the treatment using the above drugs in an attempt to cure the disease.

REFERENCES

Barsanti JA: Sporotrichosis. In Greene CE (ed): Clinical microbiology and infectious diseases of the dog and cat, Philadelphia, 1984, WB Saunders.

Burke WA: Use of itraconazole in a patient with chronic mucocutaneous candidiasis, J Am Acad Dermatol 21:1309, 1989.

Chandler FW, Watts JC: Pathologic diagnosis of fungal infections, Chicago, 1987, ASCP Press.

Dunstan RW, et al: Feline sporotrichosis, J Am Vet Med Assoc 189:880, 1986a.

Dunstan RW, et al: Feline sporotrichosis: a report of five cases with transmission to humans, J Am Acad Dermatol 15:37, 1986b.

England T, et al: Multistate outbreak of sporotrichosis in seedling handlers, 1988, Arch Dermatol 125:170, 1989.

Iwasaki M, et al: Skeletal sporotrichosis in a dog, Compan Anim Pract 2:27, 1988.

Kan VL, Bennett JE: Efficacy for four antifungal agents in experimental murine sporotrichosis, Antimicrob Agents Chemother 32:1619, 1988.

Kaplan W, Ochoa AG: Application of the fluorescent technique to the rapid diagnosis of sporotrichosis, J Lab Clin Med 62:835, 1963.

Macy DW, Small E: Deep mycotic diseases. In Ettinger SJ (ed): Textbook of veterinary internal medicine, vol 1, Philadelphia, 1983, WB Saunders.

Moriello KA, et al: Cutaneous-lymphatic and nasal sporotrichosis in a dog, J Am Anim Hosp Assoc 24:621, 1988.

Raimer SS, et al: Ketoconazole therapy of experimentally induced sporotrichosis infections in cats: a preliminary study, Curr Ther Res 33:670, 1983.

Restrepo A, et al: Itraconozole therapy in lymphangitic and cutaneous sporotrichosis, Arch Dermatol 122:413, 1986.

Rippon JW: Subcutaneous and systemic fungal infections. In Moschella SL, Hurley HJ (eds): Dermatology, ed 2, vol 1, Philadelphia, 1985, WB Saunders.

Rosser EJ: Sporotrichosis and public health. In Kirk RW (ed): Current veterinary therapy X, Philadephia, 1989, WB Saunders.

Rosser EJ, Dunstan RW: Sporotrichosis. In Greene CE (ed): Infectious diseases of the dog and cat, Philadelphia, 1990, WB Saunders.

SECTION

II

Ectoparasites

6

Flea Allergy Dermatitis and Flea Control

John M. MacDonald

Diagnostic Criteria for Flea Allergy Dermatitis

SUGGESTIVE
Clinical Features:
Dog: Pruritus and hair loss affecting the lower back and pelvic region
Cat: Pruritus and "miliary dermatitis" or hair loss in the inguinal region or dermatitis and hair loss over the lower back and thighs

COMPATIBLE
Above plus
Evidence of fleas

TENTATIVE
Suggestive or *Compatible* plus
Positive response to flea control

DEFINITIVE
Above plus
Positive reaction to the intradermal flea antigen test

Importance

Flea allergy continues to represent the most common hypersensitivity in dogs and cats. In the southeastern United States it is estimated that flea-related problems account for more than 50% of the skin conditions observed in veterinary practices. Regional variations occur, with areas having warm temperatures and high humidity posing more risk for parasite problems.

The importance of flea allergy includes both the dermatitis resulting from the allergy and the potentiation of other coexistent diseases. Flea allergy tends to aggravate atopy, and they are often observed together. Flea allergy also results in dry scaly skin (xeroderma), which may intensify pruritus. In general, flea allergy is a major reason for treatment failures or recurrence of clinical signs in cases with multiple allergies. This is exemplified by dogs that have both atopy and flea allergy satisfactorily controlled through hyposensitization therapy (for the atopy) but that relapse when exposed to fleas.

Overestimating the relevancy of flea allergy is as important as underestimating it. The combination of pruritus with evidence of fleas often evokes an assumed relationship, and other diseases are overlooked. Flea allergy is frequently diagnosed in dogs as the only or primary diagnosis when much of the pruritic problem may be caused by canine atopy or food allergy. Fleas are usually the primary reason for the addition of glucocorticoid therapy to the combined regimen in treating an atopic/flea allergic dog that is otherwise well-controlled with nonglucocorticoid therapy. This is of particular significance in cases with poor tolerance to glucocorticoid therapy. Better flea control results in less glucocorticoid requirement. Refractoriness of flea allergy to glucocorticoid treatment may also be observed in cats and is most pronounced when there is minimal flea control or coexisting food allergy.

Pathogenesis

The flea most commonly infesting dogs and cats is *Ctenocephalides felis,* although studies conducted in the southeastern United States have shown that *Pulex irritans* accounts for better than 81% of the cases. *Ctenocephalides canis* is least commonly observed. The flea is well adapted and often exists quite compatibly with the host without producing skin irritation unless an allergic reaction is induced.

The skin disease caused by fleas is now recognized as a specific hypersensitivity reaction. Without allergy there are minimal skin lesions even in cases with high flea infestation. Dogs with other allergic disease (canine atopy) are at higher risk for developing hypersensitivity to flea antigen. Eighty percent of the atopic dogs living in flea-infested areas also have concurrent flea allergy. The development of flea hypersensitivity under natural conditions is variable with regard to age. Flea allergy has been documented in dogs as young as 6 to 8 weeks. By contrast, some dogs may live with a flea infestation for many years before becoming allergic. Therefore the onset of flea allergy may be observed much later in life, unlike canine atopy, which has a typical onset between 1 and 3 years of age and rarely after 6 years. Flea allergy should be included in the differential for any pruritic dog, young or old, with potential flea exposure.

Attempts to identify the flea antigen have resulted in variable findings. Flea antigen has classically been described as a low — molecular weight hapten. More recently two additional allergens of much larger size than any previously recognized have been identified. The importance of the newly recognized high — molecular weight haptens is their increased binding to dermal collagen. In addition to the antigenic stimulation, flea saliva by itself contains histaminelike compounds and enzymes that may have an irritant effect. However, if this were a major factor, more dermatologic disease would be observed in non–flea allergic animals infested with fleas.

Experimental work performed in flea-naive dogs (Halliwell and Gorman, 1989) has demonstrated the ability to sensitize animals within 12 weeks by exposure to fleas. Intermittent exposure to flea feeding favored a hypersensitivity reaction, in contrast to more continuous exposures. Immunoglobulin response documented both an IgE and an IgG antiflea antibody production. Delayed reactions (24 to 48 hours) were also noted. The sequence of hypersensitivity reactions (immediate or delayed) was not consistent. The production of antiflea antibody was not observed or was very low in flea-naive dogs and dogs with chronic flea exposure, in contrast to dogs that had developed flea hypersensitivity. Dogs with more chronic flea exposure either failed to develop flea allergy or developed it to a lesser degree or later on in the exposure sequence. The Halliwell study suggested that continued flea exposure with an abundance of fleas may discourage the development of hypersensitivity. Interfering with the flea burden by introducing a flea control program poses an interesting concern.

Other recent evidence suggests the occurrence of different types of immunologic responses in addition to the classical immediate and delayed type of hypersensitivity. Late onset or late phase IgE-mediated response has been recognized in both canine atopy and flea allergy. This cellular response occurs 3 to 6 hours after the antigen exposure and interaction with specific IgE. Cutaneous basophil hypersensitivity reaction (CBH) has also been associated with the immunologic response to flea allergy. When this phenomenon occurs, there is an infiltration of basophils in the dermis in response to intradermal injection of antigen. Sensitization may occur from either IgE or IgG. Basophils are attracted through chemotactic response and on subsequent exposure with allergen undergo degranulation and release mediators. The end result is a response characterized by features similar to both immediate (Type I) and delayed (Type IV) reactions.

The most consistent immunologic reaction has been observed with intradermal allergy testing. (This will be discussed further in the diagnostic section of this chapter.)

CLINICAL DISEASE
History

The clinical signs and history of flea allergy may vary depending upon the reactivity of the animal and its exposure to fleas. Environmental factors affecting flea populations influence disease progression and seasonal observation. In northern climates the disease may completely resolve during the winter months. By contrast, in warmer climates (southern U.S.) the problem may persist year round but be more intense during the spring, summer, and fall. Increased flea infestation will amplify the clinical disease and decrease the response to symptomatic antipruritic therapeutics. Conventional dosage of glucocorticoids is only partially effective if a high flea burden is sustained. In addition, the use of pesticides may have only a limited effect if the climate favors flea infestation and replication. Early-onset flea allergy may be observed in young animals.

The most common complaint is pruritus with compulsive biting, chewing, and licking, particularly in the pelvic region. History questions should include previous flea control measures for the affected patient as well as contact with other animals and the environment. Documenting the number of pets in a household is important for understanding the severity of the problem and selecting the ideal treatment regimen.

A lack of commitment by the pet owner to sustained parasiticidal treatment is often the major factor of ongoing or recurrent clinical disease. Identifying the specific problem as regards the type of client is important. There are three explanations that account for the majority of failures to control flea allergy. First, the program of flea control is inadequate, from either overdependence on products based upon inaccurate descriptions of efficacy provided by manufacturers or undertreatment. Second, pet owners may not believe the clinical problem is related to the flea. Third, the owners may assume they are doing a good job of flea control even though they are not. Determining the cause of failure and counseling the pet owner are essential for satisfactory treatment.

Secondary complications may also affect the clinical response. Superficial or deep pyodermas often accompany flea allergy and contribute to the overall pruritus. Excessive use of flea control products (pour-ons or alcohol-containing sprays) may cause excessive drying (xeroderma), which adds to the pruritus.

Physical Examination

Classical flea allergy results in the formation of lesions over the tailhead region in the form of a wedge. Lesions usually will also be observed on the caudal aspect of the thighs and may include the lower abdomen and inguinal region. Erythema, hair loss, and scales are typical (Fig. 6-1). Papules are the primary lesion in experimentally induced flea allergy dermatitis, although in clinical cases they often represent coexistent pyoderma. However, they may be observed following antibiotic

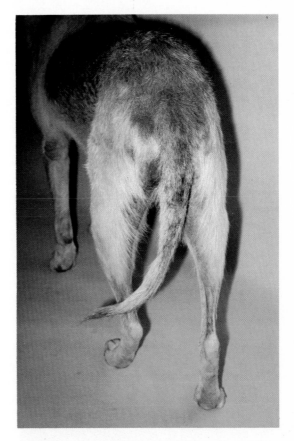

Figure 6-1. Early flea allergy dermatitis in a dog showing hair loss and erythema over the dorsal lumbosacral region and caudomedial thighs.

treatment and satisfactory response of the pyoderma. In this situation they are most likely associated with the flea allergy, despite the fact that other diseases may be associated with a papular dermatitis (scabies or food allergy). Young dogs with flea allergy will show generalized pruritus with scale formation, perhaps more accentuated over the lower back, but often without classical features early in the disease. As the condition progresses, more typical distribution patterns develop.

Secondary lesions may follow chronic flea allergy or result from the secondary pyoderma. Hyperpigmentation with thickening of skin over the pelvic limbs and inguinal region is typical of uncontrolled flea allergy. Hair loss with comparable lesions over the dorsal lumbosacral region, along with hyperpigmentation and lichenification, is observed in the chronic uncontrolled case (Fig. 6-2). Secondary bacterial folliculitis with consequential furunculosis may lead to scarring of the dorsal pelvic region and the inability to grow hair from follicle destruction.

Coexisting canine atopy will usually demonstrate otitis externa, facial dermatitis, pododer-

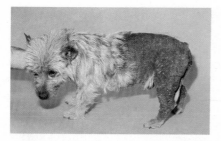

Figure 6-2. Chronic flea allergy dermatitis with minimal control of fleas. Note the dramatic distribution of lesions affecting the pelvic area with alopecia, hyperpigmentation, and thickening of the skin.

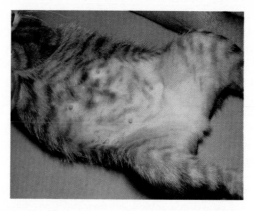

Figure 6-4. Hair loss caused by excessive licking in the inguinal region of a cat with flea allergy dermatitis. This pattern is often misdiagnosed as "feline endocrine" or "feline symmetrical" alopecia. A positive flea antigen reaction was observed on this animal by an intradermal test performed on the skin of the right lateral abdomen.

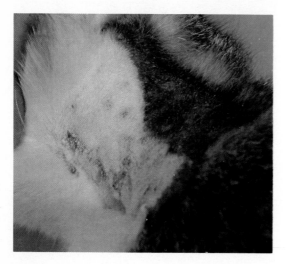

Figure 6-3. Flea allergy in a cat demonstrating a papular ("miliary") dermatitis around the cervical area. The hair has been removed for better visualization of the lesions.

matitis, axillary dermatitis, and lesions on the front legs especially cranial to the elbow region. In general, pruritus occurring cranial to the shoulders and axilla should be viewed with speculation as to the possibility that it is another disease and not flea allergy. The concurrence of flea allergy with feline atopy has also been observed.

The clinical features of flea allergy in cats are more variable than in dogs. Several patterns exist. The cat commonly develops a miliary, crusting dermatitis that has come to be referred to as "feline miliary dermatitis." Flea allergy is the most frequent, though not the only, cause of this syndrome. The occurrence of a miliary eruption around the neck is most often associated with flea allergy in cats (Fig. 6-3). Another pattern is alopecia in the inquinal region that may have minimal signs of dermatitis and no miliary crusts (Fig. 6-4). This

pattern is often misdiagnosed as an endocrine-based problem when there is no gross evidence of inflammation. Many cases have the limited dorsal lumbosacral involvement classically observed in dogs. A combination of distribution patterns may be present in an individual animal. A cat from the southeastern United States with inguinal alopecia and crusts palpable in the cervical region usually has flea allergy dermatitis. Other clinical features observed in cats include eosinophilic lesions (ulcers, plaques, or granulomas) and unusual behavior (including compulsive overgrooming).

The major differential diagnoses of flea allergy include food allergy, atopy, scabies, and cheyletiellosis. Primary keratinization defects with dermatitis and pruritus may also appear as flea allergy.

DIAGNOSIS

The diagnosis of flea allergy is often based on historical information in combination with the classical dermatologic pattern affecting the pelvic region and lower back.

Identification of fleas may be difficult and often poses a problem of diagnostic confirmation to a skeptical pet owner. Many owners will use parasiticidal therapy prior to the examination, restricting observation of fleas. Finding fleas on cats may be difficult because of their fastidious grooming habits. Identification of flea feces or *Diplydium* segments can help. The use of a flea comb will facilitate demonstrating the flea and is a recommended practice for routine examination. A variety of flea combs are available, with the primary difference being size and how close the comb teeth are to one another. The Twinco (Lambert Kay) all-metal comb is ideal for shorter coated dogs and cats since it contains approximately 28 teeth per inch. It is more difficult to use on longer coats. Combs with fewer teeth per inch are easier to use but may not be as effective in collecting fleas. The use of flea combs by the owner is an excellent method of monitoring animals for flea infestation.

Parasiticide therapy is sometimes helpful, but it may have limitations in heavily flea-infested areas demonstrating negligible response.

IMMUNODIAGNOSTICS
Intradermal Allergy Testing

The intradermal allergy test with flea antigen is a convenient, reliable, and expedient method of diagnosing flea hypersensitivity. In 90% of flea allergic animals a positive reaction occurs within 15 minutes (immediate) (Fig. 6-5). A delayed reaction may be observed in 24 to 48 hours in cases that show no immediate reaction.

A variety of flea antigens are available, but I have found the Greer Laboratory Flea Extract most reliable. The concentration obtained from the laboratory is 1:100 W/V and should be diluted to 1:1000 W/V for test purposes. The laboratory provides all material necessary (in kit form) for conducting the allergy test, including the positive control (histamine), the negative control (diluent), and

a supply of intradermal test syringes. The test is conducted by injecting 0.05 to 0.1 ml of each substance (histamine, diluent, flea antigen) intradermally. A black marker is used to identify the injection sites, which are best located in the glabrous area of the abdomen and therefore in most cases not requiring removal of hair. The procedure is frequently done in the examining room with clients present for comparison of results. Following the injection of antigen, approximately 15 minutes should be allowed for optimal recording of the reaction. The reactions are graded from 0 to 4+. The histamine wheal represents a 4+ reaction, and the saline wheal a 0. Grading is done by comparison to the histamine and saline controls.

The size of the reaction and its redness and turgidity are all useful criteria. In general, a 4+ reaction is a wheal with a mean diameter equal to or greater than the saline control wheal plus 75% of the difference between the histamine and the saline control diameters. A 3+ is equal to or greater than the saline control diameter plus 50% to 74% of the difference between the saline and histamine diameters. A 2+ is equal to or greater than the saline diameter plus 25% to 49% of the difference between the saline and histamine diameters. A significant reaction would be 2+ or greater, to indicate hypersensitivity to fleas.

For example, if the histamine wheal diameter is 12 mm and the saline control 4 mm, a 4+ reaction would be 10 mm or greater.

$$4+ = 4 \text{ mm} + 75\%(12\text{-}4) = 10 \text{ mm (or greater)}$$
$$3+ = 4 \text{ mm} + 50\%(12\text{-}4) = 8 \text{ mm (to 9.9 mm)}$$
$$2+ = 4 \text{ mm} + 25\%(12\text{-}4) = 6 \text{ mm (to 7.9 mm)}$$

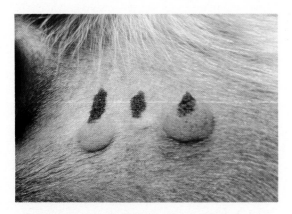

Figure 6-5. Intradermal allergy test conducted with Greer flea antigen (1:1000) on the abdomen of a flea-allergic dog demonstrating a positive (4+) reaction at 15 minutes postinjection. The histamine (positive control) is on the left, saline (negative control) in the middle, and flea antigen on the right.

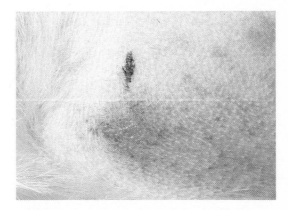

Figure 6-6. A delayed reaction to flea antigen observed 24 hours postinjection in a flea-allergic dog. The skin is erythematous and indurated at the injection site but lacks the "wheal and flare" response seen in the immediate hypersensitivity reaction. (See Fig. 6-5 for comparison.)

A 1+ reaction is not significant. A 2+ is significant only if it is indurated and erythematous **and** fits the history. A 3+ and 4+ are significant if they fit the history. In the event of a negative immediate response, the injection site should be evaluated 24 and 48 hours later for a delayed reaction. The delayed reaction will show not the typical wheal and flare but rather an area of induration and skin thickening (Fig. 6-6). It may be seen in a small percentage of flea-allergic animals. Flea-allergic animals infrequently fail to demonstrate either an immediate or a delayed positive reaction to flea antigen. Although a negative flea antigen test does not rule out flea allergy, other causes of the condition should be investigated.

Flea antigen testing can be done during therapy with glucocorticoids and/or antihistamines without medication withdrawal. Although the reaction may be somewhat suppressed, it is usually sufficient to offer diagnostic confirmation. Negative test results obtained while the animal is on medication cannot be interpreted as strictly and should be repeated after withdrawal of the medication for more accurate determination. The advantage of intradermal flea antigen testing without medication withdrawal is that it provides diagnostic confirmation without interruption of treatment. The test may be negative in young dogs early in the course of the disease. To recognize any change in reactivity, a negative test performed at one evaluation should be repeated later.

Intradermal allergy testing for flea antigen is also helpful in documenting hypersensitivity in cats. The procedure is conducted similarly to that in dogs but often requires removal of hair unless sufficient hair loss has occurred with the disease. Normally tranquilization is not utilized, although in some cases it may be necessary. Allowing the owner to stay with the cat during the test can provide a calming effect. Ketoset or xylazine hydrochloride may be used but rarely is required.

In-Vitro Allergy Test Procedures

Flea allergy testing is available with both the RAST (radioallergosorbent test) and the ELISA (enzyme linked immunosorbent assay) technique for identification of circulating anti-flea IgE. It is unwarranted, however, due to the ease and reliability of intradermal testing. The current in vitro tests available for flea allergy have variable accuracy, with both false-positive and false-negatives observed. The cost factor and the time required for reporting results are additional reasons to avoid this diagnostic procedure for flea allergy.

TREATMENT

General Concepts and Considerations

Treatment of flea allergy dermatitis often requires a combination of approaches. Elimination of the antigen source is, without doubt, the best method. Recognition of the parasite life cycle is essential to adequate therapy. The adult female *Ctenocephalides felis* is capable of significant procreation. As many as 20 to 28 eggs per day may be laid, with several hundred produced in the female's life-span of 6 months to a year. These eggs usually incubate for between 2 and 12 days depending upon the favorableness of environmental conditions. The subsequent larvae are both secretive and motile, finding areas in the environment to feed on organic material and flea waste. The larvae undergo two molts to reach the third (instar) larval stage, which produces a cocoon. The total larval stage usually lasts between 14 and 21 days but may be as short as 9 or as long as 200 days. The cocoon containing the pupa is the most resistant stage of the life cycle and is virtually immune to most environmental pesticides. It may last anywhere from a number of days to a month, also depending upon environmental factors. A humidity of 75% to 85% with an environmental temperature of 65° to 80° F is ideal. Emergence of the adult flea may occur in as short as 16 to 21 days, and the life-span of the adult is 6 to 12 months. The female flea will not produce ova unless a blood meal is attained, therapy completing the life cycle.

The restriction of most parasiticides is their limited effectiveness against only the adult stage of the life cycle. Newer products, including insect growth regulators, are targeted toward both the ova and the larvae, preventing maturation to the pupal stage and thereby interfering with the life cycle prior to the adult emergence. This type of treatment is more effective but, in an environment that is heavily infested, may require repeated applications in combination with adulticidal compounds.

Treatment should be directed toward both the animal and the premises. The adult stage has been estimated to represent only 1% of the flea population, with the balance consisting of fleas in the preadult form.

The ideal flea control product would be a compound that was active against the preadult stages and long-lasting while having minimal environmental impact. Other characteristics would include a fast mode of action, minimal mammalian toxicity, odorlessness, and being both nonabrasive and nonirritating to the skin or coat. The ideal product is theoretical; nevertheless, most clients expect such an item to be available. Their first assumption is that the veterinarian will provide a remedy that can be applied quickly and easily, is inexpensive and safe for the pet and environment, and can be used safely around people. Client education concerning flea control is often the most frustrating part of treatment. The risk:benefit ratio must be considered as well as any obstacles relating to effective treatment. Product performance expressed by the manufacturer is often overstated and almost never comes close to actual results. Data accumulated for product efficacy are generally obtained from studies performed in the laboratory rather than in the field. Analysis of results leads to presentations of statistical significance that do not consider practical limitations. An example would be a product with a "14-day" claim that demonstrated a statistical difference between the flea infestation of treated dogs on day 14 and that of a control group but still had an unacceptable level of infestation (e.g., 74 fleas vs. 185 fleas). Although residual activity might be demonstrable, the infestation would still be so great as to remain unacceptable.

Using products beyond the label restrictions (extralabel use) is a violation of EPA regulations and is not legally permissible even if the practice is routinely followed by other veterinarians. These restrictions differ from the extra-label use of drugs regulated by the FDA.

Treatment concerns must be directed toward all aspects of flea infestation, in particular the affected animal and the environment. Flea-allergic cats are more of an obstacle to successfully following a treatment regimen because of their high host appeal and increased sensitivity to pesticide products and because it is impossible to control the outside environment and the intensity of clinical disease. Bathing pets with a nonparasiticidal shampoo should be done routinely to remove any residual active ingredient and to prevent possible buildup (which might lead to intoxication).

Systems of Parasiticide Application for use on the Animal

Pour-on Insecticides (Dips)

Pour-on insecticides provide the optimal treatment for insecticidal activity against fleas. They offer more uniform distribution as well as more complete penetration of the coat, especially for pets that have a high proportion of secondary hairs. Residual activity is determined by the active ingredient(s), which also may limit the application rate. Most pour-on parasiticides have a limited period of effectiveness, and therefore a weekly ap-

plication is usually recommended. Many contain organophosphates, which restricts their frequency of application to once a week or less. It is recommended that, to avoid insecticidal buildup, residual material be removed from the coat and skin with a detergent shampoo. Repeated applications may cause either a drying effect or irritation, particularly if the product contains a high concentration of petroleum distillates. The addition of moisturizers or emollients to the prepared dip may be helpful. A routine practice is to set aside a quart of solution from the gallon of parasiticide prepared, add to this an emollient or humectant, and pour the mix over the pet. Both an insecticidal and a moisturizing effect can thus be obtained.

Insecticidal Sprays for Animal Application

Most of the sprays currently marketed contain pyrethrins in combination with pyrethroids. These provide a quick knockdown effect but are often short-acting and limited in their depth of coat penetration and completeness of body coverage. Their advantages are the ease with which they can be applied, the low toxicity of their active ingredient(s), and the fact that they may be reapplied frequently. Another advantage of sprays, even on long-coated dogs, is that they may provide a repellant effect, which retards flea reinfestation. Most sprays are effective for less than 48 to 72 hours. Although regular use does improve efficacy, there is then the increased expense.

Insecticidal Powders

Powders or dusts are utilized primarily to provide more residual effectiveness; however, they may also potentiate the buildup of insecticide. Active ingredients often either are ineffective (carbaryl) in certain geographical regions or provide increased risks by containing acetylcholinesterase depressant compounds (carbamates, organophosphates). Repeated use of powders usually increases drying of the skin and lowers cosmetic acceptability. Safety factors are also a concern, particularly if small children have contact with the pet and exposure to the insecticide.

Insecticidal Shampoos

Most shampoos have good cleansing features, and are therefore helpful for their detergent effect, but do not provide effective flea control. Limitations include incomplete dispersion and penetration of the hair coat, ineffective flea-killing activity, and difficult removal of any residual insecticide by rinsing. Insecticidal shampoos can be used prior to medicated shampoos to remove fleas as well as to cleanse the skin and hair. An often overlooked limitation of shampoos is the contact time required for insecticidal activity. Most research has shown that a pyrethrin shampoo needs 15 minutes of contact for adequate flea-killing activity. A 5-minute application is still required even at five times the concentration of pyrethrins typically used. An advantage of insecticidal shampoos is that they can be used repeatedly, since the insecticide is almost completely rinsed from the animal. Treatment of puppies or older debilitated animals with an insecticidal shampoo is recommended, because of its safety, to simply remove a flea infestation. This may also be a disadvantage, however, since there is no residual activity and reinfestation can occur soon after the shampoo if fleas are encountered. SynerKyl is an ideal flea shampoo.

Flea Collars

Flea collars are ineffective for the flea-allergic animal. Their benefit, though limited, is for the in-contact animal without flea allergy. Chlorpyrifos-containing collars appear to be the most effective on the market today. Unfortunately, they do not provide adequate control for the flea-allergic animal. They are the treatment of choice when either the client is not willing to apply or the pet will not tolerate the use of more effective formulations such as pour-ons or sprays. Because of concerns for an additive effect leading to toxicity, flea collars that contain organophosphates should not be used when a systemic medication of the same type has been administered. Additional treatment (spray or a pour-on) is usually required with flea collars for optimal effectiveness but must include active ingredients that will not inhibit cholinesterase. Electronic flea collars have been proved ineffective in multiple controlled studies, and marketing in some states has been restricted.

Systemics

Systemics have the advantage of ease of administration. They usually are organophosphates, although newer products contain insect growth regulators (benzoylphenyl ureas) in lieu of adulticidal activity. Most systemics do not provide sufficient sustained blood levels for continuous flea-killing capability. This limits their effectiveness because of incomplete control of the flea burden on animals. In addition, there is virtually no benefit to the flea-allergic animal since the insecticidal effect of systemics requires the flea to be feeding and thereby initiate the allergic response. A major concern is the additive effect of systemic organophosphates

when the animal is also exposed to environmental insecticides and topical products containing carbamates or organophosphates. This may lead to intoxication. Systemics using organophosphates should be limited to healthy animals. The control of premise flea infestation would require long-term sustained treatment with a systemic at an interval of application not approved. Usefulness has been reported through prolonged administration of systemics (e.g., fenthion) to animals confined indoors with only limited outside exposure (patio, deck, balcony). This approach seems inefficient, since premise treatment will provide more rapid results, but it may be helpful when pet owners are not willing to treat inside the house.

Active Ingredients

Achievement of the ideal formulation of a parasiticide is difficult. Consumer expectations or residual activity pose a dilemma for manufacturers. Organophosphates have traditionally been the parasiticides with greatest residual activity. This still holds true, with chlorpyrifos being the most effective. Pyrethrins and pyrethroids are popular because of their safety and the increased frequency with which they can be used, in contrast to the acetylcholinesterase depressants (carbamates and organophosphates).

Botanical Insecticides

Botanical insecticides are derived from a plant source. The two most common compounds are pyrethrins (derived from the chrysanthemum petal), and rotenone (which is extracted from the root of the *Derris* plant). The advantage of these compounds is their low toxicity and usually rapid knockdown activity. A disadvantage is that they are vulnerable to rapid degradation and thus provide only minimal residual activity. There is no acetylcholinesterase suppression. The combination of pyrethrins with synthetically prepared insecticides resembling pyrethrins (pyrethroids) is a common practice and may provide some residual activity beyond that expected from pyrethrins alone. Another enhancement to prolong efficacy is microencapsulation. (A discussion of this follows.) Pyrethrins, pyrethroids, and rotenone can be used in combination with organophosphates without concern for potentiating intoxication.

Most pyrethrins require insecticide synergists and many utilize routine insect repellents. The three repellents most commonly included in flea sprays are MGK264 (di-N-propyl isocinchomeronate), butoxypolypropylene glycol, and Deet

(N,N-diethyl-*m*-toluamide). The familiar repellent MGK 11 is no longer used due to the expiration of its EPA registration. The effectiveness of repellents has been controversial, although unpublished data from manufacturers demonstrate improved flea control when a repellent is included in the product compared to when it is not.

DuraKyl, a pour-on insecticide (made by DVM) that contains rotenone and pyrethrins, is approved for both dogs and cats. The pyrethrin dip made by Adams Veterinary Research Laboratories (Norden-Beecham-Smith/Klein) is likewise effective for on-animal application to dogs and cats and may be used repeatedly. Pyrethrin pour-ons are not expected to have residual efficacy beyond 36 to 48 hours. They were first formulated as a spray and remain a popular method of application. Early sprays contained high concentrations of alcohol (Adam's Flea Off Mist) and were noted for their rapid knockdown effect. Water-base sprays came later and are popular now because of their improved animal acceptability.

Pyrethroids

Pyrethroids are synthetic insecticides based on the chrysanthemate molecule and, in general, have comparable toxicity to pyrethrins. Most have poor flushing activity, however, and therefore are combined with pyrethrins. Their duration of activity on the animal should not be expected to exceed 3 to 5 days. Insect resistance may occur with pyrethroids more commonly than with other compounds. The most widely used pyrethroid currently is permethrin, frequently combined with pyrethrins in the formulation. The pyrethroid fenvalorate with the repellent Deet was formulated several years ago and produced as an over-the-counter product called Blockade (Hartz Mountain). Although the formulation appeared to have favorable attributes (safety and efficacy), toxicities were reported, particularly in cats and older or smaller-breed dogs. This product is currently on the market following some limited toxicity studies without major modification of its formulation. There are still anecdotal reports of toxicities, suggesting no improvement in safety. Perhaps a reason for the difference between observations in the laboratory and experience with the pet population is the heterogeneity of pets. Older dogs or those with concurrent diseases are more likely to have adverse reactions than are young, healthy research Beagles.

Premise applications of pyrethroids utilize foggers and concentrates for dilution and spraying. Variable reports of residual activity have appeared.

Examples of on-animal products currently using

permethrin and pyrethrins include Duocide LA Spray (Allerderm), SynerKyl Shampoo and SynerKyl Spray (DVM), Expar Dip (Coopers), Permectrin (Bioceutic), a pour-on product, and Mycodex 14-Day Spray (Norden-Beecham-Smith/Klein). Products containing permethrin have been shown in field studies to lose efficacy on the third day after application, including Mycodex 14. A product recently introduced is Ex Spot (Coopers/Pittman-Moore), which contains 65% permethrin and is designed to be applied as spot therapy (with claims of up to 28 days' efficacy from a single application). There are no data available supporting these claims in fieldlike conditions.

Organophosphates

Organophosphates are used primarily in two types of application. One is a pour-on product for on-animal use, and the other a premise treatment (which includes foggers, granules, and emulsifiable concentrates used for surface sprays). Organophosphates are acetylcholinesterase depressants and may have a cumulative effect with other products embodying similar mechanisms of action (including carbamates).

Organophosphate products that are most popular for on-animal application include phosmet (e.g., Paramite, made by Zoecon/VetKem) and chlorpyrifos (Duratrol, produced by 3M Animal Care Products). Studies conducted with phosmet dip in comparison to a pyrethrin dip have shown minimal enhancement of the organophosphate over that with a pyrethrin (Table 6-1). Expectation of activity with phosmet should not extend beyond 3 days. The microencapsulation of chlorpyrifos (Duratrol) increases its safety and residual efficacy, and the product is available in formulations for both premise application and on-animal treatment.

Premise applications often include diazinon, malathion, or chlorpyrifos. These are occasionally formulated in combination with short-acting insecticides such as pyrethrins or insect growth regulators. Organophosphate-containing products have but limited use on cats, older debilitated animals, or extremely young animals. Another agent such as a botanical or a pyrethroid should be selected for these situations.

Some organophosphates are used as systemics; they can thus provide a circulating blood level that produces insecticidal activity in the form of a lethal blood meal to the parasite. The two systemic active ingredients are cythioate (Proban) and fenthion (Pro Spot). Fenthion has limited effectiveness in controlling fleas in the flea-allergic patient, and field studies conducted with Pro Spot at the man-

Table 6-1. Effectiveness of a microencapsulated chlorpyrifos pour-on insecticide (Duratrol) versus a phosmet pour-on (Paramite)

COLLECTION TIMES	AVERAGE NUMBER OF FLEAS		
	Control dogs (n = 6)	Duratrol-treated dogs (n = 6)	Paramite-treated dogs (n = 6)
DAY −7	43	47	71
DAY 0	58	145	64
HOUR +6	48	0	0
DAY +1	29	0	0
DAY +3	149	0	9
DAY +7	144	7	60
DAY +14	147	14	130
DAY +20	102	25	58
DAY +24	131	98	116
DAY +28	145	128	138

ufacturer's (Haver Lockhart) recommended dosage of 10 mg/kg showed the product unable to relieve the flea burden to less than an average of 12 fleas per animal at any time following a single application. Since Pro Spot works primarily as a systemic, it can reduce the flea infestation on a particular patient by only a limited amount.

The reduction of fleas occurs only after flea feeding. There is a dosage discrepancy between previous studies (indicating 14 to 22 mg/kg as optimal) and the recommendations from the manufacturer of Pro Spot (10 mg/kg). This difference may be a factor relating to the variable efficacies reported. Incidents of human and pet intoxication by contact with fenthion have been reported and are of particular concern when small children may be exposed through pet contact or direct handling of the product. Pets treated with inaccurate dosages also are at increased risk, particularly very young, old, or debilitated animals. Extralabel use (i.e., beyond label recommendations) of Spot-On, the large animal fenthion product, or Pro Spot is a violation of the law.

ProBan (1.6% cythioate) is formulated as both a liquid and a tablet for oral administration. It has limitations with flea-allergic dogs, since it likewise requires the fleas to be feeding. Although it may effectively eliminate fleas, the allergic reaction has already been induced. Another concern with cythioate is the duration of its effective blood level. Most studies have suggested that the effective level will be sustained for a maximum of 6 to 12 hours. The manufacturer recommends an average effective dosage of 30 mg per 20 pounds of body weight once every third day or twice weekly. The liquid

is recommended at a dosage of 1 ml per 10 pounds of body weight at the same interval. A regional practice is to treat every 48 hours, which is beyond the legal use by label recommendations, and is still not effective. The difference between a 48-hour interval of treatment and the effective blood level is as much as 36 hours. The manufacturer suggests an additional need for environmental treatment. The use of cythioate may eliminate fleas that escape either the environmental or the on-animal treatment and thus augment their effect. Organophosphate intoxication can be avoided by limiting the use of products to either premise application or on-animal or systemic treatment but not combinations.

Active ingredients without cholinesterase suppression are useful for complementing organophosphates. However, concern by some manufacturers (e.g., Zoecon/VetKem) has led to the reformulation of products (Siphotrol Plus II) to remove organophosphates, although this appears to be less efficacious.

Techniques of Extending Efficacy without Potentiating Toxicity
Stabilization

Most parasiticides are vulnerable to degradation by several methods. The most common are oxidation, hydrolysis, and inactivation by ultraviolet exposure. Means of extending the efficacy period have included stabilization by the addition of antioxidants or UV light protectants and using microencapsulation.

The first approach was developed in the product Adams 14-Day Spray, which used a technique of combining antioxidants and UV protectants with the synergized pyrethrin active ingredient. Although this extended activity, it had only limited effect beyond a 5-to-7-day period.

Microencapsulation

Microencapsulation has been effective in extending the efficacy of insecticides. It was developed and used most by 3M Animal Care, applying the technique to pyrethrins or chlorpyrifos. The microencapsulation procedure uses a polyurea microcapsule 15 to 20 μm in diameter that contains the insecticide. The shell wall is permeable to the insecticide but is otherwise resistant to rupture. The insecticide contained within the microcapsule is hydrophobic; therefore in a water suspension it does not leak through the capsule wall. The microcapsules dry after the product is sprayed in the environment or applied to the animal. Once dry, a small amount of insecticide leaches from inside the microcapsule to the surface and adheres to the insect. When a flea contacts this microcapsule, there is increased adherence to the cuticle (by electrostatic charge) as well as the cohesive effect of the insecticide on the capsule surface. As the surface coating of the insecticide slowly degrades, additional product leaches from inside the capsule to the surface (Fridinger, 1984). Thus the amount of material in the environment or on the pet is limited, and only after contact with the insect is the material extruded. No more than a few microcapsules are required for an insecticidal effect, and it is estimated that the product concentrate contains as many as 50 million per milliliter.

Products utilizing microencapsulation include 3M's Sectrol (a microencapsulated synergized pyrethrin) and Duratrol (a microencapsulated chlorpyrifos).

Controlled field trials with Sectrol and Duratrol have shown enhanced efficacy. The average number of fleas was substantially reduced at day 14 and day 20 following a single application of Duratrol versus that seen with phosmet (Paramite) (Table 6-1). Duratrol is available both for on-animal application and as a house/kennel spray and a yard/kennel concentrate spray. Sectrol is available as a premise spray and for on-animal application, the latter including Two Way Pet Spray and Two Way Flea Foam. These products contain both free pyrethrins (for quick knockdown) and microencapsulated pyrethrins (for residual effect). Two Way Flea Foam is particularly advantageous on cats, since it can be applied without the usual disturbance of the animal.

Duratrol Dip has been approved only for dogs; and despite the fact that current label information restricts application to every 3 weeks, the product sponsor has demonstrated excellent safety with application every 7 days and reapplication following a shampoo. Although this interval has been shown safe, it still violates EPA restriction until label changes are made. Nevertheless, reapplication subsequent to shampooing provides a continuation of insecticidal activity. It is important that the shampoo *not* contain a cholinesterase inhibiting ingredient.

The advantages of microencapsulation include:
1. Improved residual efficacy
2. Improved safety
3. Parasite targeting
4. Improved environmental safety
5. Decreased parasiticide odor

Insect Growth Regulators

Insect growth regulators (IGRs) have been popularized as an adjunct to adulticide products. The two compounds most commonly used are methoprene (Precor) and fenoxycarb. Precor is found in the VetKem product Siphotrol Plus II. Whereas it once used a combination of chlorpyrifos and synergized pyrethrins, more recently it has been reformulated and permethrin has replaced the adulticides. There have been anecdotal reports of decreased efficacy of the new formulation compared to the older product. The combination of Precor and synergized pyrethrins is found in Ovitrol Plus. Precor has recently shown ovicidal activity as well as being a juvenoid. Juvenoids are insect growth regulators that mimic growth hormone and limit the maturation of the larval stage, which prevents maturation to the pupa. Ovitrol Plus used on the animal has some theoretical limitations, although no comparative studies have been performed. The synergized pyrethrins have only limited residual efficacy and will likely provide no more than 24 to 48 hours of adulticidal effectiveness. The Precor may have activity against eggs produced by female fleas on the animal beyond that of the pyrethrin; but, unfortunately, in the flea-allergic patient this will allow feeding of the flea, resulting in the allergic reaction. Whether there is an enhanced effect of Ovitrol over other products containing combination insecticide formulations (pyrethrins and permethrin) is questionable. The advantage of Ovitrol Plus is its safety, allowing it to be used on young animals and cats. This safety, however, can also be attained by microencapsulated pyrethrins (Sectrol), with probably more residual efficacy.

Fenoxycarb is an insect growth regulator that has been included in a number of premise application products. Ectogard contains permethrin for residual activity against the adult, in addition to pyrethrins and fenoxycarb as the insect growth regulator. The manufacturer claims prevention of adult emergence for a minimum of 21 weeks. Ultraban is a comparable product containing fenoxycarb. Cooper's Laboratory recently introduced a product called Impasse, which is a pressurized spray containing chlorpyrifos and fenoxycarb. Marketing claims for Impasse suggest up to 6 months of protection against the redevelopment of flea infestation. A 16 oz can will provide up to 1500 sq ft of treatment. Fenoxycarb is reported to have superior UV stability, in contrast to methoprene (Precor). Benzyolphenyl ureas affect the chitin production of the adult flea, rendering it vulnerable to desiccation and death. Dimilin is the benzoylphenyl urea currently marketed in international areas. Products containing this active ingredient will likely be marketed in the United States in the near future.

Inert Parasiticidal Compounds

Inert compounds are beneficial for their mechanical insecticidal effect without creating hazardous chemical intoxication and environmental buildup. The three most commonly used are diatomaceous earth, silica gel, and sodium borate (the last especially).

The product Rx For Fleas Plus Powder contains a specially polymerized borate compound that has been electrostatically charged. It is used exclusively inside the premises and is sold only through operating companies (called Flea Busters) that have technicians to perform the application. The product is guaranteed for 1 year. Research has demonstrated excellent ovicidal and larvicidal activity as early as 3 days and overall parasiticidal activity eliminating over 99% of the development to adult fleas. Research has also been conducted in a simulated premise with cats as the target host. This investigation demonstrated residual activity for 6 months from a single application of Rx For Fleas Plus Powder. The effect may have been longer, but the study was concluded at that time. The advantage of the Rx For Fleas Plus Powder is its high efficacy without intoxicating chemical composition. The house does not have to be evacuated during application. The product is odorless and can be applied to discrete areas difficult to treat with conventional sprays and foggers. A limitation is that its effectiveness is reduced if it is allowed to contact water. Thus, to maintain the 1-year guar-

antee, the owner is restricted from shampooing carpets between treatments. The product is safe for homes with small children, cats, and other sensitive pets. The only disadvantage in its application process is a small amount of dust that may collect on furniture at the time of treatment. This process has been very popular and highly successful for inside flea control in heavily flea infested areas.

FLEA CONTROL GUIDELINES
General Concepts

Successful flea control requires recognition and treatment of all infested areas. The house and yard are the most difficult but also the most important to treat. As much as 99% of the flea population is in the preadult stage and resides in the environment. This proportion of adults to preadults demonstrates the overwhelming effect that an untreated environment can have on the rate of host reinfestation. Most failures represent incomplete premise treatment resulting from ineffective product application or territories too large to treat effectively. Many professional pest control operators do not perform effective treatment for complete control although they convey assurances to the consumer that they have. Complete coverage of infested areas is not routinely achieved. Moving furniture or treating under them is often not done. Treating the seat wells is another area not addressed by pest control operators and often overlooked by "do it yourself" application. Obscure flea-infested areas are often overlooked as well. These may include carpeted closets used by cats, which are difficult to treat because of all the articles present. Removal of all items and complete coverage are imperative. Rx For Fleas provides treatment with specific pest targeting (fleas) and is the most effective method of treatment.

"Do it yourself" application is also restricted to a limited number of products (active ingredients), which likewise restricts its effectiveness. Errors in dilution or application rate may lead to failure. The licensed pest control operator may have more armamentarium but, unfortunately, does not provide more complete coverage in most cases. In addition, some of the chemicals used by professional pest control operators may be acetylcholine depressants and have an accumulative toxic effect when used simultaneously with pet treatment, resulting in pet illness. Unfortunately, the veterinarian is usually held responsible when the pet becomes ill even though it was the environmental application that exceeded the toxic limits. Developing a rapport with a reputable, cooperative, and concerned pest control operator is valuable to the veterinarian. Some individuals prefer a "do it yourself" approach and rely upon the veterinarian for proper education and product recommendation.

Because of inability to control the application area, foggers are not routinely recommended. The ideal "do it yourself" inside premise treatment is sprays. These can be purchased either as concentrates or ready for use. Hand pump pressurized sprayers are the easiest and most effective to use. Removal of pets, particularly cats, rodents, and birds is necessary, if organophosphates are used. Protecting fish from direct exposure to insecticide or indirect contact through the aeration device is also necessary.

Treatment programs must be individualized and based on the following information:

1. Number and type of pets in the household

    Cats in the household create a major concern for reinfestation. Keeping them inside is essential, since their habitat outside is usually unrestricted. Treating the house inside is necessary. Large numbers of dogs and cats in a single household pose extreme limitations for effective flea control. Long-coated dogs may complicate the problem, particularly if there is incomplete premise treatment.

2. Inside versus outside pets

    Outside territory (size, location, housing, habitat) restricts the flea control program. Dogs and cats with unlimited outside exposure are the most difficult cases to treat. Rural areas, where the habitat (grass, sand, trees, and water) is favorable for flea proliferation, are nearly impossible to treat. Access to ponds, streams, or lakes leads to removal of the insecticide and reduces any chance of on-animal control. Frequent use of botanicals or pyrethroids is often the only resource but is impractical to most pet owners. Systemics (Pro-Spot and ProBan) may be included but have minimal effect if the infested area is large. The best solution is restricting the animal to a limited area that can be treated. Unaffected in-contact household animals who serve as a continuing source of inside infestation may relieve much of the flea burden by being completely restricted to the outside while the flea allergic pet(s) remains inside.

3. Home inhabitants

    Children and the elderly are at increased risk of insecticide exposure and possible in-

toxication. Infants and toddlers are the most vulnerable because they have the closest encounters with treated surfaces (by crawling on the floor) as well as the greatest tendency for ingestion of treated articles (by placing them or their hands in their mouth).

Microencapsulated products (Sectrol or Duratrol are preferred for "do it yourself" applicators whereas inert ingredients (Rx For Fleas Plus Powder) are the ideal approach. To avoid exposure and subsequent illness, it is important to recognize individuals with known allergies or specific sensitivities. Evacuation of the premises should follow manufacturers' recommendations.

Inside Premise Control

The first step in household treatment is cleaning. If a heavy infestation is noted, thorough vacuuming of all carpeted areas followed by steam cleaning is recommended. Vacuuming upholstery, particularly the seat wells, is paramount since many pets are allowed on furniture and these areas become heavily concentrated with flea ova and developing stages. Cleaning closets is also important, especially if they are carpeted and there are cats in the household, since they are secluded and may be used for nesting. Under furniture is another area frequently overlooked. This will require moving items for proper cleaning, and the vacuum cleaner bags must be discarded to eliminate fleas collected during the cleaning. Placing flea collars or other insecticidal objects within the vacuum bag is not advised. Solid floor areas are less of a concern but still require detergent washing if there are cracks or crevices present.

"Spot" treatment of areas where pets are frequently found is recommended, even when complete application is either impractical or resisted by the pet owner. Favorite sleeping areas or heavy traffic areas inside and out may be specifically targeted and will help reduce flea population.

Parasiticidal Treatment

As previously indicated, foggers are the poorest method of inside treatment, although they are the easiest to use; hence their popularity. There is virtually no control of the area treated, and the product usually is distributed to regions where an insecticide is not wanted (tabletops, cribs, toys, articles of clothing, dishes, utensils); furthermore, it does not reach areas where application is necessary (under furniture, in closets, along baseboards, under furniture cushions, etc.).

Spray or powder application is the only sure way of complete treatment. Recommended spray products for owner application include Duratrol (microencapsulated chlorpyrifos), Sectrol (microencapsulated synergized pyrethrins), Ectoguard (synergized permethrin and fenoxycarb), Ultraban (chlorpyrifos and fenoxycarb), and Spectracide (diazinon). Treatment should include all areas mentioned in the cleaning procedures, including basements and crawl spaces if accessible. Treatment should be repeated every 2 to 3 weeks for a period of at least 6 weeks if the infestation is heavy. A maintenance regimen should include application every 4 to 6 weeks (longer only if infestation is monitored and the climate not conducive to outside flea proliferation). Most chemical sprays should not be depended upon for the effective period stated by the manufacturer.

Powders have been used for inside premise control but have not been popularized until recently, with the advent of operating companies treating homes with inert powders specifically for fleas. A specially formulated borate compound (Rx For Fleas Plus Powder) has been well-received in the southeastern United States and other areas where the operating companies (e.g., Fleabusters) are located. Research conducted in the laboratory and controlled habitat studies have shown excellent efficacy; the drug has been active against both ova and larvae. Residual efficacy is guaranteed by the manufacturer for 1 year. Application must be by the Fleabusters operating company in the area. Advantages are low toxicity, lack of odor, and excellent residual activity.

Microencapsulated sprays (Sectrol) or inert powder (Rx For Fleas Plus) should be selected for ultimate safety without compromised efficacy in treating the inside environment. Products containing insect growth regulators reduce mammalian toxicity while improving residual efficacy.

Outside Treatment

The outside area should be treated utilizing the same principles as the inside. Treatment of either inside or outside will invariably have some shortcomings. This most often is the result of a large population of pupae unaffected by the active ingredient or an incomplete application. Often the automobile that transported the flea-infested pet will be overlooked. Favorite sleeping areas may need extra attention. Removal of blankets and bedding is essential. Treating the doghouse may have been overlooked.

To control exposure factors, restriction of pet activity is necessary. Fenced-in yards are the simplest means of doing this, or dogs may be limited to an area by a chain or run.

The products used for outside treatment may be sprays or granules. Granular insecticides include the active ingredients chlorpyrifos (Dursban), diazinon, and malathion. The major caution regarding their use is the presence of young children, who may ingest or contact the compound after application. Granules provide more residual activity than nonresidual sprays do, depending upon the moisture (from natural rainfall or irrigation).

Microencapsulation (e.g., Duratrol Yard And Kennel Flea Spray Concentrate) provides more potential residual effect than conventional sprays do. The Duratrol is diluted 2 ounces per gallon of water and treats nearly 2400 sq ft with one 30-ounce container. The concentrate can be used through a conventional water hose regulator such as the Ortho 1 qt Lawn Sprayer or the Gilmore Garden Sprayer at a dilution of 4 Tbsp per gallon siphon rate. For inside kennels and doghouses the manufacturer recommends 20 fluid ounces in enough water to make 1 gallon.

Other insecticide sprays may be directly attached to a garden hose for automatic regulated dilution to ease application. Norden produces a chlorpyrifos product. Insecticide concentrates are usually found in the lawn-and-garden section of some department stores (Wal-Mart or K-Mart) or nurseries. They can be used in the same manner by prediluting or attachment to an application regulator for use with a garden hose. The outside should be treated more frequently (every 2 weeks) if there is a large flea infestation and less frequently (every 3 to 4 weeks) after several treatments and subsequent reduction of the flea population.

Monitoring Flea Infestation

The best method of determining environmental infestation is the direct evaluation of hosts inhabiting the area. The routine use of a flea comb is helpful in determining the extent of fleas. The comb should contain approximately 20 teeth per inch. Several companies make flea combs, but the one I prefer is Twinco (manufactured by Lambert Kay, a Division of Carter Wallace, Inc., Cranbury, New Jersey 08512). This device is certainly more difficult to use on long-haired or fine-coated animals or those that are matted. Due to host variability of flea appeal, all animals in the household should be combed. Recognition of animal infestation is an indication of a much larger environmental problem since the majority of organisms are in the preadult stages. Restricting cats to inside the house is an excellent method of monitoring inside infestation, particularly if in-contact dogs are also combed. There are flea traps that have been marketed, but minimal objective information is available concerning their reliability. They may be useful for determining the level of adult flea infestation in the environment. Dragging a white or red fabric along the carpet or furniture has also been described for monitoring flea infestation (but does not detect anything less than a major infestation). Abandoned homes revisited several weeks later pose minimal problem in determining the infestation level since the hungry adults will usually be attracted to people.

Pet Products

The general concept regarding treatment of pets is to use products with low toxicity and high efficacy. There is no "super" product with all the virtues and no shortcomings. Products commonly used by the editors include the following:

Pour-ons

Adams Pyrethrin Dip
Durakyl Dip
Duratrol Dip
Expar 3.4% EC
Paramite Dip
Permectin

Sprays

Aquamist
Duocide LA
Sectrol
SynerKyl

Foams

Two Way Flea Foam

Combinations of products may be required. Pour-on parasiticides applied weekly usually require supplemental treatment with a spray or foam between treatments. With the availability of effective sprays, dusts or powders are not as popular but may provide greater residual activity. Care must be exercised with treatment using multiple products each containing organophosphate compounds.

Preferred Premise Treatment Products

The preferred professional application for inside environments is Rx For Fleas Plus Powder. Preferred "do it yourself" products include Duratrol, Sectrol, Ectogard, and Siphotrol Plus II.

Treatment failure for a flea-allergic animal is usually due to ineffective flea control, although coexisting pruritic skin diseases are often part of the problem. Emphasis must be placed on determining the cause of the failure rather than looking for a substitute therapy, such as glucocorticoids. Client information sheets are necessary for proper communication. A posttreatment conference and clinical examination of the pet should be conducted 4 weeks after initiation of the program. Modification of the approach is often influenced by an owner's attitude and the extent of clinical response. Above all, encouragement and compliments for achievement are the most effective methods for ensuring success.

REFERENCES

Halliwell REW, Gorman NT: Veterinary clinical immunology, Philadelphia, 1989, WB Saunders.
Fridinger TL: Designing the ultimate weapon against fleas, Vet Med 79:1151, 1984.

SUPPLEMENTAL READING

Bevier DE: Fleas and flea control. In Kirk RW (ed): Current veterinary therapy X, Philadelphia, 1989, WB Saunders.
Moriello KA: Oh, no! not fleas again, Vet Focus 1:19, 1989.

7

Demodicosis

Kenneth W. Kwochka

Demodicosis is an inflammatory, parasitic skin disease of dogs and cats.

Canine Demodicosis

Canine demodicosis is one of the ten most common skin diseases seen in small animal practice in the United States (Sischo et al., 1989). Dermatitis develops when large numbers of the follicular mite *Demodex canis* inhabit hair follicles, sebaceous glands, or apocrine sweat glands. In small numbers, this mite is a normal inhabitant of the skin of dogs. Transmission of mites is thought to occur from dam to puppy during nursing within the first 72 hours after birth. The life cycle of the mite is spent entirely on the host. Demodicosis is not considered a contagious disease among nonneonatal healthy animals, and transmission of the mite from animals to humans has not been reported.

Canine demodicosis appears to have a complex pathogenesis that is still not completely understood. There is evidence of hereditary predisposition in certain breeds. Culling affected dams or sires has radically reduced the incidence of generalized demodicosis from individual breeding kennels. However, the genetic transmission is not known, making it difficult to provide breeders with specific recommendations.

Suppression of the immune system likely precipitates the disease in at least some cases. Generalized demodicosis has been produced in dogs by administering antilymphocyte serum or high-dose corticosteroids (Owen, 1972) and is seen in as many as 8% of adult dogs with hyperadrenocorticism (White et al., 1989). The sophisticated tests necessary to evaluate the immune system are not generally available to the practitioner, nor would they be cost-effective.

Early evidence supported the theory that an hereditary, specific T cell defect for *Demodex canis* might allow mites to multiply to large numbers and cause clinical disease and further secondary, generalized T cell suppression (Scott et al., 1974; Scott et al., 1976). This theory is plausible but a hereditary T cell defect has never been proved. More recently the role of T cell suppression has been challenged by work (Barta et al., 1983) showing that measurable immunosuppression is found only with concurrent bacterial skin infection. Similar to other mite infestations, measurable immunosuppression may be related more to absolute numbers of mites. Dogs without secondary pyoderma may have low numbers of *Demodex* while those with increasing numbers naturally are more prone to the infection. This has not been taken into consideration in any of the immune studies thus far reported in dogs.

Several predisposing factors have been either suggested or documented as initiating canine generalized demodicosis. These factors include administration of immunosuppressive drugs, serious systemic diseases, estrus, whelping, heartworm disease, and hookworm infestation. Even low doses of oral, short-acting steroids may compromise local defense mechanisms and precipitate the disease. One of the most common clinical presentations of demodicosis is an adult dog with allergies that has been receiving long-term glucocorticoid therapy.

The presence of any underlying potentially immunosuppressive or serious metabolic diseases should also be considered. These include hyperadrenocorticism, hypothyroidism, diabetes mellitus, blastomycosis and other deep mycoses, lymphosarcoma, hemangiosarcoma, and mammary adenocarcinoma.

Feline Demodicosis

Feline demodicosis is a rare cause of dermatitis. The *Demodex cati* mite is similar to *D. canis*. There is a second species of *Demodex* in cats that differs morphologically from *D. cati* by having a broad and blunted abdomen. This species is found in the stratum corneum rather than in hair follicles or glandular structures. The more superficial location may enhance response to therapy with topical agents.

No experimental studies have been conducted on the role of immunosuppression as a precipitating factor for generalized feline demodicosis. The possibility of immunosuppression is an important clinical consideration, since generalized feline demodicosis caused by *D. cati* usually is associated with systemic diseases such as diabetes mellitus, systemic lupus erythematosus, hyperadrenocorticism, toxoplasmosis, feline leukemia virus (FeLV) infection, feline immunodeficiency virus (FIV) infection, feline infectious peritonitis (FIP) infection, and neoplasia. Immunosuppressive drugs should also be considered, especially glucocorticoids and progestational compounds.

CLINICAL DISEASE
History

Extensive historical information usually is not necessary to establish the diagnosis, which is easily confirmed by deep skin scrapings. However, this information may help determine the precipitating cause of the disease. A thorough drug history should be taken to determine if any immunosuppressive drugs such as corticosteroids, progestational compounds, or chemotherapeutic agents have been administered. The owner also should be asked when the last fecal sample was evaluated for parasites, if heartworm checks have been done and preventive medication used, and what type of diet has been fed. If the affected animal is female, any relationship of the disease to estrus or whelping should be established.

Questioning should also be directed at determining if there have been signs of a more serious metabolic disease such as polyuria-polydipsia, significant increase or decrease in weight, lethargy, and weakness. In cats, the history may also give information about FeLV, FIV, and FIP status.

Presenting Signs in Dogs

Canine demodicosis is most commonly encountered in purebred dogs under 1 year of age and is observed in either of two clinical forms.

Localized demodicosis is a mild clinical condition that resolves spontaneously 90% of the time. Immunologic studies have not been performed on dogs with localized disease, and no specific recommendations are made with regard to breeding these animals. The disease usually begins with acute or gradual hair loss involving the face or extremities. Pruritus and inflammation generally are not complaints unless a secondary pyoderma, which is uncommon, has developed. Typical physical examination findings are one or more discrete, small focal areas of alopecia with varying degrees of scaling, follicular plugging, and hyperpigmentation. Lesions usually are confined to the head, neck, and forelimbs, although any area of the body may be involved. This form may occur in any breed and in either gender.

Approximately 10% of localized cases of demodicosis may rapidly or gradually progress to generalized disease. Progression in some cases may be so rapid that the localized lesions are never noticed. Generalized demodicosis is a severe, potentially life-threatening disease of purebred dogs. Breeds that appear to be at increased risk include the Old English Sheepdog, Collie, Afghan Hound, German Shepherd Dog, Cocker Spaniel, Doberman Pinscher, Dalmatian, Great Dane, English Bulldog,

Boston Terrier, Dachshund, Chihuahua, Boxer, Pug, Chinese Shar-Pei, Beagle, and English Pointer.

Generalized patchy or diffuse alopecia usually develops and may be the only abnormality early in the course of the disease. Erythema, scaling, crusting, and follicular plugging may develop quickly, resulting in the squamous form of generalized demodicosis (Fig. 7-1). Some dogs, especially adults, may develop multifocal patches of hyperpigmentation (Fig. 7-2) but still have a fairly normal hair coat. Adult Yorkshire Terriers with demodicosis may develop large patches of melanosis. Any dog with pigmentary changes should be scraped for *Demodex* mites. Occasionally an animal will have only a demodectic otitis externa or pododermatitis (Fig. 7-3).

Secondary pyoderma commonly develops with demodicosis. The pyoderma may be superficial,

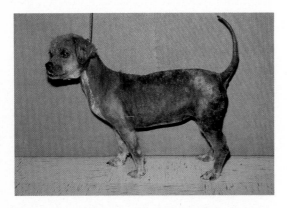

Figure 7-1. Alopecia, scale, and hyperpigmentation typical of chronic squamous generalized demodicosis.

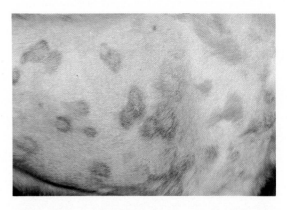

Figure 7-2. Multifocal patches of scale and hyperpigmentation on the lateral thoracic skin of a Collie with generalized demodicosis.

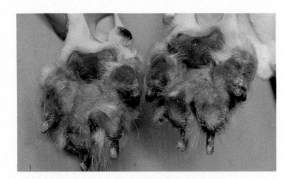

Figure 7-3. Canine pododemodicosis with interdigital erythema, alopecia, furunculosis, and footpad hyperkeratosis.

(Courtesy Dr. Patricia White, Columbus, Ohio.)

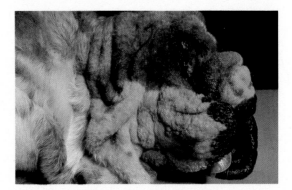

Figure 7-4. Alopecia, erythema, and furunculosis of the chin and ventral neck of an English Bulldog with generalized demodicosis.

(Courtesy Dr. Patricia White, Columbus, Ohio.)

with papules and pustules, or deep, with furuncles draining a purulent exudate (Fig. 7-4), or it may involve cellulitis, with severe pain and edema. Pruritus and a generalized peripheral lymphadenopathy are present usually with pyoderma. Animals with deep pyoderma may show signs of septicemia and may be febrile, anorexic, lethargic, and severely debilitated.

From the above description it is obvious that virtually any cutaneous lesions may be caused by demodicosis; that is why it is so important to scrape for *Demodex* mites with any dermatosis. However, the "highly suspect" lesions (where the suspicion of finding mites is high) include facial alopecia (Fig. 7-5), blepharitis, focal and multifocal erythematous scale (Fig. 7-6), focal and multifocal hyperpigmentation, comedones (Fig. 7-7), pododermatitis, folliculitis, and furunculosis.

Presenting Signs in Cats

Localized and generalized demodicosis in cats have been associated with *D. cati.* Demodicosis may be more common in purebred Siamese and Burmese cats. Pruritus may be present but usually is not. Clinical signs of localized disease include single or multiple areas of alopecia and scaling of the eyelids, periocular area, head, and neck. Signs of generalized demodicosis include macules, patches, alopecia, scaling, erythema, hyperpigmentation, crusting, and symmetric alopecia of the head, neck, legs, and trunk. Some cats will have a sparse hair coat, greasy skin surface, and hyperpigmentation with minimal scale.

Ceruminous demodectic otitis externa has been described in cats with normal skin and also in those with generalized disease. The otic exudate is dark brown. Smears from ear swabs should be examined for demodectic mites in all cats with otitis.

Signs associated with the new *Demodex* species are similar to those described for *D. cati,* but the pruritus tends to be more severe. A severe pruritic dermatitis localized to the head, neck, and elbows has been described, as has a ventral pruritic dermatitis with erythema and alopecia. Some cats with mild clinical signs may have just a symmetric pattern of truncal alopecia with normal-appearing skin.

Differential Diagnoses

An extensive list of differentials is unnecessary for this disease; mites usually are easily found with properly obtained skin scrapings.

The most common differentials for the young

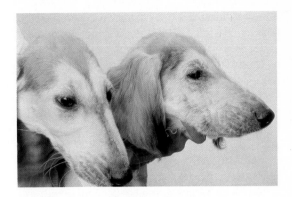

Figure 7-5. Facial alopecia and erythema associated with demodectic mange in two 3-month-old Saluki littermates.
(Courtesy Dr. Patricia White, Columbus, Ohio.)

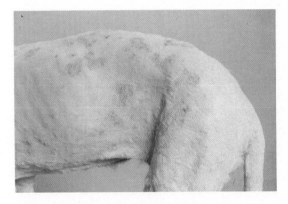

Figure 7-6. Multifocal patches of erythematous scale caused by generalized demodicosis and superficial pyoderma in a white German Shepherd Dog.
(Courtesy Dr. John Gordon, Columbus, Ohio.)

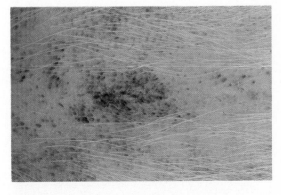

Figure 7-7. Multiple comedones on the ventral abdomen of a mixed breed dog with generalized demodicosis.
(Courtesy Dr. Patricia White, Columbus, Ohio.)

dog with localized demodicosis are dermatophytosis and bacterial folliculitis. If scrapings are negative, then a Wood's light examination, potassium hydroxide (KOH) preparation, fungal culture, bacterial culture, and biopsy should be considered.

The most important differential diagnoses for the dog with generalized demodicosis are bacterial folliculitis, bacterial furunculosis, and dermatophytosis.

Because of the extreme variability in clinical lesions reported for cats with demodicosis, many differential diagnoses should be considered, including dermatophytosis, feline atopy, food allergy, flea allergy, notoedric mange, and pemphigus foliaceus.

DIAGNOSIS

Skin Scrapings

Demodex canis and *D. cati* mites are best found by performing deep skin scrapings. Any dog or cat with a dermatosis should be scraped in two or three places and the diagnosis made. Even cats with what appears to be a pattern of symmetric alopecia with normal-looking underlying skin should be scraped. Ear swabs should be obtained for *Demodex* mites in any case of ceruminous otitis externa, especially in cats.

The deep skin scraping must be performed properly. Hair should be clipped from the area to be scraped and the skin squeezed gently to extrude mites from the follicles to the skin surface. Some dogs may need to be sedated in order to obtain proper deep scrapings, especially when sampling difficult areas such as the lips, eyelids, and interdigital spaces. The area should be scraped with a

no. 10 surgical blade or spatula until capillary bleeding is observed. Enough heavy mineral oil should be used on the skin and blade to transfer scraped material from the skin surface to the glass microscopic slide for examination under the $10 \times$ objective. Four stages of the life cycle may be observed in skin scrapings: spindle-shaped eggs (Fig. 7-8), six-legged larvae, eight-legged nymphs (Fig. 7-9), and eight-legged adults (Fig. 7-10). A large number of live adult mites or immature forms and eggs are necessary to confirm the diagnosis, since an occasional mite, especially from the face, may be a normal resident. Further scrapings should be performed if there is any question about the significance of the number of mites. Finding a small number of mites on the face warrants more extensive scrapings of the body to determine the extent of the disease.

In cats, when demodicosis caused by the more superficial mite (Fig. 7-11) is suspected, it may be prudent to perform superficial scrapings over a larger surface area to maximize chances of finding the mites.

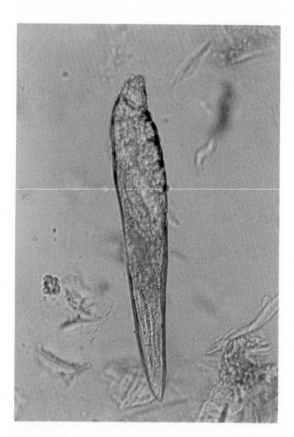

Figure 7-9. A *Demodex canis* nymph with four pairs of short, stubby legs, in mineral oil from a skin scraping.

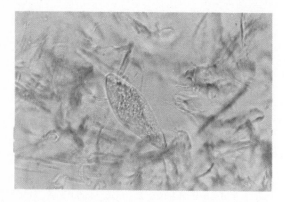

Figure 7-8. A *Demodex canis* spindle-shaped egg, in mineral oil from a skin scraping.

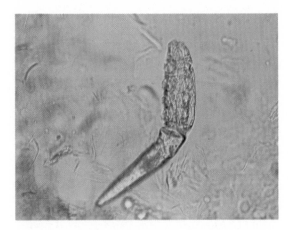

Figure 7-10. A *Demodex canis* adult with four pairs of legs, in mineral oil from a skin scraping.

Skin Biopsies

In rare instances a biopsy may be needed to confirm the diagnosis. This is especially true in chronic cases where the skin has become hyperkeratotic, lichenified, and scarred, making it difficult to squeeze mites from follicles. The hardest area from which to obtain mites is severely affected interdigital skin. Chinese Shar-Peis with truncal folliculitis should also be biopsied to rule out demodicosis definitively. Histologic examination of routine punch biopsies will reveal mites within hair follicles or within the dermis if follicles have ruptured.

Medical Evaluation

I prefer to do a complete medical evaluation on all dogs and cats with generalized demodicosis. Although this is not mandatory in the young dog that is otherwise healthy, it should be considered in all dogs over 2 years of age that develop generalized demodicosis, in dogs that are not responding to treatment or have recurrent disease, and in all cats with generalized demodicosis.

Medical evaluation of dogs should include a complete blood count (CBC), serum biochemical profile, urinalysis, fecal examination for parasites, and heartworm check. Dogs with adult-onset demodicosis should have a thyroid-stimulating hormone (TSH) stimulation test to evaluate thyroid status and a low-dose dexamethasone suppression test to evaluate adrenocortical status. Early Cushing's disease may have only cutaneous abnormalities (including generalized demodicosis) without classical systemic signs or laboratory abnormali-

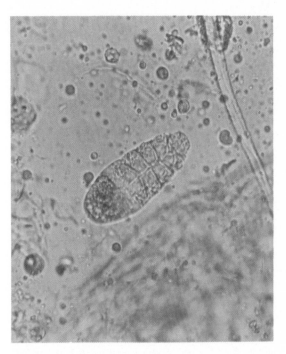

Figure 7-11. Unnamed adult demodectic mange mite from a cat, in mineral oil from a skin scraping. Note the broad, blunted abdomen.

ties. A low-dose dexamethasone suppression test is still warranted if the preliminary medical evaluation does not suggest an underlying cause for the demodicosis.

Medical evaluation of cats should include CBC, serum biochemical profile, urinalysis, fecal examination for parasites, FeLV and FIV tests, and possibly an adrenocorticotropic hormone (ACTH) stimulation test or dexamethasone suppression test.

TREATMENT
Canine Demodicosis

General Principles

Localized and generalized demodicoses require different modes of therapy, although there are some common considerations. Corticosteroids at any dosage and in any form, including topicals, are contraindicated unless the animal presented is in a life-threatening situation. They may suppress the immune system of an already compromised animal. Localized cases of demodicosis can progress to the generalized form as a result of steroid administration. Because pruritus may be associated with secondary pyoderma, treating the bacterial infection with topical therapy (antimicrobial shampoos, soaks, or whirlpools) and systemic antibiotics will usually quickly resolve this problem. Physical restraint (Elizabethan collars, T-shirts) and sedation may also be beneficial for a short period of time. The antihistamines (diphenhydramine HCl at 2.2 mg/kg q8h PO and chlorpheniramine maleate at 2 to 8 mg [total dose] q8-12h PO) will have some antipruritic and sedative effects. Drugs such as hydroxyzine and doxepin HCl should not be used with amitraz dips, because they have monoamine oxidase–inhibiting activity and may potentiate toxicity.

A secondary pyoderma, if present, must be treated according to the severity and depth of infection. A superficial pyoderma with limited distribution usually can be controlled through topical therapy with benzoyl peroxide (OxyDex, Pyoben) or chlorhexidine (ChlorhexiDerm, Nolvasan) shampoos.

Generalized superficial pyoderma requires systemic antibiotics as well as topical therapy. The antibiotic may be chosen empirically if the infection has not been treated previously, since a coagulase-positive *Staphylococcus* organism usually is isolated. Pustular contents should be examined microscopically to confirm the presence of cocci. If better assurance of clinical efficacy is desired, if the initial antibiotic fails to give good response within 7 to 10 days, or if rods are found on cytologic examination, then an aerobic bacterial culture and susceptibility test should be done. With deep pyoderma a culture and susceptibility test is mandatory.

Commonly used antibiotics include oxacillin (Prostaphlin, Oxacillin Capsules ℞) at 22 mg/kg q8h PO, trimethoprim-sulfa combinations (Tribrissen, Di-Trim, TMP-SMZ generics) at 22 mg/kg q12h PO, ormetoprim with sulfadimethoxine (Primor) at 27.5 mg/kg q24h PO, amoxicillin trihydrate with clavulanate potassium (Clavamox) at 22 mg/kg q12h PO, and cephalexin at 22 mg/kg q8h PO. Antibiotic treatment for superficial pyoderma must be continued a minimum of 3 to 4 weeks or 2 weeks after all clinical lesions have resolved. A deep pyoderma requires a minimum of 4 to 6 weeks. Aggressive topical therapy should be instituted by clipping the entire hair coat, followed by warm dilute (1:10 with water) chlorhexidine (Nolvasan Solution) or povidone-iodine solution compresses, whole-body soakings, or whirlpool baths q12h until ulcerated lesions are clean and healing. A benzoyl peroxide shampoo is also valuable following hydrotherapy.

Topical miticide therapy is started along with treatment of the pyoderma, with two exceptions: first, parasiticidal agents should not be used until the erosions and ulcers of a deep pyoderma are healed, to minimize systemic absorption and toxicity; second, parasiticidal dippings are never applied to dogs under or recovering from general anesthesia, because of possible drug interactions and toxicity.

A good plane of nutrition should be maintained in dogs with demodicosis. Even if a complete medical evaluation is not performed, these dogs should be current on vaccinations and at least checked and treated for gastrointestinal parasites. They also should be examined for *Dirofilaria immitis* microfilariae, and heartworm preventive therapy should be started if appropriate for location and season.

Localized Demodicosis

More than 90% of dogs with localized demodicosis will recover spontaneously, with disappearance of lesions in 6 to 12 weeks. Thus, the prognosis is excellent and recurrence is rare. No immunologic defect has been demonstrated, and no limitations are placed on breeding. It is not known whether localized treatment of demodicosis affects the progression to a generalized disease. Localized demodicosis often is monitored without specific acaricidal therapy. One percent rotenone ointment (Goodwinol) may be helpful when applied once a day and rubbed well into the individual lesions. However, this acaricide will usually cause more alopecia and erythema, making the lesions look worse before they improve. Benzoyl peroxide gel (OxyDex Gel, Pyoben Gel) may also be effective because of its follicular flushing activity.

Amitraz liquid concentrate (Mitaban) has been tested and proved safe and efficacious for localized demodicosis. However, *Demodex* mites are capable of developing resistance to insecticidal agents. One must question the rationale of using the only product licensed by the U.S. Food and Drug Administration (FDA) for generalized demodicosis in every localized case, when 90% of these cases self-cure, while risking possible development of resistant mite populations on individual animals. It may also be important for serious breeders to know whether they have a dog that will go on to develop generalized demodicosis, which dog should then be removed from the breeding program.

Generalized Demodicosis (Fig. 7-12)

Amitraz. Amitraz is the only drug approved for the treatment of generalized demodicosis by the FDA, and it has made management of the disease much easier for client and veterinarian. It is classified as a monoamine oxidase inhibitor, but the mechanism of its acaricidal action is not known. Clinical studies have reported results for complete, long-term cures ranging from 0% to 99%. This vast discrepancy in efficacy is probably the result of different animal populations, variations in treatment protocols, and different criteria for cured cases, including long-term follow-up periods. Actual long-term cure rates with 1-year follow-ups are probably in the range of 60% to 80% for the typical population of dogs with generalized demodicosis under 1½ years of age.

One study (Kwochka et al., 1985) reported that weekly amitraz dippings were more efficacious than dippings every 2 weeks: 78% effective as opposed to 22%. No difference was seen when the concentration of the solution was doubled and applications were done every 2 weeks. These results suggest that better cure rates may be achieved when twice the recommended frequency (weekly) of application is used. It is not known if weekly treatment decreases the time needed for a cure. Increasing the frequency of application did not result in a greater incidence of toxicity. The FDA currently approves use of amitraz at only 0.025% every 2 weeks. A more cost-effective approach is to start with biweekly applications and change to weekly in cases that do not respond or are not cleared of mites after eight to ten treatments. Cases should be reevaluated by examination and skin scrapings after every three dips. A switch from biweekly to weekly treatment should occur before eight to ten dippings if the clinical signs become worse or if mite counts either do not improve or worsen.

A recent report (Medleau and Willemse, 1991) studied the efficacy of daily amitraz therapy. A high concentration (0.125%) of amitraz solution (Taktic) was applied daily to half the body on an alternating basis. Eighty-one percent of dogs (38/47) not previously treated with amitraz were cured, as were 75% (18/24) previously treated with weekly or twice weekly applications of amitraz. The average duration of treatment was 3.7 months. Follow-ups were done for a minimum of 4 months after treatment in 15 dogs and 9 months in 56 dogs. No serious toxic reactions were seen during the study. Such use of amitraz has not been approved in the United States, but it offers a therapeutic alternative when striving for a complete cure versus clinical control.

Excellent clinical improvement is seen in most cases, even when long-term cures are not attained. Many dogs will remain asymptomatic, although still harboring mites, when treated every 2 to 4 weeks. Relapses may be seen with the development of mite resistance, but this is rare. I have successfully controlled symptoms in some cases for as long as 4 years on maintenance programs.

Other advantages of amitraz include its ease of application in the aqueous form, relatively low cost, and low reported toxicity. I recommend that all dips in the initial treatment series be performed by qualified personnel at the veterinary hospital. Most owners will not perform treatments correctly or for adequate durations. They especially have trouble with treatment of the face and feet. Those who perform the procedure should avoid direct contact with the solution or the wet animal after dipping. Reactions have been seen in people taking other monoamine oxidase–inhibiting drugs such as antihypertensive agents and antihistamines. Nausea and dizziness have been reported in such individuals who inhaled amitraz fumes during use, even though the solution did not contact their skin.

Drying and flaking of the skin are minor problems encountered on occasion, and these can be easily controlled by adding 1 or 2 capfuls of a bath oil rinse to the solution (Humilac, HyLyt*efa, Alpha-Sesame Oil). Some 8% of patients treated will show transient sedation, and 3% transient pruritus. Patients with large numbers of mites may develop vesicular and pustular eruptions with pruritus 24 hours after dipping. Other abnormalities include depression of rectal temperature and elevation of blood glucose. Seizures and acute death have been reported but are very rare. Side effects are more commonly seen in small dogs, especially the toy breeds. For these cases treatment should be started with half-strength solution, contact time should be reduced, or only half the body should be treated at one time. The concentration, contact time, or amount of body treated may be gradually increased if the initial dippings are tolerated.

The entire hair coat should be clipped on all dogs prior to the first dipping. Treatments should be preceded by a benzoyl peroxide shampoo for its follicular flushing activity to allow better penetration of the miticide. After bathing, the dog should be toweled dry to ensure that the dipping solution will not be further diluted from its optimal concentration when it contacts a wet hair coat. Another option is to shampoo the dog 12 hours before dipping, but an interval of this length may negate the desired follicular flushing activity. One vial (10.6 ml) of the concentrate should be added to 2 gallons of warm water, and the solution used immediately to ensure optimal potency, because it deteriorates

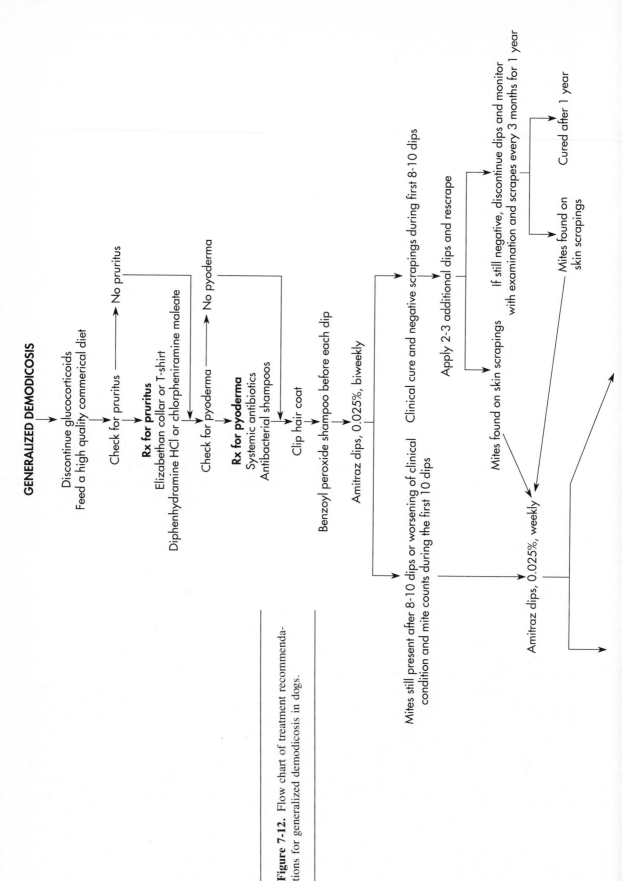

Figure 7-12. Flow chart of treatment recommendations for generalized demodicosis in dogs.

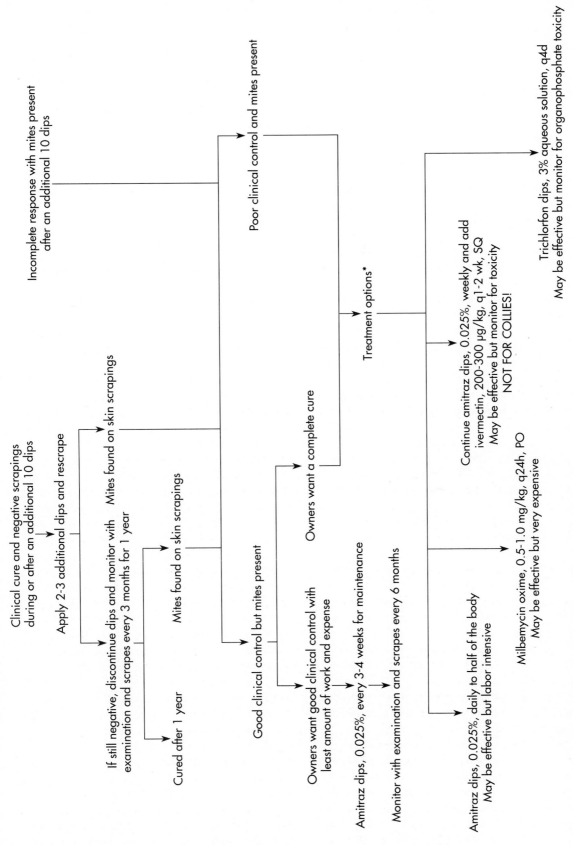

rapidly by oxidation and exposure to ultraviolet light. The solution should be continuously applied over the entire body with a sponge for 10 minutes and then allowed to air dry without rinsing or toweling. All four feet should be immersed in the solution during the 10-minute dipping procedure. The body should be kept as dry as possible between applications.

Response to therapy is monitored by physical examination and skin scrapings. Approximate ratios of live to dead mites and mature to immature forms should be noted. A favorable response to therapy is indicated by a decrease in live and immature forms. Therapy should be continued for two to three treatments after negative scrapings are obtained (no mites, no immature forms, and no eggs) and should be discontinued only after a final set of negative scrapings at that time. A minimum of ten scrapings is performed at the final visit, with special attention to previously affected areas, new lesions, and predilection areas such as the face and feet. Because many dippings may be necessary before a complete cure is achieved, I recommend biweekly dippings for ten treatments. A change to weekly treatments should be considered for ten additional applications if mites are still present. If no cure is effected after twenty dips, daily amitraz dips, an amitraz maintenance program, or another parasiticide should be considered.

Reevaluation with scrapings should be performed 4 weeks after the last dip and then every 3 months for 1 year before a case is considered cured. Owners should be called and reminded to return for reevaluation even if the dog looks normal. Frequent evaluation can often prevent the development of severe clinical lesions in relapsing cases by finding mites and reinstituting therapy prior to extensive hair loss and secondary pyoderma.

If the number of mites or the percentage of immature forms dramatically increases during initial therapy or maintenance, mite resistance may be occurring and therapeutic disaster impending. If the treatment protocol has been followed and no concurrent debilitating disease has developed, a switch to more frequent administration or a higher concentration of amitraz (or an alternate parasiticide) would be indicated.

Milbemycin. Oral parasiticidal agents have not been effective for generalized demodicosis. However, preliminary information from current studies indicates that oral milbemycin oxime (Interceptor) at high doses may be effective for amitraz-resistant cases of generalized demodicosis in dogs. Milbemycin has been used (Miller and Scott, 1991) at 0.5 to 1 mg/kg q24h PO for a **minimum** of 30 days **and** until no mites could be seen on several skin scrapings, and then for an additional 30 days. Cases were considered treatment failures if mites were not eradicated after 90 days of treatment with milbemycin at 0.5 mg/kg q24h followed by 90 days of 1 mg/kg q24h. Seventeen dogs had completed the treatment program at the time of this writing, with three failures. Of the 14 that were cleared of mites after treatment, two relapsed, four were cured after 1 year, one was still clear at 9 to 12 months, three were still clear at 5 to 8 months, and four were still clear at 1 to 4 months. Reversible neurologic signs were seen in two small dogs with very resistant demodicosis receiving doses in the range of 3 mg/kg q24h.

In a related study (Reedy and Garfield, 1991) 83% achieved negative skin scrapings; ten have remained in remission for over 1 year, six for over 6 months, and ten have relapsed. No adverse drug reactions have been seen. The final results of these studies are awaited, but it appears that milbemycin may cure 50% to 60% of amitraz-resistant generalized demodicosis in dogs. The drug is well-tolerated but, unfortunately, very expensive when used at this high dosage. It costs approximately $150 to treat a 23 kg dog for 1 month. Thus it should be reserved for cases of resistant, generalized demodicosis in which the owner wants to attempt a complete cure rather than settle for control with an amitraz maintenance program.

Additional therapeutic options. The results of ivermectin usage for generalized demodicosis have been largely disappointing. In comparison to trials conducted with other parasiticides, however, the duration of treatment with this drug has been short. One study (Gravino et al., 1985) reported efficacy at 600 µg/kg q1wk, for five treatments in 12 dogs with localized demodicosis and 8 dogs with generalized demodicosis. The editors have used ivermectin (Ivomec 1% Injection) at 200 to 300 µg/kg q1-2wk SQ **along with** amitraz in dogs with an incomplete response to amitraz when used alone. Some dogs have been cured of the disease whereas others have shown improvement of lesions while still harboring mites. The latter group has been kept on maintenance ivermectin every 3 to 4 weeks with discontinuation of the amitraz. No final conclusions can be drawn because of the low numbers of animals. Ivermectin is cheaper than milbemycin, but it has more potential for toxicity and should not be used in Collies or related breeds.

A 3% aqueous trichlorfon solution (Neguvon Pour-On) has been used successfully as a whole body dip every 4 days in some cases. No final conclusions can be drawn because of the low numbers of animals. Trichlorfon is not approved for this use, and animals must be monitored for organophosphate toxicity.

One study (Figueiredo, 1985) reported vitamin E at a dosage of 200 mg q5h PO to be curative as sole therapy in 147 of 149 cases of generalized demodicosis in dogs. The trial was based on the finding that dogs with generalized demodicosis had significantly lower serum vitamin E levels compared with normal dogs. Another study (Gilbert et al., 1990), however, did not confirm lower serum vitamin E levels in demodectic dogs, and results in the editors' practices have been largely disappointing.

Cythioate (Proban) is not an effective mode of therapy and may increase the possibility of toxicity if other organophosphates are used. Immunostimulation with drugs such as levamisole or thiabendazole does not alter the course of the disease.

Feline Demodicosis

The localized form of demodicosis in cats usually is self-limiting. Although rotenone ointment has been suggested for daily application to localized lesions, this treatment has limitations because of the good grooming habits of the cat.

Feline generalized demodicosis may resolve spontaneously, but this appears to be the exception. Treatment of generalized demodicosis in the cat usually is frustrating, and the response unpredictable because over 50% of cases have concurrent serious metabolic or viral diseases. The demodicosis may respond to even conservative topical therapy if the underlying disease can be controlled. Other cases that respond readily to conservative topical agents may have generalized demodicosis caused by the more superficial surface feeding new *Demodex* species versus the deeper follicular mite.

I prefer to first try weekly 2% lime sulfur dips (LymDyp). If there is no response after six to eight treatments, malathion (Adams Flea and Tick Dip) is next chosen. The 53% concentrate is diluted at 0.25 ounce per gallon of warm water and applied weekly. Malathion has not been approved for use in cats, and the animal must be closely monitored for organophosphate toxicity. Amitraz would be the next choice. It also has not been approved for use in cats, and it may cause anorexia, depression, and diarrhea. Dips are started weekly at half the manufacturer's recommended concentration. If the cat tolerates the amitraz well but a cure is not achieved after eight to ten dips, then the full concentration is used weekly.

Problem Situations

There are five questions commonly asked by practitioners about demodicosis:

Q1. How should unresponsive or recurrent cases of generalized canine demodicosis be handled?

A1. Many cases of suspected resistance are not truly resistant cases at all. Instead the lack of response results either because the treatment program has not been devised or followed correctly or the animal has concurrent untreated medical problems. The following treatment program checklist may be helpful:

- Have corticosteroids been avoided?
- Has any concurrent pyoderma been treated with topical therapy and systemic antibiotics?
- Has the hair coat been clipped and kept short throughout therapy?
- Has benzoyl peroxide shampoo been used before each dip?
- Has each treatment been conducted for 10 to 15 minutes, including concurrent foot soakings?
- Has the dog been kept as dry as possible between dippings?
- Have treatments been continued for two to three applications beyond negative scrapings, with a final set of negative scrapings before discontinuation?
- Is the dog on a balanced commercial diet?
- Have concurrent medical problems been explored by CBC, serum biochemical profile, urinalysis, fecal examination, and heartworm check?
- If the dog is female, has she been spayed? (Demodicosis may worsen or relapse during estrus, pregnancy, or the postpartum.)

If all the above have been considered, then therapeutic alternatives include (1) increasing the frequency of amitraz treatments to weekly or daily; (2) increasing the concentration of amitraz from 0.025% to 0.05% or 0.125%; (3) instituting a maintenance program with 0.025% amitraz dippings every 3 to 4 weeks; (4) using trichlorfon as a 3% aqueous solution applied as a whole-body dip every 4 days; (5) concurrently using vitamin E at 200 mg q5h PO; (6) continuing amitraz and adding ivermectin at 200 to 300 μg/kg q1-2wk SQ; and (7) using milbemycin oxime at 0.5 to 1 mg/kg q24h PO.

Q2. How should older dogs with adult-onset generalized demodicosis be approached?

A2. Older dogs with adult-onset demodicosis should be fully evaluated with a complete drug history, CBC, serum biochemical profile, urinalysis, fecal examination, heartworm check, and low-dose dexamethasone suppression test. If a cause cannot be found, the dog should be watched closely, since an underlying disease may become apparent weeks to months after the demodicosis is diagnosed. These cases should be treated similarly to other generalized cases, but many require maintenance dipping programs for control without complete cures.

Q3. How should dogs with pododemodicosis be handled?

A3. Dogs with pododemodicosis are especially frustrating for the practitioner. Some are presented with just pododemodicosis or at one time have had generalized disease that has cleared from all areas of the body except the feet. If weekly amitraz foot soakings do not work, then more residual activity may be achieved with 0.5 ml of amitraz added to 30 ml of propylene glycol or mineral oil and painted on the feet as needed to control the disease. Benzoyl peroxide gel applied 1 hour before the miticide may help open affected hair follicles.

Q4. What should the breeder be told about the disease?

A4. Because of the strong hereditary predisposition for generalized demodicosis, the owner must be strongly advised that the dog should never be used for breeding and should be neutered. If a juvenile dog with generalized demodicosis is to be treated without neutering, the owner should be required to sign a statement that you have explained the hereditary nature of the disease.

Q5. When should the ovariohysterectomy or castration be performed?

A5. Many dermatologists will recommend not subjecting the patient to anesthesia and elective surgery until well after the disease has been cured and therapy discontinued. The rationale is to avoid stress, which may exacerbate the disease. There is also concern that relapse may occur if the surgery is performed after therapy has been stopped or if a bitch comes into estrus during therapy or shortly after the last treatment. Patients may be neutered while still being treated, since amitraz is administered only weekly or biweekly. The current protocol I use is to get the clinical disease well-controlled and the mite counts low, skip a week of dipping if on a weekly program (or perform on the nontreatment week if biweekly), during that week perform the surgery (screen with a CBC and biochemistry profile), and then continue with dipping the following week. Thus far, no exacerbation of clinical signs, sudden increase in mite counts, or toxicity has been encountered following this protocol.

REFERENCES

Barta O, et al: Lymphocyte transformation suppression caused by pyoderma—failure to demonstrate it in uncomplicated demodectic mange, Comp Immunol Microbiol Infect Dis 6:9, 1983.

Figueiredo C: Vitamin E serum contents, erythrocyte and lymphocyte count, PCV, and hemoglobin determinations in normal dogs, dogs with scabies, and dogs with demodicosis (abstr). In Proceedings, Annual members' meeting AAVD & ACVD, 1985.

Gilbert P, et al: Serum vitamin E levels in dogs with pyoderma and generalized demodicosis (abstr). In Proceedings, Annual members' meeting AAVD & ACVD, 1990, p 12.

Gravino AE, et al: Treatment of demodectic mange natural infestations of dogs with ivermectin, Acta Med Vet 31:185, 1985.

Kwochka KW, et al: The efficacy of amitraz for generalized demodicosis in dogs: a study of two concentrations and frequencies of application, Compend Contin Educ Pract Vet 7:8, 1985.

Medleau L, Willemse T: Efficacy of daily amitraz therapy for generalized demodicosis in dogs: two independent studies (abstr). In Proceedings, Annual members' meeting AAVD & ACVD, 1991, p 41.

Miller WH, Scott DW: Milbemycin in the treatment of generalized demodicosis in the dog (abstr). In Proceedings, Annual members' meeting AAVD & ACVD, 1991, p 44.

Owen LN: Demodectic mange in dogs immunosuppressed with antilymphocyte serum, Transplantation 13:616, 1972.

Reedy LM, Garfield RA: Results of a clinical study with an oral antiparasitic agent in generalized demodicosis (abstr). In Proceedings, Annual members' meeting AAVD & ACVD, 1991, p 43.

Scott DW, et al: Studies on the therapeutic and immunologic aspects of generalized demodectic mange in the dog, J Am Anim Hosp Assoc 10:233, 1974.

Scott DW, et al: Further studies on the therapeutic and immunologic aspects of generalized demodectic mange in the dog, J Am Anim Hosp Assoc 12:203, 1976.

Sischo WM, et al: Regional distribution of ten common skin diseases in dogs, J Am Vet Med Assoc 195:752, 1989.

White SD, et al: Cutaneous markers of canine hyperadrenocorticism, Compend Contin Educ Pract Vet 11:446, 1989.

8

Scabies

Craig E. Griffin

Diagnostic Criteria
for Scabies

SUGGESTIVE
Nonseasonal ventral or pinnal pruritus
Erythematous maculopapular rash

COMPATIBLE
Suggestive plus
Poor response to antibiotics and hypoallergenic diets
Poor response to antiinflammatory doses of glucocorticoids
Epidermal parakeratosis and eosinophilic dermatitis

TENTATIVE
Involvement in approximately 50% of exposed dogs
Positive pinnal/femoral reflex without inflamed canals
Typical scabies rash in humans

DEFINITIVE
Tentative plus
Favorable response to scabicidal therapy
or
Positive identification of the scabies mite or egg

Importance

Canine scabies, commonly referred to as "sarcoptic mange," is a major differential diagnosis for any dog with nonseasonal pruritic dermatitis. This dermatosis is a contagious disease caused by the mite *Sarcoptes scabiei* var *canis*. Scabies is present throughout the country, although the incidence varies. It is more endemic in certain areas, and the incidence is influenced by how clients house and care for their pets. A recent study on the prevalence of skin diseases (Sischo et al., 1989) listed scabies as the seventh most common diagnosis in 1983.

Etiology

The adult mites are ovoid, and females are about twice as large as males. These mites are sometimes confused with *Otodectes,* which have short unjointed stalks, but *Sarcoptes* can be readily identified by the long, unjointed stalks with suckers on the front legs. The mites are relatively species-specific, although rabbits have been experimentally infected with canine and human varieties. Adult mites live approximately 4 to 5 weeks, with the egg-larva-nymph-adult cycle lasting 17 to 21 days. The entire life cycle is completed in or on the skin of the host. Canine mites can survive off the host for 19 days at 97% relative humidity and 10° C. Mites may remain infective in the typical household environment for some 24 to 36 hours (Arlian et al., 1984). As the female mite burrows into the skin, she lays as many as three to five eggs per day, which are left within the burrow along with her excretory products. The burrow is located primarily within the stratum corneum. The head of the female mite may be found in the stratum granulosum, where the mite derives its nourishment. This location may allow for better presentation of allergen.

Pathogenesis

For many years scabies has been considered a hypersensitivity reaction. Clinical observations in humans or animals that support an allergic basis include (1) the signs and severity of pruritus in infected patients vary widely; (2) initial infections have a latent period of approximately 4 weeks, with mites burrowing and no erythema or pruritus present; (3) reinfected patients have an immediate reaction; (4) experimental reinfection requires greater exposure, and the peak parasite level will be less; (5) after infection the population of mites will increase to a peak level, which does not correlate with the severity or extent of disease; (6) infections can die out spontaneously; (7) pruritus can persist for weeks following eradication of the mites; and (8) the nodular lesions seen in some patients may persist for a year despite scabicide therapy.

Laboratory evidence (Martineau et al., 1987) supporting the theory that clinical disease most likely reflects a hypersensitivity reaction also has accumulated. The histopathology of typical scabies reveals a mixed perivascular infiltrate with increased mast cells and eosinophils. Serum from scabies patients often has elevations in IgE, IgM and IgG that normalize following therapy. In both pigs and humans, scabies patients show positive immediate hypersensitivity reactions to scabies mite extracts. Among humans there has also been a cross-reaction seen in some patients to house-dust mite antigen.

CLINICAL DISEASE
History

The most consistent historical finding in cases of scabies is pruritus. There is no age, breed, or sex predilection; however, in general practice young dogs are seen more frequently, possibly because of population dynamics and the contagious nature of the disease. In one outbreak in a kennel of Dachshunds I examined, the initial sign noted by the owners was weight loss. The weight loss reflected the dogs' pruritus, which made them more active and unable to sleep.

The pruritus initially tends to involve the pinnae, extremities, and axillae. Many cases progress to the point where the client reports alopecia, crusts, and lichenification. Year-round pruritus is observed if the disease is allowed to continue. If in-contact dogs are present, over half will eventually develop signs of the disease.

Canine scabies will involve family members in 10% to 50% of cases (in my experience close to 10%), and typically only one or two family members will be affected. Lesions in humans are pruritic erythematous papules located on the arms, abdomen, or thighs.

A search for the source of infection is necessary. Questions should be asked regarding any trips to the groomer or visits to a kennel. Questions should also be asked regarding veterinary hospitals or other places that could have been a source of infectious exposure. Was the dog in for vaccinations a month or so prior to the onset of pruritus? Does the dog go to obedience school or get walked where there is a lot of dog traffic? Is there a neighbor dog that makes contact through a fence? Is the dog walked with a friend's dog, or has it visited any houses with other dogs? Even when a possible exposure cannot be determined, the diagnosis of scabies should never be totally ruled out in a dog with compatible signs.

The intensity of pruritus and the response to therapy may also be helpful in establishing a diagnosis of scabies. Scabies is usually very pruritic.

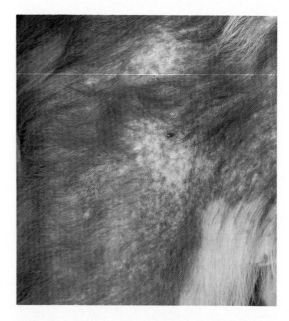

Figure 8-1. Erythematous papules and macules are the typical primary lesions found on cases with canine scabies. Alopecia occurs secondary to pruritus.

Many atopic dogs exhibit milder pruritus. Any dog that scratches considerably during examination raises the index of suspicion for scabies. Scabies should be considered if antibiotics do not affect the level of pruritus and glucocorticoid therapy is ineffective at antiinflammatory dosages.

Physical Examination

The typical case of sarcoptic mange will have a primary, erythematous, maculopapular rash (Fig. 8-1). Excoriation, crusts, and alopecia will follow. Classic cases may have yellow to honey-colored, dry, easily crumbled, adherent crusts or excessive scaling on the ear margins and elbows (Fig. 8-2). Lesions are most often seen on the pinnae, face, lateral and caudal elbows, lower extremities, axillae, ventral thorax, and groin (Fig. 8-3). The plantar and palmar aspects of the paws and interdigital areas tend to be spared until more chronic disease has developed. Although the disease can become generalized, the initial sites are most severely affected.

Chronic cases may show hyperpigmentation and lichenification. Secondary superficial pyoderma is common. Chronic recurrent aural hematomas without obvious otitis externa can occur. Patients may become emaciated, and death from severe cachexia has been described. Rare cases involving pruritus and no physical lesions that respond to ivermectin or other scabicides also suggest the diagnosis of scabies. This form has been referred to as "scabies incognito" and usually occurs in well-groomed and pampered dogs.

Peripheral lymphadenopathy is present in 50%

or more of the cases. A positive pinnal/femoral reflex is present when a dog scratches with its rear leg as the margin of the pinna is briskly rubbed or folded so that there is friction between two ear surfaces. In a study I conducted, 75% of dogs with scabies had a positive pinnal/femoral reflex. However, because false-positives occur with other causes of ear disease, the test is not specific for scabies.

A rare form of scabies has been described in dogs that is comparable to Norwegian scabies in humans. There may be no or only minimal pruritus in these cases. Crusts are heavily infested with mites, which are readily found on skin scrapings. This type of scabies occurs in dogs that are receiving systemic corticosteroids or are otherwise immune compromised (Anderson, 1981).

Differential Diagnosis

The differential diagnosis of scabies includes all nonseasonal pruritic diseases. The most commonly encountered differentials are atopic disease, food allergy, and pruritic pyoderma.

DIAGNOSIS

The skin scraping is the best diagnostic test for canine scabies (Fig. 8-4). Superficial skin scrapings should cover large areas, since the mites can be difficult to find. Scrapings should be taken from areas that have yellow crusts and papules and from the pinnal margins. Reported results of finding scabies mites from skin scrapings vary considerably. In practice, when only three scrapings are done, a definitive diagnosis is made in about 20% of the cases diagnosed by response to therapy. Examination of scrapings at low power (40×) will reveal mites and allow for rapid scanning of all the ma-

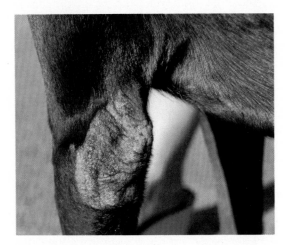

Figure 8-2. Alopecic elbow with yellow crusts that are often seen in scabies.

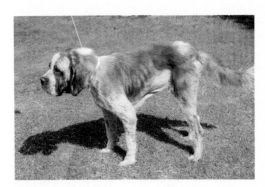

Figure 8-3. A case of scabies demonstrating the typical pattern of involvement—which is extremities, ventral, and facial.

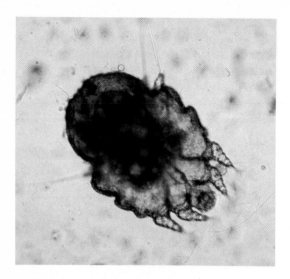

Figure 8-4. A gravid female *Sarcoptes scabiei* mite.
(Courtesy Dr. A.A. Stannard, Davis, Calif.)

terial on the slide. Negative skin scrapings **do not** rule out the diagnosis of scabies.

Fecal flotation may reveal mites or eggs in up to 27% of cases that are confirmed by positive skin scrapings (Baker and Stannard, 1974). Skin biopsies infrequently demonstrate a mite but will show a moderate to large number of eosinophils. This helps to differentiate cases of atopic disease, which have no or few eosinophils. Therefore, even though skin biopsies may not confirm a diagnosis, they can be helpful in separating a suspect scabies case from an atopic case. However, cases of insect hypersensitivity, flea allergy dermatitis, and food allergy may also have a moderate to large number of eosinophils present.

Intradermal testing to commercially available insect antigens is not very helpful in making or ruling out the diagnosis of scabies. I have found that such tests are positive to house-dust mites in 36%, and to fleas in 44%, of scabies cases when the animal was not taking corticosteroids. The major benefit of intradermal testing is to raise the clinician's index of suspicion for scabies when only fleas and house-dust mites react in a dog with scabies-compatible signs.

In vitro blood tests for allergy are usually positive in dogs with scabies. The commercially available enzyme-linked immunosorbent assay (ELISA) test and the radioallergosorbent test (RAST) (K-9 Rast) both were highly positive in over 90% of the scabies cases I tested. Positive in vitro allergy tests do not rule out scabies and do not confirm a diagnosis of atopic disease. Overlooking scabies

based on results of in vitro allergy testing may result in lifelong administration of corticosteroids to a dog with a curable disease. In some cases euthanasia is inappropriately considered when the pruritus is not controlled satisfactorily with allergy treatments.

A definitive diagnosis is made by demonstrating mites, eggs, or feces of *Sarcoptes scabiei*. A definitive diagnosis may also be made by complete cure following scabicidal therapy in a case with a tentative diagnosis. It is much wiser to err by overdiagnosing and overtreating scabies than by missing a curable disease.

TREATMENT

Ivermectin (Ivomec) is the treatment of choice in dogs other than Collies and those less than 16 weeks old. Ivermectin is administered subcutaneously 250 μg/kg and repeated at 10 to 14 days. Excellent response also has been reported with a dosage of 200 μg/kg. All dogs in contact with the affected dog should be treated or isolated from the treated dog until treatment response has been determined.

Ivermectin is preferred to topical therapy for several reasons: resistance has not been reported; injectable ivermectin is easier to administer than dips, so client compliance is not as significant a factor; ivermectin is often less expensive than topical regimens; and fewer treatments are required compared to most topical preparations.

On the negative side, ivermectin has not been approved for the treatment of scabies in dogs. **Ivermectin should never be used in Collies or Collie crosses at the scabicidal dose.** Clients should be warned of the risks even when the drug is administered to breeds other than Collies, although toxic reactions are rare. Toxic signs are primarily neurologic and include ataxia, coma, and death. The sooner signs are seen following treatment, the more severe they tend to be. Treatment of ivermectin reactions is primarily supportive. The best course involves fluid therapy, controlling seizures, and maintaining vital functions until the drug has been naturally metabolized.

Topical therapy is recommended for young dogs, Collies, and Collie crosses or when the client wishes to use an approved or possibly safer treatment. I prefer lime sulfur dips (e.g., LymDyp) because of their safety. Lime sulfur should be used at 5% for the most effective scabicidal activity. By contrast, topical organophosphates such as phosmet (Paramite) are less efficacious though regional variations have been reported. LymDyp is diluted at 8 ounces per gallon of water, and the dips are repeated at 5- to 7-day intervals. The dog is rechecked after the third dip, and in scabies cases the animal is about 50% to 70% better at this time. Many clients will feel that the dog was worse after the first dip and only started to improve after the second dip. The dips are continued until the dog is asymptomatic. Usually five or six dips are required.

Clients should be warned about the rotten egg odor and the possibility of staining jewelry, metal surfaces, and paint. Once the dog is dry, these are not problems—even the odor improves. Hair coats may become discolored (white can turn bright yellow), and the skin and hair coat may become dry; but, again, these side effects resolve following treatment. After all this has been explained, many clients still will choose ivermectin therapy.

Amitraz (Mitaban) can also be used. It is relatively safe and has fewer objectional characteristics, such as odor, than lime sulfur. However, I have found that it is not effective as a single dip. Half the dogs treated once that had positive skin scrapings before treatment had positive scrapings after one treatment by the owner. This may have reflected improper application, since the dogs were not shaved. Amitraz is mixed at its regular concentration, which is one bottle (10.6 ml) in 2 gallons of water. It is applied at 2-week intervals, and a response is usually seen after the second dip.

The major drawbacks to topical regimens are the care and effort required to apply them properly. Dogs with long, thick, or dense coats (e.g., the Chow Chow, Keeshond, Siberian Husky, and even some German Shepherd Dogs) should have a total-body clip. This is also true if the coat is particularly greasy. Most clients are reluctant to shave their dogs, especially when a diagnosis has not been confirmed. In these cases the client must be told of the importance of getting the dip to the skin surface and not just on the hair. The client must also be told how to mix and apply the dip so that the whole body is treated. I have seen many cases in which the dog was dipped for scabies but the client never applied dip to the face and sometimes even did not treat the pinnae. Therefore it should be emphasized that the whole body, including the face, muzzle, ears, and periocular region, and the entire tail, must be treated. All in-contact dogs must be treated as well or kept separated until a treatment response can be determined.

Before each dipping, the dog should be thoroughly bathed to remove grease and crusts, which could interfere with treatment. Generally, I prefer a sulfur and salicylic acid shampoo (Sebalyt). After rinsing off the shampoo completely, the client applies the diluted dip by sponge bath or pressurized pump sprayer. The dip is allowed to dry without rinsing.

In addition to scabicidal therapy, other treatments may be indicated. Cases involving moderate or severe pyoderma should be treated with 14 days of an appropriate systemic antibiotic. Mild pyoderma will resolve following resolution of the scabies. Systemic glucocorticoids (prednisone 1 mg/kg q24h) may be indicated in some scabies cases but should be used only when confirmed by positive skin scrapings; otherwise, response to therapy in a suspect case cannot be determined. The glucocorticoid may be administered to dogs with moderate to severe pruritus for the first 2 or 3 weeks of therapy.

REFERENCES

Anderson RK: Norwegian scabies in a dog: a case report, J Am Anim Hosp Assoc 17:101, 1981.

Arlian LG, et al: Survival and infestivity of Sarcoptes scabiei var. canis and var. hominis, J Am Acad Dermatol 11:210, 1984.

Baker BB, Stannard AA: A look at canine scabies, J Am Anim Hosp Assoc 10:513, 1974.

Martineau GP, et al: Pathophysiology of sarcoptic mange in swine. II, Compend Contin Educ Pract Vet 9:F93, 1987.

Sischo WM, et al: Regional distribution of ten common skin diseases in dogs, J Am Vet Med Assoc 195:752, 1989.

SUGGESTED READING

Mellanby K: Scabies, ed 2, Hampton Middlesex, England, 1972, EW Classey.

9

Cheyletiellosis

Karen A. Moriello

Diagnostic Criteria for Cheyletiellosis

SUGGESTIVE
Acute onset of mild to moderate pruritus
Mild to severe scaling with or without pruritus

COMPATIBLE
Pruritic papular lesions on owner
History of partial response to insecticides
History of contagion in other household pets
Course of disease is chronic if untreated
Older animals may be unaffected

TENTATIVE
Elimination of scaling and/or pruritus with miticidal therapy

DEFINITIVE
Identification of mite or egg

Importance

Cheyletiellosis is a parasitic skin disease of dogs, cats, and rabbits caused by infestation with *Cheyletiella* spp mites. Its incidence is unknown, because it is not a reportable disorder. However, its prevalence may be underrecognized, since many cases are diagnosed as idiopathic seborrhea or pruritus. Prevalence of the disease tends to vary with geographic region. In areas of the country with year-round flea populations, veterinarians rarely diagnose *Cheyletiella* mites as the sole cause of pruritus or scaling in dogs and cats, most likely because of the relative importance of fleas and the widespread and aggressive use of topical insecticides. By contrast, cheyletiellosis is much more common in geographic areas with seasonal flea populations—affecting mainly young animals, animals obtained from pounds, shelters, or breeding establishments, and breeds that commonly are professionally groomed.

Cheyletiellosis is noteworthy for several reasons. First, the mite is an important differential for scaling and/or pruritus in small animals. It often is difficult to isolate from the host and is much more difficult to treat successfully than was originally thought. Thus many infestations go undiagnosed and many pets, particularly Cocker Spaniels, are misdiagnosed as having idiopathic seborrhea. Second, the mite is highly contagious and an infested host will rapidly transmit it to other animals through direct contact or fomites. Finally, the mite temporarily will infest people and thus has zoonotic importance.

Life Cycle and Pathogenesis

Cheyletiella mites are very large (400 μm) and have four pairs of legs. The legs terminate in combs instead of claws, and the mite has accessory mouthparts (palpi) that terminate in hooks. These two features allow for rapid identification (Fig. 9-1).

The mites are obligate parasites that live in the keratin layer of the epidermis in pseudotunnels. They periodically feed on the host's lymph by piercing the skin with stylelike chelicera; they do not ingest keratin debris as was previously believed. Ideally, the life cycle of the mites is completed within 5 to 6 weeks. Copulation occurs on the surface of the skin or in the pseudotunnels, and eggs are deposited on hair shafts. *Cheyletiella* spp eggs (Fig 9-2) may be confused with louse eggs; however, the *Cheyletiella* eggs are smaller and less firmly attached, which tends to make differentiation possible.

Infestation with these mites results in pruritus and excessive scaling. The pruritus is believed caused by mechanical irritation and hypersensitivity to the mite. The excessive scaling may be a result of the mite's burrowing but more likely, is a host defense mechanism. Epidermal cell turnover increases in response to many infections as a mechanism by which to shed offending pathogens.

Transmission and Environmental Contagion

Cheyletiella mites are highly contagious among animals. Transmission occurs most commonly from direct contact with an infested host; however, fomite transmission and infestation from the environment are being recognized more frequently. The number of *Cheyletiella* mites present on the host is highly variable. In young, sick, debilitated, or untreated animals it may be very high; but in many cases it is surprisingly low. Combs, brushes, bedding, crates, and blankets contacted by an infested host can harbor mites, hairs with eggs or larvae serving as a source of contagion. Viable mites from contaminated bedding and brushes have been identified. Interestingly, most parasitologic references consider *Cheyletiella* spp mites to be relatively fragile and susceptible to desiccation. Early laboratory studies (Muller et al., 1989) found that male mites can live only 48 hours off the host whereas females can live for 10 days under experimental conditions. Therefore infestation from the environment was never considered an important source of contagion.

Over the last several years a markedly higher number of cases of *Cheyletiella* spp infestations have been diagnosed than in previous years. Many have not resolved until environmental insecticide treatment was instituted. Recent research on *Sarcoptes* spp host-seeking behavior and survival (Arlian et al., 1987) has concluded that dislodged mites are a source of contagion. This evidence may support environmental infestation of a host by *Cheyletiella* species. Dislodged scabies mites use odor and thermal stimuli to locate their hosts. Furthermore, canine scabies mites can survive off the host and remain infective for 3 days in warm, dry temperatures and for up to 18 to 21 days in cool, moist environments (Arlian et al., 1984). *Cheyletiella* spp mites may use similar host-seeking stimuli and be hardier than was believed previously.

Factors Affecting Susceptibility

Young animals are most susceptible to infestation. Kittens, puppies, and young rabbits from "pet

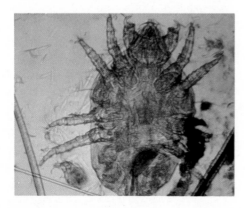

Figure 9-1. Adult *Cheyletiella* mite. Note the palpi and combs.

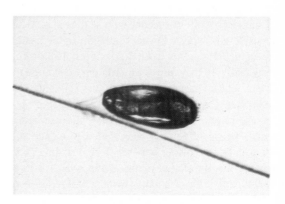

Figure 9-2. *Cheyletiella* mite egg.
(Courtesy Dr. Danny W. Scott, Ithaca, N.Y.)

mills" or pet stores are commonly infested. Debilitation, poor nutrition, starvation, poor sanitation, and overcrowding all predispose these animals to infestation. It is a clinical impression that *Cheyletiella* spp infestations are more common in small breeds of dogs that are groomed frequently, particularly Cocker Spaniels. Also, long-haired breeds of cats and dogs can be more difficult to treat.

CLINICAL DISEASE

Cheyletiella infestations in companion animals may be symptomatic or asymptomatic. The hallmark of infestation is scaling and pruritus. Scaling is the **most** consistent clinical finding, and it cannot be overemphasized that cheyletiellosis must be eliminated from the differential before a diagnosis of idiopathic seborrhea is made, especially in breeds predisposed to keratinization disorders. The amount of scaling depends on the duration of infestation, the overall health of the host (scaling is often more severe in debilitated hosts), hair length and color (excessive scaling may not be as noticeable in light-colored breeds with longer hair), and whether the owner has bathed the animal or used topical insecticides. Pruritus varies from none to severe. It is important to note that the pruritus caused by *Cheyletiella* mites is rarely as severe as that caused by scabies.

History

The most frequent client complaint is **scaling,** with or without pruritus. It is common for owners to ignore scaling in young animals, attributing it to "puppy/kitten coat." Additionally, a dry coat in an adult cat or dog may be attributed incorrectly to "low fat in the diet," decreased humidity, and a variety of other excuses. Any animal obtained from a shelter, pound, or breeder with scaling should be considered suspect. Owners may not immediately recognize that a young kitten or puppy is pruritic, especially if they are leash training the animal. Many clients assume the pet is just scratching at its collar. Clients will often report a temporary decrease in pruritus if topical insecticides are being used. If a new pet has been added to a multipet household, the owner may report that scaling and/or pruritus developed in the group over a 3 to 4 week period. Occasionally, owners will report that one or more animals in a multipet household are unaffected. However, cheyletiellosis should not be eliminated from the differential if pruritus is absent, because some animals can be asymptomatic

carriers. Finally, one of the most useful historical points is whether or not the owners are pruritic. *Cheyletiella* spp mites will temporarily inhabit the skin of people, causing a pruritic papular rash affecting the arms, abdomen, or chest.

There may be no indication of disease in a household with asymptomatic carriers until a susceptible pet is introduced. Cocker Spaniels, Poodles, and long-haired cats are most frequently found to be asymptomatic carriers. Clinical signs may develop rapidly, and the new pet often is erroneously blamed for having introduced the infestation. Infestation may be detected only after people, particularly children, are affected. Several infestations in cats have been diagnosed after clients were told by their dermatologist to have their animals examined by a veterinarian.

Physical Examination

Cheyletiella mites can infest all haired areas of a host's body. For reasons that are unknown, increased scale and pruritus are most severe on the dorsum. As mentioned earlier, the pruritus is variable in its intensity ranging from mild to severe. The intensity in dogs is not as severe as with scabies. In cats the intensity varies considerably. In several cases that I have seen the degree of pruritus was so severe that flea allergy dermatitis and feline atopy were considered much more likely differentials until the mite was isolated. In rabbits *Cheyletiella* and flea infestations can cause an almost equal degree of pruritus.

Besides being the most consistent client complaint, scaling is the most consistent clinical abnormality. It is important to note that, in general, dogs tend to have diffuse dorsal scaling; by contrast, rabbits and cats tend to have focal or multifocal patches of scaling on the dorsum. Often dogs and rabbits will show little skin reaction except for scaling. The scales may be very large and adhere to the underlying skin. Rabbits can have thick layers of scales that look like white crusts. Cats tend to have a wide range of clinical signs and may exhibit bizarre personality changes due to discomfort of the pruritis. Scaling is usually milder in cats than in rabbits or dogs. Cats may present with dorsal scaling or no skin reaction, or they may develop a papular crusted eruption (miliary dermatitis). *Cheyletiella* mite infestations have been diagnosed in cats presented for evaluation of bilaterally symmetric alopecia, miliary dermatitis, feline hyperesthesia syndrome, and psychogenic/self-trauma dermatitis.

Asymptomatic carriers may be completely free

of **both** pruritus and scaling or **just** pruritus. *Cheyletiella* spp infestations have been diagnosed in several dogs referred for idiopathic seborrhea without pruritus recognized by the owner.

There are regional differences in the prevalence of *Cheyletiella* spp infestations in the United States. Mite infestations are least common in flea-endemic areas. This is attributed to the chronic use of insecticides for flea control and their acaricidal effect. Infestations are more common in the Upper Midwest.

Differential Diagnosis

Cheyletiella spp mite infestation should be considered in the differential diagnosis of any dog presented for the clinical problems of seborrhea or pruritus. Before the diagnosis of idiopathic seborrhea is made, a trial of miticidal therapy is always recommended. This is especially important in Cocker Spaniels. Cheyletiellosis should be included in the differential of any cat presented for the clinical problems of generalized or regional pruritus, miliary dermatitis, symmetric alopecia, psychogenic/self-trauma dermatitis, and seborrhea. Mite infestations can be so severe as to mimic generalized feline dermatophytosis.

Cheyletiella infestation is one of the most important differentials for pruritus in rabbits. It should be considered whenever a client suspects he may have contracted a skin disease from his pet.

DIAGNOSIS

Definitive diagnosis of a *Cheyletiella* spp infestation requires finding either an adult mite or an egg. Ease of finding the mite is variable. Animals with asymptomatic infestations may not have a large number of mites, making it more difficult to diagnose the infestation definitively. Patients with chronic pruritus have frequently been bathed by their owners, which will remove the eggs and mites. The self-grooming of cats also removes mites, making them difficult to isolate. A diligent search for mites should always be pursued, although in some cases a positive response to therapy alone will lead to the diagnosis.

Diagnostic Tests

Direct examination of scales, acetate tape preparations, skin scrapings, and flea combing may be used to find mites. Flea combing is the **most reliable** method for finding mites in both symptomatic and asymptomatic patients.

Direct Visual Examination

Cheyletiella mites are very large and can be easily seen with a hand-held magnifying lens or loupe. They appear as moving white specks; hence the nickname "walking dandruff." They are most likely to be observed with this technique only in cases of severe infestations. Brushing epidermal debris onto a dark piece of paper may assist in recognition.

Acetate Tape Preparations

This is the classic diagnostic test for *Cheyletiella* spp. A small strip of clear acetate tape is pressed onto the hair and skin, collecting epidermal debris, and is then pressed over a drop of mineral oil on a glass slide. However, this procedure is not advocated, because it samples a relatively small area of the animal's body and is frequently negative in animals with small mite populations. It is more reliable in animals with heavy infestations.

Skin Scrapings

Superficial skin scrapings can be used. In animals with thick coats the hair should be clipped with scissors from the area to be scraped. This technique is reliable in animals with a heavy mite infestation but less when the population is low.

Flea Combing

Combing the entire coat for several minutes with a fine-toothed comb is the most reliable technique for finding mites. It is the method of choice because it is reliable, rapid, inexpensive, and acceptable to both patient and client. Also, a large volume of hair and scale can be collected in a container and examined later—an advantage in a busy practice. If positive findings are not identified during an office visit, the client should be told to comb the animal's coat several times a day for 3 or 4 days and then bring the hair samples to the hospital for inspection. A dissecting microscope is preferred for examining the samples because of the ease and speed with which mites and eggs can be found.

Response to Therapy

As with *Sarcoptes* mite infestations, clinical suspicion for a *Cheyletiella* infestation may be high but mites or eggs cannot be found. A definitive diagnosis can be made in these cases only by treating the animal and noting the response to therapy.

TREATMENT

Contrary to popular belief, *Cheyletiella* infestations are not always easily eliminated. Flea shampoos, sprays, and powders have **not** been effective as sole therapeutic agents. Successful treatment usually requires 6 to 8 weeks of therapy (as opposed to the previously recommended 3 weeks).

Treatment of the Pet

1. All furbearing pets in the household should be treated.

   Treating only suspect pets is a common error. It is important to remember that some animals may be asymptomatic carriers, especially adult animals. Regular furbearing visitors to the household also must be treated.
2. The coat of all medium-length and long-haired dogs and cats should be removed.

   This procedure is important for two reasons, although owners will often resist it. First, it enhances penetration and dispersal of topical insecticides. Second, and possibly more important, it mechanically removes mites and eggs on hairs, decreasing contagion. Animals that are clipped appear to respond to therapy more rapidly than animals not clipped.
3. Dogs and cats should be bathed in a mild hypoallergenic shampoo to remove excess scale and crusts.

   This step also serves to mechanically remove mites and eggs from the coat, and it enhances the penetration of topical insecticide. Care should be taken to prevent hypothermia in kittens and puppies.
4. All animals should be treated for a minimum of **6 to 8 weeks.**
   a. Flea shampoos, powders, sprays, and foams have proved ineffective as **sole** therapeutic agents and are not recommended.
   b. A pour-on acaricide is the treatment of choice.

      Pregnant or lactating animals, kittens, puppies, or debilitated animals. These animals should be treated weekly with warm lime sulfur (4 oz/gal) or L-pyrethrin pour-ons. Products used on cats should be approved for use on this species. Pour-ons should be diluted according to label instructions.

      Adult dogs. Weekly lime sulfur, pyrethrin, or organophosphate pour-ons, diluted according to label instruction, are very effective. Pyrethrin pour-ons are preferred, because there is less risk of toxicity.

      Adult cats. Lime sulfur or pyrethrin pour-ons are preferred in cats, to minimize the risk of toxicity.

      Rabbits and other small mammals. Lime sulfur or pyrethrin pour-ons may be used safely on these animals; however, they are predisposed to hypothermia and pneumonia. It is important to stress to clients that these animals must be kept warm and in a draft-free area until the coat dries.
5. Instruct the owner to treat the environment and decontaminate fomites.

   Environmental treatment should be included in the treatment plan. Situations have been encountered requiring environmental treatment to eliminate infestations. In one instance a pet's owner was bitten by mites every time she sat on a particular cloth couch in her home. Examination of debris vacuumed from the surface of the couch revealed live mites and eggs. In three other instances, all involving cats, lime sulfur dips appeared to be ineffective. After it was determined that client compliance was excellent and there were no untreated animals in the house, environmental insecticides were recommended and the infestation was eliminated. I currently recommend the following:
   a. If pets sleep with the owners, wash all bedding and ban the pets from beds, couches, chairs, etc. until the infestation has been eliminated.
   b. Thoroughly vacuum all floor surfaces and furniture weekly during the treatment period.
   c. Every 2 weeks use a premise spray labeled as effective for killing fleas in the environment. It is important to remove cushions from couches and treat the wells of furniture. If the animal rides in the client's automobile, instruct the client to spray the interior of the vehicle.
   d. Discard all brushes and combs used on the pet.

Treatment Failures and Alternative Therapies

Client compliance problems are common and predictable. Clients will often object to mandatory clipping of the coat, although demonstration of mites and eggs may help overcome this resistance. A permanent mount of a specimen can be used to demonstrate the mite and help convince a client to clip the pet's coat. Some clients find insecticide dips offensive, in which case lime sulfur and odiferous organophospate should be avoided if possible. Additionally, some clients cannot or will not dip their pets weekly. Therapy with amitraz (Mitaban) or ivermectin (Ivomec) is a reasonable alternative in such cases, although these preparations have not been approved for treating *Cheyletiella* infestations.

Amitraz is very effective against *Cheyletiella* mites and is a reasonable alternative to other topical parasiticides. The advantage is that the pet can be dipped every 2 weeks instead of every week. Usually only four treatments, spanning 8 weeks, are required. Amitraz may be toxic to cats and rabbits and should not be used on these species. Weekly treatment of cats with alternative acaricides is recommended.

Ivermectin is also very effective against *Cheyletiella* species. It is particularly useful in households with many pets or in kennel and cattery situations. It has been used safely in pregnant and lactating animals and in kittens and puppies less than 6 weeks of age. Ivermectin should not be used in herding breeds (e.g., Collies and Shetland Sheepdogs) because of toxicity. The recommended dosage is 200 to 400 µg/kg PO or SQ q2wk for three treatments. There is some evidence to suggest that parenteral administration is more effective. Treatment should span at least 6 weeks. Ivermectin has been used successfully as the sole therapy for *Cheyletiella* infestations. Response is greatly enhanced if the animal is also treated with a pour-on parasiticide or flea spray at least once. The only mites killed by ivermectin therapy are those that migrate to the surface of the skin and feed on the host's lymph. Theoretically, all mites eventually migrate to the skin, but a longer period may be required to kill them, in contrast to the widespread immediate kill with topical therapy.

Preventing Reinfestation

If the infestation was transmitted by a new kitten, puppy, or other pet added to the household, the risk of reinfestation is low provided no more new animals are added. Pets taken to shows, groomers, or kennels are at greater risk for reinfestation. Prophylactic application of a pyrethrin dip after shows, grooming sessions, or kennel stays may be a reasonable recommendation for clients with pets at risk. If a particular pet repeatedly becomes infested, the veterinarian should consider the following questions: Was the infestation eliminated in the first place? Is fomite transmission possible? Could asymptomatic carriers be present in the household? Is the animal frequently groomed? Are the groomer's premises contaminated? Does the animal roam?

SUMMARY

Cheyletiella infestations appear more difficult to treat now than in previous years. This may be an adaptation of the mite resulting from increased insecticide use on pets. Current recommendations include treating all pets in the household, clipping the hair coat of medium-length and long-haired animals, extending topical therapy (6 to 8 weeks), and treating the environment.

REFERENCES

Arlian LG, et al: Survival and infestivity of Sarcoptes scabiei var. canis and var. hominis, J Am Acad Dermatol 11:210, 1984.

Arlian LG, et al: Host-seeking behavior of Sarcoptes scabiei, J Am Acad Dermatol 11:594, 1987.

Muller GH, et al: Small animal dermatology, ed 4, Philadelphia, 1989, WB Saunders.

Hypersensitivity

10

Canine Atopic Disease

Craig E. Griffin

Diagnostic Criteria for Canine Atopic Disease

SUGGESTIVE

History and physical examination findings

Pruritus should be present in areas other than the dorsolumbar region

COMPATIBLE

Pruritus in one or more of the following regions: face, paw, extensor tarsus, flexor carpus, flexor elbow, axilla, pinna

Effective antibiotic therapy markedly improves the lesions so that involved areas show only secondary evidence of pruritus

TENTATIVE

Compatible plus

Exclusion of the major differentials: flea allergy dermatitis, food allergy, scabies, pruritic pyoderma, insect hypersensitivity, keratinization disorder

DEFINITIVE

Tentative plus

A positive intradermal test to one or more noninsect aeroallergens (However, by this criterion atopic disease cannot be confirmed in 10% to 18% of dogs with a tentative diagnosis.)

Importance

Atopic disease (atopy), an inherited predisposition to the development of IgE antibodies to environmental allergens, resulting in allergic disease, is one of the most common, complex, and frustrating chronic disorders encountered in veterinary practice. Canine atopy is widely accepted as the second most common allergic skin disease of dogs, with reported incidences varying from 3.3% to 85%. The reports that indicate an incidence above 15% come from dermatology referral practices. This incidence will vary depending on diagnostic criteria, local gene pools, breed popularity, and region of the country. Dermatologic conditions comprise at least 20% to 30% of disease cases presenting to small animal practitioners in Las Vegas, Nevada. Atopic disease is most common in this region, where there are no fleas (Nave, 1990). This observation supports the notion that a practice primarily diagnosing flea allergy dermatitis is overlooking atopic cases. Most likely, atopic disease occurs in 10% to 15% of the canine population. The incidence and need for management of atopic disease for the dog's whole life make a thorough understanding important.

Developmental Factors

Breed predispositions have been documented and vary in different areas of the world, suggesting a genetic basis. Breeding studies with atopic dogs have produced conflicting findings. The best results supporting a genetic basis for the disease have come from a kennel of Basenji-Greyhound crosses

(Butler et al., 1983). Some attempts to establish breeding colonies of clinically affected atopic dogs have resulted in failure (Schwartzman et al., 1983).

The conclusion from these studies is that genetic mechanisms are important but other variables also may play critical roles in the development of disease. Nongenetic factors, including environmental exposure, vaccination, and possibly infections, may be important either in the initiation of disease or in the production of antigen-specific IgE. Atopic signs have developed in unrelated dogs within the same household (Reedy and Miller, 1989). The month of birth has been associated by Van Stee (1983) with an increased incidence of atopic disease. This study showed that atopic disease occurred more in dogs born in May and December, months at the onset of specific pollen seasons, and it concluded that genetically prone dogs are particularly susceptible to sensitization during the first 4 months of life. Another study (Frick and Brooks, 1983) looked at vaccination effects on IgE production. Vaccination of puppies with modified live canine distemper virus prior to subcutaneous injection of pollen extracts caused a significant increase in pollen-specific IgE compared to what occurred in nonvaccinated littermate controls. Since most dogs are vaccinated several times between 2 and 4 months of age, the season of birth and vaccination program may both be important in the development of disease. In humans, respiratory infections are believed to be important in the development of allergic disease.

Threshold and Load

The threshold effect and allergic load are important pathophysiologic concepts to comprehend in the clinical approach to the atopic patient. Manifestations of clinical symptoms require a level of exposure to allergens that is unique to each patient. This level, referred to as the **allergic threshold,** may vary depending on nonallergenic factors (e.g., the animal's emotional or psychologic state, the presence of other diseases and/or irritants, and the weather). The allergen load is the accumulation of different allergens—food, fleas, pollen, bacteria—to which the atopic patient is sensitive. Disease will occur whenever the allergen load exceeds the allergic threshold. The allergic symptoms may not include pruritus, since it has a separate threshold and load. Other nonallergenic factors that may contribute to the pruritic load include changes such as dry skin and altered epidermal barrier function to surface toxins, bacteria, and antigens. The total contribution of allergenic and nonallergenic factors

to clinical disease is termed the **summation effect.** Although the initial hypersensitivity reaction may not have induced pruritus, these other factors can contribute to the pruritic load and eventually make an animal reach its pruritic threshold.

Pathogenesis

Recognition of canine IgE and its relationship to mast cells was the initial breakthrough in the understanding of canine atopic disease. Direct immunofluorescent studies (Halliwell, 1973) showed the binding of canine antigen-specific IgE to mast cells located in the dermis. Mast cell degranulation occurs when a multivalent antigen reaches the dermis and binds to and bridges two separate IgE molecules. During mast cell degranulation many preformed proinflammatory mediators (histamine, heparin, proteolytic enzymes) are released. Mast cell membranes altered during degranulation result in the production of other important proinflammatory mediators such as prostaglandins, leukotrienes, hydroxyeicosatetraenoic acid (HETE), and platelet-activating factor. These mediators cause a variety of cutaneous changes, including pruritus, vasodilation, edema, and inflammation.

The classic route of allergen access is through the respiratory tract—which has led to the other name for atopic disease, allergic inhalant dermatitis. However, it is also possible, as Halliwell and Gorman (1989) suggest, that some antigen is percutaneously absorbed. I believe that absorption of antigens percutaneously is of primary importance in the clinical case. The typical clinical manifestations are more compatible with percutaneous absorption. The pattern of involvement in atopic disease reflects areas where antigen can readily contact the stratum corneum or where damage to the stratum corneum is more likely to occur. This would allow for more antigen to be absorbed and trigger an allergic reaction. The improvement from frequent bathing may be due to the removal of surface antigen, which decreases the allergen load.

There is also experimental evidence (Butler et al., 1983; Rhodes et al., 1987) to support percutaneous absorption. When atopic dogs are challenged with aerosolized antigen, most develop nasal discharges, lacrimation, and respiratory abnormalities, signs not commonly seen in clinical cases. Dermatitis occurs less frequently than respiratory signs. Several studies in human allergy patients (Platts-Mills et al., 1983; Reitamo et al., 1986) have looked at skin test reactions to inhalant allergens that were applied to the skin and have shown that allergens can cause delayed reactions in patients with atopic eczema.

Chronic inflammation associated with atopic disease leads to increased transepidermal water loss, resulting in a dry epidermis. Dry skin lowers the pruritic threshold, contributing to pruritus.

Corneocytes are mature, nonnucleated, squamous cells from the surface stratum corneum. An increased adherence of *Staphylococcus intermedius* to corneocytes from atopic dogs compared to control and seborrheic dogs has been demonstrated (McEwan, 1990) and may be a factor in the predisposition of atopic dogs to pyoderma. There may also be an increased absorption of staphylococcal antigens across inflamed allergic skin (Mason and Lloyd, 1990). The combination of increased adherence and cutaneous penetration of bacterial antigen can result in more severe clinical disease.

Fatty acid metabolism abnormalities in the skin and serum have been associated with the clinical signs of atopic dermatitis in humans. The primary abnormality in these patients is thought to be associated with a defective or deficient level of delta-6-desaturase, an enzyme necessary for the metabolism of polyunsaturated fatty acids. Supplementation with gamma-linolenic acid has improved atopic dermatitis in human patients, but the exact relationship between atopic dermatitis and fatty acids is controversial.

Fatty acid supplementation and absorption studies have recently been done in dogs. In one study (White, 1990) no qualitative differences were found in the essential fatty acid levels of serum or cutaneous abrasion fluid between normal and atopic animals. In another (Horrobin et al., 1990) atopic dogs had slightly lower levels of dihomo-gamma-linolenic acid and arachidonic acid. In another (van den Broek and Simpson, 1990) resting triglyceride levels in normal and atopic dogs were no different but triglyceride levels were low in atopic dogs after a feeding of corn oil. All of this tends to imply that atopic dogs have either impaired fat absorption or altered triglyceride metabolism. Several studies have shown that gamma-linolenic acid (GLA) and eicosapentaenoic acid (EPA) supplementation will clinically improve atopic disease in some dogs.

Immune function abnormalities have been described in humans with atopic dermatitis. They include depressed cell-mediated immunity (CMI) to patch tests, depressed in vivo CMI to microbial antigens, decreased in vitro lymphocyte transformation to mitogens, and abnormalities in leukotaxis of monocytes and neutrophils. Nimmo Wilkie (1990) has demonstrated similar abnormalities in dogs with atopic disease. It was also shown that many of these abnormalities can be induced in normal dogs by causing anaphylaxis. Therefore the immune function abnormalities may be a result, and not a cause, of the atopic disease.

It is possible that atopic disease may be mediated by IgGd in addition to IgE (Willemse et al., 1985). This antibody has been produced experimentally as well as found in clinical cases. It can be compared to short-term sensitizing antibodies described in humans. Although its importance is controversial, if it is clinically relevant then in vitro tests detecting only IgE would be inaccurate. Both IgE and IgG should be detected by intradermal testing.

CLINICAL DISEASE
History

The clinical lesions of atopic disease are numerous and diverse. A thorough history is critical in making a tentative diagnosis. Pruritus is the most common historical feature of atopy. Typically there are few or no cutaneous lesions at the onset, and the disease usually becomes progressively worse. Because the owner may not recognize the early signs of atopic disease, (some will interpret the signs as normal behavior), the age of onset may be months or years prior to the clinical presentation.

Clinical signs are reported to initially occur between 6 months and 3 years of age in 75% of atopic dogs. In a review I conducted of 50 intradermal-positive allergic dogs from Southern California, 34% were symptomatic by 9 months and 10% showed signs of the disease before 6 months of age. Breeds represented in this group included Akita, Chinese Shar-Pei, German Shepherd Dog, and Golden Retriever.

It is unlikely to see atopic disease develop in older dogs and extremely unlikely for dogs to develop atopic disease after 7 years of age unless they have moved to a new environment with a different allergen load.

Numerous studies have demonstrated predisposed breeds—which include Cairn Terriers, West Highland White Terriers, Scottish Terriers, Wirehaired Fox Terriers, Dalmatians, English and Irish Setters, Golden Retrievers, Boston Terriers, English Bulldogs, Beagles, and Miniature Schnauzers. In the past, German Shepherd Dogs, Poodles, Cocker Spaniels, and Doberman Pinschers were reported at decreased risk. Cases among German

Shepherd Dogs and Cocker Spaniels have recently been described (Reedy and Miller, 1989) as increasing in frequency. I also frequently see atopy in those two breeds, as well as in many Chinese Shar-Peis. Miller et al. (1990) have reported on a survey at Cornell University that showed the Chinese Shar-Pei to be the breed at most risk for developing atopy. However, clinicians should be aware that atopy occurs in all breeds and should not inappropriately decrease their index of suspicion.

Although reports are conflicting, most show that female dogs run a greater risk of developing atopy.

Of the atopic dogs, 32% to 75% start with seasonal pruritus. Eventually 75% or more will develop nonseasonal disease. In geographic locations without true seasons, there will be more continual antigen exposure and less seasonal incidence. In my Southern California study, 24% of the animals initially presented with seasonal pruritus and 42% of this group progressed to nonseasonal pruritus, 60% started as nonseasonal, and in 16% the client could not remember how the disease started; at the time of presentation 86% were nonseasonal. The initial seasonal signs may be so mild that the client does not seek veterinary care until the problem has become perennial.

The age of onset is an important criterion in diagnosing atopic disease. The actual age of onset must be determined, not just the date when signs first prompted the client to seek veterinary care. Misleading historical information may result in an inaccurate diagnosis. Problems include the following:

1. Owner not noticing early clinical signs
2. Owner recognizing signs but associating them with another disease
3. Owner recognizing signs but interpreting them as normal behavior
4. Owner bias that signs are not significant and therefore not reported
5. Owner failing to associate signs of previous episodes or problems with the current problem

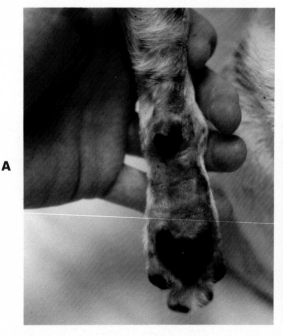
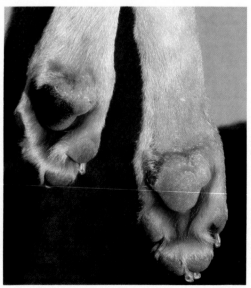

Figure 10-1. **A,** Flexor metacarpal region with alopecia, erythema, hyperpigmentation, and lichenification from chronic chewing and licking. **B,** Erythema and alopecia of the extensor metatarsal region.

Physical Examination

The major clinical sign of atopic disease is pruritus. It usually involves the muzzle, periocular region, pinnae and external ear canals, paws, axillae, groin, and abdomen. Although the face and paws are most commonly involved, many animals will have generalized pruritus by the time they are presented for evaluation.

Lichenification secondary to chronic trauma from itching of the axillae, extensor surfaces of the carpal joints (Fig. 10-1, *A*), and flexural surfaces of the tarsi (Fig. 10-1, *B*) has been seen more frequently in atopic dogs that were skin test–positive compared to those diagnosed by clinical signs alone. Lichenification of the extensor carpus and flexor tarsus went from a prevalence of 41.2% and 30.6%, respectively, in skin test–positive atopics to 0% in the skin test–negative group (Willemse and van den Brom, 1983). In this study all dogs had a history of face rubbing and paw licking, but visible clinical lesions were found on the head in only 59.4% and on the digits in 72.9%. This emphasizes that pruritus can be present with no visible lesions, a condition that seems more common in certain breeds (e.g., the Bichon Frise). The flexor surface of the elbow is frequently involved, although this area is often overlooked by the owner (Fig. 10-2).

Erythematous macules or slightly thickened plaques will be the first primary lesions found in many cases. Secondary changes characteristic of atopic disease, which include excoriations and lichenified plaques, may develop rapidly in response to pruritus. Reddish brown (rust red) discoloration of the hair may be seen with chronic licking (Fig. 10-3). Chronic licking, rubbing, chewing, or scratching can result in alopecia, lichenification, hyperpigmentation, scaling, or excoriation (Fig. 10-4). Papules are also frequently reported.

Secondary superficial pyoderma is present in approximately one third of atopic dogs (Scott, 1981; Willemse and van den Brom, 1983). This value is low compared to my experience, where 68% of intradermal-positive atopic dogs have had pyoderma. Pyoderma was the original diagnosis,

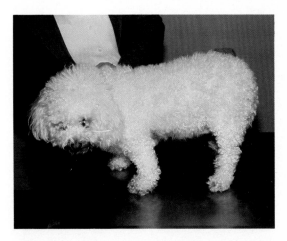

Figure 10-3. Atopic Bichon Frise with salivary staining of the paws and little other evidence of pruritus.

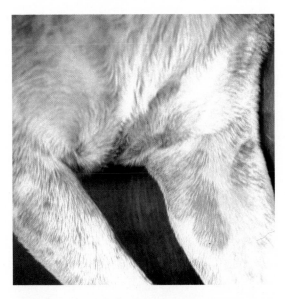

Figure 10-2. The flexor elbow is a common site for atopic dogs to lick and cause erythema and partial alopecia. Licking at this site is often not noted by the owner.

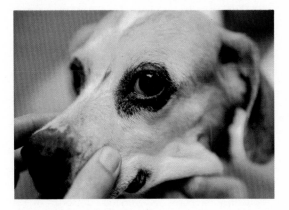

Figure 10-4. Periocular hyperpigmentation, alopecia, and lichenification from chronic rubbing around the eye.

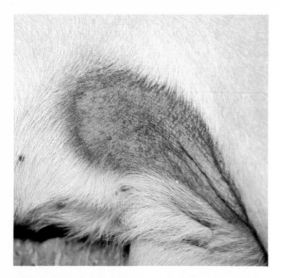

Figure 10-5. This lichenified erythematous plaque is caused by a secondary pyoderma in an atopic dog.

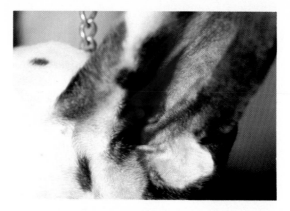

Figure 10-6. An erythematous concave pinna is a frequent sign of atopic disease.

before allergy was suspected, in 4% of the cases. Recurrence of the pyoderma may be as high as 77%. The clinical findings of pyoderma (e.g., circular crusts and crusted, lichenified plaques) are often misdiagnosed as atopic lesions and not recognized as pyoderma (Fig. 10-5). The incidence of pyoderma may be affected by chronicity of the disease and by previous corticosteroid therapy. Often cases are referred for refractoriness to glucocorticoid therapy because of an unrecognized pyoderma.

Deep pyodermas or furuncles will occasionally be seen in atopic dogs. They may be difficult to control until the atopy is treated. Bacterial pododermatitis and antibiotic-responsive "hot spots" may also be related to atopic disease. Antibiotic-responsive acral pruritic nodules, especially in Golden Retrievers and Labrador Retrievers, can be a feature of atopic disease. Signs of atopy usually are present at the time these animals develop infected lesions.

Effective treatment of the pyoderma can eliminate the pruritus in some cases, even though treatment for atopy is not given. This is the result of the summation effect, requiring both diseases to exceed the pruritic threshold.

Otitis externa is reported in 16.8% to 55% of atopic dogs (Scott, 1981; Willemse and van den Brom, 1983). If clients are carefully questioned about head shaking and previous episodes of ear disease, 50% or more will indicate some history of ear problems. Early in the course of the disease, atopics will show erythema primarily on the con-

cave surface of the pinna (Fig. 10-6). The erythema may extend down the vertical canal, and less commonly involve the horizontal canal.

Intermittent secondary bacterial or *Malassezia* infections can occur and will initially respond well to topical therapy, only to recur within weeks or months after treatment has stopped. These infections may be misdiagnosed as swimmer's ear when they occur in summer. Many such animals, in reality, have atopic disease.

Atopic disease is the most common cause of chronic otitis externa. Atopic disease should be considered in any dog with recurrent otitis, even without other signs. In Scott's (1981) study 3% of the atopic dogs had ear disease only.

Seborrhea is reported in 12% to 23% of atopics (Scott, 1981; Willemse and van den Brom, 1983). The presence of seborrhea sicca or dry skin may aggravate the pruritus by lowering the pruritic threshold. Many atopic dogs do not develop enough scales to be termed seborrhea sicca but on close examination do have dry skin.

The skin and hair coat may also be greasy. Greasy coats seem more common in certain breeds such as German Shepherd Dogs, Lhasa Apsos, West Highland White Terriers, Cairn Terriers, Basset Hounds, and Shih Tzus. Whether this reflects the atopic disease or another disorder is not known. Owners of these pets often complain about the abnormal odor. If a secondary pyoderma is also present, this odor may resolve or dramatically improve with antibiotic therapy.

Sweating or hyperhidrosis may be seen in as many as 24% of the cases but is not specific for atopic disease. Sneezing is reported in 0% to as high as 47.8% of atopic dogs (Scott, 1981; Willemse, 1984). Although the reported incidences are

CHAPTER 10 Canine Atopic Disease **105**

variable, there appears to be a correlation between sneezing and conjunctivitis. As the incidence of sneezing increases, so does that of conjunctivitis (Willemse and van den Brom, 1983; Willemse, 1984). Conjunctivitis is reported in 30% to 50% of atopic dogs.

Corneal dystrophy, cataracts, gastrointestinal symptoms, seizures, urinary tract disorders, and reproductive abnormalities have all been described as noncutaneous signs of atopic disease. However, irregular estrus cycles, urinary tract disorders, and gastrointestinal signs may also occur from previous corticosteroid therapy. Since prior treatments are not usually reported, it is difficult to determine whether these signs reflect atopic disease or treatment effects.

Atopic dogs may have concurrent allergies. Flea allergy dermatitis is often seen, with a reported incidence as high as 80%. The prevalence will vary with geographic location and flea exposure. In Southern California 60% of atopic dogs have strongly positive immediate intradermal test reactions to flea antigen. In Las Vegas, where there are no fleas, only 10% will have positive immediate reactions, and almost all of those dogs have had a history of being exposed to fleas. The presence of fleas on dogs with both atopy and flea allergy makes management more difficult and is a common reason for recurrences in controlled animals.

Insect hypersensitivities other than fleas have recently been evaluated in atopic dogs. Some 10% of non–flea-allergic animals had at least one insect reaction other than house-dust mite. Of atopic dogs in Nevada, 42% had one or more insect reactions, and 7% had three or more.

Food allergy is reported to occur in up to 30% of atopic dogs. Other reports give a lower incidence, as low as 3%; my experience has suggested about 10%. Dietary modification may help reduce the severity, type, and pattern of clinical signs or symptoms. In some dogs on dietary modification, the improvement may be imperceptible to the owner until rechallenge with the original diet. In other dogs, dietary modifications may yield improvement only after the atopic disease or fleas, insects, pyoderma, and dry skin have been controlled. This phenomenon is related to pruritic threshold and summation of effects.

The recognition of *Malassezia* dermatitis has been a relatively recent event. (See Chapter 4.) One study (Plant et al., 1991) showed that atopic dogs do not appear to be at increased risk for the development of secondary *Malassezia* dermatitis. However, the diagnosis of atopic disease was made in 25.5% of the cases, with high numbers of *Malassezia pachydermatis* found on cytologic examination of skin impressions. When this occurs, the cases become extremely pruritic and nonresponsive to conventional antipruritic drugs, including glucocorticoids. These dogs often have a greasy, yellow, crusty exudate and otitis externa.

The major differential diagnoses for atopic disease include all of the possible coexisting diseases. Flea allergy, food allergy, scabies, and pruritic pyoderma are the most commonly encountered, but any cause of pruritus can be included in the differential for atopic disease.

DIAGNOSIS

The diagnosis of atopic disease is often complicated by coexisting conditions or diseases that affect pruritus or the allergic threshold. To develop the best management plan for the atopic dog, the clinician should determine what other diseases or factors are present. Treating coexisting diseases may alleviate the clinical signs of an atopic dog by bringing a patient below the pruritic threshold. Therefore complete resolution of pruritus does not rule out atopic disease without a negative intradermal test.

The most common diseases occurring simultaneously with atopy are superficial pyoderma and, in areas where fleas are present, flea allergy. The presence of erythematous or crusted papules is not typical of atopy but is compatible with flea allergy dermatitis and superficial pyoderma. Diseases other than atopy must be pursued if appropriate antibiotic therapy does not alleviate most of the lesions. If antibiotics eliminate most lesions, and pruritus is present, then a probable diagnosis of atopic disease should be made. (Refer to Diagnostic Criteria box, p.99.) Systemic glucocorticoids cannot be utilized to help establish a diagnosis. Therefore, animals with any signs or symptoms suggesting atopy should not be given systemic corticosteroids until a diagnosis is made and safer alternative treatments have proved ineffective.

Allergy Tests

Two methods of allergy testing are readily available to practitioners. Intradermal testing has been performed for many years, and more recently in vitro tests for the detection of allergen-specific IgE have become commercially available (Appendix B). Before either of these methods is employed, however, it is best to rule out as many other dif-

Table 10-1. Treatment withdrawal times prior to intradermal testing

TREATMENT	MINIMUM DAYS SINCE END OF TREATMENT*
Oral alternate-day prednisone	14
Daily prednisone antipruritic doses	28
Triamcinolone acetonide injection	70
Methylprednisolone acetate injection	96
Diphenhydramine HCl	4
Hydroxyzine HCl	8
Acepromazine	1
Topical glucocorticoids, including eye, ear, and skin (except 0.5% hydrocortisone)	7

*Waiting longer increases the chances that there will be no interference. This is most often required when signs of iatrogenic Cushing's from long-term treatment are present. Shorter times may still have good test results, but chances of interference are greater.

ferentials or contributing diseases as possible. Although allergy testing allows confirmation of the diagnosis, it is utilized primarily to identify offending allergens so avoidance and hyposensitization can be added to a therapeutic regimen. Testing has minimal value unless hyposensitization is utilized. A strong tentative diagnosis can be made with a careful, methodical approach combining tests and trial therapies to rule out other differential diagnoses.

Prior to the utilization of intradermal or in vitro allergy tests, the patient should meet certain criteria to optimize test results and cost-effectiveness. The dog should have a compatible diagnosis of atopy. Whenever appropriate, pyoderma and scabies should be ruled out by respective therapeutic response. Pruritus should persist for more than 4 months of the year. Nonsteroidal treatments should be either proved ineffective or not preferred by the client. The possibilities of food and flea allergy should be discussed with the client; and if he or she does not prefer to treat for those first, then testing is appropriate.

Patient preparation before testing is important for the best results. Prior to intradermal testing, certain drugs must be withdrawn for appropriate times (Table 10-1). It is important to emphasize that each dog is an individual, the recommended withdrawal times are minimums, and some dogs are affected much longer. In vitro tests usually

claim that drugs do not affect their results. There are no studies in canines documenting this, and I believe that corticosteroids may have some effect. Therefore it is recommended that systemic glucocorticoid therapy be withdrawn before in vitro allergy testing, though probably withdrawal times can be shorter than those required prior to intradermal testing. For intradermal testing, the skin (generally the lateral thorax) should be as free of lesions as possible. This may call for systemic antibiotic therapy, topical shampoos, moisturizers, and physical restraint.

Practitioners must use a test, whether in vitro or intradermal, that is adapted to their region of the country. Testing with grouped allergens is not recommended. If group antigens are used, they should be limited to genetically similar plants, such as pine mix, with grasses being the exception. Grouping antigens can lead to false-positive and false-negative results, as well as to the inclusion of treatment antigens to which the patient is not allergic. A study on an in vitro ELISA test (Kleinbeck et al., 1989) showed that averages for the groups were similar to the average for the individual allergens. However, when the data are closely examined they show that a comparison of the individual allergens to the average or group score was similar only for the grasses. If one looks at the results of the allergens showing reactions that would justify hyposensitization, then for the weeds eight of 30 animals would have been hyposensitized differently and for the trees nine of 23.

Intradermal Testing

Intradermal testing is the most accepted method for making a definitive diagnosis of canine atopic disease. Intradermal testing is a procedure where a small amount of nonglycerinated aqueous allergenic extract is injected into the dermis (See Formulary.) Allergen binds with two molecules of allergen-specific IgE bound to mast cells. The binding causes mast cell degranulation and the release of proinflammatory mediators, producing an erythematous wheal in 15 to 30 minutes; this indicates a positive reaction. Intradermal testing requires considerable practice in order to gain proficiency. Two excellent references that carry a complete description of intradermal allergy testing are *Allergic Skin Diseases of Dogs and Cats,* by Reedy and Miller, and *Veterinary Clinical Immunology,* by Halliwell and Gorman.

The major advantage of offering intradermal testing in a private practice is improved client service and better patient management. Successful intradermal testing and hyposensitization also provide professional satisfaction. Intradermal testing may be a valuable source of income in a relatively busy practice that offers it.

The disadvantages of offering intradermal testing in a private practice must also be considered. The overhead expense, the work necessary to maintain adequate inventory (with testing solutions mixed every 8 weeks or more often), and the possibility of an allergen's becoming outdated are three factors. Practitioners are advised to buy treatment-strength allergen solutions and to prepare their own testing solutions every 2 or 3 months, since it is not cost-effective to buy only prepared testing solutions. A practitioner must be willing to set aside some time to learn the technique, and even then there is the time and frustration involved until the veterinarian becomes proficient. The possibility that the practice does not have an adequate volume of cases that would choose allergy testing must be considered. The editors believe the minimum volume should be an average of 2 cases a month.

Alternatives to in-house intradermal allergy testing include referring the patient to another practitioner or specialist who does intradermal testing and using an in vitro allergy test.

In Vitro Allergy Tests

Currently, in vitro allergy tests are commercially available from several companies in the United States. (See Appendix B.) Although these tests are acceptable in humans for the diagnosis and identification of potentially important antigens in allergic rhinitis and asthma, their use for atopic dermatitis has been discouraged (Hanifin, 1988). The frequent elevation of total serum IgE in persons with atopic dermatitis is associated with increased false-positive results.

The major advantage of in vitro allergy tests is their simplicity for the practitioner and patient. The practitioner collects a serum sample and sends it to a laboratory. Allergen overhead is avoided, and the work of inventorying, storing, and updating allergens eliminated. The patient does not need to be shaved and restrained for the intradermal injections. Results are reported with a numerical score, avoiding allergy test evaluation.

The laboratory incubates the serum with allergens bound to a solid medium, then rinses away the serum and unbound immunoglobulins. Next, labeled anti-canine IgE is incubated with the solid medium that has allergen and allergen-bound IgE reacted to it. The label used depends on the type of assay, and this is one of the major differences between the radioisotope label, called the radioallergosorbent test (RAST), and the enzyme-linked immunosorbent assay (ELISA). After further rinsing, the remaining labeled anti–canine IgE is detected by measuring. The amount of the reaction for anti–canine IgE for each allergen tested is compared to a standard curve established by the laboratory, and a score is assigned. The test scores are compared to normal dogs and are reported as negative, borderline, or positive. The practitioner must then correlate the results with the patient's history and decide which borderline and positive scores are significant.

The problems with in vitro testing in the canine are false-positive results and in some cases reproducibility. One study (Griffin, 1989) compared two laboratories and showed a significant difference in reproducibility, with one lab being less than 90% reproducibile. False-positive results from dogs with scabies and intradermal test–negative normal dogs have been extremely common on both RAST and ELISA tests (Griffin et al., 1990; MacDonald and Angarano, 1990). A study comparing false-positive results to total serum IgE levels (Griffin et al., 1990) documented significant correlation between false-positives for pollen reactions and IgE levels, with 45% to 47% of the positives being attributed to the level of nonspecific total serum IgE. Recently a new type of in vitro test (Veterinary Allergy Reference Laboratory) that utilizes a liquid phase technology has become commercially avail-

Table 10-2. Results of hyposensitization from intradermal and in vitro protocols

GROUP*	N†	PERCENT POOR	PERCENT FAIR	PERCENT GOOD/EXCELLENT‡
I	9	22	11	67
II	7	43	14	43
III	9	78	0	22

*See text for a description of the groups.
†The number of dogs out of the original 10 in each group that continued treatment for at least 6 months.
‡No significant difference with the nonparametric Kruskal-Wallis test.

able in limited regions of the United States (Alaba and El Shami, 1989). In humans this technique has decreased the incidence of false-positives due to background IgE. When the in vitro results are compared to results of skin tests, there still appear to be some problems with false-positives; however, the test may be more sensitive than intradermal testing. In a small study with Western Blot Analysis as the definitive reference (Alaba et al., 1991), VARL and intradermal tests had 82% and 70% sensitivity and 75% and 100% specificity, respectively; and they had 81% and 74% concordance. At present, intradermal testing is more specific for the diagnosis of clinically relevant allergens.

The comparison of in vitro with intradermal testing for clinical usefulness should be based on hyposensitization results. Several reports (Sousa and Norton, 1990) have shown the response to hyposensitization based on in vitro test results to be as effective as the hyposensitization response based on intradermal testing. All reports with both techniques showed favorable responses at 4 months' follow-up in approximately 60% of the cases.

A prospective, open study (Griffin and Rosenkrantz, 1991) compared hyposensitization results based on a commercially available ELISA test and intradermal testing. Three groups with a diagnosis compatible with atopy were evaluated. Group I dogs were positive on both the intradermal and the ELISA test but were treated according to the results of the intradermal test. Group II dogs also were positive on both tests but were treated according to the in vitro results. Group III dogs were negative on the intradermal test and positive on the in vitro test and were treated according to the in vitro results. Group I was treated with Greer allergenic extracts by my usual protocol and Groups II and III were treated with different allergens and a protocol recommended by the ELISA laboratory. Subsequent follow-up spanned 2½ years. The results,

shown in Table 10-2 indicated that intradermal testing with individual allergens and the corresponding hyposensitization protocol appeared more effective but was not statistically significant. However good results were obtained with in vitro protocols, and this approach is warranted if intradermal testing is not available. It is also tempting to speculate that group III dogs may represent a different disease or subgroup of atopic animals.

In vitro allergy testing of atopic dogs should be considered in the following situations: the intradermal test is unavailable; the client refuses to restrain or shave the dog; the test site or patient cannot be properly prepared; or intradermal injections of saline induce wheals. Optimal use of in vitro testing requires interpretation in light of the total serum IgE level, which is not currently reported by any commercial laboratories. Extra care should be taken to rule out all differentials, since in vitro testing is less specific than intradermal testing for the diagnosis of atopic disease and detection of relevant allergens.

TREATMENT

Most atopic dogs require a combination of therapeutics for optimal control of symptoms. Treatment options vary in their ease of administration, risks, efficacy, expense, and monitoring required. The treatment plan should also include the recognition and treatment of coexisting diseases.

Some problems may be permanently or temporarily eliminated (e.g., fleas and pyoderma). Atopic disease can only be controlled; it cannot be cured. Treatment is required for life and will often involve modifications. The disease may become more severe as the pet ages, requiring changes in treatment, and additional treatments may be required. Optimal management requires a familiarity with treatment options and a willingness on the part of the client to follow recommendations. Treatment goals include the use of medications that have minimal side effects and good efficacy and are accepted by the client. One aspect of treatment is client education as to expected results. In some cases the pruritus may be reduced considerably, but complete control will require additional therapy. It may be wiser in some of these to accept a low level of pruritus rather than increase the risk or costs of additional therapy. In some atopic cases with recurrent pyoderma the pruritus is mild when the pyoderma is controlled. If the relapse rate is relatively infrequent (i.e., several times a year), treating each relapse with antibiotics might be preferable to continuous long-term therapy with other agents. Selecting the best plan for individual situations is an art.

Treatment Plans

The following basic treatment plans are ones that I prefer for the management of atopic dogs. They are used in a sequence that minimizes risks to the pet over long-term use. Modifications will occur based on the individual patient's and client's circumstances. Two factors are initially considered: First, Is the client agreeable and willing to do the treatment? Second, Is the pruritus localized or widespread? When the pruritus is localized to small areas, such as the paws or pinnae, then topical glucocorticoid therapy may be sufficient. In cases that involve several body sites and require widespread coverage, the treatment plan should include a weekly bathing and fatty acid supplementation. Although these two treatments are not often satisfactory on their own, they usually are helpful and make other treatments more effective.

Additional treatments will depend on whether the pruritus is seasonal or continuous. If it is significant for only 4 months a year or less, antihistamines are recommended initially. Systemic glucocorticoids may be used if antihistamines are ineffective or the client does not wish to try them. Alternate-day prednisone for less than 4 months a year is not usually associated with significant side effects. However, the increased appetite, water consumption, urination, and behavioral changes that may occur can still make their use unacceptable. Reliance on systemic glucocorticoids should be avoided whenever possible if the pruritus is continuous.

Antihistamines or hyposensitization are the treatments of choice in cases with continuous symptoms. These are usually added to the bathing program and fatty acid supplements to achieve the additive effects. However, due to expense and work, some clients attempt to use one treatment alone. To minimize the allergic load (which often improves medication response), avoidence of the offending allergens should be attempted whenever possible. This is especially important when insect hypersensitivities are present.

In my experience, about one third of atopic dogs can be controlled without long-term use of systemic glucocorticoids or hyposensitization. It should also be stressed to the client that some pets can be well-controlled with one regimen most of the year but will require additional treatment during the pet's most severe allergy period. This period will often be associated with further exposure to fleas in dogs with concurrent flea allergy dermatitis. During such peak times concurrent antihistamines or systemic glucocorticoids may be utilized. Using hyposensitization and other techniques allows 75% of the patients to be controlled without long-term systemic glucocorticoids.

In other cases hyposensitization or antihistamines may yield only a partial response. Some cases will have residual pruritus in a localized area. Local topical therapy may now be effective instead of increasing systemic medications. Other cases will still have significant pruritus. In these cases raising the dosages or increasing the frequency of hyposensitization injections may be effective. The most difficult-to-manage cases will require systemic glucocorticoids. Systemic glucocorticoids may be preferred by some clients because of their ease, low expense, and high efficacy, and because of the perception that side effects will be slow-developing. Difficult cases may require combining several therapeutics. I have some clients who use hyposensitization, antihistamines, fatty acids, bathing programs, and systemic glucocorticoids to achieve desirable results. Stopping any one of these leads to ineffective control or undesirable increases in other treatments.

Avoidance

Avoidance requires the identification of allergens by allergy testing. Avoidance is generally impractical or unacceptable to the client. However, in some cases such as feather, tobacco, and cat allergies, exposure may be minimized. House-dust mite allergen is difficult to control, although some cases have been reported by owners to have improved by being kept outdoors more. Since bedrooms tend to contain more house-dust mite allergen than other indoor areas, limiting access to those rooms may decrease the allergen load. Mold allergens can be partly avoided by keeping dogs indoors, away from decaying vegetation, including lawns. Controlling mildew and removing indoor plants may also help minimize exposure to mold. Most dogs' atopy cannot be adequately controlled by attempts at allergen avoidance. However, when possible, it should be attempted since any reduction in allergen exposure may add to the overall improvement from a combined treatment regimen.

Topical Therapy

Topical therapy should be incorporated into treatment plans whenever possible. The major disadvantages are the time and effort needed for administration, although expense may also be an important factor. Bathing the total body or using rinses is required for regional or generalized pruritus. Treatment with ointments, creams, and lotions may be possible for localized areas. Topical therapy is often overlooked and not presented as an option to clients.

Nonsteroidal

Frequent shampooing reduces but rarely eliminates pruritus. Shampooing removes surface debris and bacterial byproducts that can contribute to the pruritic load. It may also reduce allergens on the skin surface, thereby lowering the allergic load. It may provide a temporary antipruritic effect by cooling the skin through evaporation or the use of cool water. Water will initially hydrate the stratum corneum, but repetitive applications can cause drying. Excessive drying is avoided by utilizing hypoallergenic and moisturizing shampoos and rinses (e.g., Allergroom, HyLyt*efa Shampoo and Rinse). Antibacterial shampoos may be preferred for the management of coexisting pyoderma. However, some shampoo ingredients, especially detergents, will aggravate the pruritus in certain animals. All shampoos have the potential for irritant reactions, even the hypoallergenic varieties.

Soothing rinses may be used for the symptomatic relief of pruritus, but their effect is short-acting. They are especially valuable when trying to avoid systemic drugs in preparation for intradermal testing. They are also helpful in managing acute exacerbations of pruritus.

Cold or cool water will immediately reduce and occasionally alleviate pruritus. However, the pet should be allowed to dry in a warm area (70° F or more) to decrease the chances of hypothermia. Nonprescription antipruritic products such as Aveeno Colloidal Oatmeal (Rydelle Laboratories) and Domeboro (Miles Pharmaceuticals) may be added to water to improve or prolong the effect. They should be used with cool water and may provide up to 24 to 36 hours of relief. I have found Aveeno Colloidal Oatmeal the most effective; Aveeno Oilated Oatmeal should be used for animals with very dry skin or hair. These products are available in bar or powder format with the latter preferred. Cool or tepid water (not warm, as the directions indicate) should also be used. The suspension may be poured on as a rinse, or the dog may be soaked in it. A mixture of 1 or 2 tablespoons per gallon of water is usually sufficient. Some clients have commented on a disagreeable odor with this treatment. Aveeno Colloidal Oatmeal rinses also can leave a residue in the animal's coat, which can be minimized by putting the powder in a discarded nylon stocking prior to placing it in the water.

Aluminum acetate solution (Domeboro) acts as an astringent and has antipruritic properties. It is available in tablets or packets of powder. Overall, aluminum acetate is less effective as an antipruritic agent than oatmeal but is useful when moist pruritic lesions (hot spots) are present. The duration of effect usually is shorter than with oatmeal but longer than with water alone. Also, aluminum acetate is more expensive to use than oatmeal, which limits its usefulness as a rinse. It may be used as often as needed but generally once or twice daily for hot spots.

Moisturizers help control dry skin by increasing the water content of the stratum corneum. Occlusive agents work by decreasing evaporation from the skin. Humectants moisturize by attracting water into the stratum corneum. Rehydration helps control yet another factor that contributes to pruritus. Emollients and moisturizers contain various combinations of oil (mineral, sesame), glycerin, lanolin, fatty acids, lactic acid, amino acids, urea, phospholipids, and waxes. These ingredients are incorporated into rinses, sprays, and shampoos. The occlusive (oil-based) rinses work best when applied after bathing while the skin surface is still moist. Humectants may also be applied effectively to dry skin. Humilac (a humectant spray) and HyLyt*efa (an occlusive and humectant spray) are marketed in pump devices for easy application between baths. They may also be diluted to use as an after-bath rinse.

When pruritus is localized to smaller areas, (paws, ears, periocular and perineal regions, and hot spots), numerous, more expensive, lotions, gels, creams, and ointments may be used. Most of these contain glucocorticoids, but a variety of nonglucocorticoid formulations are available.

Camphor and menthol have been used for many years as topical antipruritics in numerous nonprescription products. Their mechanism of action is not definitely known but may be related to a cooling effect. Topical antihistamines have been shown experimentally to inhibit histamine-induced pruritus and wheal and flare reactions in humans. Their clinical efficacy has not been evaluated in atopic dogs.

Witch hazel has been incorporated into lotions (PTD, Dermacool) for its antipruritic effect. It may be helpful in treating localized lesions and areas of acute moist dermatitis. With crusty or dirty lesions, witch hazel should be applied after the area has been cleansed with an antiseptic shampoo (Sulf Oxydex, Pyoben, ChlorhexiDerm, Nolvasan). Topical anesthetics can be effective when applied to eroded or inflamed areas of pruritic skin. Unfortunately, their effect is very short and with repeated use they become ineffective. Therefore they are practical only for acute problems and not for the management of chronic pruritus.

Topical Glucocorticoids

Topical glucocorticoids are valuable for treating localized reactions such as allergic otitis externa. Their antiinflammatory potency is highly variable, depending on the type of glucocorticoid and the vehicle. The vehicle is important in determining their efficacy and systemic toxicity. In general, the more occlusive and moisturizing the vehicle, the more potent will be the product. Although exceptions exist, ointments are more potent than creams and creams are more potent than lotions (assuming the glucocorticoid and concentration are comparable). Glucocorticoids produced for human use are rated for antiinflammatory activity. This has not been done for exclusively veterinary products. Ranking of the relative potencies of products that I have utilized, based on clinical experience and human studies, may be helpful in product selection (Table 10-3).

Because of variable potencies, the clinician should use and become familiar with several topical glucocorticoid preparations. Therapy usually should begin with a medium to strong product applied q12h until the inflammation has been controlled. The frequency may then be reduced to once daily. The treatment should be changed to a less potent topical glucocorticoid as the disease is controlled. The objective is to use the least potent drug that will effectively control the problem when long-term therapy (longer than 1 month) is required.

Adverse effects can be seen with topical glucocorticoid use. Most serious is the development of iatrogenic Cushing's syndrome (iatrogenic hy-

Table 10-3. Topical glucocorticoids

CLASS	GENERIC NAME	TRADE NAME	%
I	Clobetasol propionate	Temovate	0.05
	Betamethasone dipropionate	Diprolene	0.05
	Diflorasone diacetate	Psorcon	0.05
II	Amcinonide	Cyclocort	0.1
	Desoximetasone	Topicort	0.25
III	Betamethasone valerate	Valisone Ointment	0.1
	Fluocinolone acetonide	Synotic	0.01
IV	Triamcinolone acetonide	Panolog	0.1
	Dexamethasone	Tresaderm	0.1
	Betamethasone valerate	Valisone Cream	0.1
V	Hydrocortisone	Generics	0.5 to 2.5

perglucorticoidism) and secondary adrenocortical insufficiency. Iatrogenic Cushing's usually results from treating large body areas and subsequent absorption or from leaving heavy creams and ointments on the skin, where the dog licks them off. Failure to regulate refills can also lead to problems. A recent study by Morriello et al. (1988) utilized products containing triamcinolone acetonide (Panolog) and dexamethasone (Tresaderm) in dogs. The products were applied to the external ear canal, so it is unlikely that the animals experienced any systemic absorption from licking. In this study adrenal suppression and elevated liver enzymes were very significant. Another study (Zenoble and Kemppainen, 1987) looked at absorption in shaved areas of skin and also showed significant absorption with topical corticosteroids.

Proper client education about these drugs is a major factor in avoiding iatrogenic Cushing's disease. Localized adverse reactions include cutaneous atrophy, comedone formation, folliculitis, poor healing, pigment changes, and suppression of local immune responses (Fig. 10-7).

Topical glucocorticoid therapy poses another problem. Clients need to be warned about possible side effects to themselves as well as to their pets. When applying the medication, they should be instructed to wear rubber gloves, use an applicator, cover their finger with plastic wrap, or immediately wash their exposed skin. It is especially important to avoid contact with facial skin, since this area is particularly sensitive to the more potent topical glucocorticoids.

Antibiotics

Pyoderma is a frequent secondary problem in atopic disease and can add significantly to the level of pruritus. Whenever any lesions compatible with pyoderma are present, a trial of systemic antibiotics is indicated.

It is common to see atopic dogs with a history of developing resistance to a previously effective regimen of glucocorticoids, even after increasing the dosage. In most of these cases the allergy has not become "resistant" to glucocorticoids but the patient has developed a secondary pyoderma. With appropriate antibiotics and topical antibacterials, these dogs usually end up on the same or a lesser amount of glucocorticoids. The clinician should always rule out the possibility that a pyoderma is contributing to the pruritus. A trial course of systemic antibiotics is safer than a steady increase in glucocorticoids. Potentiated sulfa drugs (Primor, Ditrim), potentiated amoxicillin (Clavamox), and cephalosporins are the drugs I use most. They are given for 2 or 3 weeks in most cases. Until the atopy is well-controlled, recurrences of pyoderma are likely and repeated treatments with antibiotics will be required.

Antihistamines

The effectiveness of systemic antihistamines in canine atopy has been a subject of disagreement for years. However, it has recently been documented that antihistamines that block H_1 receptors are beneficial in controlling pruritus associated with atopic disease in dogs. Some antihistamines have other effects. The sedative effect of many may contribute to the control of pruritus. The tricyclic piperidine antihistamine azatadine and hydroxyzine hydrochloride HCl stabilize mast cells and decrease mediator release following antigen challenge in allergic patients. Controlling the portion of the pruritus that is mediated by histamine enable the patient to move further below its pruritic threshold. Some products also have antiserotonin, analgesic, and antianxiety activity, which may contribute to their effectiveness in controlling pruritus. The beneficial effect of antihistamines is reduced or eliminated when pyoderma is present. Trial antihistamine therapy can be properly assessed only after pyoderma has been eliminated.

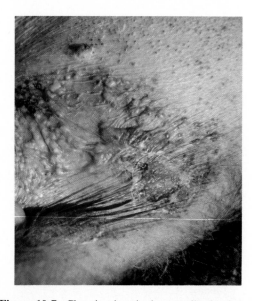

Figure 10-7. Chronic triamcinolone application has induced marked comedone formation and cutaneous atrophy. An erosion and secondary pyoderma were present, which may have partly reflected the decrease in local immune response from topical glucocorticoids.

My experience with the antihistamines diphenhydramine HCl and hydroxyzine HCl has been encouraging. In a retrospective study of 55 cases of pruritus in atopic dogs, 30% responded well enough that the clients were satisfied with the results and the dogs did not require systemic glucocorticoids. These animals were also bathed weekly. Concurrent flea and food allergy, if present or suspected, were controlled by avoidance. I currently utilize hydroxyzine HCl 2.2 mg/kg q8h, diphenhydramine HCl 2.2 mg/kg q8h, and doxepin HCl 0.5 to 1 mg/kg q12h. Generally the client is asked to try two or three of these antihistamines consecutively for 7 to 14 days.

In another open trial (Scott and Buerger, 1988) 22.2% of 45 dogs were satisfactorily controlled within 1 week by chlorpheniramine 4 mg q8h, diphenhydramine HCl 25 to 50 mg q8h, or hydroxyzine HCl 2.2 mg/kg q8h. The dogs were diagnosed with atopic disease (19), flea allergy dermatitis and atopic disease (8), flea allergy dermatitis (5), and idiopathic pruritus (13).

A double-blind, placebo-controlled study in 30 pruritic dogs has been reported (Paradis et al., 1991a). Atopic disease alone was confirmed in 21 cases. Four cases had combined allergic disease (2 food allergic and atopic, 2 flea allergic and atopic), but the nonatopic portion was avoided during the trial. One dog, only flea allergic, had fleas present throughout the trial. Four cases with idopathic pruritus were also included. All drugs and the placebo were given for 1 week, then discontinued for 2 days prior to starting the next drug. The trial was conducted over 9 consecutive weeks. The placebo was totally ineffective whereas clemastine (Tavist) at an approximate dosage of 0.05 mg/kg q12h was the most effective, with 30% of the cases responding. Astemizole (Hismanal) at an approximate dosage of 0.25 mg/kg q24h or trimeprazine (Temaril)

at approximately 0.12 mg/kg q12h was effective in 3.3% of the cases. In contrast to the editors' experience, doxepin at approximately 1 mg/kg q8h was not effective. When prednisone and trimeprazine were given in combination at the same dosage, 76.7% of cases responded satisfactorily. Prednisone at 0.2 mg/kg bid with no loading dose was effective in only 56.7% of the cases. This dosage was selected because it was equivalent to the amount of prednisone in the combination tablet of trimeprazine/prednisone. It is not the same dosage or regimen that would normally be used in clinical cases. In 75% of the dogs that responded to prednisone alone, the prednisone dosage could be reduced by 30% when trimeprazine was added.

This synergistic effect has also been documented with other nonsteroidal antiinflammatory agents. A study by Paradis et al. (1991b) compared the responses of pruritic dogs to clemastine, a fatty acid supplement (Derm Caps), or a combination of both. An effective response was noted in 10% of the failure cases when the combination was used, in contrast to either treatment alone, indicating a synergistic effect. Another study (Miller, 1989) showed a synergistic effect with Derm Caps and chlorpheniramine.

Since individual variation in response to different antihistamines is noted in humans and dogs with chronic urticaria and pruritus, several antihistamines from different classes should be tried. My typical trial therapy protocol is given in Table 10-4. Amitrypyline (1-2 mg/kg q12h), another tricyclic antidepressant with potent antihistaminic effects, may also be utilized with some success and is reasonably priced. Clemastine is not regularly prescribed, especially in large dogs, because of its cost. I have not routinely used chlorpheniramine because of frequent problems with drowsiness and a perceived poor clinical response. Anecdotal com-

Table 10-4. Protocol for trial therapy with nonsteroidal antipruritic drugs

TREATMENT	DOSAGE	WEEK(S) ADMINISTERED
Derm Caps ES	1 capsule/30 to 50 lb q24h	1, 2, 3, 4
Hydroxyzine HCl	2.2 mg/kg q8h	1 only
Diphenhydramine HCl	2.2 mg/kg q8h	2 only
Doxepin HCl	1 to 2 mg/kg q12h	3 only

Evaluate after week 4 to determine which treatment was most effective with no or acceptable side effects

ments from practitioners at educational meetings about deaths occurring at high dosages (1 mg/kg q24h) also discouraged my using the drug frequently. Astemazole and terfenadine occasionally will help but, because of cost, are not routinely prescribed.

Sedation and anticholinergic effects are the primary side effects of antihistamines. Trembling, increased pruritus, and panting have also been reported. Excitation may be seen in rare cases. Doxepin and chlorpheniramine appear to cause a higher incidence of side effects. Drowsiness may lessen or resolve with continued therapy. For other side effects and when drowsiness persists, the drug should be discontinued. Once the side effects have resolved, resuming therapy at a lower dosage may still effectively control the pruritus without the side effects.

Fluoxetine (Prozac) inhibits the uptake of serotinin and, like hydroxyzine, has an antiserotinin effect. A recent pilot study (Shoulberg, 1990) evaluated fluoxetine at 1 mg/kg once daily for 4 consecutive weeks in six atopic dogs that had been unresponsive to antihistamines and hyposensitization. Three dogs had greater than 70% reduction in their symptoms within 4 weeks. The drug was stopped in two dogs because of side effects, and one dog had a 50% reduction in signs. Side effects were seen in half the cases and included lethargy, wheals, and polydipsia-polyuria. Currently this is rather expensive treatment and should be reserved for cases refractory to other therapies. Although not germane in dogs, the practitioner should know that in humans this drug has been blamed for inducing attempts to commit suicide and questions regarding this may be raised by the client. I do not currently know of any behavioral problems in dogs treated with this drug. Due to expense, however, its use will probably be limited to occasional cases and small dogs.

Fatty Acids

A variety of cutaneous and noncutaneous inflammatory disorders may benefit from the use of fatty acid supplements in the diet. The most important fatty acids are linoleic, linolenic, gamma-linolenic, and eicosapentaenoic acid. Linolenic and linoleic are essential fatty acids required in the diet. Evening primrose oil is a good source of gamma-linolenic acid whereas eicosapentaenoic acid is found primarily in fish oils. In humans gamma-linolenic and eicosapentaenoic acid are reportedly helpful in the treatment of atopic dermatitis and psoriasis.

Free arachidonic acid released from cell membranes (mast cells, neutrophils, and keratinocytes) in allergic and other inflammatory dermatoses is metabolized to proinflammatory mediators of inflammation and pruritus. It is believed that the pruritus associated with atopic disease is decreased because of modulation of the arachidonic acid cycle. Eicosapentaenoic acid competes with arachidonic acid for metabolism and results in the formation of prostaglandins (PG) and leukotrienes (LT) that are less inflammatory. Gamma-linolenic acid is metabolized to dihomo-gamma-linolenic acid, which results in the production of the one series of prostaglandins and may also interfere with the production of the two series of prostaglandins and four series of leukotrienes from arachidonic acid. Since LTC_4, LTD_4, and LTE_4 are allergic mediators and PGE_2 lowers the pruritic threshold, decreasing their production may help alleviate the pruritus.

The importance of gamma-linolenic acid is supported by studies utilizing evening primrose oil (EPO) as the supplement. In an open study of 12 dogs with atopic disease (Lloyd and Thomsett, 1989) EPO supplementation was associated with a marked reduction in clinical signs. This response was dose-related. In a double-blind, placebo-controlled, crossover study of EPO therapy in atopic dogs Scarff and Lloyd (1990) showed a significant reduction of pruritus and erythema with improved coat condition in dogs given EPO.

A number of essential fatty acid products containing gamma-linolenic acid and/or eicosapentaenoic acid have been marketed for veterinary use. Several studies have evaluated Derm Caps in the treatment of allergic disease or pruritus in dogs. Derm Caps contain both eicosapentaenoic and gamma-linolenic acid. In an open multicenter study (Miller et al., 1989) they controlled pruritus to the client's satisfaction in 18% of 93 dogs; and in two other studies (Scott and Buerger, 1988; Paradis et al., 1991b) they satisfactorily controlled 11.1% of 45 dogs and 26.7% of 30 dogs. All the studies mentioned have shown that many more of the cases treated with Derm Caps exhibited a moderate decrease in pruritus. Another study (Lloyd, 1989) using a blend of gamma-linolenic and eicosapentaenoic acids with vitamins (EfaVet [Efamol, Inc.]) showed 18% excellent and an additional 76% good responses.

In humans with psoriasis, fish oil supplements were shown to be a good adjunctive therapy, especially when itching was a prominent symptom. Their effectiveness is enhanced when they are combined with a low-fat diet.

Since these fatty acid products are believed to work by competing with other fatty acids, especially arachidonic acid, then it would seem appropriate that the dietary manipulation of these other fatty acids might improve the effect of these supplements. This has been confirmed in a study (Harvey, 1990) that used EPO at four times the recommended dosage (150 mg/kg). Ten atopic dogs were stabilized on a commercial canned diet and EPO supplementation, and then the dogs were divided into two groups that had their diets switched to either Science Diet w/d (Hills) or a leading commercial dry dog food. After stabilization, the dogs fed Science Diet w/d continued to improve whereas the dogs fed the dry dog food worsened. Why the Science Diet w/d was more effective and dogs worsened when switched from canned to dry dog food is not known. Several possibilities—such as the fat and fatty acid content of the diets, the presence of fiber, or other factors that may affect fatty acid absorption or metabolism— need investigation. It was also noteworthy that when EPO was used at four times the recommended dosage the investigator noted a much higher response rate than when EPO was given at the clinically recommended dosage. This is in contrast to another study (Scott and Miller, 1990) that showed doubling the dosage of Derm Caps did not improve efficacy and that when improved efficacy is desired 3 or 4 times the recommended dosages may be needed.

As discussed previously, the use of Derm Caps with the antihistamines clemastine and chlorpheniramine can have a synergistic effect. In addition, Derm Caps have allowed for a reduction of approximately 50% in the dosage of alternate-day prednisone required to control atopic dogs (Miller, 1989).

Side effects from fatty acid supplements have been very limited. The most serious is the possibility of pancreatitis in animals predisposed to it. One editor (KK) had two Schnauzers that developed pancreatitis when fatty acids were added to the diet. Diarrhea is an infrequent problem and may be alleviated by reducing the amount of fat in the diet or the dosage of Derm Caps. When large dosages are utilized, the increase in caloric intake may need to be offset by feeding fewer treats, a lower–fat content diet, or a decreased total intake.

The future of fatty acid therapy in allergic and possibly other inflammatory dermatoses seems assured when one considers how benign it is. However, there is much to learn about optimizing fatty acid supplementation with regard to concentra- tions, formulations, dosages, other dietary modifications, and concurrent therapies.

Hyposensitization

Hyposensitization (immunotherapy, biologic therapy, or desensitization) is a form of treatment that attempts to modify the patient's immune response to allergenic challenge. It has been proved effective in veterinary medicine in the management of atopic patients. Its mechanism of action is not totally understood. The classic theory is that it induces the production of IgG "blocking" antibodies to the specific allergen. This IgG antibody will bind (block) allergen, making less available for binding with IgE on mast cells. In dogs the level of blocking IgG antibody produced does not always correlate with the patient's response to hyposensitization. Other mechanisms probably involve stimulation of suppressor T lymphocytes, which may then depress IgE production and induce tolerance, stabilize cell membranes, and decrease allergen-specific IgE as well as IgG.

It is not the intent of this section to adequately train the reader to become an allergist. It is also beneficial, for practical as well as economical reasons, that the practitioner have a caseload and clientele that allow frequent testing and hyposensitization. Allergen selection and hyposensitization is an art that takes time, study, and practice to learn. Using commercial kits and a casual approach will lead to poor results. The hyposensitization solution should be selected by the practitioner or specialist who has developed an interest in intradermal testing and hyposensitization. If it is the intent of the reader to prescribe hyposensitization, select antigens, and completely manage the patient without help from a specialist, then other references should be consulted for more detail (*Allergic Skin Diseases of Dogs and Cats*, by Reedy and Miller, and *Veterinary Clinical Immunology*, by Halliwell and Gorman).

The use of hyposensitization is predicated upon intradermal skin testing or in vitro testing, which determine the specific allergens to which the patient is sensitive. The results of hyposensitization are affected by several factors: the accuracy and quality of the skin test; the method of administration, type, and dose of hyposensitization extract; and the control of other environmental and intrinsic pruritic factors (fleas, pyoderma, dry skin, food allergy). No studies have been done that show whether glucocorticoids affect the response to hyposensitization. During the first 2 weeks on hyposensitization I prefer to avoid systemic glucocorticoids.

Hyposensitization has been reported effective in 50% to 80% of atopic dogs. There are differences in grading schemes, antigen sources, and treatment protocols in these studies. Only one double-blind, placebo-controlled study has been reported (Willemse et al., 1984). The placebo contained aluminum hydroxide, an immune adjuvant, which may have contributed to the 20.8% favorable response in the placebo-treated group. The treatment group had 59.3% response, which was significantly better than the placebo group.

To date, hyposensitization is the most effective alternative to treatment with systemic glucocorticoids that is available. Approximately 75% of atopic dogs can avoid systemic glucocorticoids when hyposensitization is combined with other nonsteroidal treatments. Hyposensitization is also more economical compared to many antihistamines and other treatment options, especially in large dogs. It is usually less labor-intensive than oral and topical treatments after maintenance therapy has been reached.

The client must be informed that improvement is gradual, with obvious benefit taking as long as 2 to 6 months to appear. It is important to stress that this therapy is not completely curative and most dogs need to have booster injections every 2 to 4 weeks for life. It is also best if the client is willing to learn how to give the subcutaneous hyposensitization injections so that they can be administered at home without the need for frequent clinic visits. It is imperative that recheck visits be kept, since many cases require adjustments in their hyposensitization protocol. In other cases the client may feel the hyposensitization is not helping when in reality it is, but pyoderma or another complicating factor is present.

After patients have been on hyposensitization for 4 months, they should be evaluated. Within the first 2 to 4 months clients will often notice a partial response to the hyposensitization injections. This will appear as a decrease in overall pruritus or, more commonly, a temporary reduction in pruritus for several days after the injection. In these cases the frequency of injections is increased. I increase from one injection every 20 days to as frequent as one every 10 days without changing the dose. If pruritus continues to recur earlier than 10 days following the injection, the frequency is increased further but the volume also is reduced. If pruritus increases after an injection, the dose is decreased or the pet is pretreated with hydroxyzine 30 minutes prior to the injection. In rare cases that develop pruritus following an injection, the volume of an-

tigen given may have to be lowered and may never reach the normal maintenance dose. In other reacting cases, pretreatment with antihistamines may not be effective and treatment with oral prednisone (0.5 mg/kg) 1 hour prior to the injection may be required.

Even in patients showing no response to hyposensitization, recheck appointments and phone calls are encouraged since clients usually need the support. A major cause of treatment failure is clients' discontinuing hyposensitization therapy before it has been tried long enough to achieve a response (9 months). This group of failures can be minimized with good client communication. It is most important that the clinician realize the following: hyposensitization therapy is an art, and the majority of patients are being treated with modifications made to the standard treatment protocols based on each individual patient's response.

The major economic drawback is that, compared to alternative treatments, it is more expensive to find out if it is going to be effective, since it can take 6 to 9 months before the response is determined. The expense of skin testing and initial therapy with only 60% to 80% success discourages many clients from pursuing hyposensitization. When approached carefully, the success and long-term savings usually are worth the economic risk that it may not be effective compared to lifelong systemic glucocorticoids.

Serious side effects are uncommon and usually occur in the first or second month of therapy. Anaphylaxis is the primary life-threatening side effect. Usually there will be less severe reactions to the injections preceding the development of anaphylaxis. In my experience over 10 years, two of five cases that developed anaphylaxis had had hives or angioedema previously. Other symptoms to watch for but less specific are weakness, panting, diarrhea, anxiousness, or hyperactivity. Most dermatology specialists have seen only a few anaphylactic reactions in their careers, and the vast majority of patients survive. Less serious but more common side effects are an exacerbation or worsening of the dog's clinical signs. This can usually be controlled by changing the hyposensitization protocol or pretreatment with antihistamines.

Systemic Glucocorticoids

Treatment of atopic disease requires long-term therapy; therefore short-acting oral glucocorticoids (prednisone, prednisolone, methylprednisolone) are preferred (Chastain and Graham, 1979). Methylprednisolone (Medrol) may be used when polydipsia-polyuria or incontinence is a problem, but is is not routinely used because it is more expensive. The following discussion relates to prednisone, although prednisolone or methylprednisolone may be substituted. When substituting methylprednisolone, remember that 4 mg is equivalent to 5 mg of prednisone. Prednisone should be given at approximately the same time on alternate days (morning hours preferred) to minimize adrenal suppression from long-term therapy.

The disease must be in remission before initiating alternate-day therapy. Many clinicians who try alternate-day therapy are dissatisfied and frustrated because they do not initially control the disease before starting the alternate-day therapy. Initially the daily prednisone dose should be halved and given every 12 hours until a favorable response is seen, usually in 2 days. The next step is to switch the total daily dose to once every 24 hours. This should be continued for two to three treatments. The dosage is then converted to every other day, which is done gradually by slowly decreasing the every other treatment dose while keeping the alternate treatment the same. Generally after each reduction the new dose is kept the same for two treatment cycles (4 days). On the next page is an example of how this treatment schedule would be

---

Prednisone and prednisolone are corticosteroid drugs. They have many effects on your pet's body—some are beneficial while some are not. We will attempt to use these medications so that we can minimize the undesirable effects. Common side effects include increased thirst, urination, appetite and panting. Water should be available to your pet at all times. Food intake should be regulated so that your pet does not gain weight. This is particularly important and must be emphasized to the whole family.

Occasionally these medications may irritate the stomach or intestines resulting in vomiting and/or diarrhea. If this occurs, feeding your pet with or just prior to giving the medicine may help. If vomiting or diarrhea persists or your pet appears sick, discontinue the medication and see your veterinarian. Monitoring is important for the health of your pet and reevaluations are needed.

The schedule below should be followed in administering the medication. When given once daily, the medicine should always be given at the same time. The number in the column indicates how many tablets to give at that time and day. If the problem we are trying to control returns, give the previous effective dose and call the hospital.

Medication _____ mg _____ Starting date (Day 1) _____

DAY	AM	PM	*	DAY	AM	*	DAY	AM	*	DAY	AM	*	DAY	AM	*
1				13			25			37			49		
2				14			26			38			50		
3				15			27			39			51		
4				16			28			40			52		
5				17			29			41			53		
6				18			30			42			54		
7				19			31			43			55		
8				20			32			44			56		
9				21			33			45			57		
10				22			34			46			58		
11				23			35			47			59		
12				24			36			48			60		

Continue _____ until _____.

Figure 10-8. Prednisone schedule. Marks in the asterisk column indicate that a phone follow-up or examination is needed

used to treat a 20 kg dog with atopic disease. As long as the symptoms remain controlled, the dosage is decreased until the animal is taking the original once daily dose being given only every other day. This dosage is gradually tapered until the lowest effective level is reached. A client handout may be used for dogs being given long-term glucocorticoids (Fig. 10-8). The handout is valuable and can be posted on the refrigerator or in some other obvious place, allowing checkoff of the treatment schedule. In addition, when there is a recurrence, the chart can be marked so that the clinician will know at what stage in the tapering it developed.

Many clinicians will use long-acting injections instead of the tapering regimen of oral therapy and then start alternate-day prednisone 1 to 4 weeks later. Although this may be effective for some cases, I have seen many referrals when it was not.

Optimal therapeutic dosages cannot be predetermined and depend on individual responses. The following guidelines for using prednisone (prednisolone) may be helpful: for antipruritic therapy 0.5 mg/kg q24h; for antiinflammatory therapy, 1.1 to 1.5 mg/kg q24h. The maintenance dose should be the smallest that is effective. Trial therapy with oral triamcinolone acetonide (Vetalog) is indicated for cases poorly responsive to or requiring more than 1 mg/kg/48 hr of prednisone.

Oral triamcinolone acetonide usually does not cause polydipsia-polyuria or increased appetite as often as prednisone does. Dogs that do not respond well to one type of glucocorticoid may respond better to another. Occasionally a patient will be controlled with a relatively lower dose of oral triamcinolone than with the equivalent dose of prednisone. Many references describe triamcinolone as having an antiinflammatory potency similar to that of prednisone. However, in my clinical experience it is some five to ten times as potent as oral prednisone. Thus a dose of 0.1 or 0.2 mg triamcinolone would be equivalent to 1 mg of prednisone. When oral triamcinolone is effective at 0.2 mg/kg in animals that were not controlled with prednisone at 1 mg/kg, there may be a relative steroid-sparing effect that helps alleviate some of the side effects and risks. Since oral triamcinolone suppresses the adrenal gland for 24 to 48 hours, the drug should optimally be given at a maintainence dose every 3 days (Chen, 1990). Some dogs given alternate-day oral triamcinolone had improved clinical results with fewer side effects than with the doses of prednisone needed to achieve the same effect.

Animals must be monitored for the diverse and numerous side effects that can be seen with glucocorticoid therapy. The problems I see most commonly are poor (dry) hair coat, dry skin, thin skin, muscle wasting, gastrointestinal disturbances, bacteriuria, and recurrent pyoderma. Other side effects seen less frequently include secondary infections (bacterial or fungal), demodicosis, liver disease, pancreatitis, gastrointestinal ulceration, and behavioral changes.

The most important aspect of monitoring long-term therapy is observation of the patient. Physical examinations should be done every 6 to 9 months if the client is not noticing any problems. Urine cultures should be done at least yearly, since the incidence of bacteriuria is 40% (Ihrke et al., 1985). Because recurrences are common in animals that develop bacteriuria, urine cultures may be required more often than yearly. It is not known how many dogs with bacteriuria develop clinical disease; however, it seems more appropriate to treat the bacteriuria with systemic antibiotics until we do know. Serum chemistry values should be acquired every

---

Schedule for Giving Prednisone and Converting to Alternate-Day Therapy (20 kg dog)*

Day	Number of Prednisone pills (5 mg)	
	AM	PM
1	1	1
2	1	1
3	2	
4	2	
5	1	
6	2	
7	1	
8	2	
9	0	
10	2	
11	0	
12	2	
13	0	
14	1½	

*This example utilizes a common antipruritic dose; however, some cases will require more and some less.

12 to 24 months. Elevated liver enzyme values are usually seen and should be interpreted in conjunction with physical examination findings and previous chemistry results. The patient should be reevaluated if problems are observed or the signs are recurrent.

REFERENCES

Alaba O, El Shami AS: Evaluation of non-specific IgE binding: comparison of two in vitro allergen-specific IgE assays. In El Shami AS (ed): Allergy and molecular biology, New York, 1989, Pergamon Press, p 203.

Alaba O, et al: Performance characteristics of VARL-EIA, a new in vitro canine allergen specific IgE test. Comparison with skin test and Western Blot Analysis. In Proceedings, AVA, Scottsdale, 1991, p 22.

Butler JM, et al: Pruritic dermatitis in asthmatic Basenji-Greyhounds: a model for human atopic dermatitis, J Am Acad Dermatol 8:33, 1983.

Chastain CB, Graham CL: Adrenocortical suppression in dogs on daily and alternate-day prednisone administration, Am J Vet Res 40:936, 1979.

Chen CL: Pharmacokinetics of one-day and eight-day oral administration of triamcinolone acetonide in the dog, Vet Rep 3:1, 1990.

Frick OL, Brooks DL: Immunoglobulin E antibodies to pollens augmented in dogs by virus vaccines, Am J Vet Res 44:440, 1983.

Griffin CE: RAST and ELISA testing in canine atopy. In Kirk RE (ed): Current veterinary therapy X, Philadelphia, 1989, WB Saunders, p 592.

Griffin CE, Rosenkrantz WS: A comparison of hyposensitization results in dogs based on an intradermal protocol versus an in vitro protocol. In Proceedings, AVA, Scottsdale, 1991, p 12.

Griffin CE, et al: The effect of serum IgE on an in vitro ELISA test in the normal canine. In von Tscharner C, Halliwell REW, (eds): Veterinary dermatology, vol 1, London, 1990, Baillière Tindall, p 137.

Halliwell REW: The localization of IgE in canine skin: an immunofluorescent study, J Immunol 110:422, 1973.

Halliwell REW, Gorman NT: Atopic diseases. In Halliwell REW, Gorman NT (eds): Veterinary clinical immunology, Philadelphia, 1989, WB Saunders, p 232.

Hanifin JM: Atopic dermatitis. In Middleton E, et al (eds): Allergy; principles and practice, ed 3, St Louis, 1988, CV Mosby, p 1403.

Harvey RG: Accepted for publication, Vet Rec, 1990.

Horrobin D, et al: Plasma fatty acids in dogs and their response to essential fatty acid supplementation. In von Tscharner C, Halliwell REW (eds): Advances in veterinary dermatology, vol 1, London, 1990, Baillière Tindall, p 473.

Ihrke PJ, et al: Urinary tract infection associated with long-term corticosteroid administration in dogs with chronic skin diseases, J Am Vet Med Assoc 186:43, 1985.

Kleinbeck ML, et al: Enzyme-linked immunosorbent assay for measurement of allergen-specific IgE antibodies in canine serum, Am J Vet Res 50:1831, 1989.

Lloyd DH: Essential fatty acids and skin disease, J Small Anim Pract 30:207, 1989.

Lloyd DH, Thomsett LR: Essential fatty acid supplementation in the treatment of canine atopy: a preliminary study, Vet Dermatol 1:41, 1989.

MacDonald JM, Angarano DW: Comparison of intradermal allergy testing with commercial in vitro allergy testing (ELISA) in parasitized and nonallergic Beagle Dogs. Proceedings, Annual members' meeting AAVD & ACVD, San Francisco, 1990, p 46.

Mason IS, Lloyd DH: Factors influencing the penetration of bacterial antigens through canine skin. In von Tscharner C, Halliwell REW (eds): Advances in veterinary dermatology, vol 1, London, 1990, Baillière Tindall, p 370.

McEwan NA: Bacterial adherence to canine corneocytes. In von Tscharner C, Halliwell REW (eds): Advances in veterinary dermatology, vol 1, London, 1990, Baillière Tindall, p 454.

Miller WH: Nonsteroidal antiinflammatory agents in the management of canine and feline pruritus. In Kirk RE (ed): Current veterinary therapy X, Philadelphia, 1989, WB Saunders, p 566.

Miller WH, et al: Clinical trial of DVM Derm Caps in the treatment of allergic diseases in 102 dogs, J Am Anim Hosp Assoc 25:163, 1989.

Miller WM, et al: Dermatologic disorders of the Chinese Shar-Pei: a retrospective analysis of 58 cases (1981 to 1989). Submitted, 1990.

Moriello KA, et al: Adrenocortical suppression associated with topical otic administration of glucocorticoids in dogs, J Am Vet Med Assoc 193:329, 1988.

Nave J: Personal communication, 1990.

Nimmo Wilkie JS: Cell-mediated immune function in dogs with atopic dermatitis. In von Tscharner C, Halliwell REW (eds): Advances in veterinary dermatology, vol 1, London, 1990, Baillière Tindall, p 145.

Paradis M, et al: Further investigations on the use of nonsteroidal and steroidal antiinflammatory agents in the management of canine pruritus, J Am Anim Hosp Assoc 27:44, 1991a.

Paradis M, et al: The efficacy of clemastin (Tavist), a fatty acid containing product (Derm-Caps), and the combination of both products in the management of canine pruritus, Vet Derm 2:17, 1991b.

Plant J, et al: Factors associated with and prevalence of increased Malassezia pachydermatis numbers on dog skin Proceedings, Annual members' meeting AAVD & ACVD, Scottsdale, 1991, p 22.

Platts-Mills TAF, et al: The role of dust mite allergens in atopic dermatitis, Clin Exp Dermatol 8:233, 1983.

Reedy LM, Miller WH: Allergic skin diseases of dogs and cats, Philadelphia, 1989, WB Saunders.

Reitamo S, et al: Eczematous reactions in atopic patients caused by epicutaneous testing with inhalent allergens, Br J Dermatol 114:303, 1986.

Rhodes KH, et al: Investigation into the immunopathogenesis of canine atopy, Semin Vet Med Surg (Small Anim) 2:199, 1987.

Scarff DH, Lloyd DH: Double-blind, placebo-controlled cross-over study of evening primrose oil in the treatment of canine atopy. Submitted 1990.

Schwartzman RM, et al: The atopic dog model: report of an attempt to establish a colony, Int Arch Allergy Appl Immunol 72:97, 1983.

Scott DW: Observations on canine atopy, J Am Anim Hosp Assoc 17:91, 1981.

Scott DW, Buerger RG: Nonsteroidal antiinflammatory agents in the management of canine pruritus, J Am Anim Hosp Assoc 24:425, 1988.

Scott DW, Miller WH: Nonsteroidal management of canine pruritus: chlorpheniramine and a fatty acid supplement (DVM Derm Caps) in combination and a fatty acid supplement at twice the manufacturer recommended dosage, Cornell Vet 80:381, 1990.

Shoulberg N: The efficacy of fluoxetine (Prozac) in the treatment of acral lick and allergic-inhalant dermatitis in canines, Proceedings, Annual members' meeting AAVD & ACVD, San Francisco, 1990, p 31.

Sousa CA, Norton AL: Advances in methodology for diagnosis of allergic skin disease, Vet Clin North Am Small Anim Pract 20:1419, 1990.

White PD: Evaluation of serum and cutaneous essential fatty acid profiles in normal, atopic, and seborrheic dogs, Proceedings, Annual members' meeting AAVD & ACVD, San Francisco, 1990, p 37.

Willemse A: Canine atopic disease: investigations of eosinophils and the nasal mucosa, Am J Vet Res 45:1867, 1984.

Willemse A, van den Brom WE: Investigations of the symptomatology and the significance of immediate skin test reactivity in canine atopic dermatitis, Res Vet Sci 34:261, 1983.

Willemse A, et al: Effect of hyposensitization on atopic dermatitis in dogs, J Am Vet Med Assoc 184:1277, 1984.

Willemse A, et al: Allergen-specific IgGd antibodies in dogs with atopic dermatitis, Clin Exp Immunol 59:359, 1985.

van den Broek AHM, Simpson JW: Fat absorption in dogs with atopic dermatitis. In von Tscharner C, Halliwell REW (eds): Advances in veterinary dermatology, vol 1, London, 1990, Baillière Tindall, p 155.

Van Stee EW: Risk factors in canine atopy, Calif Vet 4:8, 1983.

Zenoble RD, Kemppainen JR: Adrenocortical suppression by topically applied corticosteroids in healthy dogs, J Am Vet Med Assoc 191:685, 1987.

11

Food Allergy

John M. MacDonald

Importance

The incidence of food allergy in humans is variable, ranging from 0.3% to 7.5%. The observation of food allergy in infants is much higher than in adults and even greater in atopic children, in whom the incidence approaches 25% (Metcalfe, 1984).

The incidence of food allergy is definitely greater in people with other allergic disease.

The incidence of food allergy in veterinary medicine (dogs and cats) has also been deliberated, and much variation has been reported. Citations have varied from 1% to 23% of the population (Reedy and Miller, 1989). Most veterinary dermatologists agree that food allergy constitutes 10% to 20% of allergic responses in dogs.

Food allergy is most important, because it mimics other pruritic dermatopathies and coexists with other allergic conditions, often leading to its omission as an important differential. Yet it is one of the easier diseases to control by means of avoidance. Ignoring food allergy as a differential for a pruritic dog may either result in uncontrolled pruritus or require a high glucocorticoid dosage, posing a health risk. Evaluation for dietary hypersensitivity should be performed in all cases of intractable perennial pruritus.

Pathogenesis

Food allergy, or food hypersensitivity, is an immunologic reaction resulting from the ingestion of a food or food additive. Food intolerance is a general term describing an abnormal physiologic response to ingested food or food additives that does not include an immunologic mechanism but represents an idiosyncratic reaction involving metabolic, toxic, or pharmacologic effects of foods or food additives. Distinguishing between allergy and intolerance may be difficult and perhaps of more academic interest than clinical relevance.

The pathogenesis of food allergy has not been clarified in veterinary medicine. The most consistent pathomechanism in humans appears to be an immediate-type hypersensitivity. However, other types of immune responses have been observed with food allergy, including a delayed type of hypersensitivity.

CLINICAL DISEASE IN DOGS
History

The clinical history of food allergy in dogs is somewhat variable. The disease may start at any age, including very young and older animals. Food allergy should be strongly considered in any dog that develops pruritus prior to 6 months of age and in any dog that develops pruritus after 6 years of age with no previous history of cutaneous disease.

Nonseasonal pruritus is the most common clinical manifestation of food allergy and the reason for seeking veterinary attention in most cases. Food allergy is often associated with other pruritic dermatopathies, including canine atopy, flea allergy, and superficial staphylococcal pyoderma. Simultaneous occurrence of food allergy with canine atopy or flea allergy may cause a seasonal intensification of the pruritus, although most food allergic cases are intensely pruritic throughout the year.

The response of food-allergic dogs to conventional antiinflammatory doses of glucocorticoids is minimal in most cases. A food allergy component should be considered when a dog has been controlled by routine glucocorticoid therapy for atopy and suddenly becomes refractory to that treatment.

Historical questions may be helpful in establishing a presumptive or tentative diagnosis of food allergy, although the clinical features of the disease are comparable to other pruritic dermatoses. The association of abrupt dietary change with onset of pruritus is not a valid factor. Walton (1967) reported that 68% of patients with food hypersensitivity had been exposed to the allergen for over 2 years before becoming clinically symptomatic. The effect of specific foods may be difficult to determine without a dietary trial. On some occasions,

the owner may observe intensification of the clinical problem with introduction of certain foods, either commercial or from the table. A list of commercial dog foods, table foods, snacks, treats, and digestible chew toys should be part of the database. Specific questions regarding gastrointestinal disturbance likewise should be addressed in acquiring a history. Vomiting and diarrhea are seen with food allergy but represent a small percentage of cases. More critical evaluation of the history may reveal occasional borborygmus or flatus.

Recently a study (Frick, 1991) showed that the most common gastrointestinal change in experimentally induced canine food allergy is an increase in loose stools (to an average 3 per day).

Episodic food hypersensitivity may occur following intermittent exposure to the offensive diet from the table, predation, or eating garbage. This is especially true of cats, since owners tend to buy a wider variety of canned cat foods. Coprophagic

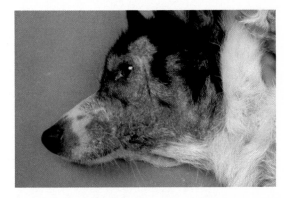

Figure 11-1. Food allergy in a dog, demonstrating extensive facial lesions from pruritus. Note the hair loss, erythema, and thickened appearance of the skin.

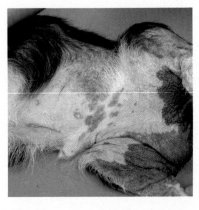

Figure 11-2. Same dog as in Fig. 11-1, showing inguinal lesions. Note the erythema and lichenified appearance of the skin.

dogs may obtain undigested material that could induce a food allergy.

Physical Examination

Although pruritus is the most common clinical sign of food allergy, it is not present in every case. Erythema with a papular eruption also commonly occurs. Urticaria and angioedema are less common clinical signs. There is much variation in the appearance and distribution of lesions, and any portion of the body can be involved. Young dogs may show generalized pruritus with no specific areas of involvement. Secondary scale and crust often appear and may be a primary owner complaint. Malodor is typically noticed when oiliness is present.

Most commonly, clinical signs mimic those of canine atopy with facial, ear, extremity, and ventral distribution (Figs. 11-1 and 11-2). In a recent study (Rosser, 1990) the ear region was most consistently involved (80%), followed by the feet (61%) and the inguinal region (53%). The axillary, anterior foreleg, and periorbital regions were nearly equal in occurrence (31% to 37%). The ear was the only area affected in 12 dogs (24%). Another pattern of clinical signs is similar to flea allergy dermatitis, affecting the lower back, tailhead region, and caudolateral thighs. A manifestation comparable to the appearance of canine scabies has also been associated with food allergy and may be more common in Labrador Retrievers (Figs. 11-3 to 11-7). A lymphadenopathy appears in some cases.

Certain breeds of dogs have a higher incidence of food allergy. In Rosser's (1990) prospective study of 51 dogs, Laborador Retrievers represented 18% of the population and Cocker Spaniels, Golden Retrievers, and German Shepherd Dogs were also overrepresented. In the Southeastern United States the Shar-Pei and Poodle may be at greater risk.

The primary differentials of food allergy are canine scabies and atopy.

DIAGNOSIS

There are a variety of proposed methods of diagnostic testing for food allergy.

Laboratory Test Procedures

Laboratory test procedures have the convenience of rapid and easy acquisition of information regarding potential allergens. Either a radioallergosorbent test (RAST) or an enzyme-linked im-

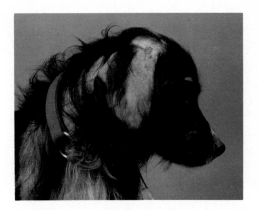

Figure 11-3. Food allergy in a dog with extensive pinnal hair loss as a result of persistent scratching. These clinical features are similar to the appearance of canine scabies.

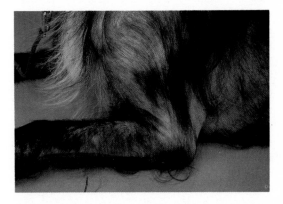

Figure 11-4. Same dog as in Fig. 11-3, showing involvement of a foreleg. The ventrum was comparably affected, as were the other legs.

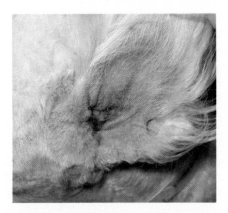

Figure 11-5. Food allergy in a Poodle, demonstrating otitis externa. Note the extension of lesions affecting most of the underside of the pinna and the increased wax buildup.

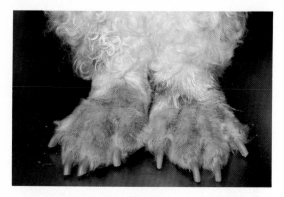

Figure 11-6. Same dog as in Fig. 11-5, showing po-dodermatitis and evidence of self-inflicted lesions from foot chewing.

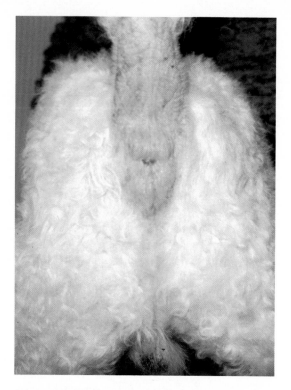

Figure 11-7. Perianal region of the dog in Fig. 11-5, showing erythema and skin thickening due to compulsive licking in this area as a result of food allergy.

muosorbent assay (ELISA) is commercially available for evaluating circulating IgE levels. Although the advantage of these tests is obvious, their correlation with actual food hypersensitivity is not known. There have been reports (Sampson and Albergo, 1984; Bjorksten, 1988) of good correlation in humans between in vitro test procedures and skin testing and food allergy. This has not been documented in veterinary medicine. Instead studies by McDougal (1987) and Jeffers et al. (1991) suggest a lack of correlation between food allergy, RAST, or ELISA results and in vivo intradermal allergy test results. Positive predictive values were recently determined to be 40% whereas negative predictive values were 60.9% (Jeffers et al., 1991). The results of intradermal allergy testing appear to be superior. The overall consensus of most dermatologists is that dietary trials are a more effective method of diagnosis. Standardizing a diet based on in vitro test results provides minimal advantage over empirical decision making without prior testing.

Intradermal Allergy Testing

Intradermal allergy testing for foods has long been utilized for identification of offending antigens in human allergy, and with some reports of good correlation. Much controversy exists in veterinary allergy. Studies that have been conducted to determine overall reliability have shown similar shortcomings with intradermal test procedures as with in vitro testing. Recent findings (Jeffers et al., 1991) indicate that, based on a positive predictive value, there is a 60% chance that a dog demonstrating clinical allergy to a food will demonstrate a positive reaction on intradermal testing. A negative allergy test to foods has a predictive value of

62.3% that the animal will not be food-allergic.

Many veterinary allergists (and I also) utilize a collection of representative food substances in the intradermal allergy test. Incorporating foods with other allergens minimizes the additional expense for this evaluation. Since many food-allergic dogs concurrently have either atopy or flea allergy, it merits evaluation with these other allergens. The exact identification of specific offending food substances may lack correlation. However, the recognition of positive food antigen reactions on an intradermal test suggests that the animal may be food-allergic. This can then be confirmed by elimination trials. The procedure is used as a screening test, with increased suspicion of a food allergy component when several food allergens show strong positive reactions. The diagnosis should be confirmed with a dietary trial. The strong possibility of several food allergens demands more complete evaluation than either skin tests or in vitro testing can provide.

Dietary Restriction

Confirmation of food allergy can be determined only by an elimination trial. The diet is restricted to a specific food determined by the animal's previous exposure and known reactions. The preferred diet is home-prepared and simplified to include a protein source and a carbohydrate source. The primary objective is to select a food combination to which the animal has minimal or no history of previous exposure. This may require reviewing the list of ingredients of commercial dog foods and treats. Although a lamb and rice combination has recently been in vogue for dietary trials, the prevalence of these substances in commercial feed is limiting its usefulness. Protein sources include lamb, fish, venison, rabbit, tofu, and pinto beans. Rice has conventionally been the carbohydrate source of choice, but it should be restricted to either whole grain brown rice or rice that has undergone minimal processing. This excludes products that have been preprocessed for rapid cooking. Another carbohydrate source that may be substitiued for rice is potato. Preparation of the potato should not include milk or butter. Three standard diets are lamb and rice (or potato), fish and rice (or potato), and pinto beans and rice (or potato). Tofu has been used successfully but has two major disadvantages: poor palatability and low caloric density (i.e., it fails to provide adequate satiety). Tofu is composed of soybean, and this restricts its use if the commercial food contains soy.

Various methods can be used to prepare the restricted diet. The food can be stewed, baked, boiled, broiled, or microwaved. Shoulder roasts or larger cuts of meat are more economical and easier to prepare. The meat may be removed from the bone prior to cooking and placed in a food processor for chopping. Meat should not be boned by the butcher and ground through a meat grinder due to the strong possibility of contamination by other meat allergens, including beef or pork. The meat should be mixed with the cooked rice at a ratio of one part meat or protein to three or four parts carbohydrate. Tofu is best boiled.

Some pet owners prefer to buy baby food for small dogs. Selection of the food type should follow the same guidelines relative to previous exposure. Some also supplement the home-prepared food with baby food. The restricted diet **must exclude** all other food sources, including table scraps, chew toys, treats, and access to other animals' food. Predation is a primary concern with cats. Dogs that are coprophagic must be carefully monitored to eliminate the undigested protein from cat litter or other dog feces. Although some veterinary allergists suggest using distilled water for drinking, it is my experience that this has but minimal effect on the large percentage of food-allergic dogs.

Chewable heartworm preventive pills should be replaced with diethylcarbamazine (in an unchewable form), ivermectin, or milbemycin. Chewable vitamins likewise should be avoided. Supplementation with a multivitamin may be used during the elimination trial, although it probably is not necessary for the length of the trial. Concern is often expressed about young growing dogs placed on a home-prepared elimination diet. An option to balancing a home-prepared diet is to select one of the commercial foods listed in Table 11-1 with protein supplementation. Any vitamin-mineral supplement during an elimination trial should be the nonchewable variety and **not** derived from a plant source. Consulting with nutritionists for advice about specific breed requirements may be helpful. I have not had any problems using a limited trial of 4 to 8 weeks with home-prepared diets containing a multivitamin-mineral supplement.

Problems encountered during a trial may include inappetance, vomiting, diarrhea, or constipation. Dogs fed fresh lamb are more likely to develop diarrhea. This can be decreased by trimming all the fat from the meat, although some animals will have persistent loose stools even with lean meat. The trial should be terminated and the diet modified if gastrointestinal disturbance continues. Another trial should be undertaken with different food after the problem has been resolved. Potato may be substituted if constipation is noted with rice. Some stool softeners contain food-derived products; these should be avoided. Occasionally a dog will not eat the desired food for the trial. It may be necessary to try other foods to find one with proper appeal.

Owners will often want to give their pets treats during the elimination diet. Using the same or similar ingredients as the main diet provides an option that does not compromise the trial. Small treats of meat may be saved during the food preparation. Rice cakes from the grocery or health food store are compatible with a rice-based diet. Some commercial foods (e.g., Nature's Recipe Lamb and Rice Kibble) have compatible biscuits for use as treats. Restricting treats to a minimum is suggested to avoid the introduction of several variables. Some pets are accustomed to receiving fruits or vegetables for treats, which I have not recognized as a major problem. The treats incriminated most often as adversely affecting the dietary trial are dog biscuits containing milk, beef jerky treats, rawhide chew toys, and other treats consisting of meat, meat by-products, or dairy products.

The most difficult part of the trial is avoiding any other food. Pitfalls include households with more than one dog, where there is access to another's food. Pets on elimination diets fed table

Table 11-1. Selected diets for food-allergic dogs

MANUFACTURER	NAME OF DIET	PRIMARY INGREDIENTS	TYPE OF FOOD
Nature's Recipe	Lamb & Rice Kibble	Ground whole wheat, lamb meat meal, rice, wheat bran, lamb and mutton fat, tomato pomace, lamb bone meal	Dry
Nature's Recipe	Rabbit & Rice	Rabbit (lungs, kidneys, spleens, livers, hearts), brown rice, potatoes, carrots, peas	Cans
Hill	d/d	Whole chicken egg and brewer's rice	Dry
Natural Life	Lamaderm	Brown rice, lamb meal, grain sorghum, oatmeal, animal fat, flaxseed, alfalfa meal, kelp	Dry
Natural Life	Lamaderm	Lamb, brown rice, peas, carrots, dried kelp	Cans
Iams	Eukanuba	Poultry by-product meal, chicken, corn, rice flour, poultry fat, beet pulp, meat meal, dried whole egg, brewer's yeast	Dry
Iams	Lamb & Rice	Lamb meat, rice flour, ground corn, whole egg, fish meal, beet pulp, animal fat	Dry
Protocol	Canine Formula 4r	Rabbit and brown rice	Cans
	Canine Formula 4c	Whole dressed chicken, brown rice, chicken liver	Cans
Wysong Medical	Anergen	Lamb meal, chicken, brown rice, flaxseed, quinoa, yeast, flaxseed oil, spirulina palentensis, kelp, garlic, dried aspergillus	Dry
Wayne (Royal Canin)	Lamb & Rice	Lamb meal, brewer's rice, wheat, poultry fat	Dry
Wayne (Royal Canin)	Lamb & Rice Puppy Formula	Lamb meal, brewer's rice, ground wheat, poultry fat	Dry
Lick Your Chops	Mutton & Rice	Mutton, mutton liver, brown rice, carrots, peas, kelp	Cans
Nutro Products	Lamb Meal & Rice	Lamb meal, ground rice, wheat flour, rice bran, safflower oil, dried whole egg, natural flavors	Dry

foods by children are also a concern, since this would invalidate the test results. Food that falls from the high chair may disrupt the dietary trial. Owners need to be coached about problem areas for optimal exclusion of extraneous food sources. Putting the dog in a transport kennel or a fenced-in backyard, utility room, garage, or some other room may help during regular family meals or when feeding other pets. Family outings, picnics, and visits to fast-food stores may lead to impulse feeding of the dog in trial. Gracious neighbors and delivery people likewise may reward the pet with snacks, interfering with the trial.

Dietary Standardization

Many pet owners resist conducting an elimination trial with home-prepared food but are willing to restrict the diet to a single commercial food. The diets listed in Table 11-1 are suitable for this purpose. Three Nature's Recipe varieties (Lamb & Rice Kibble, Rabbit & Rice canned food, and non-meat diet) and Hill's Dry d/d have been effective for this procedure. Other options include Iams Eukanuba, Natural Life Dry Lamb & Rice Dog Food, and Protocol Rabbit & Rice Diet. This approach provides a conservative means of evaluating food allergy, although it is somewhat compromised compared to home-prepared fresh food because of the several ingredients and additives present. This procedure is becoming more popular because of the labor intensiveness and cost of home-prepared hypoallergenic diets. Dietary standardization is not as useful either to confirm food allergy or to identify food allergens, but it is a practical method of evaluating a food-allergic suspect.

Length of an Elimination Trial

The duration of a food trial has been debated for some time. The most recent evidence suggests that dietary restriction should be prolonged. In the prospective study conducted by Rosser, only 25% of the food-allergic dogs showed demonstrable change of the pruritus within 3 weeks (conventionally the termination point used by many veterinarians), whereas 59% showed improvement within 6 weeks. The remaining 41% showed a response between 6 and 10 weeks. It is obvious that premature cessation of the dietary trial may lead to erroneous conclusions about food allergy.

The most difficult aspect of conducting a dietary trial of this duration is owner compliance. Not only are cost factors an important consideration, but of-

ten the irresistability of providing other dietary sources is a concern that may invalidate the dietary trial. The labor involved with food preparation likewise is a deterrent for conducting a long trial. Convincing arguments for conducting a dietary trial should be advanced before the onset. Supportive understanding of the undertaking should be shared. I routinely tell pet owners the procedure is more important than any diagnostic test I could do and may provide the solution to the problem. Coaching pet owners through the trial is essential and often the difference between success and failure.

Monitoring the Dietary Trial

Frequent evaluation of response to the dietary elimination trial is mandatory. During the time of the dietary trial, it is important to control coexistent factors that may potentiate the pruritus and obscure the results. The two most important, and often coexistent, diseases are flea allergy dermatitis and superficial pruritic pyoderma. Consistent use of parasiticides may be required to control the clinical signs of flea allergy dermatitis. Antibiotics may be required during outbreaks of pyoderma. Selection of antibiotics sometimes requires elimination of those that have known antiinflammatory activity (e.g., trimethoprim-potentiated sulfas, erythromycin, tetracycline). The coexistent use of antipruritic medication during both the elimination and challenge phase of the dietary trial should be avoided. However, glucocorticoid therapy may be needed during the first 14 to 20 days of the dietary trial to control intense pruritus and self-mutilation. After this time the steroids are terminated, the restricted diet is continued, and the patient continues to be evaluated. If the pruritus persists, medication can be reinstituted and the above procedure repeated at intervals throughout the trial period (8 to 10 weeks).

It is important to monitor both the change in pruritus and the observation of clinical lesions. This requires periodic examinations in the clinic. It is helpful for the owner to monitor the improvement during the dietary trial, but the owner's interpretation cannot be relied on as the exclusive method of evaluation. Assessment is best done by reporting the percent change in degree of pruritus. The value may vary from 0% to 100% and actually, in some situations, may be associated with worsening of the condition in a non–food-allergic dog. It is important to monitor not only the intensity of the pruritus during the trial period but also the location of the pruritus and the pet's itching habits (e.g., foot chewing, face rubbing, ear scratching, groin licking). This may be better validated by using a diary to record these observations. A placebo effect may occur in some cases. The percent of improvement may represent less than complete resolution of the pruritus. Food allergy combined with canine atopy may show partial response, but usually greater than 40% improvement occurs.

Dietary Challenge

The confirmation of food allergy can be made only after optimal improvement of the case and conducting a dietary challenge. The challenge most often uses the single most common diet fed before the elimination trial. Some owners may be reluctant to institute a dietary challenge, particularly if the improvement has been considerable. It is important to follow through with careful monitoring of the dietary challenge even when the owners may feel the improvement has been minimal. Often the improvement is so gradual that the change is not as noteworthy to the owner. There is persistent pruritus due to coexisting allergic disease, which further obscures the observation. However, when the animal is challenged, there may be a pronounced increase in the pruritic intensity, which often is a significant recognition of allergy to that food. Reversal of manifestations after return to the elimination diet provides further evidence of a causal relationship. Since most food-allergic dogs have coexistent pruritic problems, there is the likelihood of encountering this situation.

If antibiotics were administered during the elimination trial, they should be continued through the challenge. The interpretation is more difficult in cases of nonpruritic food-allergic individuals that have a chronic relapsing pyoderma as the most consistent problem. In these cases the relapsing tendency of the pyoderma is the only method of determining the association with food allergy. Observing the recurrence of the pyoderma upon food challenge is evidence of the relationship.

Cooperative clients may prefer to document food allergy by utilizing specific foods as a challenge. Fresh meat, including chicken, beef, pork, or turkey, is readily accessible from the grocery store. Since the bias of dietary challenge is not as prominent with animals as with people, the use of double-blind, placebo-controlled food challenges is not necessary. Other sources of food allergens include powdered milk, which may be added to the elimination diet to evaluate milk allergy. A variety of cereal grains (wheat, soy meal, corn, rye, oats) may be obtained from health food stores for food challenge.

It is important for the pet owner to use only one food at a time for challenge. Likewise, in the event of relapse (intensification of pruritus or dermatitis) during the challenge, the animal should be returned to the elimination diet for a time to return to the prechallenge level of clinical signs before another test food is added. Response to challenge usually does not require more than 3 to 5 days, and the return to prechallenge level requires less time than the response noted during the original trial. In general most dogs respond to the elimination diet subsequent to the challenge within 14 days. Another food may be used for challenge if there is no reaction after 7 days to the previous food challenge.

Potential cross-reactivity of food allergens with other foods or with environmental substances is also a concern. Approximately 42% of dogs allergic to either beef or milk "showed" reactions to both upon challenge whereas reactivity "observed" to both chicken meat and whole chicken egg was 33% (Jeffers et al., 1991).

TREATMENT

The treatment of choice is avoidance of the offending food antigens. The ideal diet would be commercially available, contain a simplified ingredient list, and be readily accessible, nutritionally complete, and reasonably priced. The feasibility of satisfying all these factors is slim in most cases. A selective list of dog foods that can be used is found in Table 11-1. The ingredients in these foods are quite variable. Confusion arises when different food sources are used in products with the same name. For example, the dry form of Hill's d/d contains whole chicken egg and brewer's rice, which has shown good efficacy in controlling food-allergic animals. However, the canned form of d/d contains mutton and rice. In one study (White, 1986) the canned form of this product caused pruritus in 54% of food-allergic dogs when challenged. Most food-allergic dogs are allergic to several foods. This makes formulating an ideal diet more difficult.

Another food with recognized effectiveness in controlling food allergy is Nature's Recipe Lamb & Rice Kibble, which also contains other ingredients, including wheat. Nature's Recipe also produces a rabbit and rice diet and a nonmeat diet, as does Protocol. Natural Life produces a hypoallergenic diet called Lamaderm for dogs and cats that contains lamb and rice. Protocol also makes a chicken-based dog food. Eukanuba, made by Iams, has been used for dogs, and this company now makes canned chicken for cats. Wysong's hypoallergenic dog food, Anergen, originally contained lamb and rice but recently has been modified to include chicken. Lick Your Chops is a lamb-and-rice–based canned food that has been developed for both dogs and cats.

It appears that most food hypersensitivity is derived from the protein or carbohydrate ingredients, unlike previous concerns about food additives and preservatives. Offending allergens most often incriminated in my experience are beef or cow's milk. The natural exclusion of meat or meat by-products, as well as whey, is definitely important in achieving the ideal food.

Some animals develop hypersensitivity reactions to their restricted diet over a period of time. A new elimination trial may be necessary using different food sources. The use of chromolyn has produced conflicting reports on its benefit in the treatment of food allergy in people, but it has not been evaluated adequately in veterinary medicine. Alternate-day prednisone therapy may be necessary, depending on the coexistent allergies previously discussed. Reevaluation of clinical cases depends on the control attained by diet restriction and the presence of other coexistent pruritic problems. Home-prepared hypoallergenic diets have been helpful in situations where commercial diets have failed and the owners have had the food items, time, and financial means for this procedure. Provisions for a balanced home-prepared diet have been developed by the Hill Pet Products Company, Topeka, Kansas.

CLINICAL DISEASE IN CATS

Food allergy has been recognized as a major cause of pruritus in cats. The clinical manifestations are highly variable. Food allergy is more common in cats than in dogs and should be considered a major differential in animals that are self-mutilative. As in dogs, the pathomechanism in cats has not been well-established, although immunologic hypersensitivities, including Type 1 reactions, are likely.

History

Historical findings associated with food allergy in cats may include prolonged exposure to the dietary source. The foods causing the allergy may be more difficult to determine in the cat because of the variety of food used in commercial diets. As a matter of fact, the marketing of these "banquet varieties" provides exposure to a wider variety of potentially offending allergens. Some veterinarians consider fish diets a common cause of food allergy in the cat. Practically any food can be the source of the problem, including wild animals caught by cats. A historical account of the animal's habitat and surroundings may be helpful in determining potential exposure. Identification of the animal's primary diet, as well as table scraps provided, is also an essential part of the history.

A dietary trial is often avoided due to the popular belief that cats tolerate respositol glucocorticoid therapy (methylprednisolone acetate) and it is so efficacious for many pruritic cats. Megestrol acetate is often inappropriately used if there is little or no response to the glucocorticoid regimen. Food allergy in cats is usually refractory to glucocorticoids and megestrol acetate. A combination of other pruritic diseases will also affect response to symptomatic treatment. Feline atopy, a once overlooked diagnosis, appears to be more common than at first realized and may be associated with coexistent food allergy.

Physical Examination

The clinical signs associated with food allergy in cats are quite variable, with pruritus predominating. Clinical features may resemble "feline miliary dermatitis" syndrome, characterized by excessive miliary crusting with pruritus. The face and head show the classical distribution pattern of food allergy in the cat (Figs. 11-8 and 11-9). Multifocal ulcerative lesions infiltrated with eosinophils are often observed in food-allergic animals (Fig. 11-

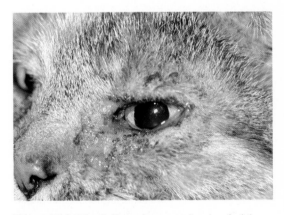

Figure 11-8. Food allergy in a cat, showing facial dermatitis and periocular excoriations.

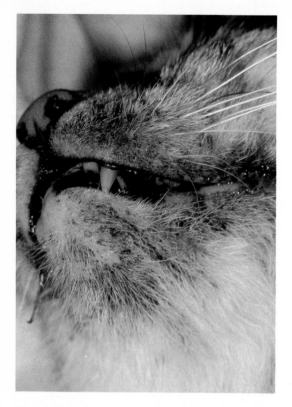

Figure 11-9. Same cat as in Fig. 11-8, showing further signs of facial pruritus affecting the chin and muzzle.

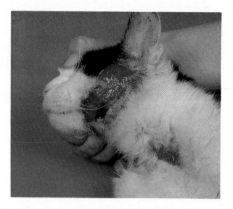

Figure 11-10. Food allergy in a cat, showing multifocal ulcerative lesions located in the region of the head and neck. These self-inflicted lesions are often misdiagnosed as "idiopathic eosinophilic plaques" because of their appearance and the dermal infiltrate of eosinophils demonstrated on dermatohistopathology.

10). Unfortunately, these lesions may be confused with the syndrome eosinophilic granuloma complex and be passed over as an idiopathic problem without the proper diagnostic pursuit. Food allergy sometimes manifests as pruritus and crusting dermatitis on the lower back with an associated alopecia of the caudal abdomen and inguinal region produced by excessive licking similar to flea allergy dermatitis. Hair loss on the medial aspects of the forelegs or in the axillae or the observation of compulsive foot licking suggests food allergy or coexistent atopy. Generalization of the pruritus and lesions may be anticipated when the problem is chronic. Some cases may reach total-body involvement.

Differential Diagnosis

Food allergy should be considered in the differential diagnosis of all pruritic cats and in particular for those with facial involvement and poor responsiveness to conventional glucocorticoid therapy. The differential diagnoses of food allergy in the cat must include feline atopy, feline scabies *(Notoedres cati), Cheyletiella* dermatitis, and dermatophytosis. Flea allergy dermatitis is often seen as a coexistent problem in the southeastern United States.

DIAGNOSIS

Diagnostic testing should include rule-out of ectoparasitic and mycotic etiologies. A routine skin scraping should be performed, as well as a dermatophyte test medium culture. Intradermal allergy testing with flea antigen is helpful to determine the presence of flea allergy. Complete intradermal allergy testing may be used to identify feline atopy. Allergen selection can include foods, although there is little known about the correlation of intradermal allergy test results and food allergy in cats. Positive reactivity to food allergen does not confirm the diagnosis of food allergy, nor does negative reaction rule out food allergy.

The diagnostic test of choice includes a restricted diet, much as in dogs. Lamb baby food has been widely used as a standard for the elimination diet in cats. A lamb diet should not be used if it has been part of the regular diet prior to the trial. The predatory nature of cats may pose difficulties in performing dietary trials. Finicky appetite associated with certain foods used in the trial or boredom with the diet after initiation of the trial are also problems. Environmental restriction of cats is mandatory during food trials. The cat must not be allowed outside, and its access to house foods from the table or garbage must be prevented. Dietary trials should be continued for a minimum of 4 to

Table 11-2. Selected diets for food-allergic cats

MANUFACTURER	NAME OF DIET	PRIMARY INGREDIENTS	TYPE OF FOOD
Nature's Recipe	Rabbit & Rice	Rabbit (lungs, kidneys, liver, spleen, heart) brown rice	Cans
Protocol	Feline Formula 4c	Chicken (whole dressed), brown rice, chicken liver	Cans
Lick Your Chops	Lamb & Rice	Lamb, lamb liver, rice gluten, brown rice, corn, whole eggs, dried kelp	Cans
Iams	Chicken Formula Cat Food	Chicken, poultry liver, whole egg, rice	Cans
Wysong Medical	Feline Anergen	Poultry, poultry by-products, brown rice, oat groats, poultry fat, lamb meal, flaxseed, spray-dried digest of liver, kelp	Dry
Hill's	Feline d/d	Lamb by-products, water, lamb liver, rice, rice flour, powdered cellulose	Cans

6 weeks, or possibly longer if tolerated by the animal. The trial may be terminated prior to this if there is enough improvement of clinical signs. The question of taurine supplementation has been controversial and remains an individual preference, although most nutritionists feel it is not likely that the cat will develop a deficiency during the time interval of this dietary restriction. Fresh meats contain sufficient taurine without supplementation. Commercial taurine supplements may be used.

In lieu of performing an elimination trial, some commercial foods may be used to standardize the diet. Foods such as Nature's Recipe Rabbit & Rice, Iams Chicken Formula Cat Food, Wysong's Hypoallergenic Cat Food, or Lick Your Chops Mutton & Rice are useful for this purpose (Table 11-2). Control of ectoparasitic diseases, such as fleas, is essential during the dietary trial to avoid the coexistence of other pruritic sources. To eliminate the coexistence of a bacterial folliculitis, antibiotics should be used (especially in cats with a crusting dermatitis) before the dietary trial. Dietary trials are best conducted without any concurrent medication, particularly those that would obscure observation of the response. Antihistamines or glucocorticoids may be needed during the initial 2 to 3 weeks of the dietary trial for symptomatic relief in the intensely pruritic cat. To create an observation window in the trial, withdrawal of **all** medication is essential. This is best performed 3 or 4 weeks after beginning the trial. The response observed may be acute, with abrupt resolution of the

lesions and pruritus over a short time. Other cases require a longer trial period, with a slower resolution observed. Monitoring the patient is critical and should include both the owner's input and intermittent clinical examinations with observation of physical lesions.

Dietary challenge may be utilized following noticeable improvement or resolution of the clinical signs. Options include identification of specific offensive allergens, which is best attained by the introduction of individual food substances (e.g., cow's milk, ground beef, poultry, fish, and other foods identified from the history). Another approach is to identify a commercial diet that is known to be an offending diet by evaluation of the commercial foods previously used before the elimination diet was started.

TREATMENT

As with dogs, the treatment of choice in cats is avoidance. Selective commercial foods may be used as "hypoallergenic diets." (See Table 11-2.) Commercially available diets are best for maintenance of cats with food allergy, although restrictions may be observed in certain animals with several food reactivities. Home-prepared hypoallergenic diets have more limitations in cats than in dogs due to the wide availability of food substances and the unique requirements of cats, as well as their finicky appetites.

The recurrence of food allergy appears to be more common in cats than in dogs, although studies have not been performed to verify this. It is not unusual to observe relapses when cats develop allergy to newer foods. At this point reevaluation by selection of a different hypoallergenic diet is necessary to provide further evaluation of the problem. Complications occur by the association of other pruritic dermatopathies, including feline atopy and flea allergy, which may be misinterpreted as a recurrence of the food allergy itself. Critical evaluation of therapeutic trials with parasiticides and antiinflammatory drugs is necessary. Treatment of coexistent problems is essential to maintaining optimal reduction of the pruritus in these animals. Allergy testing and hyposensitization therapy for atopy should be considered. Alternate-day oral prednisone therapy may also be considered, in addition to antihistamines, to provide symptomatic relief of pruritus. Reevaluation of recurrent pruritus should include acquiring a fungal culture from any animal that has been placed on glucocorticoid therapy, since dermatophytosis may result as a complication.

Long-term control of the food-allergic animal requires the persistent cooperation of the pet owner. Once the animal becomes normal after being changed to a special diet there may be more laxity in the restriction of food. Nevertheless, continued effort is necessary to maintain a standardized diet so allergenic foods are avoided and allergic symptoms do not recur.

REFERENCES

Bjorksten B: New diagnostic methods in food allergy, Ann Allergy 59:150, 1988.

Frick OL: Pathogenesis of chronic allergic reactions using the atopic dog as a model. In Proceedings, AVA, Scottsdale, 1991, p 7.

Jeffers J, et al: Diagnostic testing of dogs for food hypersensitivity, J Am Vet Med Assoc 198:245, 1991.

McDougal BJ: Correlation of results of the radioallergosorbent test and provocative testing in 20 dogs with food allergy, Proc Am Acad Vet Dermatol 3:42, 1987.

Metcalfe DD: Food hypersensitivity, J Allergy Clin Immunol 73:749, 1984.

Reedy LM, Miller WH: Allergic skin diseases of dogs and cats, Philadelphia, 1989, WB Saunders.

Rosser EJ: Food allergy in the dog: a prospective study of 51 dogs. In Proceedings, Annual members' meeting AAVD & ACVD, 1990.

Sampson HA, Albergo R: Comparison of results of skin tests, RAST, and double-blind, placebo-controlled food challenges in children with atopic dermatitis, J Allergy Clin Immunol 74:26, 1984.

Walton GS: Skin responses in the dog and cat to ingested allergens: observations on 100 confirmed cases, Vet Rec 81:709, 1967.

White SD: Food hypersensitivity in 30 dogs, J Am Vet Med Assoc 188:695, 1986.

SUGGESTED READINGS

Bahna SL: Diagnostic tests for food allergy, Clin Rev Allergy 6:259, 1988.

Metcalfe DD: Disease of food hypersensitivity, N Engl J Med 321:255, 1989.

12

Insect and Arachnid Hypersensitivity

Craig E. Griffin

Diagnostic Criteria for Insect and Arachnid Hypersensitivity

SUGGESTIVE

Pruritic dermatitis (seasonal, or seasonally more severe) that involves short or sparsely haired areas such as the bridge of the nose, pinna, muzzle, groin, and distal extremities

COMPATIBLE

A suggestive case that is not responsive to a hypoallergenic diet, that is negative on intradermal testing for common inhalant allergens, and, if nonseasonal, that is not responsive or is only temporarily responsive to treatment for sarcoptic mange

TENTATIVE

A compatible case that is positive on intradermal testing to insect allergens; the patient may improve with aggressive insect control or with changing of the environment to one relatively insect-free (e.g., boarded in a veterinary hospital) Eosinophilic perivascular dermatitis may be present in biopsy

DEFINITIVE

A definitive diagnosis requires both a tentative diagnosis and confirmation with provocative exposure

Importance

Insect and arachnid hypersensitivities other than flea allergy dermatitis are not often considered as causes of dermatitis in small animals. Many pruritic dogs, especially young ones with seasonal and nonseasonal pruritus, are diagnosed as having idiopathic pruritus after negative workups for food allergy, flea allergy, and atopic disease. About 10% of clinically diagnosed atopic dogs will have negative results on intradermal testing to pollen, flea, and house-dust mite antigen. In one Southern California study, 202 suspect canine atopics were intradermal tested; of these, 4.5% were insect/arachnid positive but negative to all the other 62 allergens tested, including fleas and house-dust mites. In Las Vegas, Nevada, where there are no fleas, 8.3% of 48 atopic suspects were positive to these organisms only and 6.3% were totally negative when intradermally tested with 62 antigens. If we assume that the 6.3% were suffering from insect/arachnid allergy then, had the offending organism not been tested for, some 14.6% of the cases would have remained undiagnosed. The diagnosis of an insect/arachnid hypersensitivity should be considered in these cases.

The response to hyposensitization in canine atopy is about 60%. It is likely that some of these failures to hyposensitization reflect our inability to detect causative allergens. It has been my experience that skin test–negative results in atopic suspects and some failures in hyposensitization therapy are due to undetected insect/arachnid hypersensitivities. These patients are usually then treated indefinitely with systemic glucocorticoids.

The diagnosis of hypersensitivity may replace one of idiopathic pruritus, and specific immunotherapy or avoidance may prevent the need for glucocorticoid therapy.

Pathogenesis

An insect/arachnid hypersensitivity is an allergic reaction (usually Type I, Type IV, or cutaneous basophil hypersensitivity) to an allergen produced by the organism. In the case of biting insects, this is often a protein present in the insect's saliva. Nonbiting insects (e.g., houseflies, cockroaches, aphids), as well as biting and stinging insects (ants, bees), may also have allergenic proteins (Reisman, 1988). This is well-documented with house-dust mites, which produce specific allergens that are also present in their fecal material (Hellreich, 1962; Platts-Mills et al., 1983).

Allergic reactions to the bites of fleas, mosquitos, blackflies, chiggers, lice, bedbugs, kissing bugs, deerflies, and ants have been described in humans. However, insects may cause disease without biting the affected patient. In humans, well-documented allergic reactions have been reported to cockroaches, caddis fly wings, and chironomids (Kino et al., 1987; Kang, 1990). Provocation tests (Kino and Oshima, 1978; Tee et al, 1985; Ostrom et al, 1986) have shown that butterfly, moth, housefly, and honeybee body dust can cause allergic asthma in humans and may be detected in rare cases as occupational allergies. Numerous nonbiting insects induce IgE responses in humans (Baldo and Panzani, 1988). Cockroach allergy may manifest as dermatitis, and in entomologists, occupational arthropod dermatitis may occur in as many as one third of workers (Kang, 1990). Similar to human atopic dermatitis associated with house-dust mite antigen, the incidence of cockroach allergy is related to the rate of household infestation (Kang, 1990). Additionally, topical application of cockroach antigen in sensitive patients induces local eosinophilia.

Besides these studies documenting allergic reaction to insect body parts without biting, there is other compelling evidence to support insect/arachnid allergies as a cause of clinical disease. It has been shown that positive skin tests are much more common in asthma patients that failed routine hyposensitization than in patients responding to hyposensitization (Hellreich, 1962). Additionally, cockroach-allergic patients that had failed pollen hyposensitization therapy were notably improved following cockroach hyposensitization therapy (Kang et al., 1988).

Depending on the organism and the environment, exposure to insect/arachnid antigens may show marked seasonal fluctuations (Kino et al., 1987). In one study (Lierl et al., 1990) moth antigen rose in April and persisted to September, but in another (Wynn et al., 1988) it peaked in June and in August-September. Insect/arachnid antigens generally peak in summer and early fall, the seasons that coincide with increased severity in many allergic dogs. Outdoor air samples contain insect allergens to ants, crickets, moths, and flies in quantities comparable to common aeroallergens of pollens and molds (Lierl et al., 1990).

CLINICAL DISEASE
History

No age, breed, or sex predilections are yet known. Similar to atopy, the disease tends to occur in young to middle-aged animals. One feature of insect/arachnid hypersensitivity that may help raise the clinician's index of suspicion is a sudden onset; this is in contrast to what happens with atopy.

The history for an insect/arachnid hypersensitivity will depend on which type of syndrome is seen. In general these disorders have a seasonal pattern, although it may be continuous. Most commonly the history is similar to that for dogs or cats with atopic disease. The abdomen, groin, legs, and face are most severely affected, but localized lesions may occur. All or some of these areas may be affected. Most of insect/arachnid hypersensitivity cases are also atopic or flea-allergic, which may modify the history. In some cases (e.g., tick bites, stable flies, chiggers, fire ants) clients may be aware of the animal's exposure to the inciting insect. However, a history of exposure may not be obtainable.

Physical Examination

Physical examination findings are variable depending on the type of organism and the pathologic mechanism involved in the reaction. The most common sign is pruritus associated with a maculopapular rash. Chronic pruritus results in alopecia, lichenification, and excoriations. Secondary pyodermas are common, characterized by crusted papules, pustules, and lichenified plaques. The abdomen, groin, ventral thorax, axilla, face, and legs are most commonly affected (Fig. 12-1). Any one or a combination of these sites may be affected in a particular case.

Nodules and papules induced by mosquito bites

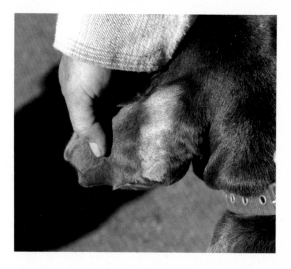

Figure 12-1. Note the erythema and discoloration in the groin, abdomen, and axilla of a Dalmatian with insect/arachnid hypersensitivity. This dog was negative to other antigens on intradermal tests and did not respond to a hypoallergenic diet.

Figure 12-2. Fly bite granulomatous plaque on the dorsal convex pinna in a German Shorthaired Pointer. Histopathology showed a multinodular lymphogranulomatous dermatitis.

in cats are usually found on the bridge of the nose and pinna. Stable flies occasionally induce a granulomatous reaction, producing nodules or plaques and varying degrees of alopecia on the most dorsal aspect of the pinna, either the convex base in dogs with pendulous ears or the apex in erect-eared dogs (Fig. 12-2). Ticks may induce nodules due to granuloma formation at the site of attachment.

Acute-onset nasal dermatitis may be observed. Pruritic papules and nodules will be found on the bridge of the nose. Chronic lesions may be ulcerated and may develop a thickened, fibrotic plaque. Secondary infection will cause these cases to mimic nasal furunculosis (Fig. 12-3).

The differential diagnoses of insect hypersensitivity in the dog are primarily atopy, food allergy, nasal pyoderma, and scabies, although any pruritic disease could be listed. In cats atopic disease, food allergy, notoedric mange, and eosinophilic granulomas would be the major differentials.

DIAGNOSIS

In both dogs and cats with a compatible history and physical examination, a diagnosis can be made in cases involving exposure to an insect or arachnid and subsequent development of clinical lesions. Tick bite reactions, chiggers, and stable fly reactions would be examples. However, such observations are not usually possible for sensitivities to biting insects such as *Culicoides* spp., mosquitos, blackflies, and ants. Additionally, the possible relationship between disease and insect parts (e.g., moths, houseflies, cockroaches, and possibly ants) is rarely considered. The client will usually be unaware of any potential problem from these organisms. Therefore, in some other cases a tentative

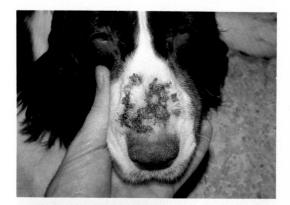

A

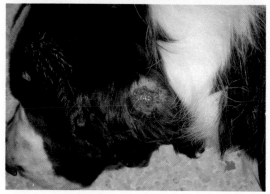

B

Figure 12-3. Crusted ulcerative nodules and papules on the bridge of the nose, **A,** and dorsal lateral pinna, **B,** of an English Springer Spaniel that was intradermal test–positive to blackfly and horsefly. The owner retrospectively noted small flies (gnats) around the dog's face. Cytology demonstrated numerous eosinophils from these lesions.

Table 12-1. Results of intradermal tests to insects and arachnids in 241 suspect atopic dogs

ANTIGEN	LAS VEGAS 48 POSITIVE (% at 3 or 4+)	SOUTHERN CALIFORNIA 193 POSITIVE (% at 3 or 4+)
Blackfly	16.7	11.4
Mosquito	10.4	7.8
Deerfly	6.3	9.3
Horsefly	10.4	17.1
Red ant	4.2	5.7
Black ant	8.3	4.2
Flea	8.3	59.7
Housefly	6.3	ND
Cockroach	6.3	ND
House-dust mite	14.6	48.7

ND, Not done.

diagnosis is made when a compatible case responds to nothing but insect control.

Cytology and histopathology may be helpful in making a diagnosis. Many of the insect hypersensitivities will have an eosinophilic infiltrate. Eosinophils are not usually seen in canine atopy.

Without known exposure, a tentative diagnosis requires positive intradermal tests to insects or arachnids. Intradermal testing has not been investigated thoroughly in dogs and cats for most organisms other than house-dust mites and fleas. I have done intradermal testing with Greer antigens for the organisms shown in Table 12-1 on more than 240 atopics. The incidence of reactions in atopic or flea-allergic dogs is also shown in the table. Dr. Karen Moriello, at the University of Wisconsin, tested at 500 and 1000 protein nitrogen units (pnu) 15 normal Beagles. The 15 were negative to all insects (housefly and cockroach not tested) at both concentrations. In addition, 5 normal dogs that were pets in Southern California were intradermal test–negative at 1000 pnu/ml.

A definitive diagnosis of a true insect/arachnid hypersensitivity requires a compatible diagnosis with a positive intradermal test to confirm that a hypersensitivity is present. In addition, at this early stage of understanding about insect/arachnid hy-

persensitivity, a cause and effect should be established to make a definitive diagnosis. Because this is usually extremely difficult to do, a definitive diagnosis is not often made and the clinician and client treat the animal on the basis of compatible or tentative diagnoses.

TREATMENT

In general, avoidance is the treatment of choice, and then, depending on the organism involved, repellents or environmental treatment may be helpful. In cases with a tentative diagnosis and an unknown organism, I use both topical repellents, such as Duocide LA (Allerderm), and aggressive environmental treatment. Aggressive environmental treatment requires weekly spraying of the yard with permethrin, chlorpyrifos, or diazinon for 4 weeks. The indoor environment should be treated with insecticidal foggers (usually containing pyrethrin or permethrin) and the floors sprayed with a residual of microencapsulated diazinon, chlorpyrifos, or pyrethrin. This is repeated in 2 weeks. Weekly baths with a moisturizing hypoallergenic shampoo are also recommended. If several pets are present, the unaffected animals are treated not with repellents but with insecticidal dips. Hopefully, this will encourage the offending organism to bite or land on the nonallergic patient and be killed by the residual insecticide left from the dip.

In cases with a compatible diagnosis that cannot be controlled with avoidance, hyposensitization, antihistamines, and systemic glucocorticoids are used.

Hyposensitization to most insect/arachnid allergens has not been evaluated in dogs. In flea allergy dermatitis, controlled studies have not shown a statistically significant benefit. However, studies of 6 to 9 months' duration have not been done. In dogs, success with the house-dust mite has been seen. Hyposensitization in humans with allergy to the house-dust mite, cockroach, caddis fly, and stinging insects is well-documented. I also have cases that appear to have responded well to hyposensitization, but controlled studies have not yet been done.

Hyposensitization with aqueous insect extracts is done in the same way as for pollens in atopic dogs. In most cases atopy and insect/arachnid hypersensitivity occur together and are treated concurrently with hyposensitization. Further studies are required before the response to this form of therapy can be adequately described.

Antihistamines, such as hydroxyzine HCl, 2.2

mg/kg q8h, are helpful in some of these cases. This is not just due to their effect on atopic disease, since cases that have reacted to insects only on intradermal testing with 70 antigens have responded to antihistamines. One ant-allergic dog repeatedly exposed to allergen by lying on ant hills will consistently improve when hydroxyzine is given following exposure. Systemic glucocorticoids are required in some cases. Similar to treating atopic disease, alternate-day, short-acting glucocorticoids are preferred, since long-term treatment is usually required.

REFERENCES

Baldo BA, Panzani RC: Detection of IgE antibodies to a wide range of insect species in subjects with suspected inhalant allergies to insects, Int Arch Allergy Appl Immunol 85:278, 1988.

Hellreich E: Evaluation of skin tests with insect extracts in various allergic diseases, Ann Allergy 20:805, 1962.

Kang BC: Cockroach allergy, Clin Rev Allergy 8:87, 1990.

Kang BC, et al: The role of immunotherapy in cockroach asthma, J Asthma 25:205, 1988.

Kino T, et al: Allergy to insects in Japan. III. High frequency of IgE antibody responses to insects (moth, butterfly, caddis fly, and chironomid) in patients with bronchial asthma and immunochemical quantitation of insect-related airborne particles smaller than 10 μm in diameter, J Allergy Clin Immunol 79:857, 1987.

Kino T, Oshima S: Allergy to insects in Japan. I. The reagenic sensitivity to moth and butterfly in patients with bronchial asthma, J Allergy Clin Immunol 61:10, 1978.

Lierl MB, et al: Concentrations of airborne insect-derived particles in outdoor air (abstr 412), J Allergy Clin Immunol 85:246, 1990.

Ostrom NK, et al: Occupational allergy to honeybee body dust in a honey-processing plant, J Allergy Clin Immunol 77:736, 1986.

Platts-Mills TAF, et al: The role of dust mite allergens in atopic dermatitis, Clin Exp Dermatol 8:233, 1983.

Reisman RE: Insect allergy. In Middleton E, et al (eds): Allergy, principles and practice, ed 3, vol 2, St Louis, 1988, CV Mosby, p 1345.

Tee RD, et al: Occupational allergy to the common house fly *(Musca domestica):* use of immunologic response to identify atmospheric allergen, J Allergy Clin Immunol 76:826, 1985.

Wynn SR, et al: Immunochemical quantitation, size, distribution, and cross-reactivity of Lepidoptera (moth) aeroallergens in southeastern Minnesota, J Allergy Clin Immunol 82:47, 1988.

Immune-Mediated Dermatoses

13

Pemphigus Foliaceus

Wayne S. Rosenkrantz

Diagnostic Criteria for Pemphigus Foliaceus

SUGGESTIVE
History and physical findings

COMPATIBLE
Suggestive plus elimination of differential diagnoses by means of negative skin scrapings, fungal culture, and response to antibiotics

TENTATIVE
Compatible plus cytology with acantholytic cells

DEFINITIVE
Tentative plus characteristic dermatopathology or positive direct intercellular immunofluorescence or immunoperoxidase

Pemphigus foliaceus is the most common autoimmune skin disease of dogs and cats (Ihrke et al., 1985b; Griffin, 1987). In autoimmune skin diseases, antibodies, or activated lymphocytes, are made against normal body components. The pemphigus complex includes a group of skin diseases that result from autoantibodies made against keratinocytes or their cellular components. All forms of pemphigus contain autoantibody deposition in the intercellular area of the epidermis. In humans the autoantibodies in pemphigus foliaceus and pemphigus vulgaris have been shown to be different (Stanley et al., 1986). The antigen in pemphigus foliaceus is most likely desmoglein, a glycoprotein component of the desmosome. (The desmosome is the site where cells attach to one another.) Desmosomes are more numerous in the superficial epidermis, which is the initial site of cell detachment (acantholysis) in pemphigus foliaceus.

The common pathologic process in all forms of pemphigus is acantholysis. Acantholysis is defined as epidermal cell-to-cell detachment resulting in intraepidermal vesicle formation. Commonly these vesicles are infiltrated with neutrophils and/or eosinophils. Acanthocytes, which are keratinocytes that have lost their cellular attachments and have "rounded up," are also present within the pustule. Clinically this results in superficial pustules that rapidly rupture, dry out, and become a superficial crust.

The initial stimulus for autoantibody formation is not known. With the prevalence of the disease in certain breeds, genetic factors are likely involved. Other stimuli may include drugs (penicillamine and phenylbutazone) and ultraviolet light

(Muller et al., 1989). A virus spread by an insect vector is suspected in an endemic form of pemphigus foliaceus seen in South America that shares many similarities with canine pemphigus foliaceus (Zone and Provost, 1985). This form of pemphigus in humans is called pemphigus endemicus. It is different from classic human pemphigus foliaceus by having an early age of onset, generalized progression, palmoplantar involvement, alopecia, and good response to glucocorticoids. These features are similar to many of the clinical features seen in canine pemphigus foliaceus. Some investigators notice seasonal exacerbation of pemphigus cases. Many cases exhibit more active flare-ups and require higher immunosuppressive drug dosages in the warmer months. In addition, there may be a higher incidence of pemphigus foliaceus in dogs with allergic skin disease (Rosenkrantz, 1991). It is unknown whether allergies may be a predisposing factor or whether the chronic drug therapy used to control allergic symptoms acts as a predisposing factor.

CLINICAL DISEASE

There is no sex predilection in dogs or cats with pemphigus foliaceus. Akitas, Doberman Pinschers, Newfoundlands, Bearded Collies, Schipperkes, Finnish Spitzes, and Dachshunds may be at higher risk than other breeds (Ihrke et al., 1985b; Muller et al., 1989). Chow Chows also may be at high risk, but this has not been compared to a control population (Griffin, 1987). In one study the mean age of onset was 4.2 years, with 65% of affected dogs developing the diseases before 5 years of age (Ihrke et al., 1985b).

The initial primary lesion is a erythematous macule that progresses rapidly through a pustular lesion and eventually leaves a dry yellow-brown crust (Fig. 13-1). Because the pustular stage is so short, the practitioner needs to be aware of all the different clinical presentations. Individual lesions can vary from micropustules (1 mm) to larger pus collections (10 mm in some cases). The pustules may develop on an erythematous base, many times with several pustules coalescing and subsequently rupturing, leaving crusted plaques. Lesions may be both follicular and nonfollicular in location. The crusts are usually easily removed, often leaving a moist, erosive, or ulcerated surface. The follicular epithelium is commonly affected, resulting in multifocal to diffuse areas of alopecia (Fig. 13-2). The signs may wax and wane, with many cases having acute flare-ups within hours or overnight.

Most lesions start on the face. In one study (Ihrke et al., 1985b) 60% of the cases generalized within 6 months and 27% remained localized for 1 to 3 years. Lesions that remain limited to the face may complicate the distinction between pemphigus foliaceus and pemphigus erythematosus. The most commonly affected localized areas of the face are the bridge of the nose and the planum nasale (Fig. 13-3). Other facial areas affected include the muzzle, periocular area (especially the dorsomedial canthus), and the pinnae.

Other localized sites are the footpads and genitals (Fig. 13-4). When the footpads are affected, lameness is common. In some cases the pads can be the only site affected (August and Chickering, 1985; Ihrke et al., 1985c). The pads may have pustules, but this is rare; more commonly they appear cracked, crusted, and hyperkeratotic. In cats,

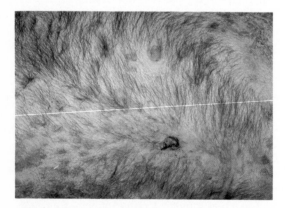

Figure 13-1. The initial primary lesion in pemphigus foliaceus is an erythematous macule that progresses rapidly through a pustular stage and results in a dry yellow-brown crust.

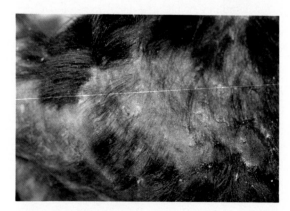

Figure 13-2. Because pemphigus foliaceus commonly affects the follicular epithelium, alopecia is often multifocal to diffuse.

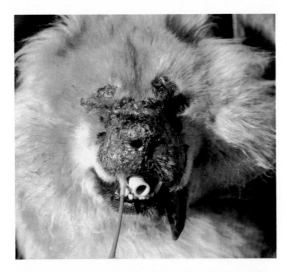

Figure 13-3. The most common initial and localized site for pemphigus foliaceus is the bridge of the nose.

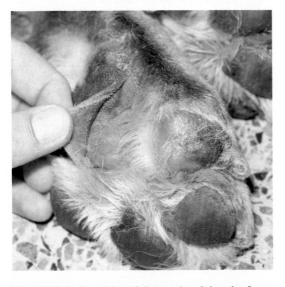

Figure 13-4. Pemphigus foliaceus involving the foot pads of an Akita.

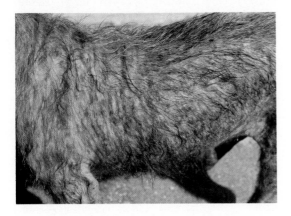

Figure 13-5. Generalized pemphigus foliaceus.

in addition to facial, periocular, and pinnal lesions, other commonly affected sites include the perimammary gland and nail bed locations (Caciolo et al., 1984). In both dogs and cats oral lesions are extremely rare. I have never seen oral involvement in any cases of pemphigus foliaceus. Some cases will develop generalized lesions (Fig. 13-5). These animals often have fevers as high as 40.5° C, depression, pruritus, lameness, pitting edema, and lymphadenopathy.

The differential diagnoses for pemphigus foliaceus include other pustular, scaling, and crusting diseases such as pemphigus erythematosus (PE), lupus erythematosus (LE), bacterial folliculitis, zinc-responsive dermatitis, dermatophytosis, demodicosis, dermatomyositis (DM), mycosis fungoides (MF), metabolic epidermal necrosis (MEN), and other sterile pustular diseases. Many of these diseases have a tendency to affect the face (PE, LE, zinc-responsive dermatitis, dermatophytosis, demodicosis, DM, MF, MEN). Some affect only the footpads (zinc-responsive dermatitis, MEN, LE). Others are commonly more generalized (bacterial folliculitis, demodicosis, dermatophytosis, MF).

DIAGNOSIS

The diagnosis of pemphigus foliaceus can occasionally be difficult to make. A careful history and physical examination are important. Major differentials such as demodicosis and dermatophytosis can easily be ruled out by skin scrapings and dermatophyte test medium (DTM) cultures. Smears from intact nonfollicular pustules are optimal. Smears can also be made by removing crusts and impressing a glass slide on the moist erosive surface. Smears may be stained with a Wright or Diff-Quik stain. The large rounded cells (acanthocytes) often can be seen in large clumps or rafts (Fig. 13-6). The most important diagnostic criterion is finding a subcorneal or intraepidermal acantholytic pustule on routine histopathology. The infiltrate is usually a mixture of eosinophils and neutrophils.

Optimally, several intact pustules with erythematous bases should be selected for histopathologic examination. Punch biopsies are an efficient way of obtaining samples. Punch biopsies (Acuderm) are available in 2 to 8 mm diameters. The most commonly used sizes for skin pathologic conditions are 4 to 6 mm. Selection depends on the size of the lesion to be sampled. Local anesthesia with 2% lidocaine without epinephrine is preferred. Usually

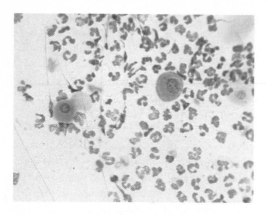

Figure 13-6. Diff-Quik–stained pustular smear from a dog with pemphigus foliaceus. Note the large rounded keratinocytes ("acanthocytes").

1 to 2 ml injected subcutaneously will produce adequate anesthesia. Samples should be handled gently and immediately placed in 10% buffered formalin. If larger elliptical sections are taken, these samples should be placed on cardboard or a wooden tongue depressor prior to formalin fixation to prevent curling. To obtain an optimal biopsy, it may be necessary to send the animal home or hospitalize it until pustular lesions appear. Another option is to biopsy crusted areas. Not all biopsy sites should be prepared. Often these overlying crusts are filled with numerous acanthocytes. Dermatopathologic examination should be performed by a veterinary pathologist who has a special interest in dermatopathology or by a veterinary dermatologist trained in dermatopathology. (See Appendix B.) A thorough history, clinical findings, and differential diagnosis should be included with biopsy samples.

Direct immunofluorescence optimally shows a diffuse intercellular deposition of immunoglobulin and possibly complement components. Reports indicate that 25% to 76% of animals with a tentative diagnosis of pemphigus foliaceus have autoantibodies (Ihrke et al., 1985b; Griffin and Rosenkrantz, 1987; Werner et al., 1983). Indirect immunofluorescence is usually negative, although in one report (Ihrke et al., 1985b) 67% of cases were positive. Antinuclear antibodies (ANAs) are not present.

For direct immunofluorescence sampling, tissue specimens should be taken from perilesional erythematous skin. Whenever possible, they should not be taken when the animal is on glucocorticoids or other immunosuppressive drugs. Samples are placed in Michel's fixative. Samples for direct immunofluorescence are commonly taken at the same time that routine biopsies are taken. They can be held in the Michel's medium for extended periods without loss of accuracy (Ihrke et al., 1985a) and only submitted to the laboratory if routine dermatopathology is not diagnostic.

Immunoreactants can also be detected by the immunoperoxidase technique. This technique may utilize routinely formalin-fixed tissues and is done with a light microscope. However, false-positive reactions have been a problem in humans and animals (Moore et al., 1987).

Since many cases of generalized pemphigus present with systemic symptoms, it is not unusual to see changes on routine complete blood counts. Many dogs can have markedly elevated white blood cell counts (as high as 80,000), with neutrophils predominating, although occasionally high eosinophil counts will also be seen.

Currently, a definitive diagnosis requires characteristic dermatopathologic findings with a compatible physical and history. It is best to have positive direct immunofluorescence results; however, this may not occur, even in cases with optimal sampling and disease staging. Therefore the practitioner should place emphasis on routine histopathology. Negative direct immunofluorescence results or even nondiagnostic dermatopathology does not rule out the diagnosis (Griffin and Rosenkrantz, 1987). On occasion, repeat biopsies may be needed to confirm the diagnosis before long-term immunosuppressive therapy is started.

TREATMENT

Many cases are complicated by secondary pyoderma; therefore, it is common to utilize antibiotics initially with immunosuppressive therapy. Antibiotic choice is usually based on empirical selection of agents effective against coagulase-positive *Staphylococcus*. Initially antibiotics are often needed for 2 to 3 weeks. It is not uncommon to use them intermittently during the treatment for pemphigus. This may be partly secondary to immunosuppression from side effects of the treatment.

Systemic Glucocorticoids

Of the various immunosuppressive agents used to treat pemphigus foliaceus, systemic glucocorticoids (in the form of prednisone) are most common. Induction dosages of 2.2 to 3.3 mg/kg q12h

(Muller et al., 1989) are generally used, although Griffin (1987) and Rosenkrantz (1989) have both had success at lower dosages, 1.1 mg/kg q12h. Methylprednisolone (Medrol) can be used in animals that have polyuria-polydipsia on prednisone. Methylprednisolone has less mineralocorticoid side effects and, particularly in smaller-breed dogs, may produce less polyuria-polydipsia. The tablets come in 4 and 16 mg sizes, equivalent respectively to 5 and 20 mg of prednisone. The induction dosage is 0.8 to 1.5 mg/kg q12h. The major disadvantage of methylprednisolone is expense; even the generics are more costly than prednisone. Cases that fail to respond by full remission at these induction dosages within 7 to 14 days are candidates for other, more potent oral glucocorticoids or combination immunosuppressive therapy. Long-term response to systemic glucocorticoids generally is favorable in 30% to 40% of the cases (Ihrke et al., 1985b). Once remission is obtained, the oral prednisone or methylprednisolone is tapered to approximately 2 to 0.5 mg/kg q48h for long-term management.

Tapering to a long-term maintenance dosage is best achieved over an 8- to 10-week period. An example for a 40 kg dog would include an initial induction of 50 mg prednisone q12h for 14 days, followed by 7 days of 100 mg once a day. In subsequent weeks the alternate-day dosages would be lowered by 20 mg a week—for example, week 1 (Mon.)100 mg, (Tues)80 mg, (Wed.)100 mg, (Thurs.)80 mg, etc.; week 2 (Mon.)60 mg, (Tues.)100 mg, (Wed.)60 mg, etc.; week 3 (Mon.)100, (Tues.)40, etc. Once an alternate-day regimen is reached, the tapering should continue, again lowering 20 to 10 mg per week—(Mon.)100, (Tues.)0, (Wed.)100, etc. for week 5; (Mon.)80, (Tues.)0, etc. for week 6; (Mon.)60, (Tues.)0, etc. for week 7. When 1 mg/kg q48h is reached, the tapering process can be much slower. Dosage reduction should be at every 2 to 4 weeks, 5 to 10 mg per week. Most cases will require a minimum maintenance of 0.5 mg/kg q48h. If cases flare up during tapering, induction needs to be restarted; or an alternative mode of therapy needs to be utilized if the flare-up occurs at too high a maintenance dosage. If glucocorticoids are used as the sole therapy, semi-yearly to yearly CBCs, chemistry screens, and urine cultures should be performed to monitor for common side effects. Periodic ACTH stimulation tests can also be utilized to monitor adrenal gland atrophy. Common "cushingoid" changes may require discontinuation of the glucocorticoid and a change in the immunosup-

pressive therapy. If significant side effects develop, alternative therapy will need to be considered.

In severely affected cases, parenteral glucocorticoids can be tried as an initial means of calming down the disease. This is referred to as "pulse parenteral glucocorticoids" (White, 1985). Success has been seen with shock dosages of dexamethasone (0.5 mg/kg) or methylprednisolone succinate (1 mg/kg) given 2 days consecutively followed by a maintenance oral prednisone or methylprednisolone dosage (White, 1985; Rosenkrantz, 1991).

Alternative Glucocorticoids

The use of other, more potent, oral glucocorticoids can also be tried at induction and maintenance regimens. Oral triamcinolone at 0.2 to 0.3 mg/kg q12h or dexamethasone at 0.1 to 0.2 mg/kg q12h can be used for 7 to 14 days for induction, with tapering to 0.1 or 0.2 mg/kg q48-72h (triamcinolone) and 0.05 to 0.1 mg/kg q48-72h (dexamethasone). As with prednisone, monitoring for side effects needs to be performed. These glucocorticoids are more potent and have a longer half-life than prednisone, and side effects can be produced more readily. For this reason it is important to strive for an every-third-day administration. However, some cases will maintain well, with minimal cushingoid complications, on a q48h administration schedule (Rosenkrantz, 1991).

Topical Glucocorticoids

Topical glucocorticoids may be valuable in the treatment of localized pemphigus lesions. The potency of the topical glucocorticoid can be geared to the severity of the lesion. Usually a minimum of 2.5% hydrocortisone cream is sufficient, but more potent topical steroids may be needed, such as 0.1% betamethasone valerate (Valisone) creams or ointments, fluocinolone acetonide (Synotic), or 0.1% amcinonide (Cyclocort). Care must be taken with topical steroids, since systemic side effects and localized reactions can occur. Using topicals q12h the first week, decreasing to q24h the second week, and to q48h by the third week is recommended. Some cases can be maintained on a application schedule of once or twice a week.

Combinations

Combination therapy with glucocorticoids and other immunosuppressive drugs is the alternative to straight glucocorticoids. The following combination regimens may be used successfully:

1. Azathioprine (Imuran) is an antimetabolite that is transformed into the active agent 6-mercaptopurine, which interferes with DNA and RNA synthesis by inhibiting the enzymes needed for purine synthesis. The immunosuppression results from inhibition of T and B lymphocytes, with primarily T lymphocytes affected. Azathioprine has a slow onset, frequently taking 4 to 6 weeks to produce clinical effects. The dosage is 2.2 mg/kg q24-48h in conjunction with standard glucocorticoid induction dosages. Once in remission, both the glucocorticoids and the azathioprine should be tapered to the lowest possible effective alternate-day dosage or less. Major side effects include bone marrow suppression, evidenced by leukopenia, thrombocytopenia, or anemia. Pyoderma, generalized or localized demodicosis, or dermatophytosis may be a therapeutic complication. Cutaneous lymphoma has occurred in some chronically treated cases, but a direct relationship to azathioprine therapy has not been documented. It is important to perform recheck visits whenever a recurrence is suspected, since the recurrence may not be pemphigus but a secondary complication. When a secondary opportunistic infection occurs, drug dosages may need to be cut in half and therapy for the secondary infection started (i.e., amitraz, griseofulvin, antibiotics). Initially a CBC and platelet count should be performed every 2 weeks for the first 10 to 12 weeks. Once the CBC is stabilized, the frequency of monitoring can be decreased to every 2 to 3 months. Periodic chemistry screens should also be performed, since some cases can develop a hepatotoxicity associated with just straight azathioprine. Cases with marked liver enzyme elevations and SGPT levels as high as 5000 μg/dl have been seen (Rosenkrantz, 1991). Most cases respond favorably to drug withdrawal. Azathioprine is not generally recommended for use in cats, since the bone marrow suppression may be marked and fatalities can occur. If used in cats, the dosage should be 1 mg/kg q24-48h.

2. Chlorambucil (Leukeran) is an alkylating agent that results in misreading of the genetic code as well as DNA breakage and cross-linking. It is the slowest-acting and least toxic of the alkylating agents and can be added to a glucocorticoid or azathioprine-glucocorticoid regimen. In cases of feline pemphigus foliaceus, success with chlorambucil may be seen on a dosage of q48h. Chlorambucil is available as a 2 mg nonscored tablet. The dosage is 0.1 to 0.2 mg/kg q24-48h used solely or with another immunosuppressive. Mon-

itoring is similar to that with azathioprine. Side effects relate to myelosuppression and mild gastrointestinal side effects (Rosenkrantz, 1989).

3. Cyclophosphamide (Cytoxan) is another alkylating agent, considered very potent, that can be used individually or in conjunction with glucocorticoids and chlorambucil. It is available in a 25 or 50 mg tablet. The dosage is 1.5 mg/kg q48h. However, I do not typically use this drug in pemphigus foliaceus cases due to its potent myelosuppression and potential for hemorrhagic cystitis and because other therapies are generally effective.

4. Chrysotherapy, the use of oral and parenteral gold salts, has been shown to have antiimmunologic and antiinflammatory effects. Its antiinflammatory effects include reduction of lysosomal enzymes, histamine, and prostaglandin; and the effect is to inhibit complement formation, chemotaxis, phagocytosis, respiratory burst–free radical superoxide release, and hormonal and cellular immunity. Two parenteral compounds are available, aurothiomalate (Myochrysine) and aurothioglucose (Solganal). An oral form, auranofin (Ridaura), is also available. Aurothioglucose is the parenteral

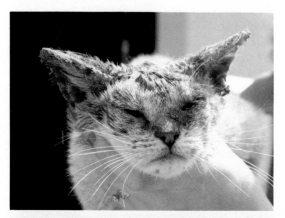

A

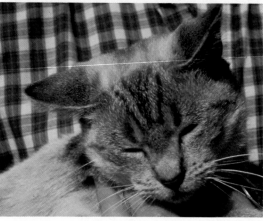

B

Figure 13-7. Pemphigus foliaceus in a cat. **A,** Prior to gold salt therapy. **B,** 14 weeks after initiation.

form preferred by many veterinarians. It is available in 10 ml vials of 50 mg/ml. The current protocol is 1 mg/kg q1wk intramuscularly. It is recommended that a test dose of 1 to 5 mg be used the first week followed by a second test dose of 2 to 10 mg the second week to rule out idiosyncratic reactions. I and some specialists do not do test dosing and start initially with 1 mg/kg q1wk. Clinical response is not expected for 6 to 12 weeks, and for this reason the drug is often used in conjunction with oral glucocorticoids initially during the lag phase. If there is no response by the sixteenth week, the dosage can be increased to 1.5 mg/kg q1wk. Once a response is seen, the injection interval may be reduced to an as-needed basis (i.e., every 2 weeks to 2 months). Occasionally the injections can be discontinued, and the disease will remain in remission. This has been seen primarily in cats. Approximately 25% of the cats treated with gold have remained in remission for longer than 2 years (Fig. 13-7). Although chrysotherapy has been helpful in dogs, the results have been less successful than in cats. Some investigators have had success with the oral form, auranofin, at 0.1 to 0.2 mg/kg q24h. Major side effects of chrysotherapy include hepatic necrosis, thrombocytopenia, toxic epidermal necrolysis, stomatitis, and proteinuria. Minor side effects are sterile abscesses at injection sites and eosinophilia. Platelet counts, complete blood counts, and urinalysis should be performed every 2 weeks during the first 16 weeks. Once remission and a maintenance dose are achieved the monitoring can be decreased to monthly and eventually quarterly.

5. Cyclosporine is a cyclic polypeptide immunosuppressive metabolite of the fungus *Tolypocladium inflatum Gams* that inhibits interleukin-2 (T cell growth factor), thus blocking the proliferation of activated T lymphocytes. It also blocks gene activation and mRNA transcription and may inhibit the interaction of T cell antigen receptor with the antigen. Cyclosporine also affects other lymphokines, including gamma-interferon. It has had limited success against pemphigus in dogs and cats (Rosenkrantz et al., 1989). Cyclosporine (Sandimmune) is available in an oral form (100 mg/ml in a 50 ml bottle). The intravenous preparation has a solubilizing agent (polyoxyethylated castor oil) that has caused anaphylactoid reactions and is not recommended. The initial induction dosage is 20 mg/kg q24h. It is often used in conjunction with oral glucocorticoids and tapered to 10 mg/kg q48h once remission has been obtained. The drug is very expensive, which is a major limiting factor in its clinical use. Its adverse reactions include gastrointestinal disturbances, pyoderma, bacteriuria, nephrotoxicity, gingival hyperplasia, papillomatous dermatitis with malignant features, and upper respiratory viral infection (the last in a cat) (Rosenkrantz et al., 1989).

6. Dapsone (Avlosulfon) and sulfasalazine (Azulfidine) are the most common sulfones and sulfonamides used in veterinary medicine. They cause antiinflammatory activity by inhibiting the neutrophil cytotoxicity system and nonspecific antiinflammatory properties on cell-mediated immunity. The dosage of dapsone is 1 mg/kg q8-12h, and of sulfasalazine 22 to 44 mg/kg q8h (Scott, 1986; Rosenkrantz, 1989). A favorable clinical response should occur in 4 to 6 weeks. A limited number of cases have been treated with these drugs, and minimal responses have been seen. Potential side effects include anemia, neutropenia, thrombocytopenia, hepatotoxicity, gastrointestinal signs, and skin reactions. Sulfasalazine can cause keratoconjunctivitis sicca, which is generally nonreversible. When this drug is being used, tear production should be checked regularly with Schirmer tear strips. Complete blood counts and chemistry screens should also be checked every 2 weeks for the first 6 weeks of therapy and reduced in frequency after the dosage has been decreased.

•   •   •

The initial treatment of choice for pemphigus foliaceus is either systemic or topical glucocorticoids. Topical glucocorticoids are best suited for small, localized lesions. Prednisone is the glucocorticoid of choice for initial and long-term maintenance therapy. If undesirable side effects develop or a poor response to prednisone is seen, alternate glucocorticoids (e.g., oral methylprednisolone, triamcinolone, or dexamethasone) may be tried. Cases refractory to initial therapy sometimes respond to pulse dosages of parenteral methylprednisolone succinate or dexamethasone, followed by a maintenance oral glucocorticoid program. Antibiotics should be used initially when secondary pyoderma is present. In cases that cannot be controlled at safe alternate-day glucocorticoid dosages, azathioprine should be added. Some investigators suggest starting azathioprine as an initial therapy in conjunction with glucocorticoids. However, the expense of the drug and monitoring are often limiting factors. In addition, 30% to 40% of the cases will not require azathioprine.

If a case cannot be controlled with combination azathioprine and glucocorticoid therapy, chlorambucil should be added to the treatment. If the response is still poor, alternative therapies such as gold salts, cyclosporine, chlorambucil, and sulfa drugs may have to be considered. In refractory cases the primary diagnosis should be reconfirmed, and consultation with a specialist may be advisable.

REFERENCES

August JR, Chickering WR: Pemphigus foliaceus causing lameness in four dogs, Compend Contin Educ Pract Vet 7:894, 1985.

Caciolo PL, et al: Pemphigus foliaceus in eight cats and results of induction therapy using azathioprine, J Am Anim Hosp Assoc 20:571, 1984.

Griffin CE: Diagnosis and management of primary autoimmune skin diseases: a review, Semin Vet Med Surg (Small Anim) 2:173, 1987.

Griffin CE, Rosenkrantz WS: Direct immunofluorescent testing: a comparison of two laboratories in the diagnosis of canine immune-mediated skin disease, Semin Vet Med Surg (Small Anim) 2:202, 1987.

Ihrke PJ, et al: The longevity of immunoglobulin preservation in canine skin utilizing Michel's fixative, Vet Immunol Immunopathol 9:161, 1985a.

Ihrke PJ, et al: Pemphigus foliaceus in dogs: a review of 37 cases, J Am Vet Med Assoc 186:59, 1985b.

Ihrke PJ, et al. Pemphigus foliaceus of the footpads in three dogs, J Am Vet Med Assoc 186:67, 1985c.

Moore FM, et al: Localization of immunoglobulins and complement by the peroxidase antiperoxidase method in autoimmune and nonautoimmune canine dermatopathies, Vet Immunol Immunopathol 14:1, 1987.

Muller GH, et al: Small animal dermatology, ed 4, Philadelphia, 1989, WB Saunders p 497.

Rosenkrantz WS: Immunomodulating drugs in dermatology. In Kirk RW (ed): Current veterinary therapy X, Philadelphia, 1989, WB Saunders, p 570.

Rosenkrantz WS: Personal observation, 1991.

Rosenkrantz WS, et al: Clinical evaluation of cyclosporine in animal models with cutaneous immune-mediated disease and epitheliotropic lymphoma, J Am Anim Hosp Assoc 25:377, 1989.

Scott DW: Sulfones and sulfonamides in canine dermatology. In Kirk RW (ed): Current veterinary therapy IX, Philadelphia, 1986, WB Saunders, p 606.

Stanley JR, et al: Antigenic specificity of Fogo Selvagem autoantibodies is similar to North American pemphigus foliaceus and distinct from pemphigus vulgaris autoantibodies, J Invest Dermatol 87:197, 1986.

Werner LL, et al: Diagnosis of autoimmune skin disease in the dog: correlation between histopathologic, direct immunofluorescent, and clinical findings, Vet Immunol Immunopathol 5:47, 1983.

White SD: Pulse therapy. In Proceedings, Annual members' meeting AAVD & ACVD, 1985.

Zone JJ, Provost TT: Bullous disease. In Moschella SL, Hurley HJ (eds): Dermatology, ed 2, vol 1, Philadelphia, 1985, WB Saunders, p 557.

SUGGESTED READINGS

Castro RM, et al: Brazilian pemphigus foliaceus, Clin Dermatol 1:22, 1983.

Halliwell REW: Skin diseases associated with autoimmunity. I. The bullous autoimmune skin diseases, Compend Contin Educ Pract Vet 2:911, 1980.

Manning TO, et al: Pemphigus diseases in the feline: seven case reports and discussion, J Am Anim Hosp Assoc 18:433, 1982.

14

Discoid Lupus Erythematosus

Wayne S. Rosenkrantz

Diagnostic Criteria for Discoid Lupus Erythematosus

SUGGESTIVE
Nasal lesion and history

COMPATIBLE
Suggestive plus elimination of differentials (fungus, demodicosis, nasal solar dermatitis, contact reaction, pyoderma)

TENTATIVE
Compatible plus routine dermatohistopathology showing a plasmacytic lichenoid dermatitis with hydropic degeneration

DEFINITIVE
Compatible plus characteristic dermatopathology or positive direct basement membrane zone immunofluorescence and negative ANA

The second most common immune mediated skin disease in dogs, after pemphigus foliaceus, is discoid lupus erythematosus (DLE). Although it is classified as a primary autoimmune disease, its antigen is not cutaneous. Instead, the antibody is directed against another body constituent and the antigen-antibody complex then localizes within the skin. There is some doubt as to the pathologic role that cutaneous localized antigen antibody complexes may play.

Discoid lupus erythematosus is considered to be a benign form or variant of systemic lupus erythematosus (Griffin et al., 1979; Scott et al., 1983a). In dogs the term generally implies cutaneous lupus affecting primarily the planum nasale and face. However, DLE is also used by many practitioners to describe other forms of cutaneous lupus. There are numerous forms of cutaneous lupus in humans, ranging from benign to severe, and it is likely that a similar spectrum will eventually be recognized in dogs.

The exact pathogenesis of lupus erythematosus is unknown. Currently in humans there is evidence (Zone and Provost, 1985) that genetics, sunlight, and viruses may all be factors. One proposed mechanism for cutaneous lupus implicates sunlight, which causes nuclear and cytoplasmic antigen expression on the surface of the keratinocyte cell membrane. Specific antibodies bind to the antigen surface of the basal cell and initiate a cytotoxic process termed antibody-dependent cellular cytotoxicity (Norris and Lee, 1985). The damaged keratinocytes release lymphocyte attractants, producing a chronic infiltrate that promotes the cellular cytotoxicity. This could explain the different type of cellular infiltrate seen in cutaneous lupus from that seen in other autoimmune skin diseases.

CLINICAL DISEASE

Discoid lupus erythematosus is considered more common in female dogs. Collies, German Shepherd Dogs, Siberian Huskies, Shetland Sheepdogs, and their crosses appear to be predisposed (Scott et al., 1983a). No age predilection has been observed, lesions having developed in dogs as young as 9 months of age (Griffin et al., 1979).

The initial lesion is often a small area of slate gray depigmentation or erythema over the planum nasale, alar fold, or lips. These depigmented macules rapidly progress to depressed atrophic areas. An early sign of the disease is when the normal rough cobblestone-like architecture of the planum nasale is lost (Fig. 14-1). Erosions, ulceration, and crusting may appear as the disease progresses. In advancing cases scarring and marked tissue loss can occur, with the rostral nasal cartilage being damaged (Fig. 14-2). It appears that the lupus is responsible for the loss of cartilage, but secondary pyoderma may also contribute to cartilage loss. Following minor trauma profuse hemorrhage can develop from the planum nasale.

Less commonly lesions are seen periocularly and on the pinnae, distal limbs, and genitalia. Lesions occurring in these locations are variable depending on the state of the disease. Early lesions appear as scaly erythematous macules. Progressive lesions may appear as crusted, eroded, depigmented, or hyperpigmented and well-demarcated patches. Alopecia is common as lesions advance. Pinnal lesions will often appear well-circumscribed with circular to wedge-shaped areas of necrosis, frequently resembling other vascular diseases that affect the pinnae (Fig. 14-3). Scrotal lesions are usually depigmented, ulcerated, and heavily crusted.

Half the cases seen are exacerbated by sunlight. For this reason the disease may have seasonal flareups and is more common in areas with consistently sunny climates.

The differential diagnosis for DLE can be divided into diseases affecting and those not affecting the planum nasale.

Diseases affecting the planum, with early depigmentation, include systemic lupus erythematosus, pemphigus complex (foliaceus and erythematosus), drug reactions, erythema multiforme, mycosis fungoides, a Vogt-Koyanagi-Harada–like syndrome, contact reactions, squamous cell carcinoma, trauma, and nasal solar dermatitis. Nasal solar dermatitis, or "collie nose," usually represents cases of DLE that have been aggravated or induced by sun exposure. Sunburn nasal lesions and true nasal solar dermatitis do exist in dogs and are described in detail in Chapter 30.

Diseases affecting the nasal area that generally do not start on the planum nasale include dermatomyositis, demodicosis, and both bacterial and dermatophyte infections.

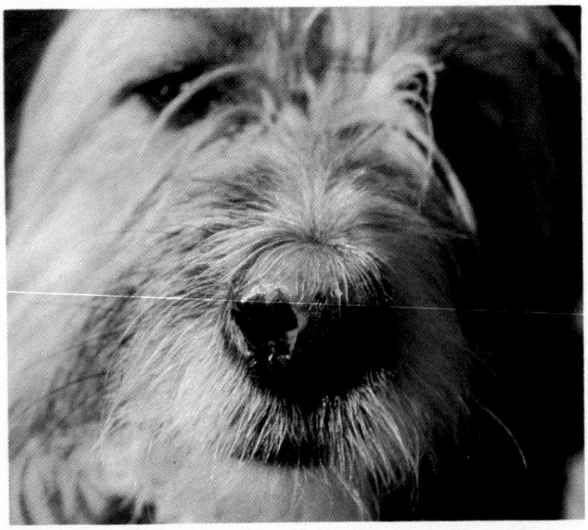

Figure 14-1. Early DLE in a dog. Note loss of the normal cobblestone-like architecture of the planum nasale with depigmentation.

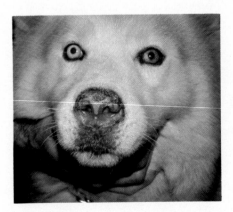

Figure 14-2. Chronic DLE in a dog. Note the loss of nasal tissue and scarring, with rostral lip involvement.

DIAGNOSIS

The diagnosis of DLE is made on the basis of a combination of clinical findings, eliminating differentials, and (ultimately) routine dermatohistopathology and immunohistopathology. The best sites for routine dermatohistopathology are nonulcerated erythematous depigmented macules and atrophic scaly lesions.

Biopsy samples for direct immunofluorescence can be taken from nonulcerated erythematous depigmented macules. In human patients direct immunofluorescence samples are more commonly positive in nonedematous lesions at least 60 days old (Weigand, 1984). It is unknown whether older sites are preferred in dogs.

Biopsy samples should be taken while the dog is sedated or under general anesthesia. If sedation is used, concurrent local anesthesia with lidocaine will be required. The lidocaine should be injected subcutaneously at approximately 1 to 1.5 ml per

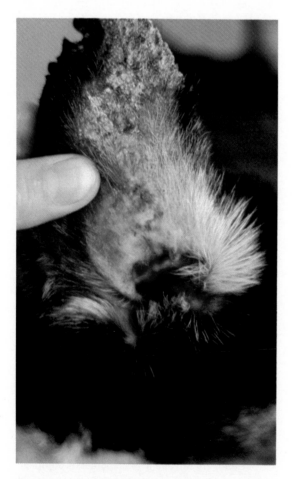

Figure 14-3. DLE affecting the pinna in a dog. The well-circumscribed hyperpigmented areas represent older damaged areas.

site. The easiest way to obtain a sample is with a biopsy punch. A 4 to 6 mm punch is the optimal size. The sample should be removed gently, and excess blood blotted and placed in formalin fixative. The biopsy site is closed with either absorbable or nonabsorbable simple interrupted or cruciate sutures.

Samples for direct immunofluorescence require special preservative solution (Michel's fixative) and can be held for extended periods without compromising results (Ihrke et al., 1985).

An alternative to direct immunofluorescence for detecting tissue immunoreactants is utilizing immunoperoxidase testing. Advantages of this technique are that routinely fixed and prepared tissues can be used and immunofluorescence equipment is not needed. However, false-positive reactions have been a problem in humans and in animals (Moore et al., 1987).

The classic changes seen with routine dermatohistopathology include epidermal and follicular hyperkeratosis, thickening of the basement membrane, vacuolar changes in the basement membrane, liquefaction degeneration of the basal cells, and apoptotic (individual, dead) keratinocytes usually located in the lower epidermis. The dermal changes may include a subepidermal bandlike infiltrate (lichenoid pattern) composed of plasma cells and lymphocytes. A similar infiltrate in a periadnexal pattern is common. Pigment incontinence in early lesions is also common since melanocytes may be damaged in the basal cell layer. Excessive dermal mucin is sometimes a feature of discoid lupus erythematosus. Special mucin stains (e.g., Alican blue) can aid in the diagnosis (Rosenkrantz et al., 1986).

Optimally, direct immunofluorescence should reveal a granular or rough band of immunoglobulin and/or complement along the basement membrane zone. In one study (Scott et al., 1987) C3 was the most common immunoreactant in dogs. IgG, IgM, and IgA have all been reported, so testing for individual immunoglobulins is recommended. Results of direct immunofluorescence in dogs with DLE have been extremely variable. Reports vary from 25% to 100% positive (Scott et al., 1983b; Werner et al., 1983). In one study (Griffin and Rosenkrantz, 1987) two separate laboratories were used to evaluate positive immunofluorescence. When either laboratory was utilized, 67% positive reactants were identified; however, the individual laboratories did not score the dogs the same. When both laboratories were utilized on the same samples, 83% positive reactants were detected. These results should suggest to the practitioner that direct immunofluorescence testing is not universally standardized.

Many normal dogs can have positive basal laminar immunofluorescence in the nasal planum to IgM and polyvalent immunoglobulin antisera (Scott et al., 1983b). Results should be interpreted in light of this finding, or samples should be taken when possible from areas other than the planum nasale.

Samples for routine dermatopathology should be sent to pathologists who have a special interest or special training in dermatopathology. (See Appendix B.) Direct immunofluorescence and immunoperoxidase testing are generally performed at veterinary university laboratories. The practitioner should check with the closest veterinary school for the availability of these tests.

Routine laboratory testing (hemogram, chemistries, urinalysis, protein electrophoresis) is usually unremarkable. LE cell tests are negative, and antinuclear antibody (ANA) is also negative or has very low positive titers.

TREATMENT

Since DLE is not a life-threatening disease, treatment is often for cosmetic purposes only. Some cases are mild and may wax and wane, requiring no treatment at all. When hemorrhage and severe ulceration are present or when the client is overly concerned, a more aggressive treatment option may be tried.

In mild cases initial therapy options include sun avoidance and use of water-resistant sunscreens with a high SPF, systemic vitamin E, and topical steroids. The most damaging UV light occurs between 10:00 AM and 2:00 PM, and clients should make an effort to keep their pet indoors during these hours. If the dog is an outside dog, shade should be available and a waterproof sunscreen with an SPF of 15 or greater applied q12-24h.

Vitamin E (DL-alpha tocopherol acetate) has been advocated as a safe therapy (Scott et al., 1983a). Others have found vitamin E to be rarely effective by itself. Most agree that vitamin E is a relatively benign drug and may reduce the need for other therapy, allowing less topical and systemic glucocorticoids to be used. Aqueous vitamin E (Aquasol E) is the form of choice, the dosage varying from 400 to 800 IU q12h PO. Anecdotal reports also exist that topical vitamin E may aid in lesion resolution.

When topical steroids are utilized, initially a potent fluorinated steroid, 0.1% amcinonide (Cyclocort) should be applied q24h for the first 10 to 14 days. When the disease is in remission, potent fluorinated steroids can be used on an as-needed basis (i.e., every 48 hours to every third day). Once in remission, switching to a less potent steroid should also be tried (i.e., hydrocortisone 0.5% to 2.5%). The practitioner should be aware of topical glucocorticoid–induced atrophy and cushingoid problems from steroids.

The combination of tetracycline and niacinamide has been described (White, 1990) as an alternative treatment for DLE. The study evaluated tetracycline and niacinamide in the treatment of pemphigus foliaceus (n = 5), pemphigus erythematosus (n = 11), and discoid lupus erythematosus (n = 14). Dogs that weighed more than 10 kg were given 500 mg of tetracycline and niacinamide q8h PO, and those weighing less than 10 kg were given 250 mg of each drug. Niacinamide and tetracycline were effective for DLE, with 65% (9/14) dogs showing an excellent response and 14% (2/14) a good response. Other practitioners' experiences with tetracycline-niacinamide in treatment of DLE have been less impressive. Only 25% of my cases have shown any response to this therapy. Side effects are uncommon but can include anorexia, vomiting, and diarrhea. If these symptoms develop, the niacinamide should be discontinued and the tetracycline continued; some cases may respond to just the tetracycline.

If lesions are unresponsive to these forms of therapy, systemic glucocorticoid therapy may be used in conjunction with one or more of the above-mentioned treatments. Prednisone dosages of 1 mg/kg q12h PO will generally put the disease into remission. On the average this may take approximately 14 days. Once in remission, the prednisone can be tapered to q48h and will usually keep the disease in remission. Many cases can be tapered off the prednisone after a few weeks and then maintained on just topical steroids, vitamin E, and sunscreens. Some cases will require systemic prednisone only during the summer months, which reduces the concern for glucocorticoid side effects.

The risk of treatment with glucocorticoids and other immunosuppressive agents should be discussed with the client. Some owners do not demand complete control of the disease, and more aggressive therapy can be avoided. If the described methods of treatment fail and a client demands complete control, azathioprine (Imuran) can be prescribed in combination with glucocorticoids. Azathioprine is usually started at 1 to 1.5 mg/kg q24h PO and requires regular monitoring for bone marrow suppression. When remission is obtained, many cases can have the azathioprine tapered to once q48-72h. Complete blood and platelet counts are recommended q2wk during the first 12 to 16 weeks of therapy. After 16 weeks most cases need a complete blood count only every 1 to 2 months and eventually this can be tapered to quarterly. Periodic chemistry screens are also recommended because occasional hepatotoxic reactions have been associated with azathioprine. If mild abnormalities are detected in the CBC or chemistry screens, the dose can be cut to once q48h. If abnormalities persist or intensify, discontinuation of the drug is needed until values normalize. Starting the dosage at half the previous level is then recommended.

In humans antimalarial drugs and thalidomide may be successfully used in the treatment of chronic DLE (Sontheimer, 1985). Although antimalarial drugs may be of some benefit, they have not been evaluated in dogs and their use should be monitored because of potential side effects. Thalidomide has sedative effects, may cause birth defects, and is not available commercially in the U.S.

In summary, DLE is a relatively benign autoimmune skin disorder. Treatment should be based on the severity of the lesions and the client's concern. Initial therapy should include client education, sun avoidance, sunscreens, oral vitamin E, and topical steroids. Tetracycline and niacinamide should be evaluated next. If lesions are still unresponsive, systemic glucocorticoids can be tried. If all treatment measures fail, azathioprine combination therapy may be utilized.

REFERENCES

Griffin CE, Rosenkrantz WS: Direct immunofluorescence testing: a comparison of two laboratories in the diagnosis of canine immune-mediated skin disease, Semin Vet Med Surg 2:202, 1987.

Griffin CE, et al: Canine discoid lupus erythematosus, Vet Immunol Immunopathol 1:79, 1979.

Ihrke PJ, et al: The longevity of immunoglobulin preservation in canine skin utilizing Michel's fixative, Vet Immunol Immunopathol 9:161, 1985.

Moore FM, et al: Localization of immunoglobulins and complement by the peroxidase antiperoxidase method in autoimmune and non-autoimmune canine dermatopathies, Vet Immunol Immunopathol 14:1, 1987.

Norris DA, Lee LA: Pathogenesis of cutaneous lupus erythematosus, Clin Dermatol 3:20, 1985.

Rosenkrantz WS, et al: Histopathological evaluation of acid mucopolysaccharide (mucin) in canine discoid lupus erythematosus, J Am Anim Hosp Assoc 22:577, 1986.

Scott DW, et al: Canine lupus erythematosus. II. Discoid lupus erythematosus, J Am Anim Hosp 19:481, 1983a.

Scott DW, et al: Pitfalls in immunofluorescence testing in dermatology. II. Pemphigus like antibodies in the cat, and direct immunofluorescence testing of normal dog nose and lip, Cornell Vet 73:275, 1983b.

Scott DW, et al: Immune-mediated dermatoses in domestic animals: ten years after. II, Compend Contin Educ Prac Vet 9:539, 1987.

Sontheimer RD: Subacute cutaneous lupus erythematosus, Clin Dermatol 3:58, 1985.

Weigand DA: The lupus band test: a re-evaluation, J Am Acad Dermatol 11:230, 1984.

Werner LL, et al: Diagnosis of autoimmune skin disease in the dog: correlation between histopathologic, direct immunofluorescent, and clinical findings, Vet Immunol Immunopathol 5:47, 1983.

White SD, et al: The efficacy of tetracycline and niacinamide in the treatment of autoimmune skin disease in 20 dogs. In Proceedings, Annual members' meeting AAVD & ACVD, San Francisco, 1990, p 43.

Zone JJ, Provost TT: Bullous disease. In Moschella SL, Hurley HJ (eds): Dermatology, ed 2, Philadelphia, 1985, WB Saunders, vol 1, p 557.

15

Cutaneous Drug Reactions

Wayne S. Rosenkrantz

Diagnostic Criteria for Cutaneous Drug Reactions

SUGGESTIVE

History of drug exposure and compatible physical signs; drug reactions can mimic any skin disease

COMPATIBLE

History of drug exposure to an agent that has been documented to cause cutaneous reactions with compatible physical signs

TENTATIVE

History of clinical improvement on discontinuation of the drug; the criteria and histopathology are consistent with one of the patterns described for drug reactions; erythema multiforme and toxic epidermal necrolysis are the best defined

DEFINITIVE

Tentative plus recurrence of clinical signs on rechallenge with the suspected agent; this is not recommended, since rechallenge can result in a fatal reaction

Importance

Cutaneous reactions are one of the most commonly observed adverse effects of drugs. A cutaneous drug reaction (CDR) can mimic many other skin disorders and can result from any orally, topically, or parenterally administered drug or biologic. Two to three percent of human hospitalized patients have a CDR. Penicillins, sulfonamides, and blood products are responsible for two thirds of the cutaneous reactions (Wintroub et al., 1987). Sulfamethoxazole and penicillins are the most common causes.

The incidence of CDR in dogs and cats is unknown. Numerous drugs have been reported to cause reactions (Table 15-1). The ones most commonly associated in dogs and cats are sulfonamides, primarily sulfadiazine and sulfamethoxazole, and penicillins such as ampicillin and amoxicillin.

Pathogenesis

The pathomechanism of drug reactions includes immunologic (Type I, II, III, and IV hypersensitivities) and nonimmunologic mechanisms. Immunologic reactions are not completely dependent on the host immune response. There is individual variation in the host's ability to absorb or metabolize a drug. Genetic makeup and age may be important factors. Molecular structure of the drug is also an important determinant of its antigenicity.

Another factor to consider in immunologic drug reactions is cross-reactivity. An example of this is the reactions to cephalosporin antibiotics in peni-

Table 15-1. Cutaneous drug reaction (CDR) patterns with associated drugs or other biologics

CLINICAL PRESENTATION	DRUGS AND BIOLOGICS
Urticaria-angioederma	Vaccines, antibiotics (trimethoprim-sulfadiazine and -sulfamethoxazole, cephalosporins, penicillins, tetracycline), stinging insects, blood transfusions, antisera, bacterins, amitraz, propylthiouracil
Maculopapular eruptions (morbilliform)	Antibiotics (penicillins, trimethoprim-sulfadiazine and -sulfamethoxazole, cephalosporins, tetracycline), shampoos (citrus-based, herbal-based, coal tar, benzoyl peroxide)
Fixed drug reactions	Diethylcarbamazine, 5-fluorocytosine, aurothioglucose
Erythroderma (exfoliative)	Shampoos (citrus-based, herbal-based, coal tar, benzoyl peroxide), dips (D-limonene, lime sulfur), levamisole, L-thyroxine
Purpuric reactions	Azathioprine, chlorambucil, cyclophosphamide, cephalexin, trimethoprin-sulfadiazine and -sulfamethoxazole, tetracycline, penicillins, chloramphenicol, levamisole, aurothioglucose, dapsone, synthetic estrogens, thiabendazole
Vesicobullous reactions (pemphigus, lupus, bullous pemphigoid–like reactions)	Triamcinolone, cephalexin, trimethoprim-sulfadiazine, and -sulfamethoxazole, primidone, distemper–hepatitis–leptospirosis-parvovirus vaccine
Lichenoid drug reactions	Cyclosporine
Superficial suppurative necrolytic dermatitis	Natural flea shampoos (citrus and herbal), coal tar shampoo
Erythema multiforme	Aurothioglucose, cephalexin, chloramphenicol, diethylcarbamazine, gentamicin, levamisole, L-thyroxine, trimethoprim-sulfadiazine and -sulfamethoxazole, ormetroprine-sulfadimethoxine, and penicillin
Toxic epidermal necrolysis	Levamisole, cephalexin, cephaloridine, trimethoprim-sulfadiazine and -sulfamethoxazole, 5-fluorocytosine, FeLV serum, ampicillin, hetacillin, aurothioglucose
Injection site reactions	Vaccines (rabies, distemper–hepatitis–leptospirosis-parvovirus, feline rhinotracheiitis–Calici–panleukopenia), glucocorticosteroid injections (methyl prednisolone acetate, triamcinolone, dexamethasone), antibiotics (penicillin, trimethoprim-sulfadiazine, amikacin), anthelmintics (praziquantel)

cillin-allergic cases. Similar molecular structure is present in both drugs. The route of administration of the drug may also influence the degree of the host's immune response and reaction. The environment can occasionally affect the host immune response. An example is the requirement of sunlight in a photo allergic reaction.

Type I immunologic reactions are IgE mediated and generally occur within minutes of exposure. The symptoms are variable, but pruritus, urticaria, and anaphylactic reactions may occur. The most common examples include penicillin, allergen therapy, vaccine, and venomous stinging insect reactions.

Cytotoxic or Type II reactions can result from a drug's attacking the tissue directly, its combining with an antibody and then attacking the tissue, or its inducing an immune response directed at the tissue. The role of cytotoxic mechanisms in CDR has not yet been determined.

Type III immunologic reactions are dependent on immune complexes that usually require circulation of antigen for longer than 6 days. This latent period is needed for synthesis of the antibody. IgG and IgM are the most common antibodies produced in this type of reaction. Type III reactions may produce arthralgias, fever, edema, and maculopapular or urticarial lesions. Type III symptoms are often characterized as serum sickness, and antibiotics are most commonly implicated.

Cell-mediated or Type IV reactions require previous exposure to induce a sensitized state and then a subsequent exposure for clinical signs to appear. Contact allergic reactions are most commonly Type IV. Some delayed reactions to systemic penicillin may occur this way in humans.

Nonimmunologic CDR occurs by a variety of mechanisms. Some reactions can cause release of mast cell and basophil mediators, stimulate complement pathways, or interfere with arachidonic acid metabolism. Overdosage and toxic accumulation can produce nonimmunologic CDR, but more commonly these result in an exaggeration of the pharmacologic action of the drug. Some drugs have secondary side effects that occur as part of their normal pharmacologic action. Examples include alopecia or purpura following administration of chemotherapeutic agents. Some drugs can disrupt normal body flora, permitting the development of opportunistic infections. For example, a cutaneous yeast infection may result from chronic antibiotics. This has been documented in humans and in dogs (Plant et al., 1991). Incompatible drugs can interact and produce CDR. Such reactions may result from alteration of metabolism or elimination by another drug. Variations in metabolism or nutritional status can also result in CDR. Lastly, preexisting skin diseases may be exacerbated by drugs.

CLINICAL DISEASE

A drug reaction can imitate any skin disease, but a good history will often suggest the possibility. Drug histories should always be taken on any case with skin disease. It is common in practice to use multiple drugs, which may increase the incidence of CDR. Many drugs and biologics often are not considered as potential causes of CDR due to their common usage. Vitamins, mineral supplements, food additives, aspirin, heartworm preventives, shampoos, dips, coat conditioners, and vaccines are all items that can cause CDR. The practitioner also needs to keep an open mind for the potential of a drug reaction. Often a dog may present with angioedema of the face or limbs and immediately a venomous insect is blamed. Without a proper

drug history the real cause, such as a reaction to an oral antibiotic, could be missed.

It may be difficult to implicate a particular agent as the cause of the cutaneous reaction. Previous experience that the drug(s) in question has at least been reported to cause CDR may raise suspicion for a particular agent (Table 15-1). The timing of the events is an important historical consideration. Most CDRs occur 1 or 2 weeks after starting therapy. However, with chronic drug administration, it may take months or even years for a reaction to develop. For example, a reaction to phenobarbital may occur in a dog with epilepsy, even though the phenobarbital has been used for several years. Additionally, reactions can occur as long as 3 weeks (even longer) after a drug has been stopped.

There are several CDR classifications. Many are based on historical, morphologic, and dermatohistopathologic features. This classification may help implicate the causative agent.

Urticaria

Urticaria is characterized by transient smooth, elevated papules or wheals that are often erythematous and may be pruritic. When deep dermal or subcutaneous tissues are involved, this is called angioedema. Clinically, affected animals present with marked edematous swelling that may or may not be pruritic and exhibit serum leakage.

Many drugs and biologics can cause urticaria, but the most common are antibiotics, stinging insect venoms, and vaccines (Fig. 15-1). Most urticarial reactions have a favorable prognosis and

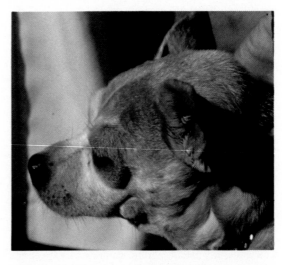

Figure 15-1. Urticarial angioedema reaction associated with an allergen injection. Note the diffuse edema, especially worse periocularly.

general health is not threatened. Angioedematous reactions, particularly those affecting the nasal passages and airways, may be fatal.

The differential diagnosis for urticarial and angioedematous CDR includes folliculitis, cellulitis, vasculitis, erythema multiforme, lymphoma, and mast cell tumors. The most confusing and common differential is short-coat bacterial folliculitis. Short-coated dogs with early folliculitis will present with a papular eruption that often is inappropriately called hives or urticaria.

Maculopapular Eruptions

Maculopapular reactions in humans are called morbilliform eruptions and are one of the more common patterns of CDR. Mild maculopapular eruptions may go unnoticed in dogs and cats due to hair coverage, so incidence is difficult to assess. Because most inflammatory skin diseases in small animals present with macules and papules, many drug-induced lesions go undiagnosed. This type of CDR is usually symmetric and truncal in its initial location. Many cases have no pruritus while others are incredibly pruritic. This reaction is usually self-limiting and generally poses no risk to life.

The differential diagnosis includes almost any inflammatory skin disease, with folliculitis, allergic skin disease, and scabies being major considerations.

Fixed Drug Eruptions

Fixed drug eruptions are characterized clinically by focal to multifocal areas of sharply demarcated erythematous lesions. In humans they tend to affect the face and genital areas. Upon rechallenge, the lesions recur in the same location. Although only a few cases have been reported in dogs, clinical lesions appear similar. Fixed drug reactions on the scrotum of male dogs exist as a result of diethylcarbamazine, 5-fluorocytosine, and aurothioglucose (Fig. 15-2) (Van Hees et al., 1985; Mason, 1988; Rosenkrantz, 1990). Scrotal lesions tend to hyperpigment. This is another feature similar to that reported with fixed drug reactions in humans. However, postinflammatory hyperpigmentation from any inflammatory skin disease may be seen in dogs.

The differential diagnosis for a fixed drug reaction includes autoimmune skin diseases (lupus erythematosus, pemphigus complex), contact allergic reaction, erythema multiforme, and toxic epidermal necrolysis.

Erythroderma

Erythroderma or erythematous drug reactions appear as diffuse pink to reddish coalescing macules or patches. They are a result of marked vascular dilation. A technique known as **diascopy** can be utilized to document that the erythema is due to vascular dilation: a clear glass slide pressed against the skin will cause blanching.

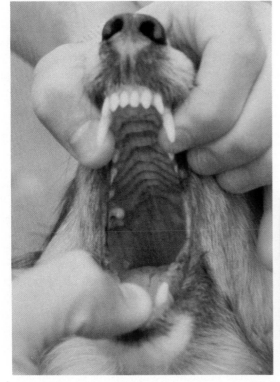

A

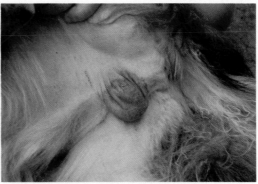

B

Figure 15-2. A, Fixed drug reaction in a dog being treated with aurothioglucose for rheumatoid arthritis. On a subsequent injection oral ulceration occurred.
B, Concurrent scrotal lesions associated with a subsequent aurothioglucose injection.

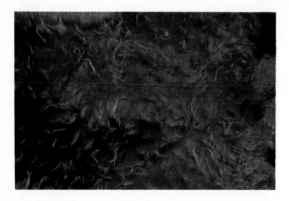

Figure 15-3. Erythroderma reaction associated with a benzoyl peroxide shampoo.

Erythroderma is usually associated with a contact-induced reaction in dogs. Shampoos or dips are the most common products responsible (Fig. 15-3). Occasionally a reaction will result from systemically administered drugs. Oral levamisole has caused two such reactions (Van Hees et al., 1985). Two cases of pruritic erythroderma have been recognized (Beale, 1991) in association with thyroid supplementation. Both were thought due to the dye in tablets that were being used. The symptoms resolved when different-colored tablets by the same manufacturer were utilized at the same dosage. Most erythroderma CDRs do not pose great danger and are unlikely to be fatal.

Major differentials include allergic skin disease, with atopy, food, and contact being the most likely possibilities. Parasitic diseases such as scabies need consideration, especially if pruritus is a major symptom. Immune mediated diseases like lupus erythematosus can present with diffuse erythema. Cutaneous T cell lymphoma in its initial phase can also produce marked erythroderma. Secondary bacterial folliculitis may be a complicating factor.

Exfoliative Reactions

Exfoliative reactions present with diffuse scaling, flaking, and variable crusting that may be indistinguishable from other keratinization defects. Erythroderma reactions often result in exfoliation. Some investigators, in fact, have combined the two as exfoliative erythroderma, with the same differential diagnosis applying as for erythroderma.

Purpuric Reactions

Purpuric reactions are a result of hemorrhage into the tissue. Clinically such lesions appear as purplish or brownish red discolorations. Diascopy

does not produce blanching as seen in erythroderma reactions. Purpuric lesions, on occasion, can appear as urticaria ulcers, or hemorrhagic blisters. A drug-induced purpura may result from immune complex vasculitis or a drug-induced thrombocytopenia, or it may be a predictable drug side effect. The latter is seen more commonly with bone marrow suppressive drugs that induce thrombocytopenia such as azathioprine, cyclophosphamide, and chlorambucil (Fig. 15-4).

Purpuric reactions associated with thrombocytopenia can be life-threatening and need immediate treatment to prevent diffuse hemorrhage. If the purpura is associated with a vasculitis, the clinical course is difficult to predict. Many cases can be self-limiting, others chronic. The outcome may reflect internal organ involvement.

The differential diagnosis for purpura includes idiopathic thrombocytopenia, other bleeding disorders, and systemic lupus erythematosus. The differential for purpura vasculitis includes other causes of vasculitides such as infections, systemic lupus erythematosus, malignancies, cold agglutin disease, or disseminated intravascular coagulation.

Vesicobullous Reactions

A cutaneous drug reaction (CDR) will often mimic vesicobullous autoimmune diseases. One case of suspected injectable triamcinolone acetonide–induced bullous drug reaction was seen by Mason (1987) in a dog. It contained many features similar to canine bullous pemphigoid. I also have seen a case of suspected cephalexin-induced lupus erythematosus (Rosenkrantz, 1990) (Fig. 15-5). This case originally was treated for an acral pruritic nodule with cephalexin and developed facial, oral, genital, and rectal ulcerative lesions while on therapy. The dermatohistopathology was consistent with lupus erythematosus. I have also seen vesicobullous eruptions associated with distemper–hepatitis–leptospirosis-parvovirus vaccine in Dachshunds. Cases were presented with severe lesional involvement of the pinnae, oral cavity, foot pads, and other mucocutaneous junctions. The dermatohistopathology consisted of an interface dermatitis and vasculitis. Although most drug-induced reactions resolve after discontinuation of therapy, some will require continual immunosuppression despite drug withdrawal and avoidance.

The differential diagnosis for vesicobullous reactions includes the pemphigus complex, particularly pemphigus vulgaris, bullous pemphigoid, dis-

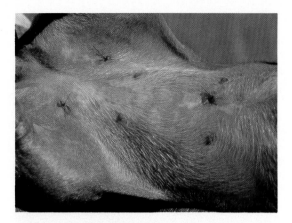

Figure 15-4. Purpuric reaction as a result of thrombocytopenia from azathioprine administration.

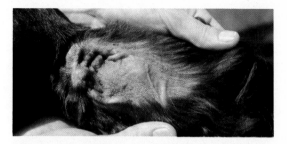

Figure 15-6. Lichenoid psoriasiform lesions in an English Springer Spaniel. Many lesions have features of lichenoid drug reactions similar to those in humans. A drug etiology should be considered.

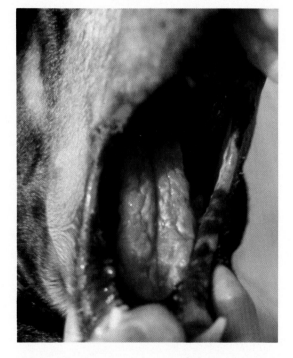

Figure 15-5. Vesicobullous reaction in a dog being treated with cephalexin. Dermatohistopathology was consistent with lupus erythematosus.

coid and systemic lupus erythematosus, erythema multiforme, toxic epidermal necrolysis, cutaneous lymphoma, candidiasis, and ulcerative stomatitis.

Lichenoid Drug Eruptions

A lichenoid drug reaction will resemble lichen planus in humans—idiopathic inflammatory skin disease with flat, violaceous, pruritic polygonal papules in circumscribed patches. In humans these reactions are most commonly associated with gold

salt therapy. Histopathologically eosinophils are abundant in drug-induced lichen planus. Although not documented to be drug induced, a lichenoid/psoriasiform dermatosis has been reported in English Springer Spaniels (Fig. 15-6) (Gross et al., 1986; Mason et al., 1986). However, it has also been seen in many other breeds. These idiopathic lesions share some morphologic and histopathologic features of lichenoid drug eruptions seen in humans: they are usually asymptomatic, symmetric, flat-topped papules that may have a scaly or hyperkeratotic surface; most contain lymphoplasmacytic lichenoid infiltrates; some have eosinophilic microabscesses; many will be self-limiting and have features of lichenoid drug reactions in humans (and therefore a drug reaction should be considered).

Cyclosporine has been reported (Rosenkrantz et al., 1989) to produce a solitary lichenoid plaque or small nodule that histologically contains a lymphoplasmacytoid infiltrate with malignant features. The cyclosporine-induced lesions responded to drug withdrawal or dosage reduction.

The differential diagnosis of a lichenoid drug reaction includes staphylococcal folliculitis, demodicosis, dermatophytosis, granulomatous reactions, and neoplastic disease.

Superficial Suppurative Necrolytic Dermatitis

Superficial suppurative necrolytic dermatitis is a recently described entity seen in four Miniature Schnauzers (Rosenkrantz et al., 1991). All cases had been bathed with either a natural flea shampoo product or a coal-tar shampoo within 5 days of lesional onset. The initial lesions appeared as er-

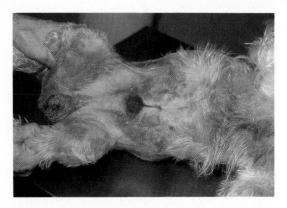

Figure 15-7. Superficial suppurative necrolytic dermatitis in a Miniature Schnauzer. Note the erythematous papules coalescing to plaques.

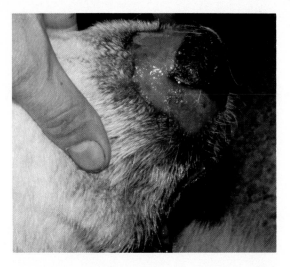

Figure 15-8. Erythema multiforme in a dog associated with trimethoprim-sulfamethoxazole administration.

ythematous papules coalescing to plaques over the ventral, lateral, and dorsal truncal areas (Fig. 15-7).

All cases were febrile and depressed and reacted painfully to touch. All contained a similar dermatohistopathology, whose major feature was a suppurative superficial necrolytic dermatitis with marked parakeratosis and epidermal edema. Three of the cases responded to antibiotic and supportive therapy. One was euthanized due to progression despite antibiotic, fluid, and corticosteroid therapy.

The clinical differential diagnosis includes other causes of drug reactions, bacterial folliculitis, erythema multiforme, and toxic epidermal necrolysis. The dermatohistopathology also has striking similarities to metabolic epidermal necrosis (hepatocutaneous syndrome).

Erythema Multiforme

Erythema multiforme (EM) as described in humans is an acute, self-limited, inflammatory condition that affects the skin and mucous membranes. It is generally characterized by distinctive iris or target lesions with central clearing. In humans the onset is usually associated with malaise and sore throats. When it affects the mucosal surfaces, it is often called erythema multiforme–major or Stevens-Johnson syndrome. Recognized causes or precipitating factors in humans include infectious agents like such as *Mycoplasma,* viral, bacterial, and fungal infections, neoplasia, collagen diseases, and drugs (Elias and Fritsch, 1987). Immune complex mechanisms are most likely responsible, but the pathogenesis is still unclear.

Erythema multiforme has been recognized in dogs in association with drugs (aurothioglucose,

cephalexin, chloramphenicol, diethylcarbamazine, gentamicin, levamisole, L-thyroxine, trimethoprim-sulfadiazine and -sulfamethoxazole, ormetoprim-sulfadimethoxine, phenobarbital) and staphylococcal infections (Scott, 1983; Goldschmidt and Wolfsdorf, 1988; Rosenkrantz, 1990; Griffin, 1991). EM has been associated with penicillin and aurothioglucose in cats.

Lesions observed in small animals include erythematous macules or papules that spread peripherally and clear centrally, producing annular target or arciform lesions. Although such maculopapular target lesions are reportedly common with EM in dogs, urticarial plaques, vesicles, or bullae can also be seen. Some investigators recognize extensive vesiculobullous and ulcerative lesions of the oral and nasal mucosa, pinnae, axillae, and groin areas as the most common lesions associated with EM and find the target lesions extremely rare (Fig. 15-8). When vesiculobullous and ulcerative lesions are present, affected animals can be systemically ill with fever, depression, and anorexia.

Erythema multiforme may run a variable course. Some cases spontaneously regress whereas others continue. Animals with severe oral and mucosal or extensive cutaneous involvement may die.

The differential diagnosis includes non–drug induced EM, bacterial folliculitis, demodicosis, dermatophytosis, urticaria, and other immune-mediated vesicular and pustular diseases.

Toxic Epidermal Necrolysis

Toxic epidermal necrolysis (TEN) is a severe cutaneous reaction characterized by widespread erythema and epidermal detachment. The affected skin often looks scalded. Toxic epidermal necrolysis shares many features with severe erythema multiforme and controversy exists on whether TEN is just a severe form of EM or is a separate entity.

A variety of etiologic factors have been implicated in humans with TEN. Drugs such as sulfonamides, butazones and hydantoins are most commonly responsible. Viral, bacterial, fungal, neoplastic, vaccination, graft vs host, and idiopathic causes have also been reported (Wintroub et al., 1987). Levamisole, cephalexin, 5-fluorocytosine, bacterial infections, liver disease and neoplasia have been reported in dogs (Van Hees et al., 1985; Scott, 1987). FeLV serum, cephaloridine, ampicillin, hetacillin, and idiopathic etiologies are reported in cats (Muller et al., 1989). An immunologic pathomechanism is suspected in TEN, but the exact nature of the disorder remains unclear (Fritsch and Elias, 1987).

The clinical signs of TEN are generally acute. Prodromal signs of a burning sensation, skin tenderness, fever, arthralgias and malaise are common in humans. A diffuse erythematous rash develops within hours to a few days. The face and extremities are commonly affected first with subsequent spread to the rest of the body. Vesicles or large bullae will usually appear next. Lesions then progress to full skin sloughing and ulceration. The mucous membranes are usually affected more severely. The disease appears and progresses very similar in small animals with the exception of some of the prodromal signs. The early erythema is often overlooked in small animals due to the hair coat. Some owners may report areas of blotchy skin in the sparsely hair sites of the groin and medial thighs. Fever and malaise are common. Many cases present with irregular patches of full thickness sloughs over the trunk with wide spread mucosal ulceration (Fig. 15-9).

Differential diagnosis includes a drug reaction, erythema multiforme, contact irritant and allergic reactions, burns, other autoimmune diseases (such as pemphigus vulgaris, lupus erythematosus, and bullous pemphigoid), lymphoreticular neoplasia, and infectious conditions. A condition called staphylococcal scalded skin syndrome in humans can appear identical to TEN. This condition is linked to the release of a destructive exotoxin (exfoliation, epidermolysin) usually by group 2, phage type 71, staphylococci (Elias and Fritsch, 1983).

The mortality rate in humans can be as high as 50%, many persons succumbing to the extensive fluid and electrolyte loss and to secondary bacterial infections. The mortality rate is more variable in

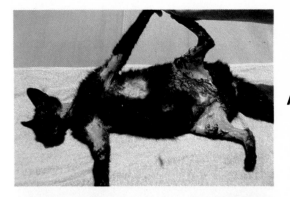

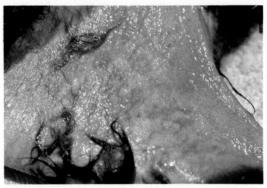

Figure 15-9. A, Toxic epidermal necrolysis in a cat. **B,** Closer view showing toxic epidermal necrolysis of the medial thigh.

small animals. Cases with extensive mucosal surface involvement and large truncal sloughs are at greater risk for dying.

Injection Site Reactions

Injection site reactions can present with either alopecia or severe crusting, ulceration, and necrosis. Glucocorticosteroid-induced reactions commonly have well-circumscribed areas of alopecia, atrophy, and either hyperpigmentation or hypopigmentation. Vaccine reactions can also have alopecia and skin pigmentation changes. Poodles are at greatest risk for rabies vaccine reactions (Schmeitzel, 1986; Wilcock and Yager, 1986). Other causes of inflammatory injection reactions that I have seen include penicillin, trimethoprim-sulfadiazine, amikacin, and praziquantel.

The time from injection to lesion development may vary from weeks to months. A careful history is necessary to correlate the site of the injection with the development of lesions. The dermatohistopathology will often show lymphocytic panniculitis and vasculitis. With glucocorticoid reactions there is also epidermal/follicular/adnexal atrophy and an occasional granulomatous nodular reaction accompanying the vehicle. Most cases are self-limiting, but it may take several months and the patient may require antibiotics or even surgical excision pending healing and the desired cosmesis.

The differential diagnosis for injection site reactions includes previous trauma, infections, alopecia areata, and traction alopecia.

DIAGNOSIS

History and clinical progression are important in making a diagnosis of a drug reaction. The following criteria suggests an immunologic CDR: (1) the reaction seen does not resemble a pharmacologic action of the drug; (2) the reaction occurs as a result of small amounts of the drug; (3) the reaction occurs within several days following initial administration of the drug; (4) the reaction is characterized by signs and symptoms generally associated with a hypersensitivity reaction; (5) the reaction reoccurs upon rechallenge; (6) the causitive agent may cross react with similar drugs; and (7) resolution may occur within several days of discontinuing the drug.

To prove that a drug reaction is immunologic in origin, it is optimal to document an immune response. The most accurate way to do this is with rechallenge, but it is often impractical and can be life-threatening. Certain in vitro immunologic tests have been devised for humans. However, the presence of a positive in vitro test does not document that a patient's symptoms are due to a drug allergy. Such tests are most accurate in IgE-dependent reactions. The presence of other antibody classes and cell-mediated immune response has a poor correlation with drug induced hypersensitivity reactions.

Laboratory findings are often unremarkable or nonspecific in drug reaction cases. It is not unusual to see elevated blood counts and, if other organ involvement is present, associated enzyme elevations related to a particular organ system.

Dermatopathology is the most valuable diagnostic tool. It aids in ruling out other differentials and helps support suspicion of a drug reaction. Less definitive changes are seen in drug-induced urticarial, morbilliform, and erythroderma reactions. Such reactions demonstrate variable degrees of edema, vascular dilation, and hemorrhage. Purpuric and vascular reactions should contain evidence of active vascular damage and hemorrhage. Fixed drug reactions are usually characterized by papillary/dermal mononuclear cellular infiltrates obscuring the dermal/epidermal junction. The associated basal cell degeneration can lead to pigment incontinence and secondary bulla formation. The diagnosis of superficial suppurative necrolytic dermatitis in the Miniature Schnauzer, and of injection sites in any breed, is based on a distinct dermatohistopathology.

The dermatohistologic features of EM and TEN are quite well-defined and would rate the highest suspicion for CDR. The most notable change in the epidermal forms of EM is the presence of prominent single cell necrosis of keratinocytes (apoptosis) and satellitosis of lymphocytes and macrophages. When the individual cell necrosis becomes more confluent, this often is associated with clinical vesiculated lesions. It is common in EM to see necrotic keratinocytes affecting the follicular epithelium. This change is often associated with a hydropic lichenoid dermatitis. The other, less commonly recognized, histologic reaction of EM is the so-called dermal form. This pattern clinically may correlate better with urticarial EM lesions. With the dermal form, dermal collagen is separated by massive amounts of edema, often with hydropic degeneration of basal cells. The subepidermal/dermal collagen may become vertically oriented and take on a weblike appearance. It is not uncommon to see subepidermal clefts or vesicles. A mixed lymphocytic mononuclear perivascular infiltrate is also not uncommon with EM reactions.

Histopathologic features of TEN include hydropic degeneration of basal cells, full-thickness necrosis of the epidermis, and minimal dermal inflammation. Dermatoepidermal separation with subsequent subepidermal vesicles is a frequent finding.

Direct immunofluorescence testing in CDR can reveal positive immunoglobulin deposition in a variety of patterns, but most often in the basement membrane zone and blood vessel walls. However, whether immunoglobulin or complement deposition is involved in the pathogenesis of the drug reaction or is a result of the drug reaction is unknown. Therefore, direct immunofluorescence testing is not considered useful for the diagnosis of CDR.

TREATMENT

Once the diagnosis of drug eruption is made, the suspected offending agent should be discontinued and avoided in the future. In some cases simply discontinuing the offending drug results in complete clearing of the skin lesions. In more severe drug reactions (EM and TEN) topical and systemic supportive therapy is necessary.

The use of topical therapy to control secondary

infection, remove scale and crust in exfoliative reactions, or to aid in resolving healing lesions is often overlooked. Products containing benzoyl peroxide (OxyDex, Pyoben), sulfur–salicylic acid (SebaLyt, Sebolux), or chlorhexidine (ChlorhexiDerm, Nolvasan) are excellent to help with secondary infection and promote healing. Such shampoos can be used daily initially. Whirlpools or soaks in chlorohexidine solutions (Nolvasan) may be utilized. Whirlpools or soaks may be better with EM and TEN because some of these cases can be quite painful and the animal will not tolerate shampoos. Clipping the hair over affected sites is recommended. With full-thickness sloughing reactions such as TEN, the affected sites may require debridement.

Although systemic antibiotics have little benefit in correcting the initial insult, their use in severe drug reactions is very important for controlling secondary pyoderma. In severe reactions with loss of epidermal barrier function and the presence of necrotic tissue, there is concern for life-threatening sepsis. It is not uncommon to see changes in the wound flora. A shift from coagulase-positive staphylococci to a gram-negative flora can occur. Cultures and sensitivities may be valuable in antibiotic selection. Care is needed in antibiotic selection to avoid those that may be on the list of ill-advised agents or chemically related antibiotics (i.e., cephalosporins can cross-react with penicillin antibiotics). Many times patients may be so ill that oral drugs cannot be given and parenteral administration is required. In this situation the aminoglycosides (gentamicin 2 mg/kg q12h IM or SQ and amikacin 10 mg/kg q12h IM or SQ) can be quite valuable. When not contraindicated by the previous drug history, wide-spectrum oral antibiotics, such as a cephalexin 20 to 30 mg/kg q12h PO and amoxicillin–clavulanic acid 13.75 mg/kg q12h PO are excellent choices.

In addition to sepsis, the other major cause of mortality in drug reactions is extensive fluid, electrolyte, and colloid losses through the ulcerated areas. For this reason intravenous fluids and electrolyte replacement and maintenance during the recovery phase are required. Initial fluid therapy in severe CDR is similar to that in treating shock or burn cases. Lactated Ringer's at 80 ml/kg for the first 24 hours is recommended. Potassium losses can be extensive, and monitoring and supplementation based on frequent electrolyte measurements are required. Some cases may require colloid supplements. Indications, types, and dosages of such supplements can be obtained from additional references (Bell and Osborne, 1989; Lippert and Armstrong, 1989) or by referring severely critical cases to internal medicine specialists.

The use of systemic corticosteroids in CDR is controversial. Generally, in severely affected cases that are progressively deteriorating the use of corticosteroids is indicated. Initial shock dosages of dexamethasone 1 mg/kg IV followed by prednisone at 2 mg/kg q24h PO for 10 days is a recommended protocol. If lesions are clearing, the prednisone is tapered to q48h and eventually discontinued. Recovery, depending on the underlying cause, usually occurs in 3 to 4 weeks. Some cases of drug reactions can induce a chronic relapsing dermatopathy that may require life-long therapy.

REFERENCES

Beale K: Personal communication, 1991.

Bell FW, Osborne CA: Maintenance fluid therapy. In Kirk RW (ed): Current veterinary therapy X, Philadelphia, 1989, WB Saunders, p 37.

Elias PM, Fritsch PO: Erythema multiforme. In Fitzpatrick TB, et al (eds): Dermatology in general medicine, New York, 1987, McGraw-Hill, p 555.

Elias PM, Fritsch PO: Staphylococcal scalded skin syndrome, epidermolysin, and pathogenesis of blister formation. In Goldsmith L (ed): Biochemistry and physiology of skin, New York, 1983, Oxford University Press, p 1037.

Fritsch PO, Elias PM: Toxic epidermal necrolysis. In Fitzpatrick TB, et al (eds): Dermatology in general medicine, New York, 1987, McGraw-Hill, p 563.

Goldschmidt MH, Wolfsdorf K: Erythema multiforme—a retrospective study of 14 cases in the dog. Proceedings, Annual members' meeting AAVD & ACVD, 1988, p 28.

Griffin CE: Unpublished observation, 1991.

Gross TL, et al: Psoriasiform lichenoid dermatitis in the Springer Spaniel, Vet Pathol 23:76, 1986.

Lippert AC, Armstrong PJ: Parenteral nutritional support. In Kirk RW (ed): Current veterinary therapy X, Philadelphia, 1989, WB Saunders, p 25.

Mason KV: Subepidermal bullous drug eruption resembling bullous pemphigoid in a dog, J Am Vet Med Assoc 190:881, 1987.

Mason KV: Fixed drug eruption in two dogs caused by diethylcarbamazine, J Am Anim Hosp Assoc 24:301, 1988.

Mason KV, et al: Characterization of lichenoid psoriasiform dermatosis of Springer Spaniels, J Am Vet Med Assoc 189:897, 1986.

Muller GH, et al: Small animal dermatology, ed 4, Philadelphia, 1989, WB Saunders, pp 474 and 539.

Plant J, et al. In Proceedings, Annual members' meeting AAVD & ACVD, Scottsdale, 1991.

Rosenkrantz WS: Unpublished observations, 1990.

Rosenkrantz WS, et al: Clinical evaluation of cyclosporine in animal models with cutaneous immune-mediated disease and epitheliotropic lymphoma, J Am Anim Hosp 25:377, 1989.

Rosenkrantz WS, et al: Superficial suppurative necrolytic dermatitis in miniature schnauzers: a retrospective analysis, Proceedings, Annual members' meeting AAVD & ACVD, Scottsdale, 1991, p 99.

Schmeitzel CP: Focal cutaneous reactions at vaccination sites in a cat and four dogs. In Proceedings, Annual members' meeting AAVD & ACVD, 1986.

Scott DW: Erythema multiforme in the dog. J Am Anim Hosp Assoc 19:453, 1983.

Scott DW: Immune mediated dermatoses in domestic animals: ten years after. II, Compend Contin Educ Pract Vet 9:539, 1987.

Van Hees J, et al: Levamisole-induced drug eruptions in the dog, J Am Anim Hosp Assoc 21:255, 1985.

Wilcock BP, Yager JA: Focal cutaneous vasculitis and alopecia at sites of rabies vaccination in dogs, J Am Vet Med Assoc 188:1174, 1986.

Wintroub BU, et al: Cutaneous reactions to drugs. In Fitzpatrick TB, et al (eds): Dermatology in general medicine, New York, 1987, McGraw-Hill, p 1353.

Keratinization Disorders

16

Overview of Normal Keratinization and Cutaneous Scaling Disorders of Dogs

Kenneth W. Kwochka

Scaling Disorders of Dogs

SCALING SECONDARY TO AN UNDERLYING DISEASE

Pruritic

Canine scabies, cheyletiellosis, flea allergy dermatitis, atopy, food allergy dermatitis, pyoderma

Nonpruritic

Demodicosis, dermatophytosis, hypothyroidism, hyperadrenocorticism, sex hormone abnormalities, pemphigus foliaceus, mycosis fungoides, chronic steroid administration, environmental factors

DIFFERENTIAL FOR PRIMARY KERATINIZATION DISORDERS

Generalized

Primary idiopathic seborrhea, vitamin-A responsive dermatosis, zinc-responsive dermatosis, epidermal dysplasia, sebaceous adenitis, follicular dystrophy, Schnauzer comedo syndrome, canine ichthyosis

Localized

Lichenoid-psoriasiform dermatosis, nasodigital hyperkeratosis, canine ear margin dermatosis, canine acne

---

Importance

One of the most common clinical presentations to the small animal practitioner is a dog with scaly skin. In a study conducted during 1983 (Sischo et al., 1989) it was the fourth commonest cutaneous abnormality in North American dogs.

Cutaneous scaling disorders challenge the practitioner with diagnostic dilemmas and therapeutic difficulties. The veterinarian must determine whether the scaling is simply secondary to an underlying dermatosis or associated with a primary keratinization defect.

Primary disorders of keratinization are dermatoses usually manifested clinically by excess scale formation. Histologically the most striking abnormalities involve the keratinizing structures of the body. The epidermis is not the only keratinizing portion of the skin. Other structures include the hair follicle outer root sheath, hair cuticle, and claw. Any of these structures may be involved either alone or in combination when a keratinization abnormality is present.

To differentiate between secondary scaling and a primary keratinization disorder requires a complete well-organized diagnostic plan, a knowledgeable cooperative owner, good client communication, and adequate finances. A complete diagnostic plan usually results in a definitive diagnosis, allowing for a more accurate prognosis and a decision on specific treatment.

When the underlying dermatosis is identified and treated, secondary scaling usually has an excellent prognosis for complete cure or control. Scaling associated with primary keratinization defects is more difficult to control and requires a lifelong clinical management program with topical and systemic therapy.

This chapter will present an overview of normal keratinization, pathogenesis of primary keratinization disorders, and the general clinical approach to dogs with cutaneous scaling. Chapters 17, 18, and 19 discuss, respectively, specific primary keratinization disorders, topical therapy of cutaneous scaling, and the use of retinoids for primary keratinization disorders. Chapter 20 deals with sebaceous adenitis, a relatively new keratinization disorder that affects several breeds of purebred dogs.

Normal Keratinization

Keratin is a very stable, tough, inert protein rich in cystine and disulfide bonds. The cells of the stratum corneum are composed primarily of this protein and form, along with the lipid-rich intercellular domain, the major protective barrier for the rest of the body. The complex process by which a mitotically active keratinocyte in the basal layer of the epidermis becomes a dead keratinized corneocyte is referred to as keratinization.

Epidermopoiesis

Like blood cell lines in the bone marrow and gastrointestinal epithelium, the epidermis is a renewable cell population. Columnar keratinocytes migrate from the mitotically active pool in the basal layer, through the spinous layer and granular layer, and finally into the stratum corneum, followed by normal exfoliation. This migration takes place in an orderly fashion. The normal canine epidermis is a very slowly renewing cell population (Kwochka and Rademakers, 1989a). Only 1.5% of epidermal basal cells are undergoing DNA replication at any point in time (labeling index), and it takes approximately 22 days for a cell to migrate from the basal layer to, but not through, the stratum corneum.

The upper external root sheath of the hair follicle has essentially the same cell kinetic growth characteristics as the surface epidermis (Kwochka and Rademakers, 1989a). Conversely, the hair root matrix of anagen hairs is the most rapidly renewing cell population of the body (Kwochka, 1990). The intense mitotic activity of an actively growing hair is reflected by a labeling index of 24%.

Sebaceous glands, which may have primary abnormalities in some scaling disorders, are holocrine glands with a slowly renewable, nonkeratinizing cell population. Their labeling index ranges from 0.4% to 1.8% in dogs with clinically normal skin (Kwochka and Rademakers, 1989a).

Keratogenesis

During the orderly cell migration process of epidermopoiesis, keratin is formed in a complex series of biochemical events (Freedberg, 1987). Keratin filaments form the cytoskeleton of keratinocytes in the spinous layer of the epidermis. Additionally, keratohyalin granules, which are visible in the granular layer, provide a cystine-rich protein and a protein called filaggrin. Filaggrin directs the aggregation of the keratin filaments, cystine-rich protein, and other proteins by disulfide bond formation into the inert keratin protein.

Other processes take place concurrently during keratinization that are essential to the formation of the stratum corneum. A thick stratum corneum cell envelope is formed when a soluble protein, keratolinin, migrates to the cell surface and is cross-linked with involucrin by the enzyme transglutaminase (Freedberg, 1987).

Intracellular lamellar organelles called lamellar bodies or membrane coating granules are synthesized in the stratum spinosum (Elias, 1987; Freinkel, 1987). These structures contain lipids, especially phospholipids. The lamellar bodies fuse with the plasma membrane and extrude their contents into the intercellular space at the level of the stratum granulosum. These lipids have a highly structured bilayer configuration, make up 80% of stratum corneum lipids, and are high in ceramides. Apocrine and sebaceous secretions also contribute to the surface lipid film.

The dead, inert cellular keratin and intercellular lipids form the two-compartment model system for the protective barrier of the body, the stratum corneum (Elias, 1991). Although there is a great degree of organization to the corneocytes and intercellular lipids, modulations of enzymatic activity continue in the stratum corneum, resulting in variations of permeability, cell cohesion, and desquamation.

The epidermal barrier protects against the loss of body fluids, macromolecules, and electrolytes; the entrance of toxic agents, microorganisms, and ultraviolet radiation; and low-voltage electric current (Blank, 1987).

Pathogenesis of Primary Keratinization Disorders

An abnormality involving any of the steps in epidermopoiesis, keratinization, apocrine or sebaceous glandular function, intercellular lipid formation, cell cohesion, or cell desquamation may result in the formation of visible scale.

Most primary keratinization disorders are familial and are probably genetic defects leading to inborn errors of metabolism. In some cases the abnormality may be a primary cellular defect of the keratinocyte. However, the epidermal keratinocyte may also be normal though responding to abnormal humoral factors that control cell maturation and proliferation. There may also be an abnormality in apocrine or sebaceous glandular function or in epidermal lipid production, which could lead to aberrations in corneocyte cohesion and desquamation and result in retention hyperkeratosis and visible scale.

Most experimental work on primary keratinization disorders has been done in Cocker Spaniels with primary idiopathic seborrhea (Kwochka and Rademakers, 1989b). The basal cell labeling indices are 3 to 4 times greater for the seborrheic epidermis, hair follicle infundibulum, and sebaceous glands, indicating that these structures are hyperproliferative. The cell renewal time for the viable epidermis is decreased from 22 to 8 days. The accelerated cell renewal results in overproduction of corneocytes and visible scale. Similar epidermal cell kinetic abnormalities have been identified in Irish Setters (Baker and Maibach, 1987).

There is evidence that the cell proliferation abnormalities in Cocker Spaniels are a result of a primary cell defect. The cells remain hyperproliferative when grown in pure cell culture without dermal components (Kwochka et al., 1987). Additionally, the seborrheic epidermis remains hyperproliferative 6 weeks after being grafted onto the dermis of normal dogs (Kwochka and Smeak, 1990). Finally, both in vivo and in vitro, the total cell cycle time of the basal epidermal keratinocyte is significantly shortened in seborrheic versus normal dogs (Kwochka, 1991). These findings suggest that the disease in Cocker Spaniels might be better termed "primary epidermal hyperproliferation" than primary idiopathic seborrhea.

The aforementioned experimental studies have had direct clinical therapeutic application and suggest the potential value of the retinoids, especially etretinate (Tegison), in helping control the hyperproliferation associated with the disease. This drug has shown good efficacy in a doubleblind, placebo-controlled study (Power and Ihrke, 1990). Its mechanism of action is currently being evaluated.

Cutaneous lipids and fatty acid production have also been evaluated in seborrheic dogs. On seb-

orrheic skin of various breeds, there was a substantial increase in the relative amounts of free fatty acids and a decrease in the amounts of diester waxes (Horwitz and Ihrke, 1977). Quantitative studies on sebum production have not been reported.

A recent study (Campbell, 1990) found elevated cutaneous levels of arachidonic acid in 21 dogs with cutaneous scaling and suggested that this might be responsible for epidermal hyperproliferation and inflammation. It also indicated that fatty acid supplements such as sunflower oil (1.5 ml/kg, q24h, PO) might be helpful treatment by altering fatty acid levels in the skin.

Another study (White, 1990), however, found no differences in omega-6 (including arachidonic acid), omega-3, or omega-9 cutaneous fatty acid profiles between a group of 20 dogs with normal skin and 6 Cocker Spaniels with primary idiopathic seborrhea.

There have been no studies published investigating keratin proteins, cell cohesion, or cell desquamation in the normal canine epidermis or in the epidermis of dogs with primary keratinization disorders.

CLINICAL DISEASE

Disorders of keratinization are characterized clinically by mild to severe dry (Fig. 17-1), waxy, or greasy (Fig. 17-2) scales. There is also some degree of "seborrheic odor" associated with the skin condition. In fact, the severe "rancid fat odor" in dogs with greasy scale and secondary bacterial or yeast infections is often the owner's primary complaint. Since hair follicles and glandular structures may also be involved, it is not unusual to see comedones and follicular casts (Fig. 20-2). Comedones are blackheads resulting from dilation of hair follicles with keratin plugs. Follicular casts are tightly adherent scale around hair shafts.

Common secondary findings include alopecia, inflammation, crusts, pruritus with secondary excoriations, and pyoderma. Unfortunately, these secondary findings are common with virtually any dermatosis.

The most difficult task for the practitioner is to determine whether a primary keratinization defect is present or the scaling and other signs are simply secondary to an underlying dermatosis. The latter is much more common and should be considered first when a diagnostic plan is being formulated. Important diseases causing secondary scaling include demodicosis, scabies, cheyletiellosis, atopy, food allergy, flea allergy, pyoderma, dermatophytosis, hypothyroidism, hyperadrenocorticism, sex hormone abnormalities, pemphigus foliaceus, mycosis fungoides, and environmental influences (e.g., low humidity).

In diseases classified as primary keratinization defects, the exact cause for the apparent keratinization abnormality is unknown or the cause is known and the primary pathophysiology involves a keratinization defect. Specific diseases include primary idiopathic seborrhea, vitamin A–responsive dermatosis, zinc-responsive dermatosis, epidermal dysplasia, sebaceous adenitis, follicular dystrophy, lichenoid-psoriasiform dermatosis, Schnauzer comedo syndrome, canine ichthyosis, nasodigital hyperkeratosis, canine ear margin dermatosis, and canine acne.

Signalment

The signalment provides some useful information in distinguishing between primary and secondary scaling. Generally, primary keratinization disorders are hereditary and appear during the first 2 years of life. This is especially true of primary idiopathic seborrhea, epidermal dysplasia, follicular dystrophy, Schnauzer comedo syndrome, canine ichthyosis, and canine acne. Infectious, parasitic, and allergic dermatoses are the most common causes of secondary scaling in this age range.

Middle-aged animals are less likely to have primary keratinization defects, more likely presenting with secondary scaling due to allergies, endocrinopathies, and autoimmune disease (especially pemphigus foliaceus). For older animals, cutaneous neoplasms such as mycosis fungoides should also be considered.

There is no characteristic sex predilection for the primary scaling disorders.

Breed, along with age of onset, is the most important part of the signalment in considering differentials for the primary keratinization disorders (Table 16-1).

History

In dogs with primary keratinization disorders a complete history will reveal that the scaling started at a young age. An **observant** owner will also indicate that the scaling or comedomes were present prior to the development of secondary signs (e.g., pruritus, pyoderma, inflammation, and alopecia). If these secondary signs were observed before the scaling, a primary keratinization disorder is unlikely.

Another extremely important aspect of the history is response to previous therapy. Many of the primary keratinization disorders and secondary causes of scaling are complicated by pyoderma and some degree of pruritus associated with the pyoderma. If the scaling resolves *completely* by treatment of the pyoderma with antibiotics, it is unlikely that a primary keratinization defect is present. Some degree of scaling, comedones, or follicular casts would still be present. The presence of these lesions after antibiotics *without* pruritus or cutaneous inflammation suggests a primary keratinization defect, an endocrine dermatosis, or environmental factors. Scale remaining after antibiotics *with* significant pruritus and inflammation is more indicative of parasitic and allergic dermatoses.

Other aspects of the history are of greater importance in diagnosis of the secondary causes of scaling. Exposure to an infected animal or environment prior to development of the scaling suggests a parasitic dermatosis (especially scabies and cheyletiellosis) or dermatophytosis. Seasonal pruritus associated with scaling suggests atopy, flea allergy dermatitis, or other insect hypersensitivities such as those due to biting flies, mosquitoes, or ants. Concurrent systemic signs with scaling (e.g., polyuria, polydipsia, lethargy, cold intolerance, and abnormalities in estrus cycle or sexual behavior) may suggest an endocrinopathy. Endocrine dermatoses are usually associated with minimal pruritus unless complicated by pyoderma or severe xerosis.

More complete clinical aspects of the individual diseases causing secondary scaling and the primary keratinization disorders are discussed in their appropriate chapters.

DIAGNOSIS

Because there is no one specific laboratory test, it can be difficult and frustrating to make a definitive diagnosis of a primary keratinization disorder. A combination of factors must be considered—including the signalment (especially age and breed) and history as described above, elimination of secondary causes of scaling by execution of a complete diagnostic plan, findings on histopathologic examination of skin biopsies, and response to appropriate therapy based on the histologic findings.

Diagnostic Flow Chart (Fig. 16-1)

A scaling dermatosis, especially if it involves large areas of skin, should never be diagnosed as a primary keratinization defect without a complete

Table 16-1. Breed incidence for primary keratinization disorders in dogs

DISEASE	BREED(S)
Primary idiopathic seborrhea	Cocker Spaniel
	English Springer Spaniel
	Basset Hound
	West Highland White Terrier
	Doberman Pinscher
	Labrador Retriever
	Irish Setter
	Chinese Shar-Pei
Follicular dystrophy	Doberman Pinscher
	Rottweiler
	Yorkshire Terrier
	Irish Setter
	Dachshund
	Chow Chow
	Standard Poodle
	Great Dane
	Italian Greyhound
	Whippet
	Silky Terrier
	Chihuahua
Epidermal dysplasia	West Highland White Terrier
Ichthyosis	West Highland White Terrier
Vitamin A–responsive dermatosis	Cocker Spaniel
	Miniature Schnauzer
	Labrador Retriever
Zinc-responsive dermatosis	Alaskan Malamute
	Siberian Husky
Sebaceous adenitis	Standard Poodle
	Akita
	Vizsla
	Samoyed
Nasodigital hyperkeratosis	Cocker Spaniel
Lichenoid-psoriasiform dermatosis	English Springer Spaniel
Schnauzer comedo syndrome	Miniature Schnauzer
Ear margin dermatosis	Dachshund
Acne	English Bulldog
	Boxer
	Doberman Pinscher
	Great Dane

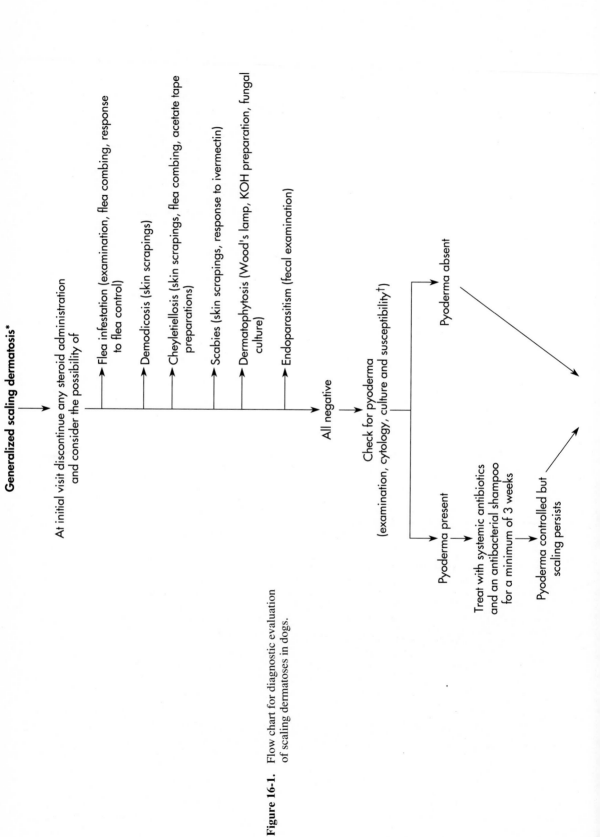

Figure 16-1. Flow chart for diagnostic evaluation of scaling dermatoses in dogs.

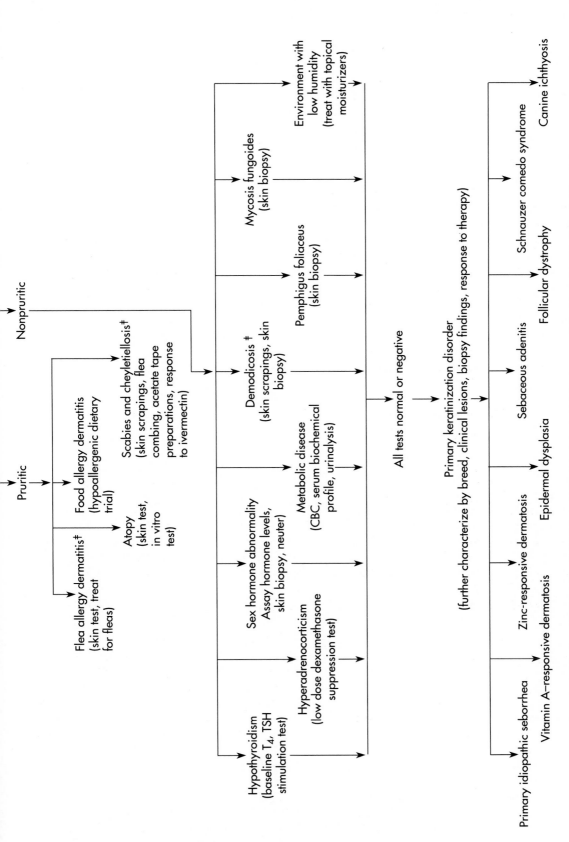

Pruritic

Nonpruritic

Flea allergy dermatitis‡
(skin test, treat
for fleas)

Food allergy dermatitis
(hypoallergenic dietary
trial)

Atopy
(skin test,
in vitro
test)

Scabies and cheyletiellosis‡
(skin scrapings, flea
combing, acetate tape
preparations, response
to ivermectin)

Hypothyroidism
(baseline T₄, TSH
stimulation test)

Hyperadrenocorticism
(low dose dexamethasone
suppression test)

Sex hormone abnormality
Assay hormone levels,
skin biopsy, neuter)

Metabolic disease
(CBC, serum biochemical
profile, urinalysis)

Demodicosis ‡
(skin scrapings, skin
biopsy)

Pemphigus foliaceus
(skin biopsy)

Mycosis fungoides
(skin biopsy)

Environment with
low humidity
(treat with topical
moisturizers)

All tests normal or negative

Primary keratinization disorder
(further characterize by breed, clinical lesions, biopsy findings, response to therapy)

Primary idiopathic seborrhea

Vitamin A-responsive dermatosis

Zinc-responsive dermatosis

Epidermal dysplasia

Sebaceous adenitis

Follicular dystrophy

Schnauzer comedo syndrome

Canine ichthyosis

*This flow chart best used for dogs with multifocal or generalized scaling. Localized scaling disorders can usually be diagnosed by clinical lesions and biopsy findings.
†Culture and susceptibility not needed for all cases, but are recommended if the pyoderma is chronic or has been treated previously.
‡Reconsidered because these may be missed at time of the initial visit.

diagnostic plan to first rule out secondary causes of scaling. A flow chart is often helpful for approaching these cases in a stepwise logical manner. This is particularly true when attempting to rule out secondary scaling for suspect cases of primary idiopathic seborrhea, vitamin A–responsive dermatosis, zinc-responsive dermatosis, epidermal dysplasia, sebaceous adenitis, follicular dystrophy, and Schnauzer comedo syndrome. The diagnostic tests utilized include skin scrapings, fungal culture, bacterial culture, intradermal allergy testing or serologic testing for allergen-specific IgE, food-elimination diet, complete blood count, serum biochemical profile, hormonal assays, fecal examination for parasites, and skin biopsies.

Unfortunately, not every case will flow through the chart easily. In very chronic cases it will often be difficult to determine whether pruritus is a primary problem or secondary to chronic skin changes. Thus some cases will need to be evaluated for allergic as well as endocrine dermatoses. Some patients may have more than one underlying disease that needs to be controlled (e.g., a dog with secondary scaling due to atopy and food allergy). Some may also have a primary keratinization disorder that is further complicated by another skin disease, which, together, make the condition of the skin especially bad (e.g., a West Highland White Terrier with idiopathic seborrhea or epidermal dysplasia complicated by severe atopy).

Lichenoid-psoriasiform dermatosis, canine ichthyosis, nasodigital hyperkeratosis, ear margin dermatosis, and canine acne are primary keratinization disorders so characteristic, either clinically or histologically, that often the diagnosis can be made using skin biopsy and minimal additional diagnostics (skin scrapings, fungal culture, bacterial culture). The diagnostic flow chart is usually unnecessary for these disorders.

Skin Biopsy

Skin biopsy is the most important diagnostic tool for primary keratinization disorders. Histologic changes will be (1) diagnostic for (sebaceous adenitis, follicular dystrophy, Schnauzer comedo syndrome, lichenoid-psoriasiform dermatosis, canine ichthyosis, canine acne), (2) compatible with (vitamin A–responsive dermatosis, zinc-responsive dermatosis), or (3) suggestive of (primary idiopathic seborrhea, epidermal dysplasia, nasodigital hyperkeratosis, ear margin dermatosis) a primary keratinization disorder. Additionally, histologic changes may suggest or help

rule out dermatoses associated with secondary scaling.

The best time to take a skin biopsy is early in the course of the diagnostic evaluation, but after secondary pyoderma has been controlled with antibiotics and topical therapy. Histologic changes associated with pyoderma make evaluation of the biopsy difficult.

Although the diagnosis is usually best made from biopsy of an early lesion uncomplicated by chronic changes, it is important to take at least three biopsies from lesions of various ages to maximize the chance of a definitive identification. Multiple biopsies also allow the pathologist to determine the stage of the disease, which may affect choice of therapy and prognosis. For example, early stages of sebaceous adenitis show inflammation centered on sebaceous glands whereas chronic changes are often associated with complete absence of sebaceous glands. The latter condition may be confused with an endocrinopathy and generally carries a poorer prognosis for successful clinical management.

Skin biopsies should be sent to a veterinary pathologist who specializes in dermatopathology. The primary keratinization disorders are unique enough that a general pathologist may not be able to make the diagnosis.

TREATMENT
General Principles

Treatment of scaling usually starts before a specific diagnosis of cause is made. In fact, treatment may start even before it is clear that the scaling is secondary or due to a primary keratinization defect, because the owner and veterinarian generally want to make the patient look and feel as good as possible as quickly as possible.

Since many dogs with scale have secondary pyoderma, initial treatment consists of antibiotics (potentiated sulfonamides, cephalosporins, amoxicillin trihydrate with clavulanate potassium) and a topical antibacterial/keratolytic shampoo (OxyDex Shampoo, Sulf OxyDex Shampoo, Pyoben Shampoo) for 3 to 4 weeks. Not only does this improve the condition of the skin and hair coat, it allows assessment of the role of infection in scaling when the patient is reevaluated.

During the course of a diagnostic evaluation, steroids should not be administered. **First,** steroids may affect the ability to control any concurrent pyoderma. **Second,** it is important to determine how much pruritus remains after the pyoderma is controlled. This information will help determine whether parasites and allergies (pruritus remains) or endocrine and primary keratinization disorders (pruritus resolved) should be considered as major differentials. The concurrent use of steroids masks signs and does not allow for such an assessment. **Third,** the use of topical or systemic steroids before a definitive diagnosis may make the condition worse by adverse effects on sebaceous secretions, keratinization, and hair production.

Secondary scaling is best treated by management of the underlying disease. However, symptomatic topical therapy is helpful in controlling scale formation until the disease is treated with more specific therapy. Specific treatments are covered in the appropriate chapters.

Topical Therapy

Symptomatic topical therapy with shampoo formulations is the major form of treatment used to manage most of the generalized primary keratinization defects. The active ingredients in these shampoos are moisturizers, keratolytics, keratoplastics (see p. 193), antibacterials, degreasers, and follicular flushers. These ingredients are also incorporated into ointments, gels, creams, lotions, and pads for some of the more localized keratinization abnormalities. Selecting proper agents depends upon the specific condition. All these products are discussed in detail in Chapter 18.

Systemic Therapy

When topical therapy fails to control a primary keratinization defect adequately or if topical therapy is too time-consuming for the owner, systemic agents can be utilized. Most work has been done with three retinoids—retinol, isotretinoin (Accutane), and etretinate (Tegison)—which have been used for idiopathic seborrhea, vitamin A–responsive dermatosis, sebaceous adenitis, Schnauzer comedo syndrome, canine ichthyosis, nasodigital hyperkeratosis, and acne. The proper use of these agents is discussed in Chapter 19.

Oral zinc is used for zinc-responsive dermatosis. Steroids may be helpful for epidermal dysplasia and sebaceous adenitis. Cyclosporine A has also been helpful in sebaceous adenitis. Antibiotics are often needed to control secondary pyoderma associated with many of the primary keratinization disorders.

These drugs are discussed in more detail in Chapter 17 with the individual primary keratinization disorders.

REFERENCES

Baker BB, Maibach HI: Epidermal cell renewal in seborrheic skin of dogs, Am J Vet Res 48:726, 1987.

Blank IH: The skin as an organ of protection. In Fitzpatrick TB, et al (eds): Dermatology in general medicine, ed 3, New York, 1987, McGraw-Hill, p 337.

Campbell KL: Effects of oral sunflower oil on serum and cutaneous fatty acids in seborrheic dogs. In Proceedings, Annual members' meeting AAVD & ACVD, 1990, p 44.

Elias PM: The special role of the stratum corneum. In Fitzpatrick TB, et al (eds): Dermatology in general medicine, ed 3, New York, 1987, McGraw-Hill, p 342.

Elias PM: Dynamics of epidermal barrier formation, function, and metabolism. In Proceedings, Forty-second annual meeting, American College of Veterinary Pathologists, 1991, p 96.

Freinkel RK: Lipids of the epidermis. In Fitzpatrick TB, et al (eds): Dermatology in general medicine, ed 3, New York, 1987, McGraw-Hill, p 191.

Freedberg IM: Epidermal differentiation and keratinization. In Fitzpatrick TB, et al (eds): Dermatology in general medicine, ed 3, New York, 1987, McGraw-Hill, p 174.

Horwitz LN, Ihrke PJ: Canine seborrhea. In Kirk RW (ed): Current veterinary therapy VI, Philadelphia, 1977, WB Saunders, p 519.

Kwochka KW: Cell proliferation kinetics in the hair root matrix of dogs with healthy skin and dogs with idiopathic seborrhea, Am J Vet Res 51:1570, 1990.

Kwochka KW: In vivo and in vitro examination of cell proliferation kinetics in the normal and seborrheic canine epidermis. In Proceedings, Annual members' meeting AAVD & ACVD, 1991, p 46.

Kwochka KW, Rademakers AM: Cell proliferation of epidermis, hair follicles, and sebaceous glands of Beagles and Cocker Spaniels with healthy skin, Am J Vet Res 50:587, 1989a.

Kwochka KW, Rademakers AM: Cell proliferation kinetics of epidermis, hair follicles, and sebaceous glands of Cocker Spaniels with idiopathic seborrhea, Am J Vet Res 50:1918, 1989b.

Kwochka KW, Smeak DD: The cellular defect in idiopathic seborrhea of Cocker Spaniels. In Von Tscharner C, Halliwell REW (eds): Advances in veterinary dermatology, London, 1990, Baillière Tindall, p 265.

Kwochka KW, et al: Development and characterization of an in vitro cell culture system for the canine epidermis. In Proceedings, Annual members' meeting AAVD & ACVD, 1987, p 9.

Power HT, Ihrke PJ: Synthetic retinoids in veterinary dermatology, Vet Clin North Am 20:1525, 1990.

Sischo WM, et al: Regional distribution of ten common skin diseases in dogs, J Am Vet Med Assoc 195:752, 1989.

White PD: Evaluation of serum and cutaneous essential fatty acid profiles in normal, atopic, and seborrheic dogs. In Proceedings, Annual members' meeting AAVD & ACVD, 1990, p 37.

Primary Keratinization Disorders of Dogs

Kenneth W. Kwochka

Differential Diagnosis of Primary Keratinization Disorders of Dogs

GENERALIZED
Primary idiopathic seborrhea, vitamin A–responsive dermatosis, zinc-responsive dermatosis, epidermal dysplasia, sebaceous adenitis, color mutant alopecia, follicular dystrophy, Schnauzer comedo syndrome, canine ichthyosis

LOCALIZED
Lichenoid-psoriasiform dermatosis, idiopathic nasodigital hyperkeratosis, canine ear margin dermatosis, canine acne

---

This chapter addresses the clinical aspects of primary keratinization disorders in dogs. I strongly recommend that it be read **after** Chapter 16, especially if the reader is looking for a practical approach to the diagnosis and management of a dog presented for a scaling dermatosis. Chapter 16 describes the normal keratinization process and pathophysiology of keratinization disorders. More important, it also details the general clinical approach to cutaneous scaling in dogs and presents an organized plan for differentiating scaling secondary to other dermatologic diseases from that due to true primary keratinization disorders. When the underlying dermatosis is identified and treated, secondary scaling usually has an excellent prognosis for complete cure or control. A primary keratinization disorder should never be diagnosed until secondary causes of scaling have first been considered.

Importance

Primary disorders of keratinization are dermatoses that usually manifest clinically as localized or generalized excess scale formation. The scale may originate from the interfollicular epidermis or emanate from hair follicles as comedones and follicular casts. Histologically the most striking abnormalities involve the keratinizing structures of the body—including the epidermis, the hair follicle outer root sheath, and the hair cuticle.

Taken individually, primary keratinization disorders are not commonly encountered; as a group, however, they represent a significant portion of the dermatologic caseload in general and specialty practice. It is therefore important to be familiar with the diagnosis and clinical management of these diseases. Most are controllable with continued therapy but carry a guarded prognosis for complete cure. To make a rational decision on whether or not to treat a pet, the owner should be aware of this. Some of these diseases are so severe that euthanasia may be a serious consideration. There are also important implications for breeders, since most of these conditions are hereditary and breeding affected animals should be discouraged.

Pathogenesis

For most of the diseases classified as primary keratinization disorders, the pathogenesis is unknown. For others the cause is known and the primary pathophysiology involves a defect in the keratinizing epithelium or cutaneous glandular function. These abnormalities are discussed, in more basic terms, in Chapter 16 and, in relation to specific diseases, in the next section.

Primary keratinization disorders include primary idiopathic seborrhea, vitamin A–responsive dermatosis, zinc-responsive dermatosis, epidermal dysplasia, sebaceous adenitis, color mutant alopecia, follicular dystrophy, lichenoid-psoriasiform dermatosis, Schnauzer comedo syndrome, canine ichthyosis, idiopathic nasodigital hyperkeratosis, canine ear margin dermatosis, and canine acne. All of these diseases (except sebaceous adenitis, which is described in detail in Chapter 20) are discussed in this chapter.

CLINICAL DISEASE

Disorders of keratinization are characterized clinically by mild to severe dry, waxy, or greasy scales. There is also some degree of seborrheic odor associated with the skin condition. In fact, the severe "rancid fat odor" in dogs with greasy scale and secondary bacterial or yeast infections is often the owner's primary complaint. Since hair follicles and glandular structures may also be involved, it is not unusual to see comedones (Fig. 7-7) and follicular casts (Fig. 20-2). Comedones are blackheads resulting from dilation of hair follicles with keratin plugs. Follicular casts are tightly adherent scale around hair shafts.

Common secondary findings include alopecia, inflammation, crusts, pruritus with secondary excoriations, and pyoderma. Unfortunately, these secondary findings are common to see with virtually any dermatosis. Secondary *Malassezia* colonization may also be associated with primary and secondary causes of scaling. Presence of these yeasts should always be evaluated by skin swabs and cytologic examination. Details on the management of *Malassezia* dermatitis are found in Chapter 4.

Most of the primary keratinization disorders are treated with various combinations of topical antiseborrheic agents and systemic retinoids. Their use is discussed in relation to each disease but the specific drugs are covered in more detail in Chapters 18 and 19, respectively.

Primary Idiopathic Seborrhea

Primary idiopathic seborrhea is the most common chronic keratinization disorder encountered in dogs. This is true partly because many breeds with generalized scaling dermatoses of unknown cause have been lumped into that category. Some of these breeds include Cocker Spaniels, English Springer Spaniels, West Highland White Terriers, Basset Hounds, Irish Setters, German Shepherd Dogs, Dachshunds, Doberman Pinschers, Chinese Shar-Peis, and Labrador Retrievers. Extensive studies on the pathophysiology of primary idiopathic seborrhea have been done only for the Cocker Spaniel. Results of these studies are discussed in Chapter 16.

Depending on the breed, clinical signs may range anywhere from dry scaling, to greasy scaling, to scaling and greasiness with inflammation and pruritus, to any combination of these clinical abnormalities. The onset of signs is usually before 2 years of age.

Seborrhea Sicca

This term is used to describe the dry scaling of several breeds with primary idiopathic seborrhea. Affected animals have dull dry hair coats with focal to diffuse accumulations of white to gray nonadherent scales (Fig. 17-1). Breeds predisposed to this form of idiopathic seborrhea include Doberman Pinschers, Irish Setters, German Shepherd Dogs, and Dachshunds.

Seborrhea Oleosa

This term is reserved for primary idiopathic seborrheic breeds with greasy skin and hair coat. Affected dogs have greasy, brownish yellow clumps of lipid material that adhere to the skin and hair (Fig. 17-2). The material on the hair shafts has been described as "nitlike" (Fig. 17-3). Concurrent

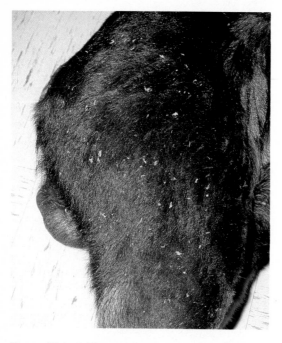

Figure 17-1. Diffuse seborrhea sicca with white non-adherent scales in a Rottweiler.

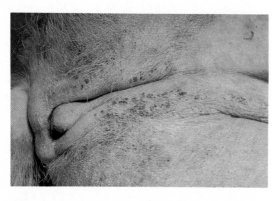

Figure 17-2. Tightly adherent brownish yellow greasy scales on the ventrum of a mixed breed dog with idiopathic seborrhea oleosa.

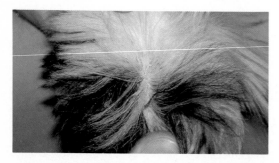

Figure 17-3. Greasy "nitlike" material adhering to the hair shafts on the leg of a Cocker Spaniel with idiopathic seborrhea oleosa.

ceruminous otitis is common (Fig. 17-4). One of the most frequent complaints is a severe rancid fat odor. Breeds predisposed to this form include Cocker Spaniels, English Springer Spaniels, Basset Hounds, West Highland White Terriers, Chinese Shar-Peis, and Labrador Retrievers.

Seborrheic Dermatitis

This presentation of primary idiopathic seborrhea appears to be a more severe variant of seborrhea oleosa since it is generally seen in the same breeds. The clinical lesions are as described for seborrhea oleosa, but additionally there is significant cutaneous inflammation, bacterial folliculitis, pruritus, and multifocal plaques of hyperkeratotic material with inflammation. The most commonly involved areas of the body are the external ear canals, pinnae, ventral neck (Fig. 17-5), chest, axillae, and inguinal and perineal areas.

Diagnosis

A definitive diagnosis of primary idiopathic seborrhea requires a number of supporting factors—including age, breed, history, elimination of secondary causes of scaling, and findings on histopathologic examination of skin biopsies. (All these elements are discussed in detail in Chapter 16.)

The most important aspect of the diagnostic plan is a full investigation for secondary causes of scaling. The primary differentials are allergic dermatitis, scabies, dermatophytosis, demodicosis, bacterial folliculitis, hypothyroidism, and vitamin A–responsive dermatosis. An additional differential in Doberman Pinschers is color mutant alopecia and adult-onset follicular dysplasia.

Biopsies are usually characterized by orthokeratotic and parakeratotic hyperkeratosis, follic-

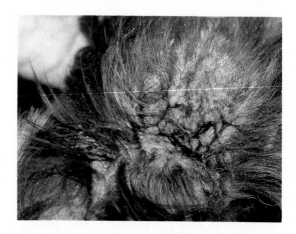

Figure 17-4. Severe ceruminous otitis in a black Cocker Spaniel with idiopathic seborrhea oleosa.

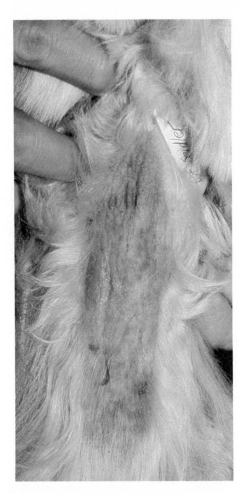

Figure 17-5. Alopecia, inflammation, and greasy scale on the ventral neck of a Cocker Spaniel with seborrheic dermatitis.

ular hyperkeratosis, and dyskeratosis. Often the follicular abnormalities are more impressive than changes in the epidermis. A superficial perivascular dermatitis with mixed cell infiltrate is also seen. Focal areas of parakeratosis over edematous dermal papillae have been reported.

Treatment

As with most primary keratinization disorders, the goal in primary idiopathic seborrhea is not to cure the disease but to control the scale formation.

When dry scaling is present, the skin and hair coat should be moisturized. This is accomplished with twice weekly moisturizing hypoallergenic shampoos (HyLyt*efa, Allergroom) and frequent moisturizing rinses (HyLyt*efa Bath Oil Coat Conditioner, Humilac). When dry scaling is severe and some keratolytic activity is needed, treatment usu-

ally consists of sulfur and salicylic acid shampoos (SebaLyt, Sebolux) followed by moisturizing rinses. Dietary supplementation with essential fatty acids (Derm Caps) may also be beneficial.

Keratolytic and keratoplastic degreasing shampoos are used to control the greasy scale and odor associated with seborrhea oleosa. Effective topical agents include coal tar (Clear Tar, NuSal-T, T-Lux, LyTar, Allerseb-T), benzoyl peroxide (OxyDex, Sulf OxyDex, Pyoben), and selenium sulfide (Selsun Blue).

The synthetic retinoid etretinate (Tegison), at 1 mg/kg q24h PO, has been effective for idiopathic seborrhea in Cocker Spaniels (Power and Ihrke, 1990), English Springer Spaniels, Irish Setters, Golden Retrievers, and mixed-breed dogs. Response was seen within 2 months and consisted of decreased scale, a softening and thinning of seborrheic plaques, reduced odor, and a lessening of pruritus. Some dogs have been maintained without signs of toxicity for several months on alternate-day therapy. (Chapter 19 provides more complete information on retinoids.)

Systemic antibiotics are recommended for patients with secondary bacterial folliculitis. A 7-to-10-day course of prednisone or prednisolone at an antiinflammatory dose may be needed during periods of severe inflammation and pruritus in dogs with seborrheic dermatitis.

Vitamin A–Responsive Dermatosis

Vitamin A–responsive dermatosis is a rare nutritionally responsive scaling disorder seen primarily in Cocker Spaniels (Ihrke and Goldschmidt, 1983; Scott, 1986). Similar syndromes have been reported in other breeds—including a Miniature Schnauzer, Labrador Retriever, and (in Europe) Chinese Shar-Peis. This is not a systemic vitamin A deficiency but probably represents a local deficiency in the epidermis, a problem with epidermal uptake, a disorder of cutaneous utilization, or a positive pharmacologic effect of high doses on the skin.

Vitamin A–responsive dermatosis usually develops within the first 2 to 3 years of life, though it may not be diagnosed until much later because the cutaneous abnormalities are often thought to represent primary idiopathic seborrhea. Clinical signs include refractory generalized scaling, a dry hair coat with easy epilation, prominent comedones, and hyperkeratotic plaques with large "fronds" of keratinous material protruding from the follicular ostia (Fig. 17-6). The plaques are usually seen

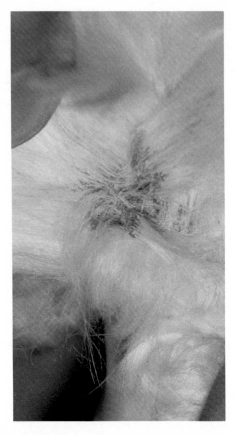

Figure 17-6. Hyperkeratotic plaque on the skin of a Cocker Spaniel with vitamin A–responsive dermatosis.

on the ventral and lateral thorax and abdomen, but the neck and face may also be involved. Other clinical features include a rancid fat odor from the skin, ceruminous otitis externa, and varying degrees of pruritus.

The condition is a rare and specific type of keratinization defect. It should not be confused with the more common primary idiopathic seborrhea of Cocker Spaniels just described. The only way to differentiate the two diseases effectively is by monitoring the response to vitamin A–alcohol supplementation.

Diagnosis

The early age of onset of refractory generalized scaling with hyperkeratotic plaques in a Cocker Spaniel is compatible with a clinical diagnosis of vitamin A–responsive dermatosis. A tentative diagnosis is made from skin biopsy findings, consisting of marked follicular hyperkeratosis with distended follicular ostia (phrynoderma-like), mild orthokeratotic hyperkeratosis of the epidermis, and mild irregular epidermal hyperplasia. Even with the

classic clinical and histologic findings, a definitive diagnosis can be confirmed only by response to supplementation with vitamin A alcohol.

The major differentials for this condition include primary idiopathic seborrhea, zinc-responsive dermatosis, generic dog food dermatosis, sebaceous adenitis, and superficial necrolytic dermatitis.

Treatment

Patients with vitamin A–responsive dermatosis are treated with 625 to 800 IU/kg q24h PO of vitamin A alcohol (retinol). Improvement is seen within 4 to 6 weeks, complete remission is obtained by 10 weeks, and treatment is needed for life. Retinol at this dosage is well-tolerated in dogs, so no clinicopathologic monitoring is necessary. Synthetic retinoids have been ineffective for this disorder and are not recommended because of their potential side effects and expense.

Keratinolytic shampoos containing benzoyl peroxide (OxyDex, Sulf OxyDex, Pyoben) have excellent follicular flushing activity. Twice-weekly usage helps remove keratinous debris from follicles and hastens recovery.

Zinc-Responsive Dermatosis

Zinc-responsive dermatosis is a rare nutritionally responsive scaling disease of several breeds of dogs (Kunkle, 1980). Its incidence seems to be decreasing; I now see only one or two cases per year. This is probably due to more selective breeding and better diets.

The disease is typically divided into two clinical syndromes—one affecting Siberian Huskies and Alaskan Malamutes, the other affecting mainly puppies on zinc-deficient diets or regimens that involve high levels of vitamin or mineral (especially calcium) supplementation.

The first dermatosis is also reported in Doberman Pinschers and Great Danes. Alaskan Malamutes have a genetic defect involving zinc absorption from the intestines (Brown et al., 1978). Thus the condition may occur even while the dog is on a well-balanced commercial diet. It may be precipitated by stress, estrus, and gastrointestinal disorders affecting absorption. Diets high in calcium and phytate (primary protein source of plant origin) may also precipitate the disorder by binding zinc in the gastrointestinal tract.

Lesions usually develop in dogs before puberty or as young adults and include alopecia, erythema, scaling, and crusting around the face (Fig. 17-7), head, scrotum, and legs. Lesions often encircle the

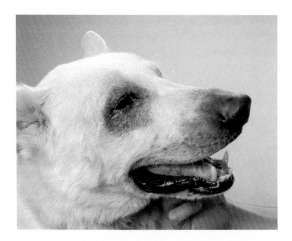

Figure 17-7. Alopecia, scaling, and hyperpigmentation involving the periocular areas and muzzle of a white German Shepherd Dog with zinc-responsive dermatosis.

(Courtesy Dr. Patricia White, Columbus, Ohio.)

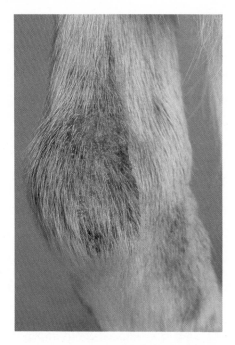

Figure 17-8. Alopecia, scaling, hyperpigmentation, and erythema of the hock of the dog in Fig. 17-7.

(Courtesy Dr. Patricia White, Columbus, Ohio.)

mouth, chin, eyes, ears, prepuce, and vulva. Thick crusts may also be found on the elbows and other pressure points of the body (Fig. 17-8), and the foot pads may be hyperkeratotic. The hair coat is generally dull and dry.

The second zinc-responsive dermatosis, in puppies being fed zinc-deficient diets or oversupplemented with vitamins and minerals (especially calcium), is also seen with diets high in phytate. Commonly affected breeds include Great Danes, Doberman Pinschers, Beagles, German Shepherd Dogs, German Shorthaired Pointers, Labrador Retrievers, and Rhodesian Ridgebacks (Kunkle, 1980; Ohlen and Scott, 1986; van den Broek and Thoday, 1986). In addition to the scaling and crusting, these dogs have secondary infections, lymphadenopathy, depression, and anorexia. The most obvious cutaneous lesions involve the head, elbows, other joints, and foot pads (Fig. 17-9).

Diagnosis

The early age of onset, dietary history, breed, and physical examination findings will be compatible with a diagnosis of zinc-responsive dermatosis. A tentative diagnosis is made from skin biopsy findings consisting of markedly diffuse surface and follicular parakeratotic hyperkeratosis and a hyperplastic superficial dermatitis. Measurements of zinc levels in hair or serum are variable and unreliable.

Important differentials for this syndrome include demodicosis, dermatophytosis, pemphigus foliaceus, generic dog food dermatosis, and su-

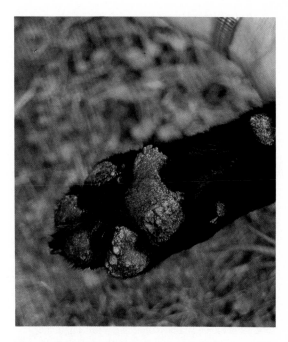

Figure 17-9. Hyperkeratotic foot pad of a puppy with zinc-responsive dermatosis.

perficial necrolytic dermatitis. Skin scrapings and fungal culture should be performed on all suspect cases in addition to the skin biopsies.

Treatment

The first syndrome of zinc-responsive dermatosis will usually respond to zinc sulfate at 10 mg/kg q24h or divided q12h PO with food. An alternative is zinc methionine (Zinpro) at 2 mg/kg q24h PO. Any dietary imbalances (high calcium and phytate) should be corrected. Symptoms resolve rapidly, but lifetime therapy is usually needed with this syndrome. Zinc may cause vomiting, in which case the dose should be lowered and the medication given with food.

The second syndrome, in puppies, will usually respond over time to dietary corrections alone. However, recovery can be hastened by supplementation as described for the first syndrome. Some puppies may need supplementation until maturity.

I have seen cases respond poorly to zinc supplementation but improve when a very low dosage of a short-acting glucocorticoid such as prednisone or prednisolone (at 0.15 mg/kg q24h PO) was added. This may have been due to some effect on zinc absorption in the gastrointestinal tract or to antiinflammatory activity on the skin lesions. A beneficial effect from combined zinc methionine and tetracycline has also been reported in a Great Dane (Fadok, 1982).

Epidermal Dysplasia

Epidermal dysplasia is an extremely severe keratinization disorder reported only in West Highland White Terriers (Scott and Miller, 1989). It appears to be a genetic keratinization abnormality, although the actual mode of inheritance and pathophysiology are unknown.

The disease develops in either sex, usually during the first year of life. Clinical signs begin with erythema and pruritus of the ventrum and extremities. These rapidly progress to a generalized disorder ("armadillo disease") with severe erythema and pruritus, alopecia, hyperpigmentation, lichenification, lymphadenopathy, greasy skin and hair coat, rancid fat odor, ceruminous otitis, and secondary bacterial infection (Figs. 17-10 and 17-11). Some dogs have secondary *Malassezia pachydermatis* colonization of the surface and infundibular keratin, which may contribute to the severity of the disease.

Diagnosis

The early age of onset of severe ventral erythema and pruritus rapidly progressing to chronic lesions in a West Highland White Terrier is compatible with a clinical diagnosis of epidermal dysplasia. A tentative diagnosis is made from skin biopsy findings consisting of a hyperplastic perivascular dermatitis with epidermal abnormalities (e.g., hyperchromasia, excessive keratinocyte mitosis, crowding of basilar keratinocytes, epidermal "buds," loss of epidermal cell polarity, and parakeratosis). Budding yeast organisms and gram-positive cocci may also be found in surface and infundibular keratin.

The real diagnostic challenge in these dogs is to determine whether the condition is due to epidermal dysplasia, some other pruritic skin disease, or a combination. Primary differentials that must be considered include atopy, food allergy dermatitis,

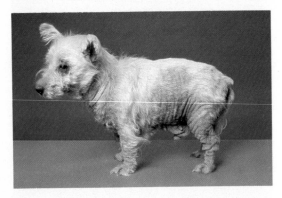

Figure 17-10. Erythema, pruritus, alopecia, lichenification, and hyperpigmentation in a West Highland White Terrier with epidermal dysplasia.

(Courtesy Dr. Patricia White, Columbus, Ohio.)

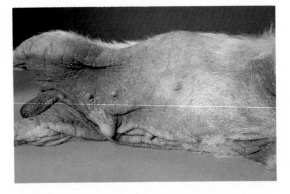

Figure 17-11. Ventral lesions of the dog in Fig. 17-10.

(Courtesy Dr. Patricia White, Columbus, Ohio.)

scabies, and primary idiopathic seborrhea. These should all be evaluated by appropriate testing or response to therapy in the diagnostic workup. A definitive diagnosis of epidermal dysplasia can be made only with characteristic clinical and histologic findings and after the foregoing differentials have been eliminated.

Another challenge is to determine how much the secondary bacterial infection or *Malassezia* colonization is contributing to the severity of the clinical condition. This can be assessed only by evaluating response after appropriate topical and systemic antimicrobial therapy.

Treatment

Epidermal dysplasia is generally nonresponsive to medical therapy with drugs including antibiotics, antiinflammatory doses of systemic glucocorticoids, antiseborrheic shampoos, vitamin A alcohol, synthetic retinoids, vitamin E, and essential fatty acids. The prognosis is poor, especially if the condition is chronic and severe secondary changes have occurred. This is one primary keratinization disorder that commonly ends with euthanasia of the pet.

Two forms of therapy offer hope in at least some of these dogs.

First, in patients with secondary *M. pachydermatis* colonization, there may be significant improvement in pruritus and skin condition with ketoconazole (Nizoral) at 10 mg/kg q24h PO and twice-weekly application of topical ketoconazole (Nizoral Shampoo) for 3 to 4 weeks. Over time, the yeast colonization will return secondary to the keratinization defect. However, this can sometimes be controlled with periodic ketoconazole shampoos. A sulfur and benzoyl peroxide shampoo (Sulf OxyDex) has also been helpful in long-term management of some cases.

I have seen patients respond to oral and topical ketoconazole in a similar fashion even when *M. pachydermatis* organisms were not present on skin swabs or biopsies. Ketoconazole has antiproliferative effects on keratinocytes in culture (Jacobs, 1991). Histologically it appears that at least part of the pathophysiology of this disease may involve a hyperproliferative basal keratinocyte population. This activity may explain the response in these dogs.

Second, in some cases seen very early in the course of the disease, before chronic cutaneous changes occur, there may be a dramatic response to immunosuppressive levels of short-acting glucocorticoids. Prednisone or prednisolone is administered at 1.1. to 2.2 mg/kg q12h PO until the condition is controlled followed by a gradual decrease in the dosage to alternate-day for long-term maintenance. Some patients will relapse while others remain in long-term remission. Before such therapy is used the patient should be evaluated for allergies and the side effects of chronic steroid administration should be explained to the owner.

Color Mutant Alopecia, Color Dilution Alopecia, Follicular Dystrophy, Follicular Dysplasia

All these terms have been used to describe hereditary alopecias with follicular dysplasia and melanization defects in a number of different breeds with various coat colors. They are included in this list of primary keratinization disorders because the keratinizing epithelium of the follicle and the hair cuticle are affected (ectodermal defects) as part of the disease process. Two general syndromes will be seen most often in practice—color mutant alopecia in many breeds and follicular dysplasia of adult black and red Doberman Pinschers. Congenital alopecias and ectodermal defects have been described in many other breeds but are rare.

Color mutant alopecia (color dilution alopecia) is a hereditary tardive alopecia seen in blue and fawn mutants of Doberman Pinschers, Miniature Pinschers, Irish Setters, Dachshunds, Chow Chows, Poodles, Great Danes, Whippets, Yorkshire Terriers, Chihuahuas, Italian Greyhounds, Salukis, Newfoundlands, and mongrels (Briggs and Botha, 1986; Carlotti, 1990; Miller, 1990a; Miller, 1991; O'Neill, 1981). It is also seen in red and occasionally in black Doberman Pinschers. The incidence of color mutant alopecia in adult blue and fawn Dobermans is between 58% and 90% (Miller, 1990a). Its pathophysiology apparently involves not only defective melanization but a primary structural defect in hair growth (Miller, 1990a).

The condition usually starts gradually within the first 3 years of life with a moth-eaten appearance (broken and stubbly hairs) to the color diluted hair coat. Hypotrichosis is complicated by dry scaling, papules and pustules (cystic hair follicles with secondary bacterial folliculitis), and eventually complete alopecia with severe scaling. The trunk is most severely affected, and the head and extrem-

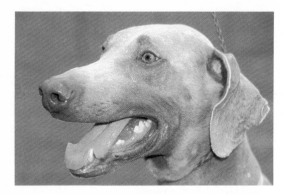

Figure 17-12. Sharp demarcation between normal tan points and alopecic areas on the face of a Doberman Pinscher with color mutant alopecia.

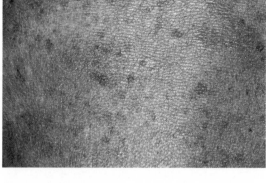

Figure 17-13. Close-up of the skin of the dog in Fig. 17-12, showing virtually total alopecia.

ities least affected. Tan points remain normal (Figs. 17-12 and 17-13). Pruritus is uncommon unless secondary bacterial folliculitis is present. Recurrent pyoderma is often the most frustrating problem in these cases and the hair loss is not reversible.

A follicular dysplasia (follicular dystrophy) has been described in four adult black and two adult red Doberman Pinschers (Miller, 1990b). Age of onset was 1 year in three dogs, 2 years in two dogs, and 4 years in one dog. In these cases the primary complaint was a slowly progressive, nonresponsive, dorsal hair loss. Hypotrichosis was first noted by owners in the lumbar regions and hair loss remained confined to the lower back and flanks. The four black dogs also had recurrent bacterial folliculitis in the alopecic areas. Although the folliculitis could be controlled with antibiotics, there was no new hair growth in the affected areas. Clinically this differs (by distribution of hair loss) from the color mutant alopecia occasionally seen in black Doberman Pinschers. A similar syndrome has been seen in Rottweilers (Griffin, 1992).

Diagnosis

The early age of onset of progressive alopecia in one of the predisposed breeds is compatible with a clinical diagnosis of color mutant alopecia. A tentative diagnosis is made from direct examination of the hair shafts (Brignac et al., 1988). Plucked hairs are prepared in mineral oil or potassium hydroxide. Large clumps of free disorganized melanin (macromelanosomes) within the hair cortex and medulla, distortion and breakage of the hair cortex along with the melanin aggregates (Fig. 17-14), and hair shafts that are devoid of cuticle may all be seen.

The definitive diagnosis is made from skin biopsy findings, including epidermal and follicular hyperkeratosis, follicular dilation, follicular cysts, and follicles devoid of hairs. Some cases show a decrease in size or number of sebaceous glands. Many hairs are dystrophic, and there are large clumps of melanin within hair follicles and in the cortex and medulla of the hair shaft. Melanin-laden cells are seen in the base of the external root sheath and hair bulb. Dermal melanophages surround the base of the follicle. Abnormal pigmentary clumping may also be seen in basal keratinocytes and melanocytes. Finally, there are variable degrees of follicular atrophy. Perifolliculitis, folliculitis, and furunculosis are present with secondary bacterial infection of the follicles.

The diagnosis of follicular dysplasia in adult black and red Doberman Pinschers is made in a similar fashion to that described for color mutant alopecia. The primary differences are the normal color of the hair coat, the fairly localized distribution of lesions to the flanks and lower back, the lack of pigmentary clumping in the basal epidermal melanocytes, and the less pronounced clumping of melanin in the follicular keratin and hair matrix cells of these dogs.

The differentials for both disorders include bacterial folliculitis, demodicosis, dermatophytosis, and idiopathic seborrhea. Hypothyroidism and other endocrine alopecias should be considered when an older dog is presented. One of the dermatoses may occur concurrently with color mutant alopecia or adult-onset follicular dysplasia. Therefore, every case should have a skin scraping, a fungal culture, and a thyroid gland evaluation with baseline T_4 or TSH stimulation test.

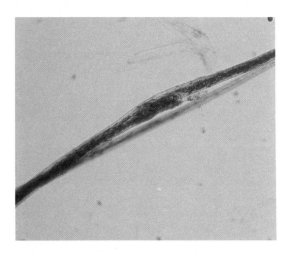

Figure 17-14. Melanin aggregates and an associated deformed hair cortex of a hair plucked from a Doberman Pinscher with color mutant alopecia.

(Courtesy Dr. John Gordon, Columbus, Ohio.)

Treatment

These diseases are chronic and poorly responsive to treatment. Hair will not regrow. The goal of treatment is to keep the follicles open, free of keratinous debris, and therefore less likely to become secondarily infected. Topical antiseborrheic agents are helpful for this, especially benzoyl peroxide shampoos (OxyDex, Sulf OxyDex, Pyoben). Benzoyl peroxide is especially effective because of its follicular flushing and antibacterial activity. Unfortunately, however, it may worsen the dry scale; thus baths should be followed by a moisturizing rinse (HyLyt*efa Bath Oil Coat Conditioner, Humilac, Veterinary Prescription Alpha-Sesame Oil Dry Skin Rinse, Micro Pearls Humectant Spray). For dogs with very dry skin the rinses can be diluted and sprayed on daily.

Systemic antibiotics are indicated when secondary pyoderma develops. Coexisting diseases, such as hypothyroidism, should also be treated since this may improve the dry skin and decrease the incidence of recurrent pyoderma. These dogs should not be used for breeding.

Lichenoid-Psoriasiform Dermatosis

Lichenoid-psoriasiform dermatosis is an extremely rare, probably inherited, keratinization defect that has been reported only in English Springer Spaniels (Gross et al., 1986; Mason et al., 1986). It has been seen in both sexes in dogs under 2 years of age.

Clinical signs include nonpruritic, erythematous, lichenoid papules and plaques involving the pinnae (Fig. 15-6), external ear canal, preauricular and periorbital skin, lips, prepuce, and inguinal region. Chronic cases have papillomatous-type lesions that may involve the face, ventral trunk, and perineum. A more generalized distribution of greasy scales and crusts may also be present. These dogs are otherwise healthy.

Diagnosis

The early age of onset of refractory plaquelike lesions involving the face, ears, and ventrum in an English Springer Spaniel is enough to make a tentative diagnosis of lichenoid-psoriasiform dermatosis. Skin scrapings and fungal culture are employed to rule out demodicosis and dermatophytosis. The definitive diagnosis is made from skin biopsy findings. Histologic examination reveals a lichenoid dermatitis (band of mononuclear cells in the superficial dermis) with psoriasiform epidermal hyperplasia, intraepidermal microabscesses, and Munro microabscesses. Advanced lesions may show papillated epidermal hyperplasia and papillomatosis. The disease has been termed lichenoid-psoriasiform because these histologic findings have features consistent with both patterns of tissue reaction.

Treatment

Lichenoid-psoriasiform dermatosis is a waxing and waning condition. Response is minimal with antibiotics, low-dose glucocorticoids, vitamin A, levamisole, dapsone, autogenous vaccines, and topical antiseborrheic agents (Muller et al., 1989). Antibiotics (especially erythromycin) may be helpful if a secondary pyoderma is present (Mason et al., 1986). Prednisone at 2.2 mg/kg q24h PO has improved lesions in some cases but has not resulted in complete remission (Mason et al., 1986).

Schnauzer Comedo Syndrome

Schnauzer comedo syndrome is a follicular keratinization defect of Miniature Schnauzers characterized clinically by multiple comedones along the dorsal midline of the back. It is probably genetic (due to its exclusive occurrence in Miniature Schnauzers). There may be a developmental defect in the hair follicle leading to abnormal keratinization, comedo formation, follicular plugging and dilation, and secondary bacterial folliculitis.

The dermatosis usually develops in young adult

dogs. Clinical signs include crusted, papular comedones (blackheads) along the dorsal midline of the back from the neck to the tail. In the early stages and in mild cases these lesions are hard to visualize through the hair coat but are more easily palpated as "bumps" down the back. In fact, some owners will present their pets for "hives". Advanced cases frequently have secondary bacterial folliculitis and in rare cases furunculosis. These lesions may be accompanied by pruritus and pain. The infection leads to alopecia with a moth-eaten appearance of the coat. The condition is chronic for the life of the dog.

Diagnosis

Gross observation of follicular comedones in a Miniature Schnauzer establishes a tentative clinical diagnosis. The definitive diagnosis is confirmed from skin biopsy showing dilated hair follicles filled with keratinous debris. There may also be dilated or cystic sebaceous or apocrine glands, folliculitis, perifolliculitis, even furunculosis.

Differentials include demodicosis, dermatophytosis, and bacterial folliculitis. Therefore all suspect cases should be scraped and fungal-cultured. A complete drug history should also be taken in Miniature Schnauzers with comedo syndrome. Glucocorticoids are comedogenic and chronic administration may precipitate or worsen the condition. I have seen older Miniature Schnauzers develop dorsal comedones with endogenous Cushing's disease.

Treatment

The majority of cases of Schnauzer comedo syndrome can be controlled with periodic application of benzoyl peroxide shampoos (OxyDex, Pyoben) to flush the follicles and control secondary bacterial folliculitis. A combination benzoyl peroxide and sulfur shampoo (Sulf OxyDex) is especially effective because of enhanced keratolytic activity. Benzoyl peroxide gels (OxyDex Gel, Pyoben Gel) are helpful to remove tightly adherent comedones. Gentle agitation with a mildly abrasive sponge (Buff-Puff) also helps mechanically remove adherent comedones. Systemic antibiotics for a minimum of 3 weeks are indicated to control secondary staphylococcal folliculitis.

If there is no response to topical therapy, isotretinoin (Accutane) at 1 to 2 mg/kg q24h PO has been quite effective. Rapid response is seen within 3 to 4 weeks. After lesions resolve, most dogs can be maintained without signs of toxicity on alternate-day therapy.

Canine Ichthyosis

Ichthyosis is an extremely rare congenital keratinization defect of dogs characterized by very severe scaling of the skin and foot pads. The canine disease seems to resemble most closely lamellar ichthyosis in children. Lamellar ichthyosis causes severe scaling with moderate to marked hyperkeratosis and a thickened granular layer histologically. It may be an autosomal recessive trait in dogs (as it is in humans) although the exact genetics have not been studied.

Ichthyosis is reported most commonly in terriers and terrier crosses (Muller, 1976; August et al., 1988). In most cases the entire body is covered with tightly adherent fine white scales. Some of these may appear as feathered keratinous projections. The ventrum may be more severely affected. There also may be extensive alopecia, hyperpigmentation, and lichenification. Large quantities of waxy adherent scales are sometimes produced, especially in the flexural creases and intertriginous regions. Severe footpad hyperkeratosis is present, with the margins of the pads more severely involved.

Diagnosis

Congenital, severe cutaneous scaling and footpad hyperkeratosis in a terrier provide a tentative clinical diagnosis of canine ichthyosis. Histologic findings—increased mitotic activity in basal keratinocytes, a prominent stratum granulosum, severe laminated orthokeratotic hyperkeratosis, vacuolated keratinocytes in the superficial epidermis, follicular hyperkeratosis and plugging—confirm the diagnosis.

Because of the congenital nature of this disorder, it is rarely confused with other keratinization defects. However, if presence at birth cannot be firmly established, the differential would include zinc-responsive dermatosis, nasodigital hyperkeratosis, primary idiopathic seborrhea, canine distemper virus, pemphigus foliaceus, lupus erythematosus, hypothyroidism, generic dog food dermatosis, and superficial necrolytic dermatitis.

Treatment

The long-term prognosis for ichthyosis is poor, not because scale formation cannot be controlled but because continual therapy will be needed for the entire life of the patient. This is especially frustrating since the condition is congenital and diagnosed in puppyhood. However, if the owner is willing to do the necessary work the condition can usually be controlled.

Topical therapy is helpful and includes warm water soaks to help remove scales, antiseborrheic shampoos (SebaLyt, Sebolux), antiseborrheic gels (KeraSolv, Retin-A) for locally severe lesions, lactic acid as a total-body rinse or spray (Humilac, Micro Pearls Humectant Spray), and a combination rinse of 75% propylene glycol and 25% humectants (Humilac). Topical therapy, other than shampoos, is used twice daily until the scale and odor are controlled and then as often as necessary for maintenance.

Excellent results have been seen with isotretinoin (Accutane) at 1 to 2 mg/kg q24h PO and etretinate (Tegison) at 1 to 2 mg/kg q24h PO. Remission is seen within 8 to 12 weeks, and some dogs can be maintained on alternate-day therapy. Etretinate may be better tolerated than isotretinoin, especially over the lifetime of therapy that will be needed to control the disease.

Idiopathic Nasodigital Hyperkeratosis

Idiopathic nasodigital hyperkeratosis is a primary keratinization disorder characterized by excess keratin accumulation on the planum nasale, foot pads, or both. It is seen most commonly in Cocker Spaniels and English Springer Spaniels although any breed may be affected. It can also occur as a "normal" physiologic process in older dogs.

Lesions may be focal or diffuse and characterized by tightly adherent thick accumulations of keratin on the planum nasale (Fig. 17-15), foot pads, or both. This material is usually extremely dry and may be accompanied by cracks, fissures, erosions, and ulcers. Severe footpad involvement causes lameness.

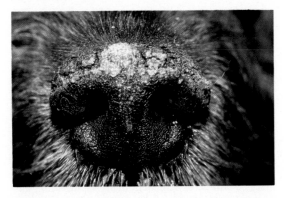

Figure 17-15. Tightly adherent thick accumulations of keratin on the nasal planum of a Cocker Spaniel with idiopathic nasal hyperkeratosis.

Diagnosis

Nasal or digital hyperkeratosis without evidence of other concurrent diseases establishes the diagnosis of idiopathic nasodigital hyperkeratosis. All diseases that can cause the lesions must be considered. Unfortunately, the list is long—and includes canine distemper virus, pemphigus foliaceus, pemphigus erythematosus, lupus erythematosus, nasal solar dermatitis (nose only), hypothyroidism, zinc-responsive dermatosis, generic dog food dermatosis, and superficial necrolytic dermatitis. In my experience pemphigus foliaceus and lupus erythematosus are the most common causes.

I recommend extensive diagnostics only when the condition is severe or if clinical signs lead me to believe that another, more serious, disease (listed above) is present. The problem is merely cosmetic for most dogs and requires neither extensive diagnostics nor treatment.

When warranted, a complete diagnostic evaluation necessitates a good history, complete blood count (CBC), serum biochemical profile, thyroid evaluation with baseline T_4 and possibly a TSH stimulation test, biopsy for histologic evaluation, and antinuclear antibody (ANA) testing. Biopsies for direct immunofluorescence are also valuable but should be taken from fresh lesions on other parts of the body. Skin from the nose and foot pads commonly shows false-positive reactions.

The histopathologic findings are most helpful in ruling out the differentials. Abnormalities for idiopathic nasodigital hyperkeratosis are nonspecific and consist of irregular epidermal hyperplasia with severe orthokeratotic and parakeratotic hyperkeratosis.

Treatment

Medical treatment of idiopathic nasodigital hyperkeratosis includes hydration of the hyperkeratotic tissue by water soakings or wet dressings followed by application of petroleum jelly as an occlusive agent to help seal moisture into the stratum corneum. Although simple hydration may be adequate for mild lesions, more severe hyperkeratosis requires a topical agent with keratolytic activity. A gel containing salicylic acid, lactic acid, and urea (KeraSolv Gel) is helpful, as is topical 0.025% or 0.01% tretinoin gel (Retin-A). These are used q12h until the condition is controlled followed by application as needed for long-term maintenance. Irritancy can be a problem, especially with tretinoin. Corticosteroid and antibiotic ointments, creams, or gels may be needed when severe inflammation or secondary infection is present.

When very severe projections of keratin are noted, especially on the foot pads and causing lameness, they may be removed surgically by trimming the dead tissue with scissors.

Canine Ear Margin Dermatosis

Canine ear margin dermatosis is a rare idiopathic keratinization defect that affects only the pinnae in a bilaterally symmetric pattern. It occurs primarily in Dachshunds. Greasy plugs adhere tightly to the skin surface and hair shafts on the pinnal margins. Alopecia may develop with time (Fig. 17-16). Pruritus is usually absent. In severe untreated cases a progression to ulceration and necrosis has been reported, due to thrombosis of the capillaries supplying blood to the pinnal margins, and may result in severe scarring with fissures.

Diagnosis

In early stages of the disease, when just scale is present, the tentative diagnosis is made from the breed and clinical signs alone. Skin scrapings and fungal culture should be performed to rule out scabies (only a consideration if pruritus is present), demodicosis, and dermatophytosis. Skin biopsies reveal prominent orthokeratotic and parakeratotic

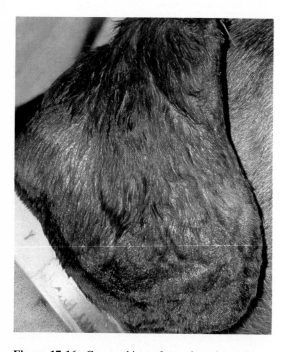

Figure 17-16. Greasy skin surface, alopecia, and hyperpigmentation involving the pinna of a Dachshund with advanced ear margin dermatosis. The other ear was equally affected.

hyperkeratosis. However, biopsy is unnecessary and the ear margin is a difficult part of the body from which to remove tissue.

The list of differentials is more extensive when the condition has progressed to ulceration and necrosis. It then includes lupus erythematosus, pemphigus complex, cutaneous vasculitis, dermatomyositis, cold agglutinin disease, frostbite, drug reactions, and lymphoreticular neoplasms. Diagnostic procedures to differentiate these diseases include a CBC, serum biochemical profile, urinalysis, skin biopsies for routine histologic examination and direct immunofluorescence, Coombs' testing, and ANA testing. Skin biopsies reveal necrosis and ulceration, and some sections may demonstrate vascular thrombosis. However, these changes are rather nonspecific and may be seen with many differentials. Therefore all these diagnostics are recommended to eliminate the differentials and establish a definitive diagnosis of canine ear margin dermatosis.

Treatment

The mild scaling form of ear margin dermatosis is usually controllable with topical therapy but rarely is curable. Periodic use of an antiseborrheic shampoo to remove the scales and waxy accumulations is all that is needed. Helpful agents include sulfur and salicylic acid (SebaLyt, Sebolux) and benzoyl peroxide (OxyDex, Sulf OxyDex, Pyoben). A topical glucocorticoid cream (e.g., 1% hydrocortisone) may be needed in severe unresponsive cases or those with severe inflammation.

The advanced ulcerative and necrotic stage is resistant to medical therapy. However, it can usually be cured by surgical removal of the affected ear margin. Tissue should be removed well into the normal portion of the pinna. This can be done to both pinnae to achieve a more symmetric cosmetically acceptable outcome. However, the full list of differentials should be considered before such aggressive surgery. The procedure will not be effective if ulceration is due to autoimmune disease, vasculitis, or dermatomyositis.

Canine Acne

Canine acne is a fairly common disorder of follicular keratinization resulting in comedones and secondary bacterial folliculitis and furunculosis. It may be similar to acne in humans—beginning during the period of sexual maturity, being self-limited or persisting into adulthood, and arising from abnormalities in sebaceous secretions that alter fol-

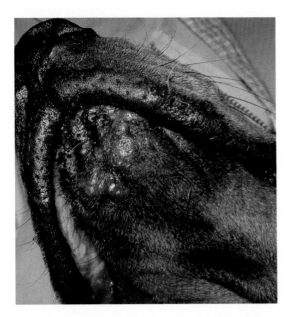

Figure 17-17. Deep pyoderma secondary to chin acne in a Doberman Pinscher.

licular keratinization, cause comedones to form, and induce secondary bacterial folliculitis. The organisms isolated are usually *Staphylococcus intermedius* and *Staphylococcus aureus*.

Acne is most common in short-coated breeds such as English Bulldogs, Boxers, Great Danes, and Doberman Pinschers. Lesions include comedones, papules, pustules, and furuncles of the chin, lips, and muzzle. In some cases lesions may be so mild as to be inapparent to the owner. In others there may be severe cellulitis with multiple draining tracts and pain (Fig. 17-17). In most dogs spontaneous resolution takes place after sexual maturity, although in short-coated breeds it may be a recurrent problem for the life of the animal, especially if not treated correctly when young.

Diagnosis

A tentative clinical diagnosis is made by history, age, breed, and clinical appearance of the lesions. Differentials include demodicosis, dermatophytosis, and bacterial folliculitis. Therefore skin scrapings and fungal culture should be performed. Cytologic examination of pustular contents or exudate from furuncles will confirm the presence of suppurative inflammation and cocci. Culture and susceptibility testing should be considered in cases with deep infection when a systemic antibiotic is to be selected. Skin biopsy findings provide a definitive diagnosis but are rarely needed.

Treatment

Mild cases of chin acne need no treatment and will spontaneously resolve with sexual maturity. In fact, aggressive topical therapy may actually worsen the condition by mechanical trauma of inflamed hair follicles.

For the more severely affected patient, treatment includes benzoyl peroxide shampoos (OxyDex, Sulf OxyDex, Pyoben) and gels (OxyDex Gel, Pyoben Gel). These are used twice per day until control and then as needed for maintenance. Benzoyl peroxide is effective because of its follicular flushing and antimicrobial activity. It may cause cutaneous irritation in some animals.

The most efficacious topical antibiobic for control of the secondary infection associated with canine acne is mupirocin (Bactoderm). It has excellent activity against gram-positive cocci, is bactericidal, works well at an acid pH, and is not systemically absorbed; it also is not chemically related to other antibiotics. In addition, it penetrates well into granulomatous deep pyoderma lesions and thus works well when furuncles and draining tracts have developed on the chin. It should be applied q12h. I often alternate it with benzoyl peroxide for the follicular flushing activity that that agent offers.

In recurrent cases or those with deep infection, systemic antibiotics and warm water soaks will be necessary. Short-term glucocorticoids such as prednisone or prednisolone at 1.1 mg/kg q24h PO may help reduce inflammation associated with foreign body granulomas secondary to ingrown hairs or keratin debris and result in a more rapid response. However, the steroids should be administered for only 7 to 10 days and the antibiotics should be continued for much longer, until the chin pyoderma has resolved.

Finally, in cases refractory to more conventional therapy, benefit may be derived from topical tretinoin (Retin-A) q12h or systemic isotretinoin (Accutane) at 1 to 2 mg/kg q24h PO.

REFERENCES

August JR, et al: Congenital ichthyosis in a dog: comparison with the human ichthyosiform dermatoses, Compend Contin Educ Pract Vet 10:40, 1988.

Briggs OM, Botha WS: Color mutant alopecia in a blue Italian Greyhound, J Am Anim Hosp Assoc 22:611, 1986.

Brignac MM, et al: Microscopy of color mutant alopecia. In Proceedings, Annual members' meeting of the AAVD & ACVD, 1988, p 14.

Brown RG, et al: Alaskan Malamute chondrodysplasia.

V. Decreased gut zinc absorption, Growth 42:1, 1978.

Carlotti DN: Canine hereditary black hair follicular dysplasia and colour mutant alopecia: Clinical and histopathological aspects. In von Tscharner C, Halliwell REW (eds): Advances in veterinary dermatology, vol 1, London, 1990, Baillière Tindall, p 43.

Fadok VA: Zinc responsive dermatosis in a Great Dane: a case report, J Am Anim Hosp Assoc 18:409, 1982.

Griffin CE: Personal communication, 1992.

Gross TL, et al: Psoriasiform lichenoid dermatitis in the Springer Spaniel, Vet Pathol 23:76, 1986.

Ihrke PJ, Goldschmidt MH: Vitamin A–responsive dermatosis in the dog, J Am Vet Med Assoc 182:687, 1983.

Jacobs P: Personal communication, 1991.

Kunkle GA: Zinc-responsive dermatoses in dogs. In Kirk RW (ed): Current veterinary therapy VII, Philadelphia, 1980, WB Saunders, p 472.

Mason KV, et al: Characterization of lichenoid-psoriasiform dermatosis of Springer Spaniels, J Am Vet Med Assoc 189:897, 1986.

Miller WH: Colour dilution alopecia in Doberman Pinschers with blue or fawn coat colours: a study on the incidence and histopathology of this disorder, Vet Dermatol 1:113, 1990a.

Miller WH: Follicular dysplasia in adult black and red Doberman Pinschers, Vet Dermatol 1:181, 1990b.

Miller WH: Alopecia associated with coat color dilution in two Yorkshire Terriers, one Saluki, and one mixbreed dog, J Am Anim Hosp Assoc 27:39, 1991.

Muller GH: Ichthyosis in two dogs, J Am Vet Med Assoc 169:1313, 1976.

Muller GH, et al: Small animal dermatology, ed 4, Philadelphia, 1989, WB Saunders, p 727.

Ohlen B, Scott DW: Zinc responsive dermatitis in puppies, Canine Pract 13:2, 1986.

O'Neill CS: Hereditary skin disease in the dog and cat, Comp Contin Educ Pract Vet 3:791, 1981.

Power HT, Ihrke PJ: Synthetic retinoids in veterinary dermatology, Vet Clin North Am 20:1525, 1990.

Scott DW: Vitamin A–responsive dermatosis in the cocker spaniel, J Am Anim Hosp Assoc 22:125, 1986.

Scott DW, Miller WH: Epidermal dysplasia and *Malassezia pachydermatis* infection in West Highland White Terriers, Vet Dermatol 1:25, 1989.

van den Broek AHM, Thoday KL: Skin disease in dogs associated with zinc deficiency: a report of 5 cases, J Small Anim Pract 27:313, 1986.

18

Symptomatic Topical Therapy of Scaling Disorders

Kenneth W. Kwochka

Therapeutic Agents for Symptomatic Topical Therapy of Scaling Disorders

ANTISEBORRHEIC AGENTS IN SHAMPOOS

Sulfur, salicylic acid, benzoyl peroxide, tar, selenium sulfide

MOISTURIZING AGENTS IN RINSES AND SPRAYS

Emollients: Coconut oil, safflower oil, sesame oil, cottonseed oil, mineral oil, vitamin E, lanolin

Emulsifier: PEG-4 dilaurate

Occlusive: Petrolatum

Humectants: Sodium lactate, glycerin, polyvinyl pyrrolidone, propylene glycol, lactic acid, urea

ANTISEBORRHEIC AGENTS IN VEHICLES FOR LOCALIZED SCALING DISORDERS

Tretinoin: Cream, gel

Lactic acid: Lotion

Salicylic acid: Gel, pads

Ceruminolytics: Earwashes

Most dogs and cats presented for cutaneous scale formation have secondary scaling that is not associated with a primary keratinization defect. The dermatoses that may result in secondary scaling include ectoparasitism, pyoderma, dermatophytosis, endocrinopathies, autoimmune dermatoses, allergic dermatoses, and environmental dermatoses. Topical therapy is important in these diseases to help control the scaling and keep the animal comfortable until the primary disease is diagnosed and treated.

Symptomatic topical therapy, especially with antiseborrheic agents in shampoo formulations, is the major form of therapy used to manage most of the primary keratinization defects. (See Chapter 17.) Ointments, gels, creams, and sprays are also useful in some of the localized keratinization abnormalities.

Because of the broad range of products available to the practitioner, topical treatment programs can be individualized for each animal. Specific products and programs are usually chosen on the basis of presenting morphologic characteristics such as mild or severe dry scale, greasy scale, inflammation, or concurrent pyoderma. However, so many companies produce the same or similar products that the practitioner should be cautioned to use a limited number and to know everything about them (including their indications, contraindications, compatibilities, incompatibilities, and time for and duration of effect).

Some of the more potent antiseborrheic products may have undesirable side effects. Frequent observations are necessary initially because of the potential for irritancy and sensitization. A milder agent should be employed first. If it does not work well, a more potent product can be tried.

Client considerations are also important factors in deciding on topical therapy. Because of the time and effort involved with most antiseborrheic shampoo programs, cooperation of the patient and owner is necessary. The characteristics of the specific products prescribed will also have an effect on compliance. For example, a high-concentration tar shampoo may be indicated once or twice a week for severe greasy scaling disorders; however, owner compliance may be a problem because such products are malodorous and can irritate skin and stain light-colored hair coats. Although a sulfur and salicylic acid shampoo may not control the scale and oil as well, it will not have the undesirable qualities of a tar product and thus better compliance can be expected, with more favorable overall results. Financial status of the owner may also be a factor, especially in chronic idiopathic scaling dermatoses in which shampoo therapy will be needed for the life of the animal.

The ability of the owner to follow instructions must also be considered. However, many problems associated with owner compliance are not a result of lack of intelligence but are client communication problems due to incomplete instructions. Directions must be kept as simple as possible and should be written out or provided in prepared client education handouts. Videotapes or demonstrations of proper bathing techniques are helpful. The ability to properly involve the client in the topical therapeutic program may actually have beneficial psychological effects by making clients feel that they are contributing significantly to the improvement of their pet. Active owner involvement in the topical therapy program is mandatory when the dog has a primary keratinization disorder that requires lifetime therapy. If the owner is not interested in participating in the treatment program, it is doomed to failure!

Veterinary dermatologists are often asked to make recommendations of shampoos that might be beneficial for a particular skin condition. Often the general practitioner will have many bottles of shampoo on the shelf with lists of ingredients and very little guidance on how these products should be used. The purpose of this chapter is to review the many active ingredients and make some general recommendations for their use in the various scaling disorders. Unfortunately, recommendations are based solely on clinical experience and studies from other species. No controlled studies have been

done on dogs or cats with any of the antiseborrheic products.

BATHING

Since scaling dermatoses are usually generalized in dogs, shampoo formulations are the best alternatives for topical therapy. No matter what specific products and active ingredients are used, the mechanical process of bathing with water is helpful in removing scales, crusts, debris, dirt, organisms, and old medications.

Water has tremendous hydrating effects if used properly. This is valuable in dry scaling disorders where the stratum corneum is dehydrated. Contact time of 10 to 15 minutes must be allowed to properly hydrate the stratum corneum. If contact time is too short and baths are being given frequently, then the continual drying actually leads to dehydration of the horny layer. After bathing or soaking and while the skin is still wet, application of an emulsified bath oil will help hold externally applied water to prolong hydration. Topical use of a humectant results in attraction of water to the stratum corneum to increase hydration. Finally, use of an occlusive agent such as petrolatum physically blocks the surface of the stratum corneum to reduce transepidermal water loss through this layer to the environment. Care must be taken not to immerse the animal in water for excessively long periods because maceration of the stratum corneum with a loss of protective barrier function can result.

Contact time for medicated shampoos varies depending on the active ingredient, the concentration of that ingredient, the vehicle, and the condition of the skin. Most products used to help control scaling have labels that recommend a 5- to 15-minute contact time. Owners should be encouraged to actually use a watch or clock to be sure that the contact is adequate. Timing should not start until the whole body is lathered, and gentle lathering should continue for the entire time. The antiseborrheic agents will not work well to reduce scale formation if they are immediately rinsed off.

Many comparable veterinary and human shampoo formulations are available to treat scaling dermatoses. I generally recommend using veterinary products because of pH differences (canine skin is less acidic than human skin), convenience, cost, and aesthetic considerations.

SHAMPOO PRODUCTS (Table 18-1)

Although some recommendations can be given for antiseborrheic shampoo therapy, these should

Table 18-1. Selected shampoos for symptomatic topical therapy of scaling disorders

TRADE NAME (MANUFACTURER)	ACTIVE INGREDIENTS	INDICATIONS	COMMENTS
Cleansing and moisturizing			
Allergroom (Allerderm/Virbac)	NaCl, glycerin, lactic acid, urea	Primary keratinization disorders with dry scale such as idiopathic seborrhea, sebaceous adenitis, ichthyosis; secondary dry scale such as with low humidity, hypothyroidism, hyperadrenocorticism, pyoderma, cheyletiellosis, atopy, food allergy, contact allergy; alternated with more drying antiseborrheic shampoos	Although not medicated may rarely cause cutaneous irritation
HyLyt*efa (DVM Pharmaceuticals)	Na-lactate, coconut oil, lanolin, glycerin, protein, fatty acids		
Sulfur and salicylic acid			
SebaLyt (DVM Pharmaceuticals)	2% Sulfur, 2% salicylic acid, 0.5% triclosan	Primary and secondary dry and waxy scaling disorders that do not respond to cleansing and moisturizing shampoos (listed above); ear margin dermatosis, zinc-responsive dermatosis, canine scabies, notoedric mange, pemphigus foliaceus	Rare cutaneous irritation, rare excess drying
Sebbafon (Upjohn)	5% Sulfur, 0.5% Na-salicylate, entsufon Na, lanolin, petrolatum		
Sebolux (Allerderm/Virbac)	2% Sulfur, 2.3% Na-salicylate		
Benzoyl peroxide			
OxyDex (DVM Pharmaceuticals)	2.5% Benzoyl peroxide	Primary keratinization disorders with greasy scale such as primary seborrhea of spaniels, terriers, Basset Hounds, German Shepherd Dogs; vitamin A–responsive dermatosis, epidermal dysplasia of West Highland White Terriers; chin acne, ear margin dermatosis, Schnauzer comedo syndrome, follicular dystrophy, pyoderma; *Malassezia* dermatosis	Excess drying, rare cutaneous irritation (especially in cats), bleaching of fabrics
Pyoben (Allerderm/Virbac)	3% Benzoyl peroxide		
Sulf OxyDex (DVM Pharmaceuticals)	2.5% Benzoyl peroxide, 2% sulfur		

Continued.

Table 18-1. Selected shampoos for symptomatic topical therapy of scaling disorders—cont'd

TRADE NAME (MANUFACTURER)	ACTIVE INGREDIENTS	INDICATIONS	COMMENTS
Tar			
Clear Tar (Veterinary Prescription)	2% Coal tar extract, collagen, lanolin, coconut oil	Primary keratinization disorders with greasy scale such as primary seborrhea of spaniels, terriers, Basset Hounds, German Shepherd Dogs; epidermal dysplasia of West Highland White Terriers; severe cases of greasy ear margin dermatosis	Rare contact irritancy, rare excessive drying; **not for use in cats**
NuSal-T (DVM Pharmaceuticals)	2% Coal tar, 3% salicylic acid, 1% menthol		
T-Lux (Allerderm/Virbac)	4% Solubilized coal tar, 2% sulfur, 2.3% Na salicylate		
LyTar (DVM Pharmaceuticals)	3% refined juniper tar, 2% sulfur, 2% salicylic acid	Primary keratinization disorders with greasy scale such as primary seborrhea of spaniels, terriers, Basset Hounds, German Shepherd Dogs; epidermal dysplasia of West Highland White Terriers; severe cases of greasy ear margin dermatosis	Strong tar odor, contact irritancy (especially of hair follicles), excessive drying, potential to stain light-colored coats; **not for use in cats**
Mycodex High Potency Tar and Sulfur (SmithKline-Beecham)	3% Coal tar, 2.5% sulfur, 2% salicylic acid		
Allerseb-T (Allerderm/Virbac)	4% Coal tar, 2% sulfur, 2% salicylic acid		
Pentrax (GenDerm)	4.3% Crude coal tar		
Selenium sulfide			
Selsun Blue (Ross)	1% Selenium sulfide	Primary keratinization disorders with greasy scale such as primary seborrhea of spaniels, terriers, Basset Hounds, German Shepherd Dogs; epidermal dysplasia of West Highland White Terriers; severe cases of greasy ear margin dermatosis; may be helpful in some cases of *Malassezia* dermatosis	Rare contact irritancy; **not for use in cats**

only be taken as general guidelines because there is a great deal of variation in individual response to products. The safest, least drying, and least irritating products should be employed first. Hypoallergenic cleansing and moisturizing agents, sulfur, and salicylic acid have minimal side effects when compared to more potent antiseborrheics such as benzoyl peroxide, tar, and selenium sulfide.

Bathing is instituted two to three times a week until good control of the scale and odor is achieved and then as infrequently as needed for maintenance. A dog with mild dry scale and no odor may be controlled after only 2 or 3 weeks and then be maintained with a bath every month. A dog with severe greasy scale and odor may require several weeks before the owner is satisfied with the response and may then still need a bath every 7 to 10 days for control. The maintenance program will vary depending on the season since extremes of heat and humidity can affect the amount of dryness or greasiness, scaling, and secondary bacterial infection.

I sometimes prefer to initially send an animal home with two or three different products, each to be used at 2-week intervals, and let the owner decide which works the best to control scaling and odor. The owner is often the best judge of efficacy, especially with regard to control of odor. This method of trying different products is not always feasible since it may be more expensive than dispensing one product at the first visit. Additionally, some owners may question the therapeutic ability of the veterinarian if more than one product is prescribed.

Several veterinary pharmaceutical companies offer therapeutic treatment packs with two or three topical products to be used together for different types of skin conditions. Although these may be helpful in a small number of cases, the combinations are often not optimal for a particular skin condition. Better efficacy is achieved by prescribing products individually on a case-by-case basis.

Cleansing and Moisturizing Agents

In dogs that have mild dry scaling, as can occur with dry heat, hypothyroidism or hyperadrenocorticism, cheyletiellosis, endoparasitism, pyoderma (usually dry scaling associated with older resolving lesions), and food allergy, all that may be needed is a mild cleansing and moisturizing shampoo for rehydration of the skin along with specific therapy for the primary disease. These shampoos are also indicated for long-term maintenance of atopy and contact allergy. They are usually mild enough not to irritate the skin of allergic dogs and cats and they help remove surface antigens from the skin and hair coat. Some caution should be exercised since even shampoos classified as being hypoallergenic may on occasion be irritating, especially to inflamed and damaged skin.

Cleansing and moisturizing shampoos may be helpful along with other more potent antiseborrheic agents in primary keratinization disorders characterized by dry scale formation such as primary seborrhea of Irish Setters and Doberman Pinschers, sebaceous adenitis, and canine ichthyosis. They are also alternated with the drying antiseborrheic agents (e.g., tars and benzoyl peroxide) to help rehydrate the skin. Finally, cleansing and moistur-

izing shampoos are useful when a dog with severe scaling cannot tolerate the more potent antiseborrheic agents.

A number of mildly medicated and hypoallergenic veterinary shampoos are used for this purpose. They clean without soap, using detergent soap substitutes and anionic/amphoteric surfactant systems. Some contain moisturizing agents (sodium lactate, natural essence of coconut oil, and essential fatty acids [HyLyt*efa]; sodium chloride, glycerin, lactic acid, and urea [Allergroom]). The moisturizing effects can be enhanced by application of a rinse containing oils or humectants after bathing.

Antiseborrheic Agents

Several well-coordinated events occur in the processes of epidermopoiesis and keratogenesis to maintain the skin in its normal state. (See Chapter 16.) Cells migrate from the mitotically active pool in the basal cell layer to the stratum corneum, followed by normal exfoliation. During this orderly migration the mitotically active keratinocyte becomes a dead keratinized corneocyte embedded in a lipid-rich domain. The intercellular lipids provide the cohesion between cells in the stratum corneum and help control exfoliation. Visible scale may result from many epidermal abnormalities including increased mitotic activity in the basal layer, abnormal cell migration, biochemical anomalies in keratin production, and aberrations in intercellular lipid production.

Antiseborrheic compounds are keratolytic and/ or keratoplastic. A keratolytic agent damages corneocytes, resulting in ballooning of the cells and subsequent cell shedding. Thus the stratum corneum is softened and removed, which promotes better control of scale formation. A keratoplastic agent "normalizes" epidermal cell kinetics and keratinization, usually by cytostatic effects on the basal cell layer. Common antiseborrheic agents include sulfur, salicylic acid, benzoyl peroxide, tar, and selenium sulfide.

Sulfur

Sulfur is commonly incorporated into antiseborrheic shampoo products. It is not only keratolytic and keratoplastic but also antifungal, antibacterial, antiparasitic, and antipruritic. Depending on the method of preparation, sulfur will be found in different particle sizes (Lin et al., 1988). Colloidal sulfur particles are smaller than precipitated particles which are smaller than sublimed sulfur. The smaller the particle size, the greater the surface area for sulfur-cutaneous interaction, and the greater the efficacy. The keratoplastic effect may be cytostatic or related to the reaction in which sulfur and cysteine combine to form cystine and hydrogen sulfide. Normal keratinization is promoted since cystine is an important constituent of the stratum corneum and the amount of hydrogen sulfide is fairly low. At higher sulfur concentrations more hydrogen sulfide is formed and breaks down keratin, resulting in the keratolytic effect. The antibacterial and antifungal activity is the result of hydrogen sulfide and pentathionic acid formation. Sulfur is drying and malodorous, though not in the concentrations found in shampoos, and is not a good degreasing agent. Therefore a sulfur-containing shampoo would be used more for a dry scaling condition and when a pyoderma was present. It has synergistic keratolytic activity with salicylic acid.

Salicylic Acid

Salicylic acid is keratolytic, keratoplastic, mildly antipruritic, and bacteriostatic. Its keratolytic effect occurs by lowering the pH of the skin, which increases hydration of the keratin and swelling of the stratum corneum cells. Also important in this desquamation is the solubilizing of the intercellular cement substance that binds scales in the stratum corneum. The synergistic activity between salicylic acid and sulfur appears to be optimal when the products are incorporated in equal concentrations (Leyden et al., 1987).

Primary scaling disorders that may benefit from the use of a sulfur and salicylic acid shampoo include primary idiopathic seborrhea (in breeds that get moderate/severe dry to waxy scale), sebaceous adenitis, ichthyosis, ear margin dermatosis, and zinc-responsive dermatosis. These shampoos will also be helpful as adjunctive therapy to control dry scale associated with parasitism (cheyletiellosis, canine scabies, notoedric mange, and endoparasites), pyoderma (usually dry scaling associated with older resolving lesions), allergies, environmental factors (dry heat), and autoimmune dermatoses (pemphigus foliaceus).

Commercial veterinary shampoos contain sulfur with either salicylic acid or its salt form, sodium salicylate. Comparative studies on these two forms have not been done in dogs. Sulfur and sodium salicylate are found in approximately equal concentrations in a veterinary shampoo (Sebolux). Another formulation (SebaLyt) contains not only sulfur and salicylic acid in equal concentrations, but also the antiseptic agent triclosan at the 0.5% level,

thereby making the product valuable when scaling is accompanied by a secondary pyoderma. Sulfur and sodium salicylate are also found in unequal concentrations (Sebbafon). This shampoo has good emollient properties by use of an entsufon sodium base, lanolin, and petrolatum.

Benzoyl Peroxide

Benzoyl peroxide (OxyDex, Pyoben) is a good keratolytic and a superior antimicrobial and degreasing agent that is useful in severe cases of greasy seborrhea, especially with a secondary bacterial component. Part of its degreasing effect is due to reduced sebaceous gland activity. Benzoyl peroxide also has flushing action, which enhances the removal of scale, glandular secretions, and bacteria from hair follicles. Sulfur has been formulated with benzoyl peroxide (Sulf OxyDex) to augment its keratolytic activity.

Benzoyl peroxide may be helpful in greasy scaling conditions such as primary seborrhea in spaniels, terriers, Basset Hounds, and German Shepherd Dogs; it also is likely helpful in epidermal dysplasia of West Highland White Terriers, vitamin A–responsive dermatosis, canine acne, greasy ear margin dermatosis, Schnauzer comedo syndrome, follicular dystrophies, demodicosis, and pyoderma. Cutaneous scaling due to any cause may be complicated by secondary *Malassezia* infection of the skin. Studies in humans (Bonnetblanc and Bernard, 1986) have shown excellent results using 2.5% benzoyl peroxide in patients with facial seborrheic dermatitis who were culture-positive for *Pityrosporum ovale*. Decreased sebaceous gland activity may play as much of a role as directly killing the fungus since it has been shown in studies that sebum exerts a permissive effect on the growth of *P. ovale* in humans. A shampoo containing ketoconazole (Nizoral Shampoo) also has excellent efficacy against *P. ovale* associated with seborrheic dermatitis in humans, but it is expensive. A low number of cases in which dogs with *Malassezia* dermatitis were treated and successfully controlled with ketoconazole shampoo in preliminary clinical trials has been reported.

Irritancy with erythema, pain, and pruritus may be a problem in dogs and cats when benzoyl peroxide is used in concentrations over 5%. Most of the human products are 5% or higher in concentration and should not be used. Due to its degreasing activity, benzoyl peroxide is very drying. Unless the animal is extremely greasy, benzoyl peroxide shampoo needs to be followed by an emollient bath oil rinse or alternated with a less drying product. Owners must be warned about the potential for bleaching of fabrics. Benzoyl peroxide has low long-term toxicity and no known oral carcinogenic effect. However, it is difficult to formulate and package and should be bought only from reputable companies.

Tar

Tar is probably the most commonly utilized antiseborrheic agent in veterinary and human dermatology. In fact, it is probably overused in cases with dry or mild greasy scale formation when a sulfur and salicylic acid shampoo would be equally effective with less potential for irritancy. Tar is keratoplastic, antipruritic, degreasing, and vasoconstrictive. Its keratoplastic effect occurs by suppression of epidermal growth and DNA synthesis in the basal cell layer of the epidermis. The superior keratoplastic activity of tar over other antiseborrheic agents has not been demonstrated in dogs. It is usually added to the treatment program when degreasing activity is desired.

Crude coal tar is the product of the distillation of bituminous coal. Thousands of components are produced, making standardization of final formulations difficult. Plant-derived tar extracts, including pine and juniper tar, are also incorporated into topical formulations. It is interesting to speculate that the tar components that give the best clinical efficacy may not be the ones responsible for the smell and other undesirable qualities. Different production techniques, especially variations in temperature and type of coal or wood, affect the degree of refinement and efficacy of the final preparation. Because of this and potential packaging problems, labels should be followed carefully and only products from reputable companies should be used. Other potential problems include irritancy, odor, staining, and photosensitization. Tar products should not be used on cats and are unnecessary since scaling in cats usually responds well to sulfur and salicylic acid shampoos. Tars are generally formulated with sulfur and salicylic acid.

Many veterinary and human tar shampoos are available, the primary difference among them being the concentration of tar. Care must be used in interpreting labels with regard to tar concentration. Tar solution is not the same as tar extract or refined tar. A shampoo containing 2.5% tar solution actually contains only 0.5% tar since the solution contains but 20% tar. Also the type of refinement used for an individual tar product may be important since the pharmacologically active components are altered in the final products. Other dif-

ferences include whether sulfur and salicylic acid are added and their concentrations.

It is generally believed that a higher tar concentration will result in superior suppression of epidermal growth and DNA synthesis and thus better clinical efficacy. However, this is not always the case and is certainly not totally predictable. Tar probably exerts its effect in many other ways than simply suppression of DNA synthesis. The higher concentration formulations demonstrate better efficacy for the severe oily scaling disorders. Tar shampoos are usually reserved for severe, greasy, primary idiopathic seborrhea that has not responded to products with sulfur, salicylic acid, and benzoyl peroxide.

There are three tar shampoos now available (Clear Tar, NuSal-T, and T-Lux) that have been formulated in an attempt to retain the desirable keratoplastic and degreasing characteristics of tar while minimizing the undesirable side effects. These products lather well and have a surprisingly pleasing odor. Although 3% and 4% products may have better clinical efficacy in severe cases of greasy seborrhea because of their better degreasing activity, these tar products have a higher degree of owner compliance. However, no comparative clinical efficacy studies have been done on these shampoos and information is also not available on the particular tar extracts utilized.

A 2% solubilized coal tar extract shampoo (Clear Tar) is one of these aesthetically pleasing veterinary tar formulations. It is a clear amber liquid with both a pleasant smell and good clinical activity, and its parent tar extract has performed well in laboratory DNA synthesis suppression assays (Lowe et al., 1982). It also contains lanolin and coconut oil extract as emollients to minimize drying. Another elegant refined tar extract shampoo (NuSal-T) is equivalent to 2% crude coal tar along with 3% salicylic acid and 1% menthol. The enhanced concentration of salicylic acid is to attain greater keratolytic activity. Menthol is included for cooling and antipruritic effects. A 4% solubilized coal tar shampoo (T-Lux) also contains 2% sulfur and 2.3% sodium salicylate for enhanced keratolytic and keratoplastic activity.

There are two 3% veterinary tar shampoos (LyTar, Mycodex High Potency Tar and Sulfur) on the market that also contain sulfur and salicylic acid. Both are dark brown opaque suspensions and have a strong odor. They are used for moderate to severe oily seborrhea when sulfur and salicylic acid shampoos, benzoyl peroxide shampoos, and lower concentration tar products are not effective.

For even more severe oily seborrhea and when the 3% tar products do not work, a 4% veterinary tar shampoo (Allerseb-T) is available. A human product (Pentrax) containing 4.3% crude coal tar is available but is aesthetically unpleasing and should be reserved for severe recalcitrant cases of waxy or oily seborrhea.

As the tar concentration increases, the chances for excessive drying, staining, and follicular irritation also increase. Owners should be advised to apply the higher-concentration tar products with care, to massage into the hair coat very gently in the direction of hair growth, and to follow by a thorough rinse. Excessive drying may necessitate the use of an emollient bath oil rinse after each shampoo or alternating with a lower-concentration tar product, a sulfur and salicylic acid shampoo, or a hypoallergenic moisturizing shampoo. Follicular irritation should be considered if the client calls complaining that the animal has suddenly developed "hive-like" lesions with pruritus after bathing.

Tar is also incorporated into spray formulations including a 1% refined tar solution in an oil in water emulsion with essential fatty acids (LyTar*efa Therapeutic Bath Oil Spray Conditioner). A 3.5% coal tar topical solution also contains liposome-encapsulated lactic acid (humectant) in an oil-free base (Micro Pearls Coal Tar Medicated Spray for Dogs). These sprays may be used after bathing or on a dry coat between baths. They should be rubbed or brushed in well to help control scale formation with more residual activity between baths. One problem with these sprays is their offensive strong tar odor, which is much worse than tar shampoo formulations. This makes client compliance difficult. A second problem is that it is hard for the spray to penetrate down to the skin surface through a thick hair coat. Thus, these sprays are better used on short-coated dogs. I have found the topical tar solutions to be particularly useful in Doberman Pinschers with primary seborrhea characterized by waxy scale.

Selenium Sulfide

Selenium sulfide is keratolytic, keratoplastic, and degreasing. It works to control scale by depressing epidermal cell turnover rate and interfering with hydrogen bond formation in the keratin. It is reported to have some residual adherence to the skin. This is one of the older antiseborrheic products, with limited usage because it is both staining and drying and it may be irritating, especially to mucous membranes and the scrotum. It is usually considered only in severe cases of oily seborrhea that are nonresponsive to sulfur and sal-

icylic acid, benzoyl peroxide, and tar. Some Cocker Spaniels with primary idiopathic seborrhea seem to do surprisingly well on this product when all other forms of therapy have failed. Several veterinary selenium-containing shampoos are available, but in my experience they are much more irritating than the human product (Selsun Blue). This shampoo is the same concentration as the veterinary products and is in a pleasant-scented detergent vehicle. Selenium at 2.5% works well to control *P. ovale* in humans but has limited clinical efficacy at 1.0% in shampoo formulations against *Malassezia* in dogs.

Pyrithione Zinc

Pyrithione zinc (Head & Shoulders) is a good keratoplastic agent that works by reducing cell turnover in the epidermis. However, it should not be used on dogs because it has been associated with experimentally induced retinopathies.

Principles of Shampoo Therapy

There are some general recommendations given for antiseborrheic shampoo therapy.

1. In a dog with a scaling dermatosis and long hair coat, it may be beneficial to clip the hair and keep it short. This makes the frequent baths easier to administer, results in the use of less shampoo, and usually leads to better control of scale and secondary pyoderma.

2. If there is a large amount of extremely greasy scale formation, bathing with a detergent (Ivory Liquid, Palmolive Liquid) prior to the use of an antiseborrheic shampoo will allow use of less of the medicated formulation, better contact with the skin surface, and thus enhanced efficacy.

3. Scaling dermatoses are generally best controlled by starting aggressively with antiseborrheic shampoos two to three times a week. After control, the frequency should be gradually decreased with determination of the optimal interval for long-term maintenance.

Mild dry scaling may respond to a moisturizing, hypoallergenic shampoo (HyLyt*efa, Allergroom). If the dry scaling is more severe and does not respond to a moisturizing shampoo, a sulfur and salicylic acid combination (Sebolux, SebaLyt, Sebbafon) may next be considered. Bath oil rinses or humectants should be applied after the skin has been hydrated by bathing. These moisturizers may also be effectively applied between shampoos using a plant mister bottle.

If the dry scaling is severe and still nonresponsive, a tar product may be necessary. However, since tars are degreasing, further drying can result even though scale formation from the epidermis is being better controlled. After-bath moisturizing rinses are mandatory in these dogs. Additionally, the tar shampoo may need to be alternated with a cleansing and moisturizing shampoo to prevent excess drying.

For cases of oily or greasy scaling, benzoyl peroxide (Pyoben, OxyDex), benzoyl peroxide with sulfur (Sulf OxyDex), tars (Clear Tar, NuSal-T, T-Lux, LyTar, Allerseb-T, Pentrax) and selenium sulfide (Selsun Blue) are useful alone or alternating in combination. However, high concentrations of these products may be irritating and very drying. Thus, after the severe problem is controlled, switching to a more innocuous agent to control the condition is indicated. For greasy seborrhea complicated by pyoderma, alternating a tar and a benzoyl peroxide product is useful. An emollient antibacterial shampoo with 0.5% chlorhexidine (ChlorhexiDerm, Nolvasan) would be preferred to benzoyl peroxide in the case of a dry seborrhea with pyoderma.

Since spaniels, Basset Hounds, terriers, and German Shepherd Dogs tend to develop a pruritic, greasy scaling disease, they seem to benefit most from benzoyl peroxide, benzoyl peroxide and sulfur, and higher-concentration tar shampoos without moisturizing bath oil and water rinses or soakings. Doberman Pinschers usually have a heavy accumulation of dry or waxy scale and so do better with a less drying agent such as a sulfur and salicylic acid–containing shampoo. The skin must be rehydrated using frequent moisturizing bath oil and water rinses and moisturizing sprays between bathings. Irish Setters present a therapeutic challenge. Some will have very dry scaling, others will be greasy, and others may have areas of both dry and greasy scaling on the same animal. Thus, two shampoos may be needed at each bathing: a moisturizing one for dry areas and a degreasing one for oily areas.

Dogs with vitamin A–responsive dermatosis benefit from benzoyl peroxide and sulfur shampoos (Sulf OxyDex), which help clean the "fronds" of keratinous material from the follicular ostia. The same is true of the follicular hyperkeratosis associated with follicular dystrophies and Schnauzer comedo syndrome.

Sebaceous adenitis tends to cause focal to diffuse dry scale formation; thus moisturizing shampoos and sulfur and salicylic acid shampoos followed by bath oil rinses are helpful. Sulfur and salicylic acid and tar shampoos are helpful for ca-

nine ichthyosis and locally for ear margin dermatosis.

MOISTURIZING AGENTS (Table 18-2)

Moisturizing agents are used to lubricate, rehydrate, and soften the skin. There are several categories (Wehr and Krochmal, 1987)—including emollients, emulsifier-emollients, occlusives, and humectants.

Emollients, Emulsifiers, and Occlusives

Emollients smooth the roughened surfaces of the stratum corneum by filling in the spaces between dry skin flakes with oil droplets. Used alone, they are not occlusive (unless in very high concentrations) and they provide only temporary symptomatic relief. Emollients include oils, animal fats, and hydrocarbons used for their local effect in protecting and softening the skin, increasing pliability, and serving as vehicles for drugs. Emollient oils include olive, cottonseed, corn, almond, peanut, persia, coconut, sesame, and safflower. Lanolin is animal fat from the wool of sheep. Hydrocarbons include paraffin, petrolatum, and mineral oil.

Emulsified bath oils are highly dispersible agents that have emulsifiers to distribute the emollient oil in water. Common emulsifiers include PEG-4 dilaurate, stearic acid, stearyl alcohol, cetyl alcohol, laureth-4, and lecithin. With an emulsifier-emollient combination (Veterinary Prescription Alpha-Sesame Oil Dry Skin Rinse) externally applied water can be held in the stratum corneum to prolong hydration.

Petrolatum is not only an emollient but is also occlusive. Occlusive agents block the surface of the stratum corneum and reduce transepidermal water loss to the environment. This results in increased water content in the stratum corneum.

Humectants

Humectant sprays and rinses use components of the natural moisturizing factor (NMF), such as carboxylic acid, lactic acid, and urea, to rehydrate the skin without oil. Other humectants include sodium lactate, glycerin, propylene glycol, and polyvinyl pyrrolidone. These agents hydrate the stratum corneum by attracting transepidermal water to it, not by attracting water from the environment.

Lactic acid is used in its free form and has also been incorporated into liposomes. These round structures made up of concentric lipid bilayers with a central hollow core for drug storage release the

Table 18-2. Selected moisturizers for symptomatic topical therapy of dry scaling disorders*

TRADE NAME (MANUFACTURER)	ACTIVE INGREDIENTS		
	EMOLLIENTS	HUMECTANTS	EMULSIFIERS
Humilac Dry Skin Spray and Rinse (Allerderm/ Virbac)	—	Glycerin, lactic acid, propylene glycol, urea	—
HyLyt*efa Bath Oil Coat Conditioner (DVM Pharmaceuticals)	Lanolin, mineral oil, safflower oil	Na-lactate, polyvinyl pyrrolidone	—
Micro Pearls Humectant Spray (Evsco Pharmaceuticals)	—	Lactic acid (encapsulated)	—
Veterinary Prescription Sesame Oil Spray (Veterinary Prescription)	Sesame oil, vitamin E	—	—
Veterinary Prescription Alpha-Sesame Oil Dry Skin Rinse (Veterinary Prescription)	Cottonseed oil, lanolin, sesame oil	—	PEG-4 dilaurate

*Also indicated to counteract the drying effects of benzoyl peroxide shampoos, tar shampoos, selenium sulfide shampoos, and flea-control products.

active ingredient over a period of time and thus result in more residual activity. Liposomes are used in a humectant spray formulation (Micro Pearls Humectant Spray).

Glycerin, propylene glycol, and urea are humectants and are also classified as demulcent polyhydroxy compounds. A demulcent is a high–molecular weight compound that forms aqueous solutions with the ability to alleviate irritation by coating the skin surface and protecting the underlying cells from stimuli. Glycerin, a trihydric alcohol, is miscible with water and alcohol and is a popular vehicle for many cutaneous drugs.

Propylene glycol is a clear colorless viscous liquid that is miscible with water and dissolves many essential oils. In low concentrations it is an effective humectant because it is hygroscopic. At 40% to 50% it is antibacterial and antifungal and serves as an excellent vehicle because of its ability to enhance percutaneous penetration of drugs. Above 50% it denatures and solubilizes protein and is therefore keratolytic. It is found in veterinary bath oil rinse formulations and has reported efficacy when mixed as a 75% rinse in water or a humectant (Humilac) for ichthyosis and sebaceous adenitis.

Urea promotes hydration and removal of excess keratin and is beneficial with dry, hyperkeratotic skin. At concentrations below 20%, urea acts as a humectant by its hygroscopic action. Above 40% it is keratolytic due to proteolytic activity on keratin and prekeratin. It is found in a veterinary bath oil rinse formulation (Humilac).

Principles of Moisturizer Therapy

Commercial moisturizers are beneficial for cases of dry scaling and after use of potentially drying agents such as benzoyl peroxide, tar, and topical flea products. It is impossible to determine, for an individual animal with a scaling dermatosis, whether an emollient (Veterinary Prescription Sesame Oil Spray), an emollient-emulsifier (Veterinary Prescription Alpha-Sesame Oil Dry Skin Rinse), or a humectant (Humilac) will give better results. One preparation (HyLyt*efa Bath Oil Coat Conditioner) contains a combination of three emollients and two humectants. I have found that emollients work well with all types of coat length and texture. Humectants seem to work better on dogs with short hair than on long-haired, thick-coated breeds. Some owners may not enjoy using emollient products because they perceive an oily consistency to the coat after it is dry. This is usually not a problem if there is strict adherence to the recommended dilutions. However, the oil-free humectants offer an alternative in these situations.

The maximum hydrating effect is best achieved when a rinse is applied after bathing while the stratum corneum is still moist. The rinse should be diluted with water according to label directions and then poured or sponged over the entire body and allowed to air dry. Moisturizing rinses may also be diluted with flea dips to minimize the drying effects of insecticides and petroleum distillates. They may also be diluted in plant mister bottles and sprayed on the skin and hair coat between baths as needed. However, emollients are less effective than humectants when used in this manner since the stratum corneum has not been hydrated prior to their application. Finally, they may be sprayed directly from the bottle at full strength for severe local hyperkeratotic lesions such as those seen with calluses, nasodigital hyperkeratosis, and ear margin dermatosis.

Three products, besides having emollient effects, are potentially beneficial when an essential fatty acid deficiency is suspected (Veterinary Prescription Sesame Oil Spray, Veterinary Prescription Alpha-Sesame Oil Dry Skin Rinse, HyLyt*efa Bath Oil Coat Conditioner). Topical application of essential fatty acids has been shown to be an effective way to correct epidermal changes associated with the deficiency. Some 4 to 6 weeks of daily application is needed to assess efficacy. Such frequent application may make the skin and hair coat too oily and limit usefulness.

TOPICAL FORMULATIONS FOR LOCALIZED SCALING
Tretinoin

Topical 0.05% tretinoin cream (Retin-A) increases the epidermal turnover rate and reduces cohesion of keratinocytes, making it useful in localized follicular or epidermal hyperkeratotic scaling disorders. It has efficacy for chin acne in dogs and cats when given daily until remission and then as needed for maintenance. In some acne cases it is alternated with topical benzoyl peroxide gel (OxyDex Gel, Pyoben Gel). Tretinoin will also help control idiopathic nasal hyperkeratosis when used along with an occlusive emollient such as petrolatum.

Allergic or irritant cutaneous reactions may be a problem in some cases. Tretinoin is available in lower concentrations (0.025% and 0.01%) in gel formulations for these patients. Alternating the retinoid with a 1% hydrocortisone cream may also help control such reactions.

Lactic Acid

Lactic acid has hygroscopic activity at low concentrations and is keratolytic at higher percentages. A high-concentration lactic acid lotion (LactiCare) is useful for idiopathic nasal hyperkeratosis, calluses, and ear margin dermatosis. It should be applied daily until the condition is controlled and then as needed for maintenance. It is a nonprescription human product that is well-tolerated by dogs.

Salicylic Acid

In addition to its incorporation in shampoo formulations, salicylic acid at 6% has been formulated with 5% urea and 5% sodium lactate as a keratolytic humectant gel (KeraSolv). This product is also used for idiopathic nasal hyperkeratosis, calluses, ear margin dermatosis, and acne. It should be applied daily until the condition is controlled and then as needed for maintenance.

Salicylic acid (0.5%, 2%) and alcohol pads (Stri-Dex Pads, Regular and Maximum Strength) are helpful when used daily for chin acne to remove comedones from hair follicles, but they may be irritating for some animals because of the alcohol content. They are also helpful in cases of Schnauzer comedo syndrome.

Ceruminolytic Agents

Some dogs with scaling dermatoses may have focal areas of severe greasy scale that are poorly responsive to degreasing shampoos such as high-concentration tars and benzoyl peroxide. The best example is the Cocker Spaniel with idiopathic seborrhea and severe oily scaling of the ventral neck and trunk, axillae, and interdigital areas.

These problem areas may be more easily managed by application of a ceruminolytic agent before bathing. Fifteen minutes prior to each bath a topical ceruminolytic agent such as dioctyl sodium sulfosuccinate (Clear-X Ear Cleansing Solution, Adams Pan-Otic) is applied to the affected areas. It is washed off during the shampoo, but it promotes resolution of the accumulated greasy material as well as control of the associated odor.

REFERENCES

Bonnetblanc JM, Bernard P: Benzoyl peroxide in seborrheic dermatitis. (Letter to the Editor.) Arch Dermatol 122:752, 1986.

Leyden JJ, et al: Effects of sulfur and salicylic acid in a shampoo base in the treatment of dandruff: a double-blind study using corneocyte counts and clinical grading, Cutis 39:557, 1987.

Lin AN, et al: Sulfur revisited, J Am Acad Dermatol 18:533, 1988.

Lowe NJ, et al: New coal tar extract and coal tar shampoos, Arch Dermatol 118:487, 1982.

Wehr RF, Krochmal L: Considerations in selecting a moisturizer, Cutis 39:512, 1987.

SUPPLEMENTAL READINGS

Gilman AG, et al: Goodman and Gilman's The pharmacological basis of therapeutics, ed 7, New York, 1985, MacMillan Publishing.

Kunkle GA: Managing canine seborrhea. In Kirk RW (ed): Current veterinary therapy VIII, Philadelphia, 1983, WB Saunders, p 518.

Kwochka KW: Rational shampoo therapy in veterinary dermatology. In Campfield WW (ed): Proceedings of the 11th Annual Kal Kan Symposium for the Treatment of Small Animal Diseases, 1988, Vernon Calif, Kal Kan Foods, p 87.

Manning TO: Topical therapy. In Kirk RW (ed): Current veterinary therapy VIII, Philadelphia, 1983, WB Saunders, p 462.

Miller WH: Antiseborrheic agents in dermatology. In Kirk RW (ed): Current veterinary therapy IX, Philadelphia, 1986, WB Saunders, p 596.

19

Retinoids and Vitamin A Therapy

Kenneth W. Kwochka

The term "retinoids" refers to the entire group of naturally occurring and synthetic vitamin A derivatives. The three major naturally occurring compounds are retinol, retinal, and retinoic acid. Retinol (the most potent analogue, the main dietary source, and the main transport and storage form of vitamin A) is metabolized to retinal and retinoic acid. General functions of the retinoids include growth promotion, differentiation and maintenance of epithelial tissue, and maintenance of normal reproductive and visual functions (Peck and DiGiovanna, 1987).

The importance of vitamin A for the maintenance of normal skin was first discovered in the 1920s. Epithelial changes due to abnormal keratinization were identified in vitamin A–deficient animals. This led to the use of high doses of oral vitamin A and topical vitamin A for a number of different dermatoses involving keratinization abnormalities.

In the last 20 years many retinoid derivatives have been synthesized and tested to develop compounds with a better therapeutic index and less toxicity than naturally occurring retinoids. There are two commercially available synthetic retinoids for human usage: **isotretinoin** (13-*cis* retinoic acid, Accutane), which is efficacious in severe recalcitrant cystic acne, Darier's disease, pityriasis rubra pilaris, and other disorders that affect the hair follicle and sebaceous gland; and **etretinate** (Tegison), the trimethyl-methoxyphenyl analogue of retinoic acid ethyl ester, which is used for psoriasis, lamellar ichthyosis, and other disorders of keratinization characterized by hyperproliferation of the epidermis and follicular epithelium. When available, etretin (Soritane), the active metabolite of etretinate, will largely replace etretinate since it is stored in body tissues for a shorter period and is thus associated with less toxicity.

Importance

Although there have been some important advances in understanding the pathophysiology and treatment of keratinization disorders in dogs, most of these dermatoses are still considered controllable and not curable. This is true of primary idiopathic seborrhea, epidermal dysplasia, ichthyosis, sebaceous adenitis, lichenoid-psoriasiform dermatosis, Schnauzer comedo syndrome, ear margin dermatosis, and acne. Together these diseases represent a significant portion of the dermatologic caseload in general and specialty practice.

Conventional drugs used in the management of primary scaling disorders include topical keratolytic and keratoplastic agents, fatty acids, antibiotics, and topical and systemic glucocorticoids. Management with groups of these medications is inconvenient, labor-intensive, and expensive for the pet owner. This as well as a less than favorable response may result in euthanasia of otherwise healthy animals. Effective medications for localized and generalized primary scaling disorders would significantly simplify management for the owner and veterinarian. The topical and oral retinoids have revolutionized treatment of a number of different scaling dermatoses in dogs and cats.

Pharmacokinetics and Mechanisms of Action

The naturally occurring retinoids (Goodman, 1981) are derived from dietary precursors of animal and vegetable origin. Retinyl esters are obtained from animal fats and fish-liver oils whereas the beta-carotene precursor comes from yellow and green leafy vegetables. Retinyl esters are hydrolyzed in the digestive tract to retinol, which is absorbed into the mucosal cells. Beta-carotene undergoes oxidative cleavage to retinal, which is reduced to retinol in the intestinal mucosa. Retinol is then esterified, complexed with long-chain fatty acids into chylomicrons, and transported to the liver via the lymphatics and blood. Retinol is stored in the liver as retinyl ester.

When needed, retinol is released from the liver in a 1:1 ratio with serum retinol-binding protein (RBP). This complex, in turn, binds to a serum prealbumin protein termed transthyretin (TTR), which also binds thyroxin but at a different binding site (Goodman, 1981).

The RBP-retinol-TTR complex circulates in the blood to deliver retinol to vitamin A–requiring tissues, such as the skin. The mechanism by which the vitamin is transferred from RBP to target cells is not known. It has been generally accepted that the delivery of retinol from RBP is mediated through a specific cell-surface RBP receptor (Torma and Vahlquist, 1984). However, definitive demonstration of this receptor has not been accomplished. Other data (Hodam et al., 1991) support a mechanism for retinol delivery from RBP to keratinocytes that does not involve cell-surface RBP receptors; instead, it is suggested that the vitamin is first slowly released from RBP and then becomes cell-associated from the aqueous phase.

In the cell, retinol binds to a specific cytosol-binding protein called cellular retinol-binding protein (CRBP). Translocation to the nucleus is then thought to occur with other nuclear receptor proteins (retinoic acid receptor [RAR] alpha, RAR gamma). Retinoic acid has its own distinct cellular binding protein (CRABP). CRABP is differentially expressed during squamous differentiation of keratinocytes so may control the effective concentration of retinoic acid in the cell and therefore indirectly regulate gene expression.

At the molecular level, retinoids work directly on the cell genome as steroid hormones do. They may affect RNA synthesis, protein synthesis, post-translational glycosylation of protein, prostaglandin synthesis, and the lability of membranes; they have also been shown (Orfanos, 1985; Hodam et al., 1991) to induce tissue transglutaminase, inhibit epidermal transglutaminase, inhibit cornified envelope formation, inhibit cholesterol sulfate synthesis, inhibit phorbol ester-induced ornithine decarboxylase activity, inhibit collagenase production, and modulate keratin expression. These effects explain the ability of retinoids to influence cellular proliferation, differentiation, and surface composition in normalizing the keratinization process.

Toxicity

Numerous adverse clinical conditions have been associated with retinoid usage in humans—including cheilitis, inflammation and xerosis of the skin and mucous membranes, pruritus, facial dermatitis, epistaxis, thinning of the hair, palmoplantar desquamation, conjunctivitis, headache, ataxia, lethargy and fatigue, psychologic changes, and visual disturbances. Other abnormalities may include transient minor elevations in liver enzymes (which return to normal even with continuation of therapy), hyperlipidemia, increased platelet count, hypercalcemia, arthralgias, photosensitivity, and teratogenicity.

Teratogenicity is a serious problem in women who take retinoids during pregnancy (Shalita, 1988). Abnormalities have included spontaneous abortions and birth defects (hydrocephalus, deformed external ears, and abnormalities of the thymus, skeletal system, and cardiovascular system). Women of childbearing age are not allowed to take retinoids unless on a supervised birth control program. There are vast differences in body storage and elimination of the synthetic retinoids (Shalita, 1988): isotretinoin and etretin are eliminated rapidly, and teratogenic effects are gone 1 month after discontinuation of therapy; but etretinate has a 100-day elimination half-life, and the length of time for teratogenic potential after stopping therapy is not known because of its storage in body fat.

Chronic hypervitaminosis A has been associated with demineralization and thinning of the long bones, cortical hyperostosis, periostitis, and premature closure of the epiphyses (Kilcoyne, 1988).

Dogs generally tolerate the retinoids better than humans do, with minimal side effects. However, retinoids should not be used in breeding animals because of teratogenicity and possible inhibition of spermatogenesis. The persistence of teratogenic effects for the various retinoids is not known in dogs. Therefore, the safest recommendation is that retinoids not be used in intact females. **Clients must also be warned about the serious potential risks from accidental human ingestion of any of the retinoids.** There is little information pertaining to the effects of retinoids at therapeutic doses on the skeletal system. Other side effects in dogs will be discussed as they relate to each specific retinoid used in the various scaling dermatoses.

CLINICAL APPLICATIONS
(Table 19-1)

The practitioner must determine when natural or synthetic retinoids may be helpful in the management of primary scaling dermatoses. This may be difficult due to variations in response and the relatively low numbers of cases treated. These agents should be reserved for cases in which there are clinical and histologic abnormalities most consistent with primary keratinization disorders of the surface and/or follicular epithelium or abnormalities of the sebaceous glands. Other causes of clinical scaling (ectoparasitism, allergies, infections, endocrinopathies) should first be eliminated from the list of differential diagnoses.

The synthetic retinoids may be prohibitively expensive for some clients. It costs $1.50 to $2.50 per day to use isotretinoin or etretinate in most dogs with a primary keratinization disorder. However, after the disorder has been brought under control, it appears that alternate-day or even less frequent administration is possible for long-term maintenance. Although $1.50 to $2.50 per day sounds expensive, it may actually be cheaper than trying to control the disease with regular shampoos, antibiotics, dietary supplements, and glucocorticoids. In the future, costs of retinoids may decrease as new synthetic analogues are approved for human usage and current products are relabeled for use in dogs and cats.

In addition to concern for cost, until these drugs are used more extensively in veterinary medicine we will not know the full range of potential toxicity. Retinoids should be used when topical keratolytic and keratoplastic agents have a limited effect or require too frequent application to be practical for long-term management. Since natural vitamin A alcohol (retinol) is less expensive than the synthetics and appears to be well-tolerated in dogs, it should be considered prior to using isotretinoin, etretinate, or etretin for a **nonspecific** epidermal scaling disorder. When any of the retinoids are used for keratinization disorders, treatment should be continued for 8 to 12 weeks before a determination of efficacy is made.

Vitamin A Alcohol (retinol)

The primary indication for vitamin A alcohol in veterinary dermatology is vitamin A–responsive dermatosis in Cocker Spaniels. Similar syndromes have been reported in a Miniature Schnauzer and a Labrador Retriever. A small subset of seborrheic Cocker Spaniels will have this disease, which responds to retinol given at 625 to 800 IU/kg q24h PO (Ihrke and Goldschmidt, 1983; Scott, 1986). This is not a dietary deficiency of vitamin A; rather, it may represent a local vitamin A deficiency in the epidermis, a problem with uptake in the skin, or a disorder of cutaneous utilization. Clinically the dermatosis is characterized by refractory seborrheic skin disease with marked follicular plugging and hyperkeratotic plaques with surface "frondlike" plugs from the follicles. These lesions

Table 19-1. Topical and systemic retinoids used to treat primary keratinization disorders

RETINOID	TRADE NAME (MANUFACTURER)	DOSE	INDICATIONS	MAJOR SIDE EFFECTS*	HOW SUPPLIED
Vitamin A alcohol (retinol)	Generics (various)	625-800 IU/kg q24h PO	Vitamin A–responsive dermatosis (seen primarily in Cocker Spaniels but occasionally also in other breeds)	Very well-tolerated	Over-the-counter in liquid and 10,000 IU capsules; by prescription in 25,000 and 50,000 IU capsules
Tretinoin (all-*trans* retinoic acid)	Retin-A (Ortho)	Applied topically q12-24h to control; then decrease frequency for maintenance	Severe unresponsive chin acne in dogs and cats, idiopathic nasal hyperkeratosis, idiopathic ear margin dermatosis, acanthosis nigricans	Irritant reaction	By prescription as 0.05% cream and 0.025% or 0.01% gel with 90% alcohol
Isotretinoin (13-*cis* retinoic acid)	Accutane (Roche)	1-2 mg/kg q24h PO for control (8-12 weeks); then try to decrease to alternate-day therapy	Schnauzer comedo syndrome, sebaceous adenitis (especially short-coated breeds), lamellar ichthyosis	Keratoconjunctivitis sicca; mild elevations in cholesterol, triglycerides, and alanine aminotransferase; pain in legs and joints	By prescription as 10, 20, and 40 mg capsules
Etretinate (trimethyl-methoxyphenyl analogue of retinoic acid ethyl ester)	Tegison (Roche)	1-2 mg/kg q24h PO for control (8-12 weeks); then try to decrease to alternate-day therapy	Idiopathic seborrhea in Cocker Spaniels (also Springer Spaniels, Golden Retrievers, mixed breeds; not West Highland White Terriers, Basset Hounds, Collies), sebaceous adenitis (may be beneficial in long-coated breeds), lamellar ichthyosis	Same as for isotretinoin but with less ocular and skeletal abnormalities so may be better for prolonged use; extended teratogenic effect due to long tissue storage (actual length of effect not known)	By prescription as 10 and 25 mg capsules

*Retinoids should not be used in breeding animals because of the potential for teratogenicity. Clients must also be warned about the serious potential risks from accidental human ingestion.

are present primarily on the ventral and lateral thorax and abdomen.

The histologic abnormalities are quite distinct, consisting of orthokeratotic hyperkeratosis and dilation of hair follicles contrasted with mild orthokeratotic hyperkeratosis of the epidermis and mild irregular epidermal hyperplasia. Response to medication is seen within 4 weeks, and complete clinical remission usually occurs by 10 weeks. Treatment is needed for life, but retinol at this dosage appears to be well-tolerated in dogs.

It is important to stress that this syndrome has very distinct clinical signs and histopathologic abnormalities and represents only a small portion of Cocker Spaniels with seborrhea. However, it is logical to try a 4-to-8-week course of retinol in dogs with ventral hyperkeratotic plaques that do not respond well to topical therapy and antibiotics.

No adverse effects were reported in 9 dogs treated with retinol at dosages ranging from 10,000 IU q24h PO (Cocker Spaniels and a Miniature Schnauzer) to 50,000 IU q24h PO (a Labrador Retriever) for periods of 6 months to 4.5 years. I do not do clinicopathologic monitoring of dogs treated with retinol.

Tretinoin (all-*trans* retinoic acid, Retin-A)

In general, because of cost, the systemic retinoids would not be considered practical for localized follicular or epidermal keratinization disorders. However, topical 0.05% tretinoin cream may be useful in these cases. This synthetic retinoid is effective though, if used systemically, it has a high incidence of side effects.

Chin acne in dogs and cats is most likely due to a follicular keratinization disorder with comedo formation and secondary bacterial folliculitis. Topical tretinoin has been used successfully to manage some of these cases, which do not respond to topical benzoyl peroxide, topical antibiotics, alcohol scrubs, or systemic antibiotics. Daily application of tretinoin to the affected area is recommended until remission, followed by a decrease in frequency for maintenance. Benzoyl peroxide washes (OxyDex Shampoo, Pyoben Shampoo) and gels (OxyDex Gel, Pyoben Gel) have been used concurrently for their antibacterial effects. Allergic or irritant cutaneous reactions will occasionally be a problem, especially in cats. Tretinoin is available in lower-concentration (0.025% and 0.01%) gel formulations for these cases. However, even these lower concentrations may not be tolerated because of the high (90%) alcohol content.

Since tretinoin increases the epidermal turnover rate and reduces cohesion of keratinocytes, it may be useful in other localized hyperkeratotic scaling disorders. It is effective when used with topical emollients for calluses and idiopathic nasal hyperkeratosis. I have also found it useful for idiopathic ear margin dermatosis and, when alternated with topical steroids, in severely lichenified lesions such as those associated with acanthosis nigricans.

Gloves should be worn by the owner when applying tretinoin, and pregnant women should neither use nor apply this preparation.

Isotretinoin (13-*cis* retinoic acid, Accutane)

Isotretinoin is a synthetic retinoid that appears to have best activity in skin diseases where the hair follicles and sebaceous glands are the primary structures involved.

Idiopathic Seborrhea

Since it has had beneficial effects on sebaceous gland abnormalities and keratinization disorders in humans, isotretinoin seemed the logical compound for idiopathic seborrheic syndromes in dogs. Unfortunately, results have been disappointing. In a double-blind, placebo-controlled, crossover study, Fadok (1986) used isotretinoin at a dosage of 3 mg/kg q24h PO for 2 months. Only one dog showed 100% improvement, with relapse after discontinuation of therapy and improvement with readministration of isotretinoin. Three dogs showed less than 50% improvement.

I used (1989) isotretinoin at 1 mg/kg q12h PO for 5 months to treat four Cocker Spaniels with idiopathic seborrhea. One dog showed slightly decreased scale production while on therapy. Abnormal histologic findings and epidermal cell migration rates remained unchanged throughout the study.

Poor response has also been seen when isotretinoin was used at 1 mg/kg q12h PO in West Highland White Terriers with greasy seborrhea characterized histologically by epidermal dysplasia.

These treatment failures should not preclude the use of isotretinoin for idiopathic seborrheic syndromes in other breeds and at various dosages. One Cocker Spaniel with idiopathic seborrhea (Bates, 1984) was reported to respond to this drug at 0.25 mg/kg q12h PO for 4 weeks. No adverse reactions were seen. The dog had not responded to vitamin A alcohol prior to the isotretinoin.

Schnauzer Comedo Syndrome

Schnauzer comedo syndrome is a seborrheic disorder of certain predisposed Miniature Schnauzers characterized by multiple comedones along the back that present as follicular papular lesions. Clinical management is usually achieved with topical antiseborrheic agents, the follicular flushing agent benzoyl peroxide, or systemic antibiotics. However, refractory cases occur that may not respond to topical therapy. Also, continued topical therapy may not be practical for all clients. These Schnauzers have been managed successfully with isotretinoin at doses ranging from 1 to 2 mg/kg q24h PO. Rapid response is seen within 3 to 4 weeks. Most dogs can be maintained without signs of toxicity on alternate-day therapy.

Sebaceous Adenitis

Sebaceous adenitis is a dermatosis characterized by severe (localized or generalized) seborrhea sicca and granulomatous inflammation with destruction of sebaceous glands (Chapter 20). Treatment includes high doses of systemic glucocorticoids, topical antiseborrheic agents, topical propylene glycol–humectant rinses, and high doses of fatty acids.

Isotretinoin is a therapeutic option for cases that do not respond to more conservative therapy. It may work by various mechanisms and at more than one stage of the disease. There may be a beneficial effect from altering lipid production in the epidermis or sebaceous glands, suppressing sebum production, or normalizing a follicular keratinization abnormality.

Excellent responses to isotretinoin at 1 to 2 mg/kg q24h PO have been seen in some poodles (Power and Ihrke, 1990) although others showed no response. The investigators stated that a higher initial dosage (2 to 3 mg/kg q24h PO) might be helpful. They also reported that it was mainly the primary hairs that regrew, resulting in a coarser, flatter coat. Two poodles have been maintained without signs of toxicity on 10 mg three times per week for up to 2 years.

Stewart et al. (1991) reported on two Vizslas with granulomatous sebaceous adenitis that were successfully treated with isotretinoin. The drug, given at 1 mg/kg q24h PO, resulted in rapid clinical response over a 2-to-3-month period. Recurrence of lesions was noted in one of the dogs 1 month after discontinuation of therapy. However, it again had a normal hair coat after another 8 weeks of treatment and after discontinuation of isotretinoin a second time has remained in remission for

1 year. No side effects of the medication were noted in either of these dogs.

Less favorable responses using isotretinoin have been reported for Akitas, Samoyeds, and Boston Terriers. My experience with isotretinoin for sebaceous adenitis has been that it is more efficacious when used in short-coated than in long-coated breeds and also that response is better when used early in the course of the disease, before massive sebaceous gland destruction has occurred.

Lamellar Ichthyosis

This rare hereditary congenital disorder of dogs is seen primarily in terrier breeds and characterized clinically by tightly adherent, verrucous, tannish gray scales and feathered keratinous projections on all or large portions of the skin. Skin biopsy reveals extreme orthokeratotic hyperkeratosis, follicular keratosis and plugging, a prominent granular layer, and many mitotic figures.

This disease in terrier breeds has been successfully managed with isotretinoin at 1 to 2 mg/kg q24h PO. Remission is seen within 8 to 12 weeks, and some dogs can be maintained on alternate-day therapy.

Toxicity

The incidence and severity of side effects associated with isotretinoin in companion animals appear to be lower than in humans. However, this may be somewhat misleading since most cases have been treated only for short periods and clinical pathological evaluations have not been performed in many cases.

One review article (Kwochka, 1989) described a low incidence of toxicity in 29 dogs treated with isotretinoin. Four dogs developed a conjunctivitis that was reversible upon discontinuation of the therapy. Other abnormalities, seen in single cases, included hyperactivity; ear pruritus; erythema of mucocutaneous junctions and feet; lethargy with vomiting, abdominal distension, and erythema; and anorexia with lethargy, collapse, and a swollen tongue. All these abnormalities were reversible or transient upon discontinuation of the therapy.

One case had an increased platelet count, three had hypertriglyceridemia, two had hypercholesterolemia, and three had transient elevations in alanine aminotransferase. The biochemical abnormalities were not associated with clinical signs. Therapy can be continued if elevations are mild. Triglyceride and cholesterol elevations have been decreased and controlled using fat-restricted diets.

During treatment, in addition to a complete

physical examination, the following should be monitored: CBCs, serum biochemical profiles (with cholesterol and triglycerides), urinalyses, and tear production. Monitoring is best done monthly for the first 4 to 6 months and then every 6 months while on maintenance therapy.

Radiographic skeletal changes have not been reported with long-term use of isotretinoin at therapeutic dosages in companion animals. However, increased pain sensitivity of legs and joints has been seen in a few cases. Those seen by me have been reversible upon discontinuation of therapy. Until more dogs on long-term maintenance therapy have been evaluated, it would be prudent to palpate long bones every 6 months and radiograph if any sensitivity is detected or reported by the owner.

It is worth repeating that isotretinoin should not be used in breeding animals because of teratogenicity and possible inhibition of spermatogenesis. **Clients must also be warned about the serious potential risks from accidental human ingestion of isotretinoin.**

Etretinate (Tegison)

Because of the profoundly beneficial effects of using etretinate on a hyperproliferative epidermal disorder (psoriasis) in humans, there has been a considerable degree of excitement over its use in dogs. Idiopathic seborrhea, like psoriasis, at least in Cocker Spaniels and Irish Setters, is partially characterized by a hyperproliferative epidermis.

Idiopathic Seborrhea

Recently (Power and Ihrke, 1990) etretinate was evaluated in 15 Cocker Spaniels with primary seborrhea. The dogs were treated for 4 months at a dosage of 0.75 to 1 mg/kg q24h PO. All showed a good to excellent response, with decreased scale, a softening and thinning of seborrheic plaques, reduced odor, and a lessening of pruritus. Most showed some response within the first 2 months and continual improvement over the next 2 months. Some severely affected dogs were treated for 6 months. Unfortunately, etretinate did not improve the ceruminous otitis externa. Clinical signs returned upon discontinuation of therapy although they decreased again with readministration of the drug. Some dogs have been maintained without signs of toxicity over several months on alternate-day therapy.

I have had similar results with etretinate used at 1 mg/kg q24h PO in an additional seven Cocker Spaniels. Response was seen within 2 months, and

four dogs have now been maintained on daily therapy for several months without toxicity.

Beneficial responses have also been seen in English Springer Spaniels, Golden Retrievers, Irish Setters, and mixed-breed dogs with idiopathic keratinization disorders. However, the drug has not been effective in seborrheic West Highland White Terriers, Basset Hounds, or Collies.

Sebaceous Adenitis

Compared to isotretinoin, there is little information available on the use of etretinate for sebaceous adenitis in dogs. Power and Ihrke (1990) reported no response in three Poodles. Three long-haired dogs (White et al., 1991) were recently treated with etretinate at 0.8 to 1.8 mg/kg q24h PO for 2 to 3 months. Two dogs at the upper end of the dosage range manifested greater than 50% resolution of clinical signs. Many more dogs will need to be evaluated before definitive recommendations can be made. However, etretinate may be a desirable alternative for long-haired dogs with sebaceous adenitis since they typically do not respond well to isotretinoin.

Lamellar Ichthyosis

Etretinate is effective for ichthyosis in terriers at 1 to 2 mg/kg q24h PO and may be better tolerated than isotretinoin, especially over the lifetime of therapy that will be needed to control this disease.

Toxicity

The same general comments about retinoid toxicity and patient monitoring apply to etretinate as to isotretinoin. Although there is little information on long-term use of the retinoids in dogs at therapeutic doses, it is believed that etretinate is associated with fewer skeletal and ocular abnormalities than isotretinoin is. However, because of storage in body fat with etretinate the teratogenic effects may last for an extended (and unknown) period after discontinuation of treatment. Etretinate should not be used in breeding animals. It is teratogenic and also may inhibit spermatogenesis. **Clients must also be warned about the serious potential risks from accidental human ingestion of etretinate.**

REFERENCES

Bates JR: Treatment of idiopathic seborrhea in a dog, Mod Vet Pract 65:725, 1984.

Fadok VA: Treatment of canine idiopathic seborrhea with isotretinoin, Am J Vet Res 47:1730, 1986.

Goodman DS: Vitamin A transport and delivery and the mechanism of vitamin A toxicity. In Orfanos CE (ed): Retinoids—advances in basic research and therapy, New York, 1981, Springer-Verlag, p 31.

Hodam JR, et al: Comparison of the rate of uptake and biologic effects of retinol added to human keratinocytes either directly to the culture medium or bound to serum retinol-binding protein, J Invest Dermatol 97:298, 1991.

Ihrke PJ, Goldschmidt MH: Vitamin A–responsive dermatosis in the dog, J Am Vet Med Assoc 182:687, 1983.

Kilcoyne RF: Effects of retinoids in bone, J Am Acad Dermatol 19:212, 1988.

Kwochka KW: Retinoids in dermatology. In Kirk RW (ed): Current veterinary therapy X, Philadelphia, 1989, WB Saunders, p 553.

Orfanos CE: Retinoids in clinical dermatology: an update. In Sauret JH (ed): Retinoids: new trends in research and therapy, Basel, 1985, Karger, p 314.

Peck GL, DiGiovanna JJ: Retinoids. In Fitzpatrick TB, et al (eds): Dermatology in general medicine, ed 3, New York, 1987, McGraw-Hill, p 2582.

Power HT, Ihrke PJ: Synthetic retinoids in veterinary dermatology, Vet Clin North Am 20:1525, 1990.

Scott DW: Vitamin A–responsive dermatosis in the cocker spaniel, J Am Anim Hosp Assoc 22:125, 1986.

Shalita AR: Lipid and teratogenic effects of retinoids, J Am Acad Dermatol 19:197, 1988.

Stewart LJ, et al: Isotretinoin in the treatment of sebaceous adenitis in two Vizslas, J Am Anim Hosp Assoc 27:65, 1991.

Torma H, Vahlquist A: Vitamin A uptake by human skin in vitro, Arch Dermatol Res 276:390, 1984.

White SD, et al: Isotretinoin and etretinate in the treatment of benign and malignant cutaneous neoplasia and in sebaceous adenitis of longhaired dogs, in Proceedings, Annual members' meeting of the AAVD & ACVD, 1991, p 101.

20

Sebaceous Adenitis

Edmund J. Rosser Jr.

<table>
<tr><td>

Diagnostic Criteria for Sebaceous Adenitis

SUGGESTIVE
Age, breed, and distribution pattern of lesions; presence of follicular casts on physical examination

COMPATIBLE
Negative skin scrapings, negative fungal culture, and negative bacterial culture or poor response to systemic antibiotics and antibacterial/antiseborrheic shampoo therapy

TENTATIVE
Compatible plus biopsies consistent with an endocrine dermatosis (nonscarring alopecia), especially with lack of sebaceous glands and normal results on endocrine function tests

DEFINITIVE
Compatible plus biopsies showing middermal granulomatous or pyogranulomatous inflammation at the level of the sebaceous glands

</td></tr>
</table>

Sebaceous adenitis is an inflammatory disease process directed against the sebaceous glands of the skin and has shown certain breed predispositions (Rosser et al., 1987; Griffin, 1988; Muller et al., 1989; Rosser and Sams, 1991; Rosser, in press). Studies are currently being considered to examine the mode of inheritance in Standard Poodles due to an increased incidence in this breed in the United States. Other breeds that may be predisposed include the Akita, Samoyed, and Vizsla. The pathophysiology of sebaceous adenitis is currently unknown, but speculations include the following: (1) Sebaceous gland destruction is a developmental and genetically inherited defect. (2) Sebaceous gland destruction is an immune mediated or autoimmune disease directed against a component of the sebaceous glands. (3) The initial defect is a keratinization abnormality with subsequent obstruction of the sebaceous ducts resulting in sebaceous adenitis. (4) The sebaceous adenitis and keratinization defects are the result of an abnormality in lipid metabolism affecting keratinization and the production of sebum (Scott, 1986; Rosser et al., 1987; Rosser, in press).

CLINICAL DISEASE

The majority of cases reported thus far have been in young adult and middle-aged dogs, with no evident sex predisposition. There appear to be two forms of the disease, with differences in both clinical presentation and histopathologic changes.

The first form occurs in long-coated breeds, including the Standard Poodle, Akita, and Samoyed.

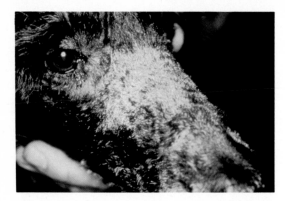

Figure 20-1. Sebaceous adenitis in a Standard Poodle with alopecia and tightly adherent scales on the dorsal planum of the nose.

(From Rosser EJ Jr, et al: J Am Anim Hosp 23:341, 1987.)

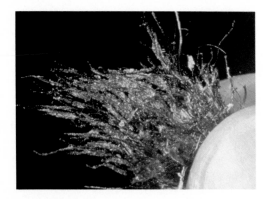

Figure 20-2. Follicular casts on hair shafts plucked from a Standard Poodle with sebaceous adenitis.

(Courtesy Dr. Kenneth Kwochka, Columbus, Ohio.)

The disease has been most closely studied in the Standard Poodle. It was first reported in black and apricot colors but is now recognized in all color variants. The first signs noted are a symmetrical and partial alopecia with excess scaling and dull, brittle hairs. Lesions are usually first observed along the animal's dorsal midline. Specific areas that may be affected include the dorsal planum of the nose, top of the head, dorsal neck and trunk, tail and pinnae. The patient is usually nonpruritic at this stage and there is no complaint of an offensive odor. In some mild forms, the disease never progresses beyond this stage. Progression of the disease results in the formation of tightly adherent silver-white scale (Fig. 20-1), follicular casts around hair shafts (Fig. 20-2), and small tufts of matted hair (Fig. 20-3). At this stage the dog is predisposed to the development of secondary bacterial folliculitis and subsequent pruritus and malodor. The condition may have a cyclic pattern (i.e., periods of spontaneous improvement and worsening independent of any treatments) and some dogs may have concurrent idiopathic epilepsy (Power, 1990). The condition in Akitas is often more severe and accompanied by chronic or recurrent secondary bacterial folliculitis with signs of systemic illness (Power, 1990).

The second form of sebaceous adenitis occurs in short-coated breeds (Fig. 20-4). Vizslas appear to be predisposed. The earliest signs are a moth-eaten, circular, or diffuse alopecia with mild scaling that affects the trunk, head, and ears. This form is usually nonpruritic, and the development of a secondary bacterial folliculitis is rare.

Two of the more common diseases initially sus-

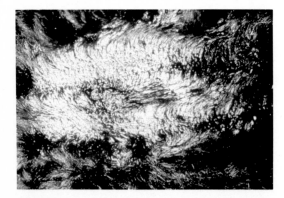

Figure 20-3. Sebaceous adenitis in a Standard Poodle with alopecia, scales, follicular casts, crusts, and tufts of matted hair with a secondary pyoderma over the dorsolumbar region.

(From Rosser EJ Jr, et al: J Am Anim Hosp 23:341, 1987.)

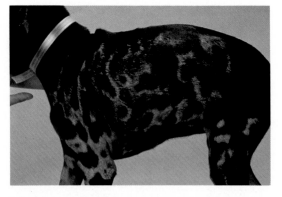

Figure 20-4. Sebaceous adenitis in a Miniature Pinscher showing characteristic circular to serpiginous alopecia and scaling.

(From Carothers MA, et al: J Am Vet Med Assoc 198:1645, 1991.)

pected in the patient with sebaceous adenitis are a seborrheic skin disease (primary keratinization disorder) and bacterial folliculitis. Therefore careful review of the history of response to treatment is often helpful. Previous treatments may have included the use of antiseborrheic shampoos, antibacterial shampoos, systemic antibiotics, and antiinflammatory dosages of glucocorticoids, with a poor or partial response to therapy. Additional differential diagnoses include demodicosis, dermatophytosis, and endocrine skin diseases.

DIAGNOSIS

A tentative diagnosis of sebaceous adenitis is based on breed, history, and physical findings. Confirmation of the diagnosis is by the histopathological examination of several skin biopsies taken from lesions representing different degrees of severity. Sites selected for biopsy should include both clinically normal skin and areas mildly as well as severely affected. The most common histologic finding is a nodular granulomatous to pyogranulomatous inflammatory reaction at the level of the sebaceous glands. Special stains and cultures for bacteria and fungi are usually negative. The exception is when a secondary bacterial folliculitis has developed, most often due to *Staphylococcus intermedius*. Moderate to marked orthokeratotic hyperkeratosis and keratinous follicular cast formation is present in long-coated breeds. Hyperkeratotic changes are mild or absent in short-coated breeds. There is a complete loss of the sebaceous glands with periadnexal fibrosis in the advanced stages of the disease. On rare occasion the entire hair follicle and adnexal structures will be destroyed.

TREATMENT

Response to therapy varies depending on the severity of the disease at the time of diagnosis. The prognosis is poor when sebaceous glands have been completely lost. The use of antiseborrheic shampoos, conditioners, emollients (Chapter 18), and essential fatty acid dietary supplements may be useful in mildly affected animals but is of little benefit in the more severe and chronic forms of the disease. In these instances two other treatments should be considered. The first (Griffin, 1988) is the use of a 50% to 75% mixture of propylene glycol and water applied once daily as a spray to the affected areas. The propylene glycol acts as a hygroscopic lipid solvent to penetrate the horny layer and in-

crease its water content. The second (Marshall and Williams, 1990; Power, 1990) is to use essential fatty acids at high dosages. One protocol employs the following empirical regimen: essential fatty acid dietary supplement (Derm Caps ES), one capsule q12h PO, and evening primrose oil, 500 mg orally q12h PO. Possible side effects include vomiting, diarrhea, and flatulence.

In general, this condition appears to be relatively refractory to treatment with either antiinflammatory or immunosuppressive dosages of glucocorticoids. A synthetic retinoid, isotretinoin (Accutane), at a dosage of 1 mg/kg q12-24h PO once to twice daily (Stewart et al., 1991) may be effective in refractory cases. (See Chapter 19 for a discussion of side effects and toxicities.) Results have been extremely variable. Isotretinoin should be started at an initial dosage of 1 mg/kg q12h PO for the first month and the patient reevaluated for response. If improvement is noted, the dosage should be reduced to 1 mg/kg q24h for another month. If further improvement is observed, the long-term goal is to control the disease with either 1 mg/kg q48h or 0.5 mg/kg q24h.

Cyclosporine (Sandimmune) has also been used in the treatment of refractory cases of sebaceous adenitis at a dosage of 5 mg/kg q12h PO (Carothers et al., 1991). Side effects may include vomiting, diarrhea, gingival hyperplasia, B-lymphocyte hyperplasia, hirsutism, papillomatous skin lesions, and increased incidence of infections (pyoderma, lower urinary tract infection, upper respiratory viral infection). Potential toxic reactions include nephrotoxicity and hepatotoxicity, which usually subside upon cessation of the drug.

Treatment should also include the use of an appropriate systemic antibiotic (Chapter 1) and a keratolytic, antibacterial, and follicular flushing shampoos (Sulf OxyDex) when a secondary bacterial folliculitis has developed. In general, the response to therapy is quite variable from one patient to the next, with the Akita being most refractory.

REFERENCES

Carothers MA, et al: Cyclosporine-responsive granulomatous sebaceous adenitis in a dog, J Am Vet Med Assoc 198:1645, 1991.

Griffin CE: Common dermatoses of the akita, shar pei, and chow chow. Presented at the AAHA general session of the AAVD & ACVD, 1988.

Marshall C, Williams J: Re-establishment of hair growth, skin pliability and apparent resistance to bacterial infection after dosing fish oil in a dog with sebaceous adenitis. In von Tscharner C, Halliwell

REW (eds): Advances in veterinary dermatology, London, 1990, Baillière Tindall, p 446.

Muller GH, et al: Small animal dermatology, ed 4, Philadelphia, 1989, WB Saunders, p 555.

Power HT: Personal communication, 1990.

Rosser EJ: Sebaceous adenitis in dogs and cats. In Kirk RW (ed): Current veterinary therapy XI, Philadelphia, WB Saunders, In press.

Rosser EJ, Sams A: Scaling dermatoses. In Allen DG (ed): Small animal medicine, Philadelphia, 1991, JB Lippincott, p 679.

Rosser EJ, et al: Sebaceous adenitis with hyperkeratosis in the standard poodle: a discussion of 10 cases, J Am Anim Hosp Assoc 23:341, 1987.

Scott DW: Granulomatous sebaceous adenitis in dogs, J Am Anim Hosp Assoc 22:631, 1986.

Stewart LJ, et al: Isotretinoin in the treatment of sebaceous adenitis in two Vizslas, J Am Anim Hosp Assoc 27:65, 1991.

Pigment Disorders

21

Uveodermatologic Syndrome in the Dog

John M. MacDonald

Diagnostic Criteria for the Uveodermatologic Syndrome

SUGGESTIVE
Signalment and history, uveitis and depigmentation

COMPATIBLE
Suggestive plus poliosis and nasal or oral ulcers

TENTATIVE
Compatible plus negative ANA, negative skin scrapings, negative fungal culture and mycotic titers, absence of infectious organisms in aqueous/vitreous fluid, with predominantly lymphocytes

DEFINITIVE
Tentative plus characteristic dermatohistopathology

Importance

The uveodermatologic syndrome is a unique systemic disorder of dogs characterized by both dermatologic abnormalities (hypopigmentation) and ocular manifestations (uveitis). It is somewhat similar to the human condition known as Vogt-Koyanagi-Harada syndrome (VKH). Although it has been recognized in veterinary medicine since 1977 (Asakura et al., 1977), there have been only sporadic reports of it since then.

The disease is not a common problem, but it has clinical relevancy due to its ocular component, which may ultimately lead to irreversible blindness. If early treatment is instituted, the disease is controllable. Although its cutaneous manifestations are less significant than its ocular component, early treatment may be effective in controlling their progression. The depigmenting changes are usually the indicator for a complete ophthalmic evaluation, despite the fact that the ophthalmic problem is most often the presenting complaint. The name **uveodermatologic syndrome** has been accepted as a descriptive term for the condition in dogs (Boldy et al., 1989).

There are similarities between this disease in dogs and VKH in humans, but there are also major differences. VKH in humans is associated with a uveomeningeal problem. The early phase is a meningoencephalitis characterized by fever, malaise, headache, nausea, and vomiting. This is usually followed by the ophthalmic phase, which includes a uveitis. Finally, there is a convalescent stage in which ocular manifestations may subside but poliosis (graying), hair loss, and leukoderma remain.

The uveodermatologic syndrome in dogs rarely presents with meningoencephalitis, and a convalescent stage is not seen. Ocular and cutaneous changes are usually encountered together. The cutaneous signs, characterized by depigmentation (vitiligo) and poliosis, are similar to those in humans. However, in dogs poliosis often progresses to leukotrichia (whitening of hair). Although the depigmentation is often present during development of the uveitis, ocular disease may precede any noticeable cutaneous changes. Intraocular depigmentation is more common in dogs than in humans (Boldy et al., 1989). Lesions not typically seen in humans but present in dogs include oral mucous membrane ulceration, erosions, and ulcers of the planum nasale.

Pathogenesis

The pathomechanism in humans has received a number of causal theories—viral, fungal, and autoimmune. The primary inflammatory reaction seems attributable to a cellular response to melanocyte cell surface receptor and melanin (Okubo et al., 1985). The resulting lesion is a granulomatous lymphocyte-induced reaction against melanin and melanocytes affecting organs that contain melanocytes (Maezawa et al., 1982). The initiating cause of the cellular response is not known although loss of immunological tolerance to melanocytes has been postulated. There has been no confirmation of pathomechanism documented in the dog.

CLINICAL DISEASE
History

The history in most cases begins with the owner's observing ophthalmic changes. Corneal edema, blepharospasm, conjunctivitis, and serous ocular discharge may be noticed. Some cases will already have progressed to impaired vision or blindness before veterinary attention is sought, and this may constitute the major part of the history. Depigmentation may be subtle but noted concurrently with ocular changes by an owner who is unusually watchful. Symptomatic therapy, including ophthalmic medication, sometimes will have but limited effect on the disease unless glucocorticoids in effective concentrations or systemically administered are part of the regimen. Cutaneous changes are usually gradual and ultimately include graying of the coat. Historical questions should be directed toward both the ophthalmic and the dermatologic problem.

There does not seem to be any geographic predilection for the uveodermatologic syndrome. The age of onset in dogs is most often 6 months to 6 years (Boldy et al., 1989). Breeds usually affected are Akitas, Samoyeds, and Siberian Huskies. The disease has also been recognized in Australian Shepherds, Old English Sheepdogs, German Shepherd Dogs, Standard Poodles, Shetland Sheepdogs, Basenjis, Golden Retrievers, Chow Chows, St. Bernards, Irish Setters, Dachshunds, and mixed breeds (Muller et al., 1989).

Physical Examination

The hallmark of uveodermatologic syndrome is bilateral anterior uveitis with cutaneous depigmentation (Fig. 21-1). However, the ocular disease (including anterior segment signs such as blepharospasm, conjunctival inflammation, corneal edema, serous discharge, aqueous flare, iris swelling, and miosis) usually precedes noticeable cutaneous changes. Retinal hemorrhage or degeneration may be observed, in addition to an exudative retinal detachment with pigmentary mottling. Optic disc hyperemia and hemorrhage are also at times present. Secondary ocular disease will include glaucoma and cataracts (Romatowski, 1985). Unless effective therapy for the eyes has been used, significant ocular changes usually occur by the time cutaneous lesions are observed (Fig. 21-2). In these instances the eyes may appear relatively nor-

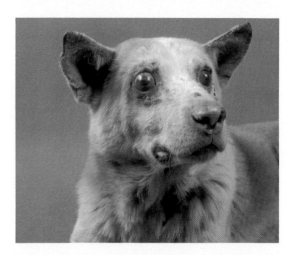

Figure 21-1. An adult Akita showing cutaneous signs of nasal depigmentation and poliosis with anterior uveitis characterized by corneal edema, miotic pupils, and iritis. The dog was blind at the time of examination.

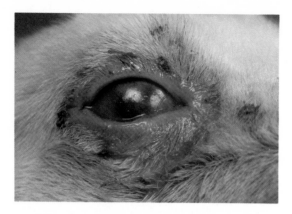

Figure 21-2. A closer view of the Akita in Fig. 21-1 showing periocular depigmentation, poliosis of the coat, and ocular changes.

mal and the cutaneous signs prominent. The disease is usually progressive for both ocular and cutaneous changes if no treatment has been used.

The dermatologic changes include depigmentation and whitening of the hair (poliosis), which first affect the nares and facial area respectively. Early changes are observed on the planum nasale and mucocutaneous junctions of the mouth and lids (Figs. 21-3 and 21-4). Alopecia may be noticed on the muzzle, particularly in the dorsonasal region. Oral and nasal erosions or ulcers can occur in chronic untreated cases (Figs. 21-5 and 21-6). Crusted lesions will sometimes develop at the cutaneous junction of the planum nasale and areas of alopecia. Poliosis is usually seen later on in the disease development. Footpad hyperkeratosis with detachment may be seen but is much less common

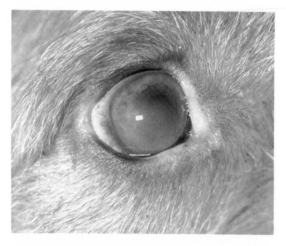

Figure 21-3. Early presentation of the uveodermatologic syndrome in a young dog. Note the depigmentation of the lid margins and the corneal edema secondary to anterior uveitis.

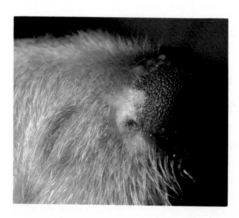

Figure 21-4. Same dog as in Fig. 21-3 with early depigmentation of the nose (at the junction with the skin).

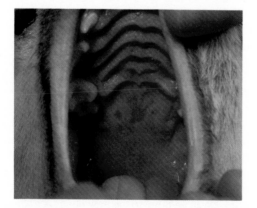

Figure 21-5. Oral cavity of the Akita in Fig. 21-1, showing ulceration of the soft palate mucosa.

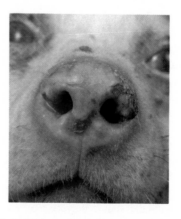

Figure 21-6. Ulcerated and depigmented nares of the Akita in Fig. 21-1.

than other features (Fig. 21-7). Evidence of secondary infections is usually not observed.

Neurologic signs have not been as well documented in dogs as ocular and cutaneous changes have. There rarely is any evidence of meningoencephalitis, and a convulsant stage is not seen. In humans dysacusis (hearing deficit) has been observed, as well as head and neck pain, but this symptom would be difficult to determine routinely in most dogs. Abnormal neurologic signs have been reported in a dog showing changed temperament in addition to a head tilt. The cerebrospinal fluid did not demonstrate pathologic findings and, likewise, examination of central nervous system tissue at necropsy did not show characteristic lesions.

Differential Diagnosis

The differential diagnosis of uveodermatologic syndrome includes autoimmune dermatoses, in particular the pemphigus complex and lupus erythematosus. Idiopathic vitiligo, neoplastic disease (epitheliotropic lymphoma), and deep mycoses (blastomycoses) are also considerations.

The uveodepigmentation syndrome is most often confused with autoimmune dermatopathies, although when cutaneous and eye disease occur together it is most likely the uveodermatologic syndrome. Other differentials more commonly causing combined depigmentation and ocular disease are mycotic infections (blastomycosis) and neoplastic disease (lymphoproliferative disorders). Idiopathic vitiligo would not be associated with ocular disease and would not demonstrate erosive or ulcerative lesions typical of uveodepigmentation unless complicated by photosensitivity.

DIAGNOSIS

The routine diagnostic data base from skin lesions should include skin scrapings and dermatophyte test medium (DTM) cultures. Crusts should be removed and an impression smear prepared from their undersurface. This should then be stained with a rapid laboratory stain and viewed under oil immersion for evidence of acantholytic cells. (See Fig. 13-6.)

Diagnostic laboratory tests should include a CBC and a panel of selected serum chemistries representative of major organ system function. A platelet count may be included if not routinely performed with the standard profile for the possible association of systemic lupus. Likewise, an ANA titer, a Coombs test, and a rheumatoid factor should

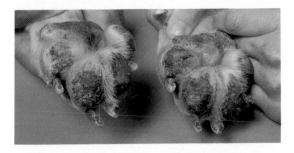

Figure 21-7. The foot pads of the Akita in Fig. 21-1 show evidence of erosion and ulcerations, with slight hyperkeratosis in some areas.

be obtained for the possible association of lupus. Positive ANA titers have been observed with the uveodermatologic syndrome (UDS) and are certainly not specific for lupus. Cytologic examination of aqueous or vitreous aspirates will frequently reveal lymphocytes with some PMNs (neutrophils). CSF cytologic examination has not contributed to the diagnosis in selected cases in which the procedure was done and is therefore not indicated unless neurologic signs are present.

Skin biopsies from affected areas are necessary for reaching a definitive diagnosis. The classical description includes an interface dermatitis (lichenoid infiltrate) consisting predominently of large histiocytic-type cells. Epidermal changes may also be observed, including hyperplasia and parakeratotic hyperkeratosis. Decreased numbers of epidermal melanocytes may be evident. Direct immunofluorescent testing is not very valuable in differentiating UDS from lupus, since both may be positive or negative for dermal junction staining.

Ocular abnormalities determined by histologic examination, either at necropsy or following enucleation, include a nonsuppurative keratitis with lymphocytic and proteinaceous material usually filling the anterior chamber. Retinal pathology may include degeneration and detachment. Various stages of optic nerve degeneration may also be seen. Uveal tracts are infiltrated with a heterogeneous population of mononuclear cells—histiocytes, macrophages, and plasmacytes. Loss of uveal melanocytes may be observed.

Case findings consistent with a diagnosis of uveodermatologic syndrome include history, signalment, the age of onset, and the combination of ocular manifestations with depigmentation. Compatible findings include ocular changes consistent with UDS in addition to the preceding. A definitive diagnosis requires compatible dermatohistopathologic changes in addition to the other described findings. The greatest concern prior to initiation of therapy is the rule-out of infectious diseases from bacterial, viral, or mycotic agents. Skin biopsies combined with cytology and culture of aqueous fluid are necessary. Serum titers from mycotic infections *(Blastomyces dermatitidis)* may be performed but provide only complementary data. Dogs with mycotic disease may not demonstrate positive titers. Likewise, noninfected dogs may have positive titers by exposure without contracting the disease. Titers, at best, help only to supplement other laboratory findings. An ophthalmic examination will often help differentiate infectious diseases from noninfectious inflammatory causes. Neoplasia, likewise, can be ruled out in most cases by dermatopathology and cytology of aqueous fluid. Epitheliotropic lymphoma (mycosis fungoides) may have some dermatohistopathological changes easily confused with UDS. In suspect cases an ophthalmic examination should be done early on to aid the diagnosis and provide a basis for proper therapy before irreversible pathology occurs.

TREATMENT

The prognosis for a dog with the uveodermatologic syndrome is variable depending on the progression of disease. When irreversible blindness has developed, euthanasia may be elected. The reversal of early ophthalmic disease provides a good outlook for control of the problem. Early recognition of clinical signs and the attainment of a tentative diagnosis for early initiation of therapy are primary objectives. Utilization of referral ophthalmologists is to be encouraged due to the complexity of the ocular pathology. The dermatologic diagnosis provides a convenient means of initiating treatment. Control of the depigmentation is a secondary priority. It is likely that the owner will accept persistent dermatologic manifestations, and thus eliminate the concern for aggressive systemic therapy (immunosuppressive treatment) in achieving cosmetic ends. Nevertheless, periodic reevaluation is paramount in the follow-up of these cases, primarily for adequate control of the ocular component.

Treatment is directed toward reducing or alleviating the inflammatory reaction. This requires glucocorticoids and possibly other immunosuppressive drugs. However, aggressive systemic immunosuppressive therapy for the achievement of cosmetic goals should be avoided. The risk factors of drugs must also be weighed against their benefits.

Both ocular and systemic therapies will be included in the typical case.

Ocular Therapy

The reader is advised to refer to other sources for more complete details concerning ophthalmic therapy. In general, ocular antiinflammatory drugs containing glucocorticoids are conventionally (and most effectively) used for the anterior uveitis. These include 0.1% dexamethasone and 0.1% prednisolone. In severe cases subconjunctival injections of a triamcinolone (0.1 ml of a 40 mg/ml suspension) may be used. If miosis or hyphema is present, pupillary dilation with topical 1% atropine or 10% phenylepherine is recommended. Intraocular pressures should be monitored, due to the possibility of secondary glaucoma. More specific ophthalmic therapy will be based on the particular ophthalmic abnormalities present. Referral to an ophthalmologist may be necessary.

Systemic Therapy

Systemic therapy should begin with prednisone orally at 2.2 mg/kg q24h for several weeks, followed by a gradual reduction over several months. This may be indicated in cases with severe ocular involvement but withheld in less severely affected animals. The regimen of glucocorticoids is comparable to that used for autoimmune dermatopathies. (See Chapter 13.) Azathioprine at 1.1 to 2.2 mg/kg q24h may be included if the response to ocular and systemic glucocorticoids is insufficient to stop progression of the disease. Any modification of systemic therapy should be specifically tailored to the individual animal.

If therapy is started early in the disease progression, cutaneous lesions may be reversible. In most cases treatment of the ophthalmic component without systemic antiinflammatories will not affect the progression of cutaneous signs. The management of cutaneous progression usually requires maintenance therapy with antiinflammatory agents. Prednisone and azathioprine are conventionally utilized. Although it is tempting to include azathioprine in most cases, a better course is to determine the glucocorticoid response before adding other immunosuppressants. The goal for prednisone therapy should be to attain a dosage of 0.5 to 1 mg/lb (2.2 mg/kg or less) administered q48h. Azathioprine should likewise be used q48h, administered on the alternate day from the prednisone. Monitoring CBCs and thrombocyte counts is necessary when azathioprine is used, and should be done at least three times a year. Control of the disease usually requires long-term therapy. Reevaluations are recommended for ocular examination every 6 months or sooner if clinical signs intensify, even though the cutaneous component is controlled.

REFERENCES

Asakura S, et al: Vogt-Koyanagi-Harada syndrome (uveitis diffusa acuta) in the dog, Jpn Vet Med 673:445, 1977.

Boldy KL, et al: Uveodermatologic syndrome in the dog: clinical characteristics and treatment of a disorder similar to human Vogt-Koyanagi-Harada syndrome, Vet Focus 1:112, 1989.

Maezawa N, et al: The role of cytotoxic T lymphocytes in the pathogenesis of Vogt-Koyanagi-Harada's disease. Ophthalmologica 185:179, 1982.

Muller GH, et al: Small animal dermatology, ed 4, Philadelphia, 1989, WB Saunders, p 542.

Okubo K, et al: Surface markers of peripheral blood lymphocytes in Vogt-Koyanagi-Harada disease. J Clin Lab Immunol 17:49, 1985.

Romatowski J: A uveodermatological syndrome in an Akita dog, J Am Anim Hosp Assoc 21:777, 1985.

SUPPLEMENTAL READING

Bussanich MN, et al: Granulomatous panuveitis and dermal depigmentation in dogs, J Am Anim Hosp Assoc 18:131, 1982.

22

Nasal Depigmentation

John M. MacDonald

Differential Diagnosis of Nasal Depigmentation

Autoimmune diseases
  Discoid lupus erythematosus
  Systemic lupus erythematosus
  Pemphigus foliaceus
  Pemphigus erythematosus
  Bullous pemphigoid
Vasculitis
Cold agglutinin disease
Allergic contact dermatitis
Drug reaction
Toxic epidermal necrolysis
Uveodermatologic syndrome
Neoplastic diseases
  Epitheliotropic lymphoma (mycosis fungoides)
  Pagetoid reticulosis
  Squamous cell carcinoma
Infectious diseases
  Mycotic
  Bacterial
Idiopathic vitiligo
Acquired idiopathic hypopigmentation
Actinic (sunburn)
Physical/chemical causes

Importance

Nasal depigmentation is a condition that affects pigmentary cells (melanocytes) or melanin production and is limited to the area of the planum nasale. It can be helpful in developing a list of differential diagnoses. However, since many diseases with nasal depigmentation have a similar appearance, with only subtle historical and clinical variations detectable among them, distinguishing the correct diagnosis may be difficult, albeit necessary for prognostic purposes and the establishment of optimal therapy.

The importance of nasal depigmentation is that it can arouse concern in the pet owner, particularly if it is erosive and changes the nasal architecture. There are many causes of nasal depigmentation; and, although many are glucocorticoid-responsive, a definitive diagnosis should be pursued before empirical therapy is initiated. There are some conditions that do not respond to glucocorticoids, others (infectious) in which glucocorticoids are contraindicated, and still others that have safer alternative forms of therapy.

Pathogenesis

Pathomechanisms include the specific destruction of melanocytes, postinflammatory lesions (interface dermatitis), enzyme abnormalities, and physical/chemical insults. Some diseases are primary genodermatoses, specifically affecting the melanocyte; others are the result of an autoimmune disease or a combination of autoimmune mediation with concurrent photointensification. The uveodermatologic syndrome results from a direct effect on the melanocyte whereas the more common causes of depigmentation are a result of inflammatory disease indirectly affecting the melanocytes. Such disease can occur from a number of specific factors and is usually associated with pathology at or near the basal cell layer of the epidermis (referred to as interface dermatitis). Its effect on the melanin system is merely coincidental with the histologic location of the inflammatory lesion. Noninfectious diseases producing an interface dermatitis that may result in depigmentation are epitheliotropic lymphoma (mycosis fungoides), discoid lupus erythematosus and pemphigus erythematosus. Allergic contact dermatitis often demonstrates nasal depigmentation early as a result of the inflammatory process. Atopic or food-allergic dogs may lose pigment through chronic nasal rubbing or inflammation. Chronic purulent nasal discharge from any cause can accumulate on the lower lateral aspect of the nose, forming crusts and ultimately causing local depigmentation.

Infectious diseases in the vicinity of the basal epidermal layer may also cause depigmentation. Some mycotic infections, especially blastomycosis, have been associated with nasal depigmentation. Rarely a bacterial facial disease (e.g., due to *Staphylococcus* spp) will have nasal depigmentation. Diseases affecting the nasal area can simultaneously involve other regions, including the eyes, oral cavity, skin, foot pads, and mucocutaneous junctions. Determining the progression of lesion evolvement in these areas may provide useful diagnostic clues.

CLINICAL FINDINGS
History

The historical account of most cases is a gradual progression from normally pigmented nares to depigmentation. However, acute depigmentation may be observed in some autoimmune diseases and contact allergies. When black areas turn blue-gray, it indicates pigment release into the dermis (pigmentary incontinence). This is most commonly observed with interface dermatitis. It is also helpful to determine whether the lesions have progressed from pigmented to white without any pink or redness being observed. Although most causes of nasal depigmentation are associated with inflammation, vitiligo and tyrosinase deficiency are not. The nose may be affected in some dogs, especially Australian Shepherds, that are initially born with de-

pigmented areas and then subjected to solar damage and that subsequently develop erosions, ulcers, crusts, or scars as a result. Occasionally the inflammation will then slowly involve adjacent pigmented areas. Determining the location of early lesions may be helpful in prioritizing the differentials. Lesions of autoimmune diseases often start near the junction of the nares and haired region and then progress to the nares proper. Contact irritant or allergy usually starts on the rostral nares and maxilla. Breed and age of onset may be helpful in diagnosing a particular case. Lupus would be more suspicious in a Collie over 1 year of age whereas dermatomyositis would be more likely in a 3-to-4-month Collie. A history of erosions, ulcers, or crust formation should be established.

Historical information about concurrent constitutional signs, including weakness, lethargy, inappetence and problems with ambulation, should be acquired. Diseases such as systemic lupus erythematosus may be accompanied by a stiff gait or intermittent lameness suggesting either arthritis or affected foot pads. Concurrent changes in coat color should be determined. Whitening or graying (leukotrichia or poliosisis) may be observed in the uveodermatologic syndrome (UDS), vitiligo, and metabolic disorders of melanin production (tyrosinase deficiency). Previous ocular problems should be determined since they may be associated with the UDS or systemic mycoses (blastomycosis).

Documenting specific drugs that the dog has received, including dosages and duration of therapy, should always be done. Response to therapy is sometimes helpful, although improper dosages and combined drug therapy often obscure the interpretation.

Physical Examination

The presenting clinical signs are variable depending on the stage and chronicity of the disease and previous therapeutic intervention. Complete nasal involvement may be observed in advanced cases. Focal or multifocal ulcerative lesions are sometimes present with crust formation. Cutaneous lesions in other areas are expected in some autoimmune conditions such as the pemphigus complex or systemic lupus erythematosus. (See Chapters 13 and 14.) Complete examination of all integument, mucocutaneous junctions, and pedal regions is essential. Clues obtained from distribution patterns and the appearance of the nasal region are often helpful in narrowing the differential diagnosis. Lupus erythematosus often has depigmentation and loss of nasal markings. Swelling, deformity, and depigmentation may be seen as early features of mycosis fungoides. By contrast, pemphigus foliaceus generally has crust formation preceding any loss of pigment or nasal markings. There is usually no crust formation or loss of nasal makings in idiopathic vitiligo. UDS may or may not have loss of nasal markings with the loss of pigment. Deformities, depressions, and scars are most common with inflammatory diseases.

Other helpful features may be observed. Hyperkeratotic foot pads are often associated with pemphigus foliaceus; and ulcerative, detached footpads can occur with pemphigus vulgaris, bullous pemphigoid, systemic lupus erythematosus, drug reactions, toxic epidermal necrolysis, and some cases of epitheliotropic lymphoma and UDS. There are no pathognomonic lesions, although there often are features that favor a specific disease or group of diseases.

DIAGNOSIS

The procedure of most diagnostic value is the skin biopsy. Although histopathology may not provide definitive confirmation of a specific condition, it is still important for disease rule-outs. Small, elliptical excisions of affected nasal tissue at or near the junction of haired skin are the easiest to acquire, although small punch specimens may be obtained from the center of the lesion. Tissues should be handled gently and submitted in 10% buffered formalin to a pathology laboratory that has expertise in dermatohistology. Tissue imprints should be collected routinely for cytologic examination prior to placing the biopsy specimens in formalin. Submission of specimens for direct immunofluorescent testing is not routinely done.

Due to the association of nasal depigmentation with autoimmune diseases and/or systemic problems, tests occasionally helpful in the etiologic diagnosis of nasal depigmentation are a CBC, serum chemistries, and urinalysis. Immunologic testing, including ANA titers, Coombs test, rheumatoid factor, and evaluation for cryoglobulinemia may also be done. Direct immunofluorescent testing of the skin and/or other organ systems can be included, although negative results do not exclude the possibility of autoimmune dermatoses. Most common causes of nasal depigmentation (vitiligo, mycosis fungoides, discoid lupus erythematosus, pemphigus foliaceus) are not diagnosed by ancillary blood testing.

Ruling out infectious cause[...] always performed, although e[...] ulcerative lesions affecting the [...] ing tissue should evoke concer[...] cobacterial disease. Tissue sho[...] ted in Stuart's transport medium[...] culture. Examination of tissue [...] is ideal for both infectious and [...] processes. Acquiring antimyc[...] may be helpful, although not c[...] ologic diagnosis. Demonstratio[...] tissues is diagnostic, but may b[...] the rare cases that have an infe[...]

AUTOIMMUNE DISEASE[...]

Autoimmune diseases accou[...] ber of cases of depigmenting nas[...] diseases include both systemic and discoid lupus erythematosus, the pemphigus complex, and bullous pemphigoid.

Discoid Lupus Erythematosus

Perhaps one of the more common causes of restricted nasal depigmentation is discoid lupus erythematosus (DLE). Discoid lupus usually occurs in Collies and German Shepherd Dogs and breeds related to them. Lesions are limited to the integument, without systemic manifestations, and usually consist of erythema with depigmentation and secondary areas of scaling, erosions, ulcers, crusts, and hair loss. The planum nasale, nares, and bridge of the nose are most commonly involved, although areas around the lips, eyes, ears, and oral cavity

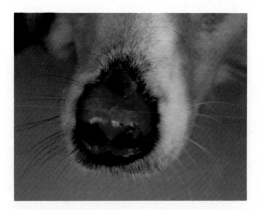

Figure 22-1. Discoid lupus erythematosus in a dog, demonstrating lesions restricted to the nasal area. There is a loss of pigment with erythema. Early erosive lesions are developing, with the loss of nasal markings.

may be affected. Many cases of discoid lupus have lesions restricted to the nares, with depigmentation the most prominent feature (Fig. 22-1). The reader is referred to Chapter 14 for more specific details.

Pemphigus Foliaceus and Pemphigus Erythematosus

Clinical Findings

Pemphigus foliaceus usually affects the facial area of dogs and is characterized by a crusting dermatopathy. Nasal depigmentation may be observed but usually follows crusting (Fig. 22-2). The reader is referred to Chapter 13 for a more detailed discussion of disease presentation, diagnosis, and therapy.

Pemphigus erythematosus has the same general pathomechanism as pemphigus foliaceus. Nasal involvement with depigmentation is commonly observed. Nasal lesions can appear similar to those of DLE, and, additionally, these cases often have crusting lesions elsewhere on the face, suggesting pemphigus foliaceus. Although there is no age, breed, or sex predilection, Collies may be predisposed. Erosions, ulcers, and crusts are usually present, particularly if there is exposure to sunlight (which intensifies the lesions). Lesions affecting the face and ears are comparable to those of pemphigus foliaceus.

Diagnosis and Treatment

Findings from direct smears and skin biopsies are comparable to those for pemphigus foliaceus and may include some of the changes seen in discoid lupus erythematosus. Immunofluorescent testing of the skin may reveal evidence of immuno-globulins with or without complement at the basement membrane zone in addition to a diffuse intercellular pattern in the epidermis. Dogs with pemphigus erythematosus often have positive ANA titers. Treatment is similar to that utilized for lupus erythematosus and pemphigus foliaceus, and the reader is referred to Chapters 13 and 14 for a more detailed discussion.

Bullous Pemphigoid

Clinical Findings

Bullous pemphigoid is an autoimmune disease observed far less commonly that discoid lupus erythematosus and the pemphigus complex. Doberman Pinschers and Collies appear to have a higher predilection. The pathomechanism is the formation of antibody against antigen at the basement membrane zone of the skin and mucosa. Although the initiation of an immune response is idiopathic, drug provocation may be involved.

Bullous pemphigoid rarely causes nasal depigmentation as the only observable lesion. True vesicles may be observed transiently in the skin, but more commonly erosions and ulcers are present. The inguinal and axillary areas are predilection sites, in addition to the face, muzzle, and oral cavity. Foot pad ulcerations and detachment may also be observed. Severely affected dogs sometimes show signs of depression, inappetence, and pyrexia.

Diagnosis and Treatment

Bullous pemphigoid is characterized histologically by subepidermal vesical formation (clefts) with a normal to acanthotic epidermis. There is no acantholysis. Inflammatory features of the dermis are variable, from a mild superficial perivascular infiltrate to a marked lichenoid pattern, and may include neutrophils with mononuclear cells. Biopsies have the most diagnostic value. In contrast to pemphigus, impression smears of bullous pemphigoid (vesicular contents or the ulcer surface of ruptured blisters) do not reveal acantholytic cells.

The preferred initial therapy is combined immunosuppressive agents. Glucocorticoids are rarely effective at levels that the dog can tolerate but may be tried when the client does not wish to utilize more expensive and labor-intensive combination regimens. Drugs that may be useful include azathioprine (Imuran) 2.2 mg/kg or chlorambucil (Leukeran) 0.1 mg/kg q24h for induction and then q48h for maintenance. Other options are dapsone 1 mg/kg q8h through remission and as

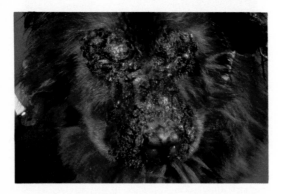

Figure 22-2. Pemphigus foliaceus in this adult Chow Chow has caused a loss of pigment in the nasal region. Note the erythema and erosive changes.

needed. More details of immunosuppressive therapy are to be found in Chapters 13 and 14.

ALLERGIC DISEASES
Allergic Contact Dermatitis

Allergic contact dermatitis is uncommon today compared to a decade ago. The classical condition was an allergy to plastic dishes, but in recent years this has become quite rare. Although other contactants can produce disease, it may be difficult to differentiate a true allergic reaction from irritancy. Exposure to petroleum distillates can cause contact lesions. Dogs kept in and around garages or chemical sources are more at risk. The classical pathomechansim of contact allergy is a delayed-type hypersensitivity involving sensitized lymphocytes. Current thoughts are that an immediate hypersensitivity reaction is involved as well.

Clinical Findings

Allergic contact dermatitis causing nasal depigmentation should have coexistent lesions affecting the skin on the rostral muzzle and tip of the mandible, unless the contactant is a medication applied directly to the nose. Variable itchiness may be observed. Early depigmentation can occur without erosions, ulcers, or crusts (Fig. 22-3). Lesions will typically begin on the end of the nose rather than the dorsal aspect near the haired area. Progression may be rapid in some cases, with subsequent erythema and erosive changes.

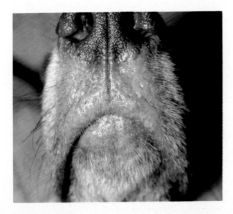

Figure 22-3. Allergic contact dermatitis developed from lying against a plastic dish. Note the inflammatory response affecting the rostral portion of the mandible, with early depigmentation of the nares. The depigmentation begins at the junction of the skin and nasal mucosa.

Diagnosis and Treatment

The diagnosis of allergic contact dermatitis is ususaly based on history and physical examination findings as well as response to avoidance. Removal of suspected sources of allergen is advised when practical, or the pet may be confined to exclude exposure. Challenge testing is necessary to confirm suspect items but is not always performed because of owner reluctance to risk recurrence of the lesion. Although commercial standardized patch test kits are available (Olivry et al., 1990), limited experience with and availability of patch testing appropriate for small animals make them impractical for routine use. Assuming the offensive agent can be recognized and eliminated, the treatment of choice is avoidance.

Atopy

Canine atopy does not cause direct pathology of the nasal area, but in some cases intense facial and muzzle pruritus will actually induce nasal lesions from aggressive nose rubbing. Although this is an uncommon association with nasal depigmentation, it may merit some consideration in selected cases with consistent clinical signs of atopy. (See Chapter 10.)

DRUG ERUPTIONS

Ulcerative lesions on the planum nasale with hypopigmentation are commonly observed in cases of drug eruptions. Cutaneous lesions with a variety of distributions patterns are usually observed in combination with nasal depigmentation. More complete details of drug eruptions, including diagnosis and treatment, are to be found in Chapter 15.

UVEODERMATOLOGIC SYNDROME

The uveodermatologic syndrome (UDS) is characterized by depigmentation or hypopigmentation and almost always includes the planum nasale. It is recognized most commonly in the Akita, Samoyed, and Siberian Husky, although other breeds have been reported. The reader is referred to Chapter 21 for more detail regarding the disease characteristics and diagnosis.

VASCULITIS

Vasculitis is an uncommon disease that may cause nasal lesions including depigmentation.

There is frequently ulceration with necrotizing lesions affecting the skin in other areas. The pathomechanism of most cutaneous vasculitides is thought to include an immune complex (Type III) hypersensitivity reaction, although a Type I (immediate) reaction may also be important, particularly during initiation of the disease. Etiologic factors include drugs, chemicals, vaccinations, hyposensitization therapy, infections (bacterial, viral, mycotic, *Ehrlichia, Rickettsia*), parasitic (*Dirofilaria immitis*), neoplasia, or coexistent diseases such as systemic lupus erythematosus. Vasculitis is often categorized by the histology (neutrophilic, lymphocytic, granulomatous, or mixed).

Physical Examination

Cutaneous lesions caused by vasculitis include erythema, discoloration, and palpable purpura. Annular lesions with sharply demarcated borders are typical. Early lesions may appear as a hemorrhagic bullae that progress to ulcerative lesions. Lesions that are cut or traumatized often bleed poorly as a result of the impaired vasculature. Wedge-shaped areas of necrosis on ear margins may be observed. The tail may also demonstrate swelling, erythema and ulceration. Oral mucosal or lingual ulcers are frequently present. Foot pads may show detachment, erosions, or ulcers. Nasal lesions in combination with foot pad, pinnal, or oral lesions should arouse suspicion of vasculitis and the potential of multietiologic factors.

Diagnosis and Treatment

Diagnostic confirmation requires histologic examination of skin biopsies. The diagnosis is not easily made in chronic cases and depends to quite an extent on the stage of the lesion at the time of biopsy acquisition. Early lesions within 24 hours of development are the most diagnostic. Histopathology may show a variation of lesions compatible with vasculitis. In some cases these changes will suggest an underlying etiology. Chronic lesions may show only remnants of vessels with minimal evidence of active inflammation.

Once a diagnosis of vasculitis has been determined, a search for an underlying etiology should be pursued. Evaluation for systemic disease should always include a CBC, serum chemistries, and urinalysis. Evidence of infectious disease should be pursued with representative cultures (blood, urine, skin, etc.). Serologic testing for parasitic and infectious diseases (e.g., *Dirofilaria immitis, Rick-*ettsia rickettsii* [Rocky Mountain spotted fever], *Ehrlichia*) should be considered in high-risk areas or in animals that have traveled in those areas. Immunodiagnostics may include ANA titer, Coombs test, and cold agglutinin tests.

Empirical treatment with glucocorticoids should be avoided until a complete workup has been attained for underlying disease. Infectious processes may be compounded by the antiinflammatory effect of glucocorticoids. Trial therapy with antibiotics is usually the first treatment utilized while awaiting results of tests to determine the primary cause. Treatment of the underlying problem is the first priority of clinical management. Immune mediated diseases with concurrent vasculitis may be responsive to prednisone or prednisolone 2 to 3 mg/kg q24h. Avlosulfon (dapsone) 1 mg/kg q8h or sulfasalazine 20 to 40 mg q8h has been used when no underlying etiology is identified.

COLD AGGLUTININ DISEASE
Physical Examination

Cold agglutinin disease is a rare immune mediated disorder in which animals develop a specific immunoglobulin (IgM class) that reacts with red blood cells at temperatures below 32° C. The condition is restricted to colder climates. Although most cases have no specific etiology, the disease has been associated with both infectious and neoplastic conditions. Review of history and organ system involvement is necessary in determining the possible role of coexisting or underlying problems. The distribution of lesions involves areas where tissue temperature may reach that of erythrocyte reactivity such as extremities (tail, ears, digits, and nares). The typical lesions are areas of focal erythema with necrosis and ulceration. Presence of hemoglobinuria may be suggestive of cold agglutinin disease.

Diagnosis and Treatment

The diagnosis is attained by confirmation of a positive Coombs test at 4° C. Skin biopsies reveal necrosis and ulceration with secondary features of opportunistic infection. Biopsies may demonstrate vascular thrombosis.

Immunosuppressive doses of glucocorticoids conventionally have been the treatment of choice, although avoidance of cold is helpful in diminishing clinical signs.

LYMPHOPROLIFERATIVE DISORDERS

Physical Examination

Neoplastic diseases associated with nasal depigmentation are usually lymphoproliferative disorders. The condition referred to as epitheliotropic lymphoma, which resembles mycosis fungoides in humans, has frequently been associated with depigmentation of the planum nasale. It usually occurs in older dogs, and early lesions often include nasal depigmentation (Fig. 22-4). Pruritus may be present and potentiated by dry scaling skin (xeroderma). Other cutaneous lesions observed are erythema (diffuse or macular), plaques, ulcers, scales, and crusts. Mucocutaneous junctions often have ulcers and crusts comparable to those in some autoimmune diseases. Ulcerative stomatitis may also be present. The disease slowly progresses unless treatment is given but is not life-threatening in its early stage (which may last for years). Invasion of vital organ systems occurs much later in the disease and this is eventually fatal.

Pagetoid reticulosis is an epitheliotropic lymphoproliferative disease that may be a variant of mycosis fungoides, although the exact relationship is not well-understood. Clinical signs may be comparable to those of mycosis fungoides (in which erythroderma and scale are the most prevalent lesions). Predilection for distal extremities may be found. However, lesions are expected in other areas besides the nasal region and often affect the foot pads, oral mucosa, and mucocutaneous junction.

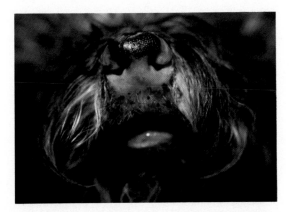

Figure 22-4. Epidermotrophic lymphoma resembling mycosis fungoides frequently results in nasal depigmentation. Coexisting cutaneous lesions were present in this case.

Diagnosis and Treatment

A tentative diagnosis may be made by cytologic examination of tissue imprints, but confirmed diagnosis requires dermatohistopathology. The distinction between mycosis fungoides and pagetoid reticulosis is frequently made on the basis of histologic variability. In pagetoid reticulosis the most prominent difference is sparing of the subepidermal area. The pathology is usually limited to intraepidermal invasion. The cell type is also somewhat different due to its monomorphic appearance, in contrast to that of the mycosis fungoides cells, which usually have a more polymorphic appearance. Diagnosis of this disease is comparable to that of mycosis fungoides, requiring both histologic and cytologic examination. Evaluation of a complete blood cell count and peripheral smear for evidence of circulating mycosis cells is necessary. Diagnostic overview of organ system function is, likewise, essential due to the possibility of parenchymal invasion later in the disease.

Alternative forms of therapy are available, although the prognosis is guarded. The initial therapy currently used for early cases of epitheliotropic lymphoma is retinoid therapy. Variable success has been reported, with the expectation of improving the condition and quality of life but not achieving a clinical cure. Isotretinoin (Accutane) has been evaluated, with some success at a dosage of 1 mg/kg q24h but improved results at 3 mg/kg q24h. Side effects of isotretinoin include cheilitis, blepharitis, and (with long-term therapy) anorexia and lethargy. Power and Ihrke (1990) have used etretinate (Tegison) in several cases, with equivocal results, at a dosage of 0.75 to 1 mg/kg q24h. Side effects included transient pruritus, vomiting, conjunctivitis, joint stiffness, and reluctance to chew. Because of cost and the potential for side effects, treatment with retinoids should be limited to cases that have a confirmed diagnosis. A complete review of product use is advised before implementing treatment. (See Chapter 19.)

Chemotherapeutic agents, either topical (mechlorethamine hydrochloride) or systemic, have been utilized with a combination of drugs. Mechlorethamine (Mustargen) is applied topically as an aqueous solution or an ointment base. The solution is prepared by combining 10 mg of mechlorethamine with 50 ml of tap water. The ointment is prepared by mixing 90 mg of mechlorethamine with 10 ml of absolute alcohol and further combining enough xipamide (Aquaphor) to prepare 900 g of ointment (Price et al., 1983). Removal

Table 22-1. Chemotherapy protocol for canine lymphosarcoma

Drug	Dosage
Vincristine	0.5 mg/m² IV once weekly on first day of each treatment week for 8 weeks
Cytosine arabinoside	100 mg/m² IV or SQ on first 4 days of *first treatment week only*
Cyclophosphamide	50 mg/m² PO in morning on first 4 days of each treatment week for 8 weeks
Prednisone or prednisolone	40 mg/m² PO daily for first week, then 20 mg/m² PO every other day for 7 weeks

Based on Brewer W (1991).

Table 22-2. Initiation of maintenance therapy* for the treatment of canine lymphosarcoma

Drug	Dosage
Vincristine	0.5 mg/m² IV every other week
Cyclophosphamide	50 mg/m² PO days 1-4 of each week that vincristine is given
Prednisone or prednisolone	20 mg/m² PO every other day

*Initiated at the end of induction therapy and continued for 16 weeks.
Based on Brewer W (1991).

Table 22-3. Long-term maintenance therapy* for the treatment of canine lymphosarcoma in remission

Drug	Dosage
Vincristine	0.5 mg/m² IV every third week
Cyclophosphamide	50 mg/m² PO for days 1 through 4 of each week that vincristine is given
Prednisone or prednisolone	20 mg/m² PO every other day

*Initiated at the end of the first maintenance regimen and continued for 24 weeks. Chemotherapy is discontinued in all animals still in remission at the end of this regimen.
Based on Brewer W (1991).

of existing hair is necessary before commencing topical therapy. The material is applied once daily or every other day. Application must be done with gloves and maximum protection since mechlorethamine is carcinogenic and can induce contact hypersensitivity in people. Disposal of the drug is also a major concern because of the biohazard and should be done in accordance with regulations. Response to this therapy is variable and often only palliative.

Systemic chemotherapy is not as efficacious against epitheliotropic lymphoma (T cell) as it is against B cell lymphoma. A chemotherapeutic protocol (Brewer, 1991) combining vincristine, cytosine arabinoside, cyclophosphamide, and prednisone may be used for the treatment of canine lymphosarcoma (Table 22-1). A CBC should be done weekly at the time of the vincristine injection. The cyclophosphamide is discontinued if the neutrophil count falls below 2500 to 3000 cells/μl and is resumed at 75% of the original dose when the count rises above 3000 cells/μl. CBCs may be discontinued if the neutrophil count remains above 2500 to 3000 for 3 consecutive weeks. The dog's temperature should be monitored daily by the owner for at least the first 3 weeks of therapy and reported to the clinician if it exceeds 39.7° C. Complete evaluation of major organ systems will then be necessary to determine possible infections or other complications.

At the end of the initial 8-week induction period maintenance therapy is started for all dogs in complete remission (Table 22-2). This is continued for 16 weeks, and at the end of the 16-week period all animals in complete remission are started on long-term maintenance (Table 22-3). A CBC should be done every 2 to 4 weeks during maintenance, following the same guidelines as with the induction therapy. Any animal still in remission at the end of the second maintenance period is taken off chemotherapy. Any animal relapsing during maintenance or while off chemotherapy is placed again on the induction therapy. Any animal that relapses on, or does not respond to, the induction therapy is started on doxorubicin 30 mg/m² IV q3wk. Premedication consists of dexamethasone 0.1 mg/kg SQ and an antiemetic (e.g., prochlorperazine or metaclopramide) given subcutaneously 20 minutes prior to the doxorubicin. The doxorubicin is diluted to 0.5 mg/ml in sterile physiologic saline and administered via an indwelling intravenous catheter over a 15-minute period. The rate of infusion should be slowed if pruritus or urticaria is observed. The infusion is stopped and fluid therapy initiated with lactated Ringer's if more severe reactions (e.g., hypotension or collapse) occur. Doxorubicin is usually limited to a cumulative dose of 240 mg/m² (eight treatments) due to cardiotoxicity.

INFECTIOUS CAUSES OF NASAL DEPIGMENTATION

Deep mycoses (in particular, *Blastomyces dermatitidis*) are the most common cause of nasal depigmentation from an infectious agent. The lesions often result in craterlike ulcers and are not necessarily restricted to the planum nasale (Fig. 22-5). Frequently they will extend to other areas of the body. This disease should be more suspect in animals living where deep mycoses are more prevalent. Early lesions may be papules, ultimately ending in a nodule with surface erosion. Coexistent diseases such as staphylococcal pyoderma or demodicosis have been observed coincidentally with the mycotic disease.

Diagnostic testing should include skin scrapings and fungal culture, in addition to histologic examination of biopsy specimens. The use of macerated tissue specimens for fungal and bacterial culture will help assure more reliable results. Organisms are not always demonstrable by India ink preparation or on tissue examination. Laboratories should be alerted for differentials that include deep mycoses when performing fungal cultures. The use

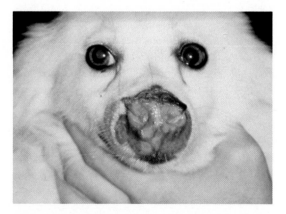

Figure 22-5. Cutaneous blastomycosis has caused extreme disfigurement and nasal depigmentation with erythema in this Samoyed. Note the punctate ulcers typical of blastomycosis.

of serologic testing for antibody production may be helpful, but negative results do not exclude a fungal disease.

Sporotrichosis has, likewise, been affiliated with nasal lesions that affect the muzzle in addition to the nares proper. Zoonotic transmission to veterinarians and technicians has been reported. Therefore protective gloving should always be worn. (See Chapter 5.)

Treatment of intermediate or deep mycoses may include the use of imidazoles (ketoconazole) and/or amphotericin B.

VITILIGO
Clinical Findings

Vitiligo is a genodermatosis affecting the production of melanin in skin and hair. It results in hypopigmentation, typically on the planum nasale and the lips and eyelids of affected dogs. In the United States, canine idiopathic vitiligo is most commonly observed in Rottweilers and Doberman Pinschers, although it has also been recognized in Newfoundlands, Belgian Sheepdogs, German Shepherd Dogs, and Collies as well as in a Belgian Tervuren and a Bull Mastiff.

The disease is characterized by the gradual development of depigmentation. Lesions usually appear before the age of 3 years and are noninflammatory. In contrast to DLE and other inflammatory diseases, nasal markings are unaffected. Leukotrichia or poliosis, either focal or regional, may be observed (Fig. 22-6). Unlike the association of poliosis with hypopigmentation in the uveodermatologic syndrome, there is no ocular counterpart in vitiligo. Periocular involvement may be observed with depigmentation of the eyelids. Foot pads and nails may depigment. The lesions observed do not include erosions or ulcers as seen with other inflammatory disease processes. The secondary development of solar aggravated lesions may result, thereby producing more destructive lesions. Most cases have permanent depigmentation, although some have been observed to spontaneously repigment.

Diagnosis and Treatment

The diagnosis is best determined by histologic examination, which characteristically shows absence of melanocytes with minimal or no evidence of inflammatory disease. A mild perivascular dermatitis, if present, is the most common inflam-

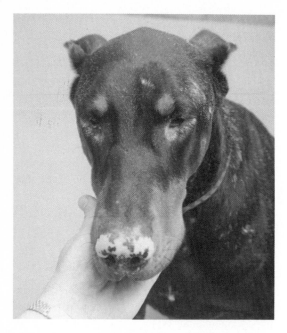

Figure 22-6. Idiopathic vitiligo in a Doberman Pinscher. Note the lack of erythema in depigmented areas and the preservation of nasal markings without erosive lesions. Leukotrichosis is also demonstrated on the head and over the shoulders.

(Courtesy, Dr. D.W. Angarano, Auburn, Ala.)

matory reaction and is primarily mononuclear. All other skin structures are essentially normal. The diagnosis of idiopathic vitiligo is strongly suggested when a gradual loss of pigment of the nares is observed in either a Doberman Pinscher or a Rottweiler prior to 3 years of age. The change is from dark pigment to white without significant erythema. However, secondary solar damage may produce inflammatory signs later in the disease progression. Rule-out of other diseases is necessary. No treatment is helpful, short of tattooing or the application of black marker.

TYROSINASE DEFICIENCY IN CHOW CHOWS

A variant of metabolic disease comparable to idiopathic vitiligo has been observed in Chow Chows that were normal at birth but developed hypopigmentation affecting the nares and tongue as well as leukotrichia. The mechanism involves a deficiency in tyrosinase, which prevents the formation of melanin. Histologic examination shows melanocytes without melanin. There is no evidence of inflammatory disease. Treatment of the condi-

tion is limited (since the metabolic defect is not amenable to therapy). Idiopathic causes of the hypopigmentation are treated with black marking pens or tattooing of affected areas. High–protective factor sunscreens may be used to prevent secondary solar damage. As with other causes of nasal depigmentation, the greatest concern is for cosmesis.

ACTINIC NASAL DEPIGMENTATION

Actinic or solar induced lesions of a primary cause are uncommon in dogs and cats, although many other diseases result in photointensification. The use of photosensitization is less common today due to the recognition of underlying disease processes. The "collie nose" so commonly assessed some years back is now recognized as an immune mediated problem with photointensification. The reader is referred to Chapter 30 for more complete discussions of photodermatitis.

ACQUIRED IDIOPATHIC HYPOPIGMENTATION

Idiopathic causes of nasal depigmentation have been reported to affect specific breeds, including Golden Retrievers, German Shepherd Dogs, Poodles, Siberian Huskies, and Samoyeds. These dogs are usually born with a pigmented nasal planum and gradually lose pigmentation throughout their life. Rarely the end point is complete depigmentation with pink coloration of the nares. The majority only hypopigment, which fortunately still provides photoprotection. The rostral nasal planum is most commonly affected. Some of these cases have recognized cyclic changes, which suggests the lack of melanocyte destruction but may result from disturbances of metabolic processes. There is little means of confirming this disease process, although histologic examination and complete workup may rule out other differentials. Treatment restrictions are much like those of other idiopathic causes without any inflammatory component.

PHYSICAL/CHEMICAL HYPOMELANOSIS

Both physical and chemical causes may result in depigmented lesions that affect the nasal area. Ultraviolet light, burns, mechanical injuries, and radiation can cause a leukoderma or leukotrichia by destruction of melanocytes. This effect usually has a known historical finding. Results may be permanent, with only artificial repigmentation procedures (tatoos or ink markers) available for treatment.

Chemical hypomelanosis can be caused by a number of contactant agents that may have antioxidant activity. Some causes include dihydroquininone and monobenzyl ether. Other reactions to corticosteroids or progestational compounds injected subcutaneously have been reported. Mechanisms associated with chemical hypomelanosis include production of free radicals that can destroy melanocytes or compete with the tyrosinase necessary for the formation of melanin. These problems are relatively rare, representing concern only in high-exposure situations. Historical information should provide a basis for suggested diagnoses. Variability of histologic findings is possible depending on the stage of disease at the time of biopsy.

SUMMARY

There is no general treatment for nasal depigmentation, short of preventing photoaggravation by restricting exposure to direct sunlight and the application of high SPF sunscreens. The exact diagnosis is the prerequisite to successful management, requiring the diagnostic procedures previously outlined. Glucocorticoid therapy provides the basis for many of the immune mediated problems, but should not be selected empirically in response to observed nasal lesions. Recognition of patterns affecting other cutaneous regions is certainly helpful, thereby providing suggestions for specific diagnostic pursuit. The reader is advised to refer to other sections covering specific diseases for more comprehensive information regarding therapeutic options.

REFERENCES

Brewer W: Personal communication, 1991.

Olivry T, et al: Allergic contact dermatitis in the dog-principles and diagnosis, Vet Clin North Am 20:1443, 1990.

Power HT, Ihrke PJ: Synthetic retinoids in veterinary dermatology, Vet Clin North Am 20:1525, 1990.

Price NM, et al: Ointment-based mechlorethamine treatment for mycosis fungoides, Cancer 52:2214, 1983.

SUPPLEMENTAL READING

Angarano DW: Dermatoses of the nose and the footpads in dogs and cats. In Kirk RW (ed): Current veterinary therapy X, Philadelphia, 1989, WB Saunders, p 616.

Griffin CE: Differential diagnosis of nasal diseases. In Kirk RW (ed): Current veterinary therapy VIII, Philadelphia, 1983, WB Saunders, p 480.

Guaguere E, Alhaidari Z: Disorders of melanin pigmentation in the skin of dogs and cats. In Kirk RW (ed): Current veterinary therapy X, Philadelphia, 1989, WB Saunders, p 628.

Kwochka K: Retinoids in dermatology. In Kirk RW (ed): Current veterinary therapy X, Philadelphia, 1989, WB Saunders, p 553.

23

Hyperpigmentation

John M. MacDonald

Differential Diagnosis of Hyperpigmentation

Genetic hypermelanoses
  Lentigenes
  Nevi
Metabolic or nutritional
Postinflammatory hypermelanosis
Hypermelanosis associated with ectoparasitism
Endocrine melanosis
Tumor melanosis
Miscellaneous hypermelanoses
  Acanthosis nigricans
  Acral melanism

Importance

Hyperpigmentation is a common observation associated with a variety of dermatologic problems in pets. The clinical relevancy of this problem is usually a concern of the owner regarding appearance (cosmetic concerns), or the possibility of neoplastic disease. Since appearance is one of the primary reasons for particular breed selection, concern for increased pigmentation may be inflated in contrast to clinical relevancy. There are many reasons for alterations in melanin production which determines hyperpigmentation. These include causes relating to genetic, metabolic, nutritional, endocrine, infectious, inflammatory, neoplastic or other miscellaneous etiologies. The following will represent a listing of differential diagnoses for the various causes of hyperpigmentation according to the basic presentation of melanin production. The clinical significance of hyperpigmentation is related to (1) the association of other disease processes, (2) concerns regarding the clinical appearance, and (3) the potential for neoplastic diseases.

Pathogenesis

Hyperpigmentation is the increased production of melanin and has generally been categorized into two areas: **melanoses,** which may be either circumscribed or diffuse and develop without preceding inflammatory skin disease, and **melanodermas,** which are associated with or follow inflammatory disorders or lesions. The majority of hyperpigmentation in dogs is due to a postinflammatory reaction (melanoderma). Endocrine disorders with hyperpigmentation are referred to as "melanoses" since they were not the direct result of an inflammatory process. They are certainly more prevalent among the most commonly encountered noninflammatory causes of hyperpigmentation in dogs.

Melanin Production

Melanin is the pigment responsible for the dark brown to black coloration of the skin. It is produced by the melanocyte, which is a specialized cell presumed to derive from the neural crest during embryogenesis. Although this cell is present in many tissues, the highest numbers are found in the epidermis, mucous membrane epithelium, and hair follicle epithelium. Two types of melanocytes are present (dendritic and nondendritic), both of which synthesize the organelle responsible for melanin production, called the **melanosome.** Only the cells containing dendrites are capable of pigment transfer to other cells. In humans the number of active melanocytes has been shown to decrease in both skin and hair follicles with increasing age. Melanocytes can be stimulated to increase in number by several factors, including exposure to ultraviolet light.

The melanosome is the subcellular structure within the melanocyte that contains the enzyme, tyrosinase, necessary for melanin synthesis. The melanosome is also the vehicle for melanin transfer from dendritic melanocytes to the surrounding keratinocytes. It is currently felt that melanosome synthesis involves intricate relationships between premelanosomal components and various subcellular organelles.

Melanin is developed from the amino acid tyrosine, which undergoes a biosynthetic change to DOPA (dihydroxyphenylalanine) by the interaction of tyrosinase. A second reaction utilizing tyrosinase converts DOPA to dopaquinone. From dopaquinone a number of reactions occur leading to the ultimate production of melanin. Actually two types of melanin are recognized in humans: pheomelanin (which is a red-yellow pigment) and eumelanin (a brown-black pigment).

The epidermal melanin unit has been used to describe the association of melanocyte with keratinocyte. In humans it has been estimated that 20 to 36 keratinocytes are serviced by a single melanocyte. Clinical pigmentation is due to the amount and organization of melanosomes in the keratinocytes that have been transferred from the melanocyte to the keratinocyte. The keratinocyte is thought to participate in the transfer process by phagocytizing the melanosome-laden dendritic tips of the melanocyte. Keratinocytes may also participate in the regulation of melanosome production by several mechanisms. Thus there appears to be a close relationship among melanin production, hyperpigmentation, and the role of keratinocytes and melanocytes. In fact, melanosome production may depend to some extent on the rate at which it is affected by the proliferating keratinocyte population.

Although factors that regulate pigmentation are numerous, the diseases related to pigmentation can be categorized into two areas. The first, referred to as "constitutive" skin color, involves melanization generated according to the inborn cellular genetic programming. (This is often referred to as the baseline pigmentation.) The second, "facultative" skin color, is an induced increase in pigmentation typically influenced by ultraviolet light, hormones, inflammation, or other primary problems.

CLINICAL DISEASE
Genetic Hypermelanoses

Genetic causes of hypermelanosis are uncommonly reported in dogs and cats, although their occurrence is probably greater than described in the literature. There are two types of genetic hypermelanotic conditions.

The first is referred to as **lentigo.** Canine lentigo is a macular melanosis usually producing dark black areas in multiple regions that increase in number and size during maturation of the animal. Lentigines are benign and have minimum significance other than the overt concern they arouse regarding neoplastic disease. They are typically not raised but, for the most part, are recognized as a pigmented macule or patch. Their most common location is the ventrum, where the hair is more sparse. The lesions usually reach a maximum number and then become static. Occasionally some will develop hyperkeratotic changes on the surface. Lentiginosis profusa is a condition observed in Pugs with a heritable basis presumed autosomal recessive in nature (Briggs, 1985).

The histologic features of lentigines reveal increased melanocytes and basal cell melanin. There are no structural changes in the epidermis, although it may thicken as lesion progression is observed. The most noticeable feature is increased epidermal pigmentation and overrepresentation of melanin granules in keratinocytes. The greatest significance of lentigo is its role in the differential diagnosis of pigmented tumors. Occurrence of malignancy following lentigines has not been observed in dogs but has been in man. Rule-out of neoplastic disease by cutaneous biopsy and dermatopathology may be indicated depending on the owner's concern. No other treatment is really necessary.

Lentigo simplex has been observed in orange cats and is similar to human lentigo simplex (Scott, 1987). This condition is recognized by asymptomatic macular hyperpigmentation typically affecting the area of the lips, gums, eyelids, and nose. The macules, which are not true lentigenes according to some (Guaguere and Alhaidari, 1989), usually develop earlier than 1 year of age and may progress to the point of maximal intensity and then remain static throughout the life of the animal. The lesions are primarily a concern of the owner for neoplastic disease. The lesions are of minimal concern and no treatment is recommended, nor is there any that is effective.

The second type of hypermelanotic condition with a genetic basis is **nevi**. The term "nevus" actually is a general one used in reference to a circumscribed congenital abnormality resulting in the faulty production of nearly mature or fully mature structures. Nevus also refers to a benign tumor of pigment cells. Epidermal nevi result from the overproduction of surface or adnexal epithelium. Melanocytic nevi have been observed in both dogs and cats. They may be single or multiple and usually have a truncal distribution. Color varies from brown to black, and the nevus may actually have a macular appearance (junctional type) or look like a papule, plaque or pedunculated lesion. It represents a hyperplastic change of melanocytes that produces excess numbers of cells in the epidermis or dermis. These lesions are benign and have never been reported to become malignant in domestic animals.

Epidermal nevi have also been recognized in dogs and represent a change more suggestive of an epidermal condition. The Schnauzer is a breed often associated with epidermal nevi frequently referred to specialists for a provisional diagnosis of melanoma because of the similarity in appearance between the two (Fig. 23-1). The lesions are characterized as raised, rough to smooth, black plaques. These may in fact have hyperpigmentation confused with melanocytic nevi. Histologic differences aid in the differentiation of the respective diseases.

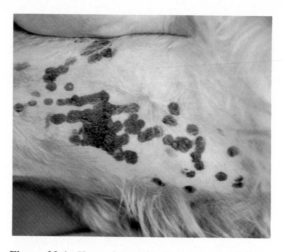

Figure 23-1. Hyperpigmented plaques on the abdomen of a Miniature Schnauzer that histologically are epithelial nevi.

(Courtesy Dr. CE Griffin, San Diego, Calif.)

Metabolic or Nutritional Hypermelanosis

There are few nutritional causes of hyperpigmentation in dogs and cats. Protein deficiency, likewise, is rarely encountered in veterinary practice, although it has been reported as a cause of epidermal hyperpigmentation associated with hyperkeratosis and loss of hair pigment. Loss of hair may also be observed in chronically deprived animals and results in patchy alopecia and hairs that are dry, dull, and easily broken.

Most metabolic causes of hyperpigmentation involve aberrations of endocrine function or are related to genetic traits resulting in the excess production of melanin. Proper dietary management is certainly advised as a conservative approach to the hyperpigmentation although it rarely results in a positive response since it is rarely the cause.

Postinflammatory Hypermelanosis

Postinflammatory hypermelanosis (melanoderma) is the most common cause of hyperpigmentation in dogs. A variety of etiologies can be associated with the phenomenon. Although physical insults such as radiotherapy, friction, or intertriginous abrasion may be a factor, the commonest cause is usually an allergic or infectious phenomenon. Most melanodermas result in macular hyperpigmentation, although chronicity and protracted pruritus with subsequent self-inflicted trauma may result in more diffuse areas. Melanodermas are different from melanoses (noninflammatory), particularly in the early phase of development, since they often have a lace or lattice pattern whereas melanoses are usually more homogeneous and diffuse. These conditions in humans are not generally accompanied by increased numbers of melanocytes, and the hyperpigmentation is restricted to areas where the inflammation was observed. The classic illustration is the tanning that follows sunburn in humans. Photosensitizing chemicals will greatly enhance this type of pigmentation, and may extend or modify the action of the spectrum of radiation involved. Sun-induced hyperpigmentation has been recognized in dogs and may be observed secondary to hair loss from endocrine disease or from self-inflicted causes (pruritus). Protection from direct sun exposure is recommended in dogs with a sparse hair coat. Sunscreens may provide an alternative when sun exposure is more intense (e.g., in southern climates).

The most common cause of hyperpigmentation of this type is allergic dermatoses and superficial staphylococcal pyoderma. Any inflammatory disease can result in pigmentary change, as seen in cases of nodular panniculitis, sebaceous adenitis, dermatomycosis, demodicosis, contact-allergic dermatitis, contact-irritant dermatitis, and other miscellaneous inflammatory diseases. Occasionally conditions such as lupus erythematosus or phemphigus will result in hyperpigmented lesions. Recognition of the primary cause is principal to properly resolving the problem. Features of the inflammatory disease, such as erythroderma, may be recognized in areas peripheral to pigmented regions. The presence of other epidermal changes, including scale and crust, is also an associated sign of underlying inflammatory disease, as is a papular or pustular condition. The specific diagnostic approach should be directed toward clinical patterns observed. Canine atopy and flea allergy are commonly recognized inflammatory diseases with hyperpigmentation in patterns suggestive of pruritus affecting either the lower back (as in flea allergy) or the face, axillae, inguinal region, and extremities of the atopic/food allergic dog (Figs. 23-2 and 23-3). These conditions are most commonly misinterpreted as endocrine-based problems. (See Chapters to 10 to 12.) Most postinflammatory hypermelansosis cases are misdiagnosed as hypothyroidism by the finding of low normal thyroxine levels and are inappropriately placed on thyroid supplementation. The observation of bilaterally symmetric lesions affecting the ventrum in combination with inflammatory disease and pruritus,

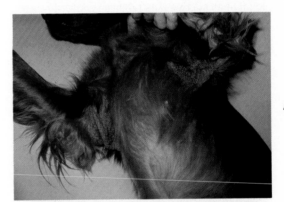

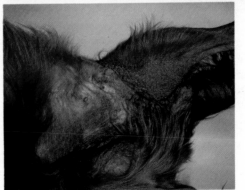

Figure 23-3. **A,** Axillary hyperpigmentation in an Irish Setter due to chronic inflammation and pruritus from canine atopy. Because of the location of the lesions, this distribution is often misdiagnosed as acanthosis nigricans. **B,** The inguinal region of this dog. Note the hyperpigmentation and lichenification, suggesting an endocrine basis although the cause is postinflammatory.

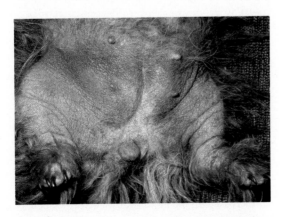

Figure 23-2. Regional hyperpigmentation affecting the inguinal area of a Scottish Terrier with chronic pruritus from atopy and food allergy. This bilateral hyperpigmentation is often misdiagnosed as an endocrinopathy. Note the presence of erythema adjacent to the hyperpigmentation.

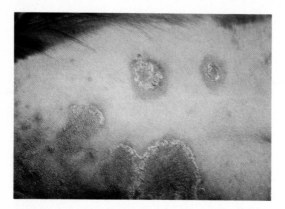

Figure 23-4. The abdomen of an Irish Setter demonstrating various stages of lesions caused by a staphylococcal pyoderma. The coalescing hyperpigmented lesions represent the resolving stage of the infection. An underlying disease should be suspected in association with the pyoderma.

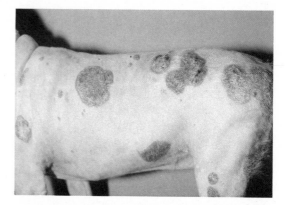

Figure 23-5. Adult-onset demodicosis with multifocal hyperpigmented macules and patches. Skin scrapings were positive for adult and immature forms of *D. canis*. The hair was shaved for better visualization of the lesions.

as previously described, should arouse one's suspicion of an allergic rather than an endocrine-based problem.

Multifocal macular lesions (or patches) of hyperpigmentation are most commonly associated with superficial staphyhlococcal pyoderma-folliculitis (Fig. 23-4). They usually follow the inflammatory phase of papules or macules and subsequently terminate in a healing lesion that shows central hyperpigmentation with a collarette of scale on the border. These lesions tend to be well-circumscribed, although they may become confluent and produce larger areas of diffuse involvement. Since lesions with this appearance can be due to dermatophytosis, its rule-out by culture procedures is mandatory. Specific therapy for the underlying problem is necessary for resolution of the pigmentary change. The reversal of these lesions may take upwards of months to years depending on their intensity and chronicity.

Hypermelanosis Associated with Ectoparasitism

Hypermelanosis (melanoderma) is associated with some ectoparasitic disease, in particular canine demodicosis (Fig. 23-5 and 23-6). Early lesions may represent a slate blue/gray pigmentary change that upon closer inspection suggests early comedone formation. Lesional development is most often seen in the adult form of demodicosis, although it may also be observed in the juvenile form. Skin scrapings of affected areas are mandatory and should be included in the assessment of any macule or patch of hyperpigmentation, re-

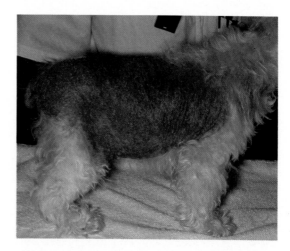

Figure 23-6. Demodicosis and secondary staphylococcal pyoderma associated with hyperpigmentation in a dog receiving chronic glucocorticoid therapy for canine atopy and flea allergy.

gardless of the animal's age. Coexistent pyoderma may be present and contribute to the melanoderma with postinflammatory hyperpigmentation. Treatment for the problem is discussed in greater detail in Chapter 7.

Endocrine Hypermelanosis

Increased pigmentation has long been associated with endocrine diseases and is usually bilaterally symmetric. Unfortunately, bilaterally symmetric postinflammatory hypermelanosis is frequently confused with endocrine-induced hypermelanosis for this reason.

Growth hormone–related diseases and sex hormone imbalances are the most common endocrine

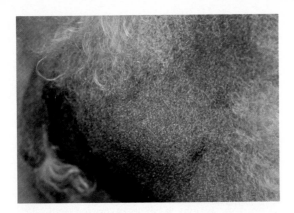

Figure 23-7. Hyperpigmentation on the thigh of an older Poodle with spontaneously occurring hyperadrenocorticism. Note the absence of erythema (dermatitis) and primary lesions. The hair epilated easily from the area surrounding the alopecia.

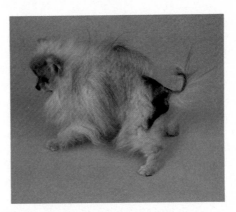

Figure 23-8. Hyperpigmentation in the pelvic region of an adult male Pomeranian with castration-responsive alopecia. Adult-onset growth hormone–responsive dermatosis has been cited as the cause of similar lesions in this breed, although specific hormonal relationships have not been confirmed.

conditions associated with hyperpigmentation. Growth hormone–responsive dermatosis is a somewhat obscure condition not completely defined. It has been reported in the Chow Chow and Pomeranian, characterized by early hyperpigmentary changes and associated alopecia. No inflammatory lesions are present prior to or during evolvement of the hypermelanosis (Fig. 23-7). Other types of endocrine problems have been associated with pigmentary disturbance, including castration-responsive dermatoses, Sertoli cell tumors, and ovarian imbalances (Fig. 23-8). Cushing's disease has been listed and is observed with some hypermelanoses, particularly in a diffuse pattern on the ventrum. Increased pigmentation may be seen in humans with ACTH therapy or chronic glucocorticoid treatment. Hypothyroidism is a disease frequently overdiagnosed and improperly recognized as the cause of many pigmentary problems in dogs. Resting levels of thyroxine (T_4) are often abnormal due to coexisting or underlying diseases, thereby leading to the erroneous conclusion. Although empirical treatment with T_4 may transiently improve the problem, the response is often limited and incomplete. Once again, postinflammatory hypermelanosis is most commonly confused with endocrine-based problems. A complete review of major endocrine diseases is available in Chapters 25 to 28.

Tumor Hypermelanosis

Tumor hypermelanosis is usually related to a melanoma in dogs, although a condition referred to as malignant acanthosis nigricans has been observed. Melanomas may have a variety of biologic

behaviors that, for all practicality, should be viewed as protentially malignant. The tumors arise from melanocytes or melanoblasts but do not necessarily pigment (e.g., the amelanotic melanoma). Breeds reported with a predilection include Cocker Spaniels, Boxers, Irish Setters, Chow Chows, Scottish Terriers, and Poodles. Distribution sites include face, trunk, scrotum, and feet as well as the oral cavity. Lesions may be solitary or multiple and have a variety of color ranging from normal pink-white to brown to intense black. It is important to remember that not all melanomas are pigmented. Malignant melanomas frequently metastasize early to the lungs, kidneys, liver, and bone. The prognosis is based on the size and duration of lesional development. Location of tumors has also been viewed as a prognostic indicator, with oral, scrotal, and digital locations being more malignant and having a higher metastatic rate. Early biopsy of pigmented lesions is helpful to differentiate melanomas from other causes of pigmentation.

In dogs benign melanomas arising from the junction of the dermis and epidermis are often called melanocytic nevi. This classification differs from the human since it also includes junctional and compound types (Muller et al., 1989). Recognition of different cell origins has been used to classify the lesions in humans. Basically it is thought that nevus cells have a dual origin from either epidermal melanocytes (as in the case of superficial lesions) or Schwann cells (as in the more deeply located lesions). They are further classified (Caro and Bronstein, 1985) by location of the nevus cells in the skin. Junctional nevi are confined to epidermal/dermal locations, intradermal nevi have clusters of cells located in the dermis only, and compound nevi have nevus cells in both locations. Benign dermal melanomas in dogs are further subcategorized as cellular or fibrous and collectively called blue nevi. Most produce a macular lesion, although some may be solid nodules. Pigmented papillomas are sometimes confused with melanocytic nevi, particularly in Rottweilers and German Shepherd Dogs. They seem to be more prevalent in flea-infested areas and may be caused by viral inoculation through flea feedings.

The occurrence of malignant acanthosis nigricans is rare in humans and is associated with a variety of malignant neoplasms. These include hepatic carcinoma, ovarian and testicular tumors, mammary adenocarcinoma with pulmonary metastasis, thyroid adenocarcinoma, and primary pulmonary carcinoma. The relationship of tumor evolvement and pigmentary changes has not been confirmed, although in humans approximately 20% of the cases of acanthosis nigricans are associated with visceral cancer. The proposed mechanism is a result of glandular hypersecretion of peptides that tend to affect epidermis and epidermal melanosis.

Miscellaneous Hypermelanoses

Acanthosis Nigricans

Acanthosis nigricans is a condition recognized rarely and is often misdiagnosed in dogs with postinflammatory melanosis affecting the axillary area, most frequently from either allergy (atopy or food allergy) or intertriginous irritation. It has been diagnosed in Dachshunds and may represent a primary idiopathic form of the disease. It has also been described in Lhasa Apsos (Scott and McGrath, 1973), and it may occur in other breeds as well. It starts at an early age in Lhasa Apsos and tends to progress throughout life. Unfortunately, "secondary canine acanthosis nigricans" is a term that has been used for postinflammatory causes, therefore complicating the association of terminology. Hyperpigmentation resulting from endocrinopathies has also been called acanthosis nigricans, although it would be best to describe this secondary change as melanoses and avoid the use of acanthosis nigricans.

The differential diagnosis of primary idiopathic acanthosis nigricans should be avoided since there is no way to reliably differentiate this condition from hyperpigmentation caused by a variety of other diseases. Axillary and inguinal hyperpigmentation most often is secondary, which also may be seen in Dachshunds. The rule is to suspect post-inflammatory causes or endocrine disease before considering idiopathic acanthosis nigricans. If inspected closely, most of the lesions will have a border of erythema surrounding the hyperpigmentation. Although the erythema may be from a secondary complication, it usually implies that the hyperpigmentation is secondary to inflammatory disease. Histologic examination of skin from both primary and secondary acanthosis nigricans may show similarities. The lack of inflammatory disease would be more compatible with primary idiopathic canine acanthosis nigricans, although many inflammatory lesions have been treated with glucocorticoids (which may result in minimal to no dermatitis).

Melatonin is the conventional treatment for idiopathic canine acanthosis, although in our experience it has almost never been used because the condition was either secondary or a benign problem not calling for this extent of treatment. It has been postulated that melatonin, a pineal gland hormone, may be a physiologic antagonist to melanocyte-stimulating hormone (MSH). The standard treatment is 2 mg q24h administered subcutaneously for 3 to 5 days and then weekly or monthly as needed. Vitamin E (DL-alpha tocopheral acetate) has demonstrated beneficial effects in limited trials (Scott and Walton, 1985). The dosage is 200 IU q12h PO. Glucocorticoids have also been a routine therapy, with some demonstrated success, which may be more a response to the underlying inflammatory disease than an effect on the pigmentary problem. The most efficacious therapy of axillary and inguinal hyperpigmentation is early recognition and institution of proper treatment.

Acral Melanism

Acral melanism is a physiologic condition observed in certain cats, particularly Siamese, Himalayan, Balinese, and Burmese breeds. Kittens are usually born white and develop dark points as adults, which is an influence of the lower external temperature. Temperature is responsible for the dark hair and may also be associated with color changes of the skin in these respective areas. The phenomenon appears to be associated with a temperature-dependent enzyme utilized in the melanin synthesis.

DIAGNOSIS

Diagnostic procedures for hypermelanosis should be influenced strongly by a consideration of several etiologies. Signalment, history, and dermatologic examination are critical for a proper diagnostic plan. Congenital problems may be recognized, and this suggests a genodermatosis as the basis, which should raise minimal concern and not call for therapeutic modification. Acquired diseases are more commonly associated with hypermelanosis and accompanied by other lesions or changes such as pruritus. Identification of pruritic habits should be part of history taking and correlated with the disease. Many allergic phenomena occur between 1 and 3 years of age, therefore placing the younger dog at risk for the development of secondary changes. Dogs older than 6 years are more likely to have endocrine causes if there is no accompanying pruritus or history of it prior to the onset. Breeds with a predilection for allergic manifestations more likely have melanoderma than a true melanosis. Chinese Shar-Peis are a good example of a breed that shows hyperpigmentation secondary to an allergic problem, particularly in the facial area. This may occur early on in the disease and disguise an inflammatory lesion.

The minimum database obtained for evaluation of hypermelanosis should include skin scrapings (for ectoparasites), a fungal culture (dermatophyte test medium), and cytology (for pyoderma or *Malassezia*). A complete blood cell count and differential should also be included whenever there is the possibility of a coexistent or underlying systemic problem. A routine panel of serum chemistries should be obtained; abnormal findings may be just coincidental and lack a cause-and -effect relationship, but they should be interpreted carefully nevertheless.

If an endocrinopathy is highly suspect, ancillary diagnostic testing usually involves hormonal assays. Pitfalls include the previous use of thyroid hormone or glucocorticoids that may interfere with the accurate evaluation of respective endocrine systems. Chapters describing endocrine based problems (Section VIII) should be reviewed for more complete presentation of diseases and diagnostic tests.

Skin biopsies and cytologic examination of tissue imprints are helpful in ruling out neoplastic disease and providing a basis for the hyperpigmentation. Features are usually present to differentiate an inflammatory process from a noninflammatory melanosis. Exact identification of the underlying disease associated with a melanoderma is **unlikely** from the dermatohistopathologic examination. Questionable lesions relating to melanoma should be routinely biopsied, but the clinician must be cautious about overinterpreting histologic results relative to acanthosis and melanosis. Mistaking hyperpigmentation due to an inflammatory reaction as a case of acanthosis nigricans is commonplace.

If neoplastic diseases are suspect, additional diagnostic procedures may include fine needle aspirate of the lymph node and cutaneous nodules for cytologic examination. Radiography of the thorax is advisable in cases with concern for malignant melanoma.

TREATMENT

Treatment of hypermelanosis is based on the primary problem. The most important challenge is to determine treatable versus untreatable conditions.

The owner's concern for hyperpigmentation may constitute an overreaction; and in this case education is the best treatment. Some genodermatoses are untreatable and of minimal significance. Others (e.g., a growth hormone–responsive dermatosis) that are acquired may be impractical to treat. The clinician is cautioned against overtreatment of an endocrine-appearing problem not definitively diagnosed. The most common pitfall is to misdiagnose postinflammatory hyperpigmentation as an endocrine-related lesion. Treatment of more common conditions should be considered first, with further diagnostic pursuit dependent on response.

REFERENCES

Briggs OM: Lentiginosis profusa in the pug: three case reports, J Small Anim Pract 26:675, 1985.

Caro W, Bronstein BR: Tumors of the skin. In Moshella SL, Hurley HJ: Dermatology ed 2, Philadelphia, 1985, WB Saunders, p 1533.

Guaguere E, Alhaidari Z: Disorders of melanin pigmentation in the skin of dogs and cats. In Kirk RW (ed): Current veterinary therapy X, Philadelphia, 1989, WB Saunders, p 628.

Muller GH, et al: Small animal dermatology, ed 4, Philadelphia, 1989, WB Saunders, p 931.

Scott DW: Lentigo simplex in orange cats, Compan Anim Pract 1:23, 1987.

Scott DW, McGrath CJ: Acanthosis nigricans in the Lhasa apso, Vet Med Small Anim Clin 68:676, 1973.

Scott DW, Walton DK: Clinical evaluation of oral vitamin E for the treatment of primary acanthosis nigricans, J Am Anim Hosp Assoc 21:345, 1985.

Diseases of the Ear

Factors and Causes of Otitis Externa

PREDISPOSING FACTORS
Conformation
  Stenotic canals
  Hair in canals
  Pendulous pinnae
  Hairy, concave pinnae
Excessive moisture
  Swimmer's ear
  High-humidity climate
Treatment effects
  Trauma from cotton applicators
  Irritant topicals
  Superinfections by altered normal
  microflora
Obstructive ear disease
  Neoplasms
  Polyps
Systemic disease
  Pyrexia
  Immune suppression/viruses
  Debilitation
  Negative catabolic states

24

Otitis Externa and Otitis Media

Craig E. Griffin

PRIMARY CAUSES

Parasites
  Otodectes cynotis
  Demodicosis
  Sarcoptic/notoedric mange
  Otobius megnini
  Eutrombicula (chiggers)
Microorganisms
  Dermatophytosis
  Sporothrix schenckii
Hypersensitivity diseases
  Atopy
  Food allergy
  Contact
  Drug reactions
Keratinization disorders
  Primary idiopathic seborrhea
  Hypothyroidism
  Sex hormone imbalance
  Abnormal cerumen production
  Foreign bodies
  Plant
  Hairs
  Foxtails
Glandular disorders
  Apocrine hyperplasia
  Sebaceous hyper- or hypoplasia
  Altered secretion rate
  Altered secretions
Autoimmune diseases
  Lupus erythematosus
  Pemphigus foliaceus
  Pemphigus erythematosus
Viral diseases
  Distemper virus
  (?) Juvenile cellulitis

PERPETUATING FACTORS

Bacteria
  Staphylococcus intermedius
  Proteus spp
  Pseudomonas spp
  Escherichia coli
  Klebsiella spp
Yeasts
  Malassezia pachydermatis
  Candida albicans
  Miscellaneous
Progressive pathologic changes
  Hyperkeratosis
  Acanthosis
  Epithelial folds
  Edema
  Apocrine gland hypertrophy and/or
    hyperplasia
  Hidradenitis
  Fibrosis
  Calcification
Otitis media
  Simple purulent
  Casseated/keratinous
  Choleasteatoma
  Proliferative
  Destructive ostomyelitis

Modified from August JR. In Solvay Veterinary Inc:
The complete manual of ear care, Trenton NJ, 1986,
Veterinary Learning Systems USA.

Importance

Otitis externa is defined as inflammation of the external auditory canal. It is a symptom of many diseases, not a specific diagnosis, and may be present in as many as 10% to 20% of the canines brought to a small animal hospital. In cats it is much less common than in dogs and is most often related to a parasitic etiology.

Management of otitis externa is a major aspect of small animal practice. Poor response to therapy is the source of much client dissatisfaction, resulting in many clients' seeking the services of another veterinarian or specialist.

In 50% of chronic cases the tympanic membrane may be or may have been ruptured, allowing extension of infection into the middle ear. Extension across a ruptured tympanum into the middle ear is the most common cause of otitis media. Once present, the otitis media is a major source of otitis externa or failure in the treatment of otitis externa. It is also the most common cause of poor results when a surgical procedure (the modified Lacroix Zepp) is utilized.

Etiologies

There are numerous causes of otitis externa. In the majority of chronic cases more than one is present. A new classification scheme (August, 1986) for the causes of otitis externa has been proposed. In it causes are broken down into predisposing, primary, and perpetuating. The box presents a modification of August's classification. The clinician should always try to recognize which factors are contributing to the otitis in an individual case.

Predisposing Factors

Predisposing factors alone may not cause otitis externa, but they increase the risk of development. These factors work in conjunction with either primary causes or perpetuating factors to cause clinical disease. The most successful management of otitis externa requires that they be recognized and wherever possible controlled in a treatment plan. The most common predisposing factors I treat are hair in the external canals or on pendulous concave pinnas, moisture, and the effects of inappropriate treatment. Clients, technicians, and groomers should be extremely careful when mechanically cleaning ears. The use of cotton applicators should be avoided or limited. Animals prone to swimmer's ear often have nonclinical atopy or food allergy. The Chinese Shar-Pei is particularly prone to ste-

notic ear canals and conformational problems in which the pinna is tightly folded over the external orifice, which may have increased skin folds. The extra or unusually deep folds become sites for fold dermatitis and infections. Systemic disease is often listed as a predisposing factor for the development of otitis externa but actually is rarely encountered.

Primary Causes

Primary causes are usually the actual inciting agent or etiology that directly causes the otitis externa. These can occur alone and induce otitis externa without predisposing or perpetuating factors. The most common causes seen in a dermatology referral practice are atopy, food allergy, keratinization disorders, and ear mites. It is critical to successful long-term management that a primary cause be found.

Parasites. *Otodectes cynotis, Demodex canis, Demodex cati, Sarcoptes scabiei, Notoedres cati,* and various species of ticks have been associated with otitis externa in dogs and cats.

The ear mite, *Otodectes cynotis,* is most common, being responsible for up to 50% or more of the otitis externa cases diagnosed in cats; in dogs its incidence is controversial, but most authors agree that it is responsible for 5% to 10% of otitis externa cases. Evidence exists that ear mites may initiate otitis externa but remain undetected in many dogs. Two explanations for this have been proposed.

One (Frost, 1961) suggests that the reported incidences are low because of difficulty in demonstrating the mites. As few as two or three mites can cause clinical otitis externa and, as with cases of sarcoptic mange, the mites can easily be missed. This theory is further supported by work in cats (Weisbroth et al., 1974; Powell et al., 1980) showing that the pathophysiology of ear mites in otitis externa involves an arthus-type and an immediate-type hypersensitivity reaction.

The second suggests that mites initiate otitis externa and then, if the inflammation becomes severe enough, they leave the canal or are destroyed.

In recurrent cases of otitis externa the possibility that other in-contact animals act as asymptomatic carriers should be considered. The asymptomatic carrier of ear mites can be a source for the affected pet. Due to variation in time of transmission from carrier to affected patient and time from onset of hypersensitivity until development of clinical signs noticeable by the owner, these cases can recur rapidly or intermittently.

Demodex cati in felines may present with just otitis externa. The cases typically show a mildly inflamed waxy otitis and are often otherwise asymptomatic.

Microorganisms. In most cases bacteria are perpetuating factors and not primary causes of otitis externa. Some rare exceptions are seen and usually relate to less common infections of pathogenic organisms. Dermatophytes are relatively common causes of pinnal disease and in rare cases may involve the external ear canal. Most studies showing bacteria to be pathogenic inoculate ears with liquid media. When controls are utilized, it is common for the liquid vehicle–treated cases to also develop clinical disease. One study looking at the pathogenicity of *Malassezia pachydermatis* (Mansfield et al., 1990) showed that inoculation with sterile Sabouraud broth resulted in a higher prevalence of gross lesions and positive *Malassezia* recovery than did inoculation with *Malassezia pachydermatis* suspended in saline.

Hypersensitivities. Atopy, food allergy, and contact-allergic dermatitis can all cause otitis externa. The otitis externa may be secondary to self-trauma, or the allergic reaction may involve the external ear canal.

Because of its high incidence, **atopy** is more frequently associated with otitis externa than are the other allergic diseases mentioned. No additional evidence of atopic disease is discovered in 3% to 5% of atopic-induced otitis externa cases. One common feature of allergic otitis is erythema of the pinna and vertical canal while the deeper horizontal canal remains relatively normal (Fig. 24-1). Chronic inflammation may eventually lead to secondary bacterial or yeast infections.

Over 20% of **food allergy** cases start with otitis externa alone and ear disease is present in up to 80% of allergic cases. When allergic otitis externa is suspected and there is no additional historical or physical evidence of allergic disease, food allergy is most likely (Rosser in Bigler and Merchant, 1990).

Contact allergic dermatitis can result from medications (especially neomycin) used to treat otitis externa. In addition, vehicles such as propylene glycol can be responsible for irritant reactions in the ear. Therefore just changing medications based on major medication ingredients may not alleviate a treatment reaction. In other cases the ear medications may cause damage only

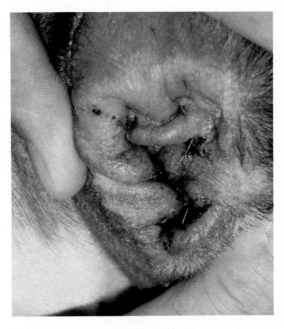

Figure 24-1. Otitis externa with secondary *Malassezia* in an atopic Boxer. The erythema of the pinna and external orifice is typical of atopic otitis externa. The moist brown discharge also is typical of the yeast or mixed cocci/yeast infection.

to already inflamed skin. Whenever a case of otitis externa fails to respond or worsens after therapy has been initiated, a contact-allergic dermatitis should be suspected.

Keratinization. The keratinization disorders generally present as chronic ceruminous otitis externa. Breeds prone to primary idiopathic seborrhea tend to have otitis externa. Endocrinopathies such as hypothyroidism, male-feminizing syndrome, Sertoli cell tumors, and some ovarian imbalances may result in chronic ceruminous otitis externa, most likely by altering keratinization and possibly glandular function. Hypothyroidism is the most commonly encountered endocrinopathy involving the ear. Many times the primary cause of the otitis externa is a disease that has some other historical or physical examination findings as a clue.

Foreign bodies. Foreign bodies such as plant material, dirt, sand, and dried medication are frequently responsible for otitis externa. In short-coated breeds loose hairs may become lodged in the ear canal. Their pointed tips can penetrate the epidermis and stimulate inflammation.

Glandular disorders. Any disorder that alters sebaceous lipid secretions can lead to otitis externa. The apocrine glands appear hypertrophied, and hidradenitis may be present. However, hidradenitis is more likely secondary to inflammation-induced alterations and not a primary cause of otitis externa. Recently, increased numbers of apocrine glands have been associated with breeds at risk for the development of otitis externa (Stout-Graham et al., 1990).

Autoimmune disease. Pemphigus foliaceus and lupus erythematosus are more common causes of autoimmune skin disease. Both frequently affect the pinna and less commonly the ear canal. However, to date I have never seen a case of pemphigus with only otitis externa.

Viral diseases. In human viruses are important agents of otitis externa. They are rarely considered in veterinary medicine, although earlier reports related otitis externa to distemper. It would seem likely that viral induced otitis externa occurs in dogs. Although juvenile cellulitis has an unknown cause, some speculate that a virus may be important. This disease of young dogs often manifests with a markedly edematous, purulent otitis externa.

Perpetuating Factors

Perpetuating factors are those that prevent the resolution of otitis externa/media. In chronic cases one or more of these factors will be present. In early cases treating the primary cause may be sufficient to control a case, but after the establishment of some perpetuating factors treatment must be directed at them. Perpetuating factors may be the major reason for poor response to therapy regardless of the predisposing factors and primary causes.

Bacteria. Bacteria are rarely primary causes, so a diagnosis of bacterial otitis externa is rarely complete. When seen, it is usually a gram-negative rod such as *Pseudomonas* spp that probably comes from exposure to contaminated water and therefore may be a combination of excessive moisture with the bacteria. *Staphylococcus intermedius* and the gram-negative organisms *Pseudomonas* spp, *Proteus* spp, *Escherichia coli,* and *Klebsiella* spp are most commonly isolated as secondary pathogens. Although the four gram-negative organisms are not routinely cultured from normal ears, once they establish infection they significantly contribute to the inflammation and epidermal damage.

Yeast. *Malassezia pachydermatis* is the most common perpetuating yeast that contributes to otitis externa. It is a budding organism with a peanut or bottle shape that may be found in as many as 36% of normal canine ears. It grows best on brain/heart infusion agar with penicillin G and streptomycin sulfate added and then incubated at 37° C (Trettien, 1987). It is a common complication with allergic otitis and may result as a superinfection following antibiotic therapy. Recently it has been shown (Mansfield et al., 1990) to be pathogenic when it or fluid is put in the ear canal. The pathologic mechanism is still unknown and controversial but probably relates to metabolic by-products of yeast growth and death.

Progressive pathologic changes. Chronic inflammation stimulates the skin lining the ear canal to undergo several changes. These include epidermal hyperkeratosis and acanthosis, dermal fibrosis, edema, and apocrine gland hyperplasia and dilation. Hidradenitis, or inflammation of the apocrine glands, may also occur. A recent study (Stout-Graham et al., 1990) found that sebaceous glands do not atrophy as had been previously reported. It was also shown based on morphometric analysis that breeds predisposed to otitis externa had more apocrine glands than sebaceous glands and those with otitis externa had an even greater area of apocrine glands. An occasional case may have sebaceous hyperplasia.

These progressive changes cause a thickening of the skin, which eventually extends to both sides of the auricular cartilage. The swelling leads to stenosis of the canal lumen. More importantly the skin is thrown into numerous folds, which inhibit effective cleaning and the application of topical medications (Fig. 24-2). These folds also act as sites for the perpetuation and protection of secondary microorganisms. The epidermis becomes thickened, and the hyperkeratotic stratum corneum increases the keratin debris that is exfoliated into the canal lumen. The increased secretions and epithelial debris may favor the proliferation of bacteria and yeast. A combination of microbial metabolic by-products, secretions, and debris trapped within the folds and ear canal from the stenosis further contributes to the pathologic changes.

Otitis media. Otitis media is inflammation of the middle ear. Exudate within the tympanic cavity is difficult to treat with topical therapy and often remains as a source for infection and proinflammatory toxins and debris to reach the external ear canal. In more advanced cases I have found keratin plugs developing within the tympanic cavity (Fig. 24-3). The keratin may serve as a reservoir for bacteria and a source of inflammation. Eventually calcification may occur, which can be observed radiographically.

It has been theorized that the tympanic membrane may dilate and extend into the tympanic cavity. Otitis media may be present with an intact tympanic membrane. In one study (Little et al., 1991a) in which eight dogs were necropsied, rup-

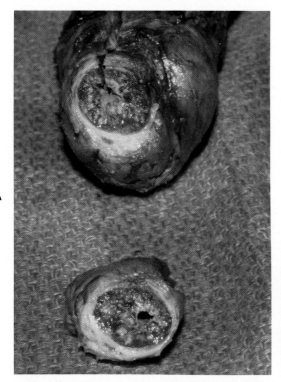

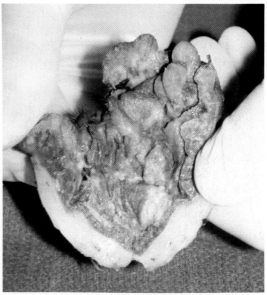

Figure 24-2. A, Chronic proliferative changes lead to stenosis of the ear canal lumen. The lower section shows a cross section of the canal about 1 cm from the tympanic membrane. Note the reduced size of the canal lumen. **B,** External ear canal with chronic proliferative changes, cut open along the longitudinal axis, demonstrating numerous folds. The brown zone represents glandular hyperplasia.

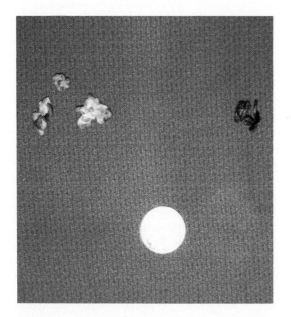

Figure 24-3. Several pieces removed from the middle ear following extensive tube flushing of the external and middle ear. Histological examination revealed the material to be lamellae of keratin. The bright spot is a dime.

tured tympanic membranes were identified in only 2 of 14 ears with otitis externa and media. However, out of the 62 middle ear specimens examined histologically a definitive tympanic membrane could be only recognized in 26%. Tissue, including adnexal structures that originated from the external ear canal, could be found in the middle ear cavity even when the tympanic membrane appeared intact. The auditory tube was patent in all cases in which it was examined at necrospy. The tympanic membrane commonly thickens in response to inflammation and may develop polyploid extensions of granulation tissue into the middle ear cavity, which in some cases formed adhesions with middle ear mucosa.

These changes may lead to the development of aural cholesteatoma in 11% of cases with chronic otitis media (Little et al., 1991b). Aural cholesteatoma is a keratinous filled epidermoid cyst within the middle ear cavity. This syndrome may also be associated with temporomandibular joint disease resulting from extension beyond the middle ear.

Little and his group (1991b) have proposed that cholesteatomas occur as a result of a pocket of tympanic membrane forming within the middle ear cavity. One predisposing factor might be spontaneous occlusion of the external ear canal from chronic proliferative changes, leading to external ear canal stenosis, which would result in a false form of otitis media. A pocket would form that still allowed for the impaction and sequestration of material from topical therapy. This theory might explain why some dogs appear to rapidly regrow their tympanic membranes after flushing of the false middle ear. In contrast to dogs with ruptured tympanic membranes, these cases could not be flushed through the eustachian tube and would be less susceptible to ototoxicity.

CLINICAL DISEASE

History

The most common and earliest indication of otitis externa is aural pruritus or head shaking. As the otitis progresses, a mild to marked exudate may develop. This is most often the point at which a client brings the pet to the veterinarian.

It is often helpful to establish whether the pruritus or a discharge was the earliest sign. In many cases the client may not know for sure but some may indicate that when pruritus was first noted there was no discharge. In many early cases, especially when the primary cause is a hypersensitivity reaction, the ear canal will look normal or have erythema limited to the pinna. Foreign bodies often start with pruritus prior to the development of an exudate. Parasitic diseases usually begin with pruritus but are more variable, (e.g., ear mites in cats often initially cause a dark discharge). Once pruritus has been established as the initial sign, the history should be directed for other evidence of hypersensitivity diseases. (See Chapters 8, 10, and 11.) Questions regarding possible exposure to foreign bodies and ear mites should be asked. Was there a rapid onset after the pet was outside? Is there exposure to roaming dogs or cats in the vicinity that could be a source for ear mites? In most hypersensitivity cases of otitis externa, odor and discharge will occur following development of a secondary infection.

Keratinization, glandular disorders, viral diseases, and autoimmune diseases typically have excessive ceruminous or scaly discharges before pruritus develops (Fig. 24-4). An odor may be noticed early in the development of disease.

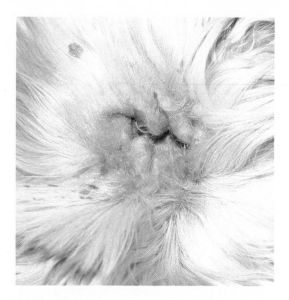

Figure 24-4. Ceruminous exudate in a hypothyroid Cocker Spaniel.

Otitis due to foreign bodies develops suddenly with intense pruritus and rapid progression. These cases are often unilateral; however, parasitic and allergic disorders can also present with unilateral secondarily infected otitis externa. Atopic disease usually is of slower onset and progression, although secondary infections may cause acute exacerbation and make these cases appear as recurrent seasonal or nonseasonal otitis. Many cases previously diagnosed as "swimmer's ear" are, in reality, atopic dogs. Food allergy may be acute or have a gradual onset.

The history should include a thorough search for predisposing factors. This includes questions regarding exposure to water, foreign bodies, and parasites. Does the client or groomer remove hair in breeds predisposed because of hair in the canals? Was hair plucked in a relatively normal ear just prior to the onset of otitis? Have powders or other treatments been applied to the ear canals? If recurrent or chronic, what previous treatments were utilized? What was the response? If initially good and then while on treatment the condition worsened, a contact or drug reaction should be suspected.

In the majority of chronic ear cases I can find historical or physical evidence of the primary disease. The owner may report that the case began with just otic disease but progressed to other areas of the body. If a case does not initially present with other signs, it usually develops them with natural progression of the disease. It is imperative that a thorough history, both general and dermatologic, be taken. If this is not done, many cases will be unnecessarily misdiagnosed. Failing to acquire a good history may postpone the institution of an optimal management plan. The common indications that an underlying problem is a hypersensitivity reaction are seasonality and pruritus in other body locations. Keratinization disorders historically may produce scale formation or changes in coat quality, color, and density.

Head shyness is sometimes seen with otitis externa. Most cases of otitis media will have signs typical only of otitis externa. Head tilt, ataxia, and Horner's syndrome may be seen when otitis media has progressed to involve tissues surrounding the tympanic bulla or inner ear. Pain when eating may be noticed in dogs with severe disease that has progressed to involve the temporomandibular joint (Little et al., 1991b).

Physical Examination

Changes indicative of otitis externa include erythema, swelling, scaling, crusting, alopecia, broken hairs, head shyness, and pain on palpation of the auricular cartilage or tympanic bulla. These changes most commonly involve the pinna, but they may be seen caudal to the pinna on the head or the lateral face over the vertical canal or ventral to this location. Aural hematomas and acute moist dermatitis of the face are also common with aural pruritus, although clinical otitis externa may not be noticeable.

Palpation of the external ear canal and tympanic bulla can provide additional information. The thickness, firmness, and pliability of the vertical and horizontal canal should be determined. Thicker, firmer, and less pliable canals are associated with proliferative changes and support a more guarded prognosis. Calcified canals rarely can be returned to normal or successfully managed with medical therapy. Pain while the temporomandibular joint and region around the tympanic bulla are being palpated implies the presence of otitis media.

Erythema of the concave pinna, with a normal convex pinna, is strongly suggestive of atopy or less likely food allergy. Early cases may have minimal erythema of the vertical canal with a normal horizontal canal. Cases that started only with ear canal disease and then, following treatment, spread peripherally in rostral and ventral directions should make one suspicious of topical therapy reactions (Fig. 24-5).

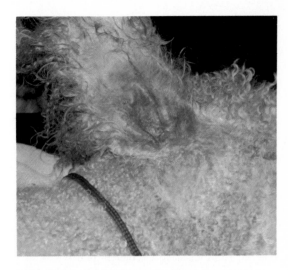

Figure 24-5. Topical-induced unilateral erythema multiforme in a Poodle treated with multiple aminoglycoside preparations (3 neomycin, 1 gentamicin). Note the extension of lesions rostrally and ventrally, a pattern typical for contact reaction.

Emphasis should be placed on looking for primary causes as well as evidence of otitis externa. A thorough dermatologic examination may show signs of pruritus in other body locations. The paws, flexor surface of the elbows and carpus, extensor tarsus, and axillae are all suggestive of atopy or food allergy. Scaly skin or poor hair coat suggests a keratinization disorder or systemic disease. Primary idiopathic seborrhea often has keratinous plugs or crusts around the nipples, interdigital wax accumulations, or perineal and ventral tail comedones. Autoimmune diseases rarely present with just pinnal or external ear canal disease. Usually facial, nasal, oral, or digital lesions will also be present. Juvenile cellulitis may manifest otitis externa as the earliest sign visible to the owner. In my experience these cases have had marked lymphadenopathy in addition to a swollen erythematous otitis externa or pinnae.

If the physical and dermatologic examinations are normal, foreign bodies, *Otodectes* mites, and swimmer's ear are highly suspect or a combination of predisposing and perpetuating factors may have initiated the otitis externa. However, other primary causes cannot be ruled out without appropriate tests.

Otoscopic Examination

The otoscopic examination is used to detect foreign bodies, determine whether otitis media is present, and assess what type of lesions, exudate, and progressive pathologic changes have occurred. If bilateral disease is present, the good ear should be examined first. This will decrease the possibility that the dog will resist examination of the second ear. Examining the good ear first also decreases the likelihood of spreading an infectious agent from the bad ear to the good ear. Having several otoscopic cones of varying sizes placed in cold sterilization containers is a good idea. A problem often encountered in practice is the extremely painful, ulcerated, swollen ear that cannot be adequately examined. Even with anesthesia adequate examination is not possible, and it becomes necessary to treat the animal, reduce the swelling and inflammation, and then have the patient return in 4 to 7 days so that an otoscopic examination can be properly performed.

A record of lesions should be kept. Proliferative changes, the amount and type of discharge, and the presence of erythema or ulcers are noted. An assessment of the tympanic membrane should also be made and recorded.

The degree of canal stenosis must be determined, since changes in lumen size can be used to help monitor treatment. Is proliferation the result of diffuse thickening, or does the canal epithelium have a cobblestone appearance? The location of the stenosis should also be noted. Does it involve the horizontal canal, vertical canal, or both?

The type of discharge may be a clue as to what primary or perpetuating factors may be involved. Debris resembling dry coffee grounds is typical of ear mites. Moist brown discharge tends to be associated with cocci and yeast infections (Fig. 24-1). Purulent creamy to yellow exudates are most often seen with gram-negative infections (Fig. 24-6). Waxy, greasy, yellow to tan debris is typical of ceruminous otitis (Fig. 24-4), sometimes seen with *Malassezia*. Ceruminous discharge most often occurs with keratinizing, glandular, and chronic allergic disorders.

It is easy to misinterpret the competency of the tympanic membrane. The membrane becomes opaque, gray, or brown due to disease and thickening and therefore loses its characteristic opalescent, fish-scale appearance. This makes it resemble a keratin plug. Middle ear changes or the medial wall of the tympanic bulla may be interpreted as a diseased but intact tympanic membrane. In one study (Little and Lane, 1989) an evaluation consisting of tympanometry, otoscopy, and palpation revealed that in inflamed ears only tympanometry was accurate for determining the integrity of the

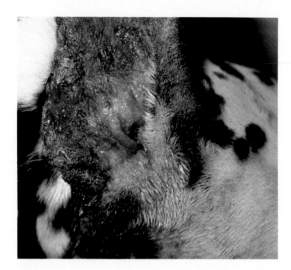

Figure 24-6. *Pseudomonas* complicating atopic otitis externa.

tympanic membrane. This study also showed that, even following lavage of the ear canal, a satisfactory view of the tympanic membrane could be obtained in only 28% of the cases otoscopically examined while the pet was anesthetized.

DIAGNOSIS

A diagnosis of otitis externa is easily made from the history and physical examination. Otitis media is much more difficult to diagnose, since many cases present with only symptoms of otitis externa. Evidence of inflamed tissues surrounding the middle or inner ear usually indicates that otitis media has occurred. Even with otoscopic examination, many cases of otitis externa may not be detected and in animals with apparently intact diseased tympanic membranes otitis media may be present. Radiology is indicated when otitis media is suspected, and especially prior to surgical procedures involving the middle ear. However, radiology is helpful only when it demonstrates middle ear pathology; normal radiographs do not rule out the presence of otitis media. Tympanometry appears valuable for diagnosing a ruptured tympanic membrane. Its usefulness in clinically inflamed ears and ears with otitis media needs to be determined, although it seems preferable to previously described techniques (Little and Lane, 1989).

Evaluation of the tympanic membrane by probing with a blunt instrument has been shown (Little and Lane, 1989) to be inaccurate and can cause significant damage to the tympanic membrane. I have described a technique of palpation and posi-

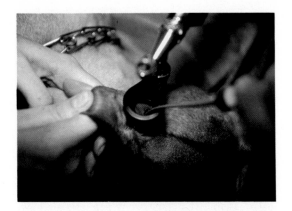

Figure 24-7. Feeding tube attached to a syringe. The other end has been passed through the surgical otoscope and down the vertical canal. Traction on the pinna allows visualization of the horizontal canal.

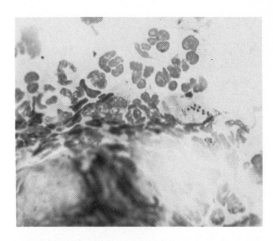

Figure 24-8. Cytologic examination of smear demonstrating wax and keratin debris at the bottom of the photograph. Neutrophils as well as cocci and rods can be seen.

tioning a soft feeding tube to help determine the presence or location of the tympanic membrane. This technique also may reveal false middle ear cavities. Under visualization with a surgical otoscope, the feeding tube is passed down the ear canal to the level where the tympanic membrane is expected to be (Fig. 24-7). In a normal ear the tip of the tube will remain visualized. In animals with false middle ears or ruptured tympanic membranes, the tube will pass beyond view and ventrally below the normal plane of the horizontal canal. Markedly proliferative changes decrease one's ability to assess whether the tube is progressing into the middle ear. However, with practice this procedure can still yield useful information.

Cytologic Evaluation

Cytologic examination of discharge usually does not establish a definitive diagnosis, but it is valuable in determining what infectious agents are present in the ear. If a sample appears representative of the discharge deeper within the canal, it can be collected with a cotton swab from the external orifice or from the tip of the otoscope cone. Alternatively, it may be collected by an ear loop passed through a cone under visualization down the ear canal so the sample selected is most representative. The sample is then smeared on a glass slide. With waxy discharges, heat fixation of the slide with the sample on it will help prevent the sample from being washed away during staining. Modified Wright's stain (Wright's Dip Stat) is a rapid method for adequately staining specimens and has two colors to help differentiate stained items. Its dis-

advantage is that all bacteria stain blue and therefore gram properties cannot be determined.

Cytologic examination reveals any cocci (*Staphylococcus* and/or *Streptococcus*), rods (*Pseudomonas* and/or *Proteus,* other gram-negatives), budding yeasts (*Malassezia* and *Candida*), or mixed infections. The presence of white blood cells, as well as phagocytosis of bacteria, suggests that the body is responding to the infection and treatment for the bacteria is warranted (Fig. 24-8). Toxic neutrophils indicate that the ear canal must be flushed to remove the toxins (Fig. 24-9).

For two reasons cytologic evaluation is the preferred method of ascertaining the role of *M. pachydermatis* in a particular case (Fig. 24-10):

1. In a study I conducted 18% of the cases that had *M. pachydermatis* detected by cytology were sterile when cultured specifically for *Malassezia* at 37° C by a commercial laboratory.

2. Cytologic examination is a crude method of quantifying the relative number of organisms present; a finding of five to ten yeast organisms per high-power field (HPF) is significant and represents yeast overgrowth (Macy, 1989). This rule must be interpreted carefully, because one study that quantified yeast in normal ears (Merchant, 1988) did find high numbers in some normal dogs. I use relative numbers of yeast organisms as a guide but also consider whether they are the major organism present. Mixed infections with numerous cocci and five to ten yeast

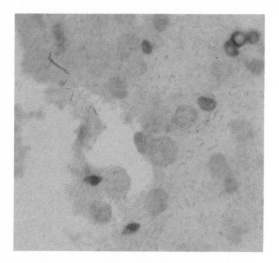

Figure 24-9. Cytology demonstrating swollen toxic neutrophils and numerous rods.

per HPF will often respond to treatment without antifungal activity. In ceruminous otitis externa with only yeast on cytologic examination, even less than five organisms per HPF may require treatment.

The cellular makeup of the exudate can also be determined, and this may help establish a diagnosis. Ceruminous otitis externa is more commonly seen with endocrinopathies and seborrhea; the discharge in this condition is keratin and glandular secretions.

Culture and Sensitivity

Culture and sensitivity should **not** be done without cytologic evaluation. **Nor** should they be per-

formed unless cytologic evaluation demonstrates that bacteria and white blood cells are present in the discharge. When therapy is going to be limited to topical treatment, a culture and sensitivity is rarely cost-effective. The primary indication for doing culture and sensitivity testing is otitis media with bacterial rods, when systemic therapy is to be prescribed. In these instances the sample should be collected with a sterile microculturette swab that is passed through a cone into the horizontal canal or preferably the middle ear.

Obviously many other tests may be needed to make a definitive diagnosis. Which tests are most cost-effective and indicated will depend on the history and complete physical examination findings.

TREATMENT

Therapy of otitis externa is dependent on identifying and controlling the predisposing and primary diseases whenever possible. In addition, cleaning the ear canals and middle ear, topical therapies, and systemic medications may be required for the effective elimination or control of primary causes and perpetuating factors. The box lists ma-

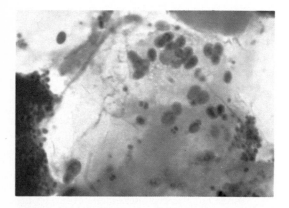

Figure 24-10. *Malassezia pachydermatitis* with some cocci and nuclear strands.

Otitis Externa Treatment Plan

1. Identify and control primary diseases and predisposing factors.
2. Perform a cytologic evaluation to determine which perpetuating microorganisms are present.
3. Clean the ear canal and false middle ear if present or the tympanic bulla if otitis media is present.
4. Allow an appropriate disinfectant to remain in the canal for 3 to 5 minutes.
5. Dry the ear canal.
6. Prescribe topical therapy that will decrease inflammation and treat whichever organisms were identified on the cytologic evaluation.
7. Prescribe systemic therapy if otitis media is present or if potent antiinflammatory effects are required.
8. Reexamine in 1 to 2 weeks to determine whether therapy has been effective and if further cleaning in the hospital or by the client at home will be indicated.

jor components of a successful treatment plan for otitis externa.

Client compliance is critical to the successful management of an otitis externa case. The effort expended in explaining the treatment plan so that the client understands and concurs is the single most important step in managing these cases. Using ear diagrams may help educate the client (Fig. 24-11). It is also important to try to anticipate whether several multiple cleaning procedures will be needed and explain this to the client beforehand. Repetitive cleaning, done while the patient is sedated or anesthetized, is usually necessary in cases with stenotic ear canals resulting from epidermal and dermal proliferation. This is because the acanthosis and hyperkeratosis cannot be reversed immediately and further keratinous secretions are likely to build up, especially in the cobblestone, heavily folded canals.

Examination and adequate cleaning may be accomplished only with appropriate patient restraint. Sedatives such as xylazine HCl or ketamine and diazepam may be sufficient for most cases. Others will require a general anesthetic. Many clients are reluctant to have their dog anesthetized but are often more understanding if the need for getting the ears cleaned and completely examined is explained in detail. It also helps to explain that some procedures are painful, as well as the problems that might occur if the patient moves while instruments are in the ear. Clients feel better knowing that with sedatives or anesthetics their pets will be spared the unnecessary pain and possible damage that could occur from uncontrolled movement during cleaning.

For cases with intact tympanums and small amounts of debris or foreign bodies, a topical anesthetic may be effective restraint. Proparacaine 0.05% (Ophthaine Solution) is usually sufficient. When combined with a sedative, the topical may eliminate the need for a general anesthetic. Two to five drops of proparacaine should be applied every 5 minutes for three treatments. In very waxy and dirty ears the topical anesthetic may not reach the complete ear canal, and sedatives are best.

Cleaning

Thorough cleaning of the ear canal is extremely important for the effective management of otitis externa. In chronic cases with otitis media, this includes cleaning the bulla. Cleaning is valuable for several reasons. Mainly it promotes effective therapy. The presence of an exudate interferes with

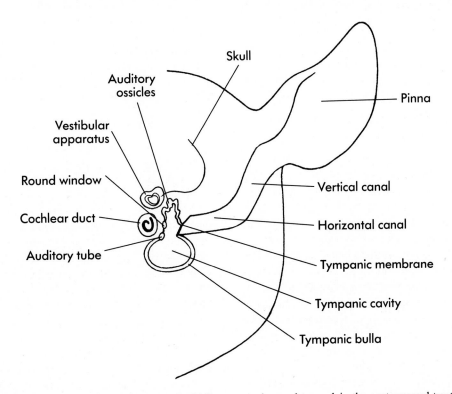

Figure 24-11. This diagram of the external and middle ear may be used to explain the anatomy and treatment objectives to clients.

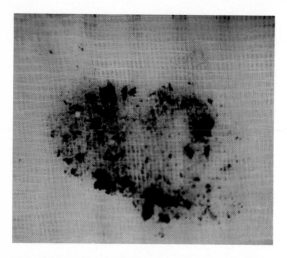

Figure 24-12. The keratinous waxy material on this gauze pad was flushed from the ear canal. If it had been left in the canal, topical therapy might have been blocked from the lower portions of the canal.

adequate examination until cleaned out. Foreign bodies, especially very small ones, are also eliminated when ears are adequately cleaned. Wax or purulent exudate prevents topical medications from reaching the skin lining the canals (Fig. 24-12). Medications are not able to reach the bacteria or yeast present beneath the exudate. Pus and inflammatory debris can inactivate some medications. Thorough cleaning removes bacterial toxins, cellular debris, and free fatty acids, reducing the stimulation for further inflammation. In proliferative ear canals thorough cleaning is one of the most valuable steps in management, just as it is in treating fold dermatitis.

Ceruminolytic Agents

Ceruminolytic agents greatly facilitate and expedite the cleaning procedure. Numerous ceruminolytics are on the market and include surfactants and detergents that act by emulsifying the waxes and lipids, which are then more readily flushed from the ear canal. Dioctyl sodium sulfosuccinate (DSS) and calcium sulfosuccinate, marketed as Surfack and Cerusol, are effective wax and debris emulsifiers. (These products should not be used at all in cats with ruptured tympanums.) Carbamide peroxide is a slightly less potent ceruminolytic that acts as a humectant by releasing urea when activated. It also releases oxygen, creating a foaming action that helps break down or dislodge larger clumps of debris. Carbamide peroxide is particularly helpful with more purulent exudates. The ceruminolytic Clear-X Cleanser combines DSS and

carbamide peroxide, utilizing the surfactant simultaneously with the humectant and oxygen-producing effects of both ingredients. It is an effective one-step ear cleanser for either waxy or purulent exudates.

Other less potent ceruminolytic agents that may be found in products are squalene (Cerumene), triethanolamine polypeptide oleate condensate (Cerumenex), and hexamethyltetracosane (Sebumsol). This group is milder than the detergents and DSS and works best with light waxy buildup. Propylene glycol, glycerin, and oil have a mild ceruminolytic effect and are best utilized for relatively normal, slightly dirty ears.

In general, all the ceruminolytics should be applied 5 to 15 minutes prior to cleaning. Gentle massage improves their effect. Most ceruminolytics and detergents are contraindicated with ruptured tympanums (Mansfield et al., 1990). Some disinfectant cleansers such as chlorhexidine and iodophor are also contraindicated with ruptured tympanums (Galle and Venker–van Haagen, 1986; Igarashi and Oka, 1988). Frequently the condition of the tympanic membrane cannot be determined until after the ear canal has been cleaned. The probability of ototoxicity may be decreased by using ceruminolytics and flushing with water. Additional detergents or disinfectants are not used in the flushing water unless an intact tympanum is noted. If the tympanum has been ruptured, thorough rinsing of the ceruminolytics is mandatory. Ear loops and flushing with water or the use of a suction apparatus will be the least ototoxic method of cleaning if a ruptured tympanum is suspected.

Cleaning Techniques

A variety of instruments are required to adequately clean the majority of ear canals presented. The items listed in the box are those I use.

Several methods for removing pus, debris, and emulsified waxes and lipids have been described. One of the easiest to set up, implement, and clean up after is the rubber ear bulb syringe. After a ceruminolytic agent has been instilled, repeated flushing with lukewarm water will remove most of the exudate. When the tympanic membrane is known to be intact, use of a detergent or disinfectant solution may improve results. A space should always be left between the rubber nipple and the canal orifice. This allows back flow and helps prevent excessive pressure on the tympanic membrane. This procedure is not effective for cleaning false middle ears or the tympanic bulla.

A feeding tube and a 12 ml syringe are very

Ear Cleaning Instruments

Alligator forceps
Ear curettes or ear loops (various sizes)
A 12 ml syringe
Feeding tubes cut to varying lengths to fit
on the syringe
Rubber ear bulb syringes
Ceruminolytic agents
Halogen otoscope with surgical head and a
variety of cones in different sizes
Suction apparatus
Frazier suction tip

---

effective for flushing the ear canal. Several different-diameter feeding tubes cut to differing lengths can be kept in cold sterilization. One attached to a water-filled syringe is passed through a surgical otoscope head and cone and down the ear canal. Once the tip is located where desired, the water can be infused and aspirated back out, along with any debris that has broken up. In severe cases and whenever the tympanum is ruptured, flushing with a syringe and feeding tube is the most effective technique and is usually preferred. This is also the method of choice for drying the ear, especially when there is no tympanum present.

Once the residual fluid has been removed, the ear canal is thoroughly examined. Any remaining wax or debris should be removed by repeated flushing or the use of an ear loop or curette. Ear curettes are effective in several situations: after flushing, in milder waxy/crusty cases, when there are small foreign bodies, and for removal of leftover wax. When larger foreign bodies or keratin plugs are present in the middle ear, an alligator forceps may be used; however, the ear curette is usually preferred.

In this technique the curette or loop (rather than a cotton swab) is gently pulled along the epidermis of the ear canal to break loose any debris. It is passed down the canal through a surgical otoscope head, moved along the canal epithelium until the wax to be extracted is reached, and then rolled over the debris and gently pulled out of the canal. In this way the risk of damaging an intact eardrum will be minimized.

Using a suction apparatus is possibly the most effective method of cleaning ears when there is thick pus or keratin plugs in the middle ear. The Frazier suction tip works well. It can be positioned to exactly the desired location prior to initiating suction. When ceruminolytics must be avoided, the suction apparatus is very effective for rapidly cleaning the external canal and middle ear cavity. However, it has three important disadvantages: (1) the lack of infusion liquid, (2) limited access to the middle ear, and (3) the time needed to clean the equipment.

Some clinicians use a dental water propulsion device (Water-Pik), which rapidly cleans the ear with multiple rapid pulses of water. However, it has no suction, and the time needed to set up and clean the equipment negates the advantages it seems to offer. It is not as effective for cleaning the middle ear as the syringe and feeding tube. Care must also be taken to avoid directing the pulsating stream directly onto a damaged tympanic membrane. Using a curved water current diffuser will help avoid damage to the tympanic membrane (Anthony Products).

Once flushing has been completed, the ear canal is dried or, in cases complicated by bacteria, a disinfectant may be applied. When the tympanic membrane is intact, a chlorhexidine solution (e.g., ChlorhexiDerm Otic or Nolvasan Otic) is extremely effective. If the tympanum is ruptured, acetic acid at 2% or 5% strength may be preferred; however, at 5%, acetic acid can cause a slight burning sensation when applied to inflamed, eroded, or ulcerated epithelium so this should be done while the patient is still sedated.

A vestibular syndrome or deafness may develop after ear flushing, even when no ototoxic drugs have been utilized, but is quite uncommon. However, when it occurs, it is generally permanent. Compensation usually occurs, especially in cats, which may be able to do so well that they appear almost normal.

Drying Agents

After the ear is cleaned and relatively dry, topical medications or drying agents can be used. Most contain isopropyl alcohol and one or more of the following: boric acid, benzoic acid, salicylic acid, acetic acid, sulfur, silicone dioxide. Veterinary products of this type include Clear-X Treatment Dryer, Oticare B, Panodry, and Otic Clear. These products can be used at home for prophylactic treatment of swimmer's ear and as a deodorizer. Alcohol and higher concentrations of the acids may be irritating or cause a burning sensation in ulcerated ears.

Combination Products

Another group of ear cleansers are actually combination products. These are utilized most effectively in ears that appear slightly dirty at examination but are not the presenting complaint. They may be helpful in ears that have a mildly objectionable odor, but they are not indicated for the treatment of clinical otitis externa. They have been utilized in the long-term management of milder recurrent waxy otitis externa after the initial episode was controlled. They tend to have less drying ingredients and to be more antimicrobial and mildly ceruminolytic than the standard desiccants. Some are primarily mild cleansers with disinfectant and drying agents added. A variety of ingredients are combined with the drying agents to achieve these effects—propylene glycol, lanolin, glycerin, lactic acid, parachlorometaxalone, chlorhexidine. Some veterinary products in this group include Epi-Otic, Oticlens A, Oti-Fresh, Nolvasan Otic, and ChlorhexiDerm Otic. An advantage of these products is their lack of antibiotics or potent glucocorticoids, which might induce bacterial resistance or adrenal suppression.

Home Flushing

Animals with especially waxy or exudative ears may need to have their ears cleaned so that topical medications can be properly applied. In most chronic cases the combination cleanser-dryers are not sufficient. For these the client should be instructed in home flushing with a ceruminolytic and the ear bulb syringe.

Home flushing is helpful for dogs with ceruminous otitis from keratinization disorders (box) or allergic diseases. Cases for home flushing must be carefully selected. In general, the tympanum should be intact if a ceruminolytic is going to be used, because the client may not be able to rinse all the drug away adequately and repetitive application could be dangerous, especially if some drug remains. The client must be willing and able to try flushing, and the dog must be tolerant of the procedure. Many dogs will tolerate home flushing after the initial inflammation and pain have resolved. Therefore this procedure is only rarely recommended in acutely inflamed or ulcerated ears. Dogs with chronic allergies and ketatinization disorders require frequent bathing, and this is when the ears should be cleaned. A ceruminolytic agent is applied just prior to the bath. Which type will depend on the severity and nature of the ear disease and exudate. After the body is lathered with shampoo, the ears are flushed and rinsed with equal amounts of white vinegar and water. Detergents should not be used for home flushing. The flushed-out debris is rinsed away with the shampoo. At the end of

---

Treatment Plan for Chronic Ceruminous Otitis Externa

1. Control perpetuating factors with appropriate antibiotics, antifungals, and glucocorticoids.
   a. Long-term home flushing will be required at weekly, bimonthly, or monthly intervals.
   b. Until the tympanic membrane is determined to be intact, use carbamide peroxide and flush with water or white vinegar and water in equal amounts.
2. In cases with intact tympanic membranes, clean with Clear-X Cleanser and rinse with water or vinegar and water.
3. Clean the external orifice and concave pinna with topical antiseborrheic tar shampoo.
4. Once or twice weekly apply drying, mildly antiinflammatory disinfectant and keratolytic agents (e.g., Clear-X Treatment Dryer) to the ear canals.

---

the bath the ears should be given a final rinse and drying solution applied. Clients should use cotton balls or swabs only in the external orifice, not down the ear canal.

Procedures that induce drainage and ventilation may be helpful. Simple ones include clipping the hair off the pinnae and plucking hair from the canals. Taping or mattress suturing the pinnae up over the head can be beneficial. Some dogs do not tolerate having their ears taped up, and an Elizabethan collar or bucket may be needed to prevent further trauma.

Surgical procedures that can be done to promote drainage or ventilation are described in most surgical textbooks. It should be emphasized that these procedures do not replace a thorough diagnostic workup and case selection should be done carefully. Surgical debridement is indicated in cases with marked proliferative changes of the medial wall.

Topical Therapeutic Agents

There is no one perfect topical otic treatment or product. The clinician should prescribe topical therapeutics for each ear based upon the desired effect. As the case progresses, the patient should be monitored and products changed accordingly.

Numerous topicals for the external ear canal are available. Most contain various combinations of glucocorticoids, antibacterials, antifungals, and parasiticidals. Each of these types of ingredients will be discussed, but the clinician should also be aware of the vehicle. The base or type of vehicle should be considered when selecting a treatment for otitis externa. In general, dry, scaly, crusty lesions are benefited by oil or ointment bases, which help moisturize the skin. Moist, exudative ears should be treated with solutions or lotions, not occlusive ointments or oils. Creams are often poor choices because the client may have difficulty getting the medication to the horizontal canal. In addition, many clients find it esthetically more pleasant to apply fluid drops than to have to insert an applicator with viscous materials into the ear canal.

Active Ingredients

Glucocorticoids have antipruritic, antiinflammatory effects and decrease exudation and swelling. In addition, they cause sebaceous atrophy and decrease glandular secretions. They may also reduce scar tissue and proliferative changes, thus helping to promote drainage and ventilation. There are many different types of topical glucocorticoids available, and it is best to choose several products of differing potency and become familiar with them. Otic products containing triamcinolone acetonide (Panolog) or dexamethasone (Tresaderm) are absorbed systemically (Moriello et al., 1988). In the study by Moriello et al. (1988), treated dogs had elevated liver enzymes and suppressed adrenal response to ACTH stimulation. The systemic absorption of more potent topical glucocorticoids should make the clinician cautious of long-term treatment. Initial therapy or treatment during acute exacerbations may require a potent topical glucocorticoid (e.g., fluocinolone, betamethasone, dexamethasone); but once the inflammation or allergic reaction is controlled, prophylactic or long-term therapy should utilize the least potent topical glucocorticoid possible. Fluocinolone acetonide in 60% dimethyl sulfoxide (Synotic) is the most potent veterinary solution available. In cases of allergic otitis externa, long-term topical glucocorticoids may be utilized as indicated in the box. Long-term therapy is safer with products containing 1% or 0.5% hydrocortisone such as HB101 and Clear-X Treatment Drying Solution. In cases of atopy or food allergy–induced otitis externa the pinna is frequently affected and should also be treated. An-

---

Treatment Plan for Allergic Otitis Externa

1. Control perpetuating factors with appropriate antibacterial or antifungal therapy.
2. Apply a potent topical glucocorticoid (e.g., fluocinolone, betamethasone, or dexamethasone) to the concave pinna and external ear canal until inflammation is gone. If antibiotics are not needed, Synotic or a mixture of 7.5 ml dexamethasone phosphate (4 mg/ml) is added to 22.5 ml of propylene glycol or Burow's solution (HB101), or PTD Lotion may be used.
3. After inflammation has resolved, decrease the frequency of application to every other day or less.
4. Switch to topical prophylactic therapy with 0.5% to 2.5% hydrocortisone at every-other-day or less frequency. (Products include HB101, PTD-HC, Cortispray, Epi-Otic HC, and Clear-X Treatment Dryer.)
5. Occasionally a disinfectant or stronger glucocorticoid may be needed, especially when clients temporarily discontinue prophylactic treatment.

---

tibiotic agents are present in many topical ear products. Uncomplicated cases of allergic or ceruminous otitis externa may be managed by topical glucocorticoids alone; however, remember that inappropriate use of combination products with topical antibiotics can cause a secondary superinfection.

Clients should be cautioned not to let their own skin contact topical glucocorticoids. At the very least they should wash their hands after contacting these medications. Human facial skin is especially sensitive to potent topical glucocorticoids, and clients should be cautioned especially against allowing these products to contact their face. To prevent any contact, topicals can be applied with applicators or protected fingers. Gloves or plastic wrap should be used to cover the fingers.

Topical **antibacterials** are indicated for cases of otitis with bacteria present, whether primary or secondary.

The aminoglycosides neomycin (Tresaderm), neomycin-polymyxin (Forte-Topical), and gentamicin (Gentocin Otic) are potent antibiotics with good activity against the pathogens usually found in otitis externa. Gram-negative gentamicin-resistant infections may be successfully treated with injectable amikacin, 50 mg/ml (3 to 5 drops each ear) q12h. However, the aminoglycosides can be ototoxic with prolonged use or in animals with a ruptured tympanum. Presoaking the ear with edetate trisodium (*tris* EDTA) or mixing gentamicin at 3 mg/ml with *tris* EDTA will increase the efficacy of these antibiotics against gram-negative organisms. *Tris* EDTA, a chelating agent, is made by mixing 6.05 g of edetate disodium with 12 g of tromethamine (Trizma base) and bringing to 1 L by the addition of double-distilled water. The mixture is then pH adjusted to 8, usually by adding an acid such as hydrochloric. The pH-balanced solution should be autoclaved so that it will be sterile.

Chloramphenicol (Liquichlor with Cerumene) is also effective, but it may stimulate excessive granulation tissue formation in the middle ear. Also clients should be careful not to contact chloramphenicol, due to the possibility of bone marrow suppression. Utilizing topical antibiotics that are not likely to be needed as systemic drugs may impede the development of resistant cases of otitis media. The more potent and broad-spectrum antibiotics (gentamicin, chloramphenicol) should not be used as first-choice treatments, lest we unnecessarily create resistant strains of bacteria. I prefer neomycin-polymyxin combinations as first-line topical antibiotics. Most topical antibiotics also contain a glucocorticoid, and it may not always be the desirable strength.

Topical antiseptics such as povidone, chlorhexidine, and acetic acid are also helpful in the treatment of bacterial otitis externa. Acetic acid has been shown very effective in the treatment of otitis externa in humans. It is believed that its activity is not completely due to the pH, because other acidic products are not as effective in killing *Pseudomonas* and *Staphylococcus*. Acetic acid is most effective against *Pseudomonas,* with a 2% solution being lethal within 1 minute of contact. *Staphylococcus* and *Streptococcus* can be killed within 5 minutes of contact with 5% acetic acid. However, this concentration is occasionally irritating. Recently Thomas (1990) reported 1% silver sulfadiazine to be an effective antimicrobial in cases of otitis externa. It is made by mixing 1 gm of silver sulfadiazine with 100 ml of sterile water; 0.5 ml of the mixture is applied to the ear twice daily. *Pseudomonas* infections are particularly frustrating to treat. (See box for treatment options.)

Treatment Options for *Pseudomonas* Infection

1. Gentamicin*
2. Amikacin* 50 mg/ml (injectable applied undiluted) 3 to 5 drops/ear q12h and not mixed with other ear drops
3. Neomycin-polymyxin combination* (requires clean ear at all treatments)
4. *Tris* EDTA, used for 15 minutes prior to an aminoglycoside
5. Chlorhexidine 1%*
6. Silver sulfadiazene 1% (or use Silvadene Cream diluted with an equal amount of water for a 0.5% solution)
7. Acetic acid 2.5% (requires at least a 1-minute soak)
8. Injectable enrofloxacin (Baytril) or carbenicillin as an ear drop†
9. Systemic enrofloxacin, gentamycin, amikacin, carbenicillin

*These ingredients are known to be ototoxic if they reach the inner ear.
†Safety with a ruptured tympanum is not known.

Antifungal agents are required in any case complicated or caused by the yeasts *Malassezia* or *Candida* and/or dermatophytes. In vitro testing has shown cuprimyxin (Unitop) and nystatin (Panolog) to be effective against *Malassezia*. Thiabendazole (Tresaderm), although not effective in vitro, may work in vivo. In cases not responsive to the other antifungals or when *Malassezia* eradication is the primary objective, topical 1% miconazole (Conofite Lotion) has been very effective. Resistant *Candida* cases can be treated with topical amphotericin B (Fungizone). For dermatophytosis, topical miconazole or thiabendazole is usually effective.

Parasiticidal drugs that are frequently used for *Otodectes* mites include pyrethrins (Cerumite, OtiCare M), rotenone (Canex), thiabendazole (Tresaderm), and carbaryl (Mitox).

In addition to utilizing an effective parasiticidal agent, two important points should always be considered: First, many animals may be asymptomatic carriers of *Otodectes;* because of this, all in-contact animals, both dogs and cats, must be treated. Second, *Otodectes* can be found on other body areas and therefore whole-body treatments with effective parasiticidals must be done. (See "Systemic Therapy," below.) The life cycle of *Otodectes* requires that otic and body treatment be continued for at least 3 weeks, a month being required in some cases.

Office Combinations

Many practitioners formulate their own topical otic products. However, care should be taken when mixing commercial products since incompatibilities are possible. Many ingredients are effective at a narrow pH range, and mixing can affect this. Some need to be present at a specific concentration, and mixing lowers the concentration delivered. Other combinations such as Synotic and amikacin may cause a precipitate. Most commercial otic products contain many ingredients other than the active ones, such as vehicles and preservatives, that may not be compatible with other active ingredients.

The advantage of office formulating is that the practitioner can select all the ingredients that will be needed for a specific case. If only two products are going to be mixed, there is another way to achieve the same or better effect. Both products are dispensed, and the client is instructed to treat with both products but at different times of the day. For example, when both *Pseudomonas* and *Malassezia* must be treated, Conofite Lotion is used once daily in the afternoon and Gentocin Otic is applied in the morning and at bedtime. Allergic otitis externa with gentamicin-resistant *Pseudomonas* may be treated with once-daily Synotic for the potent antiinflammatory effect and twice-daily amikacin injectable as eardrops.

Systemic Therapy

Systemic therapy is indicated if otitis media is present. Appropriate antibiotics or antifungals should be used until 1 week after there is no clinical or otoscopic evidence of disease. Antibiotics known to penetrate bone or to have a good history in treating otitis media should be selected and given at dosages that are on the high end of recommended. Antibiotics that are useful for otitis media include ormetoprin-sulfadimethoxine (Primor), 27.5 mg/kg q24h; trimethoprim-sulfas, 25 mg/kg q12h; clindamycin (Antirobe), 7 to 10 mg/kg q12h; cephalexin, 22 mg/kg q12h; and enrofloxacin (Baytril), 2.5 mg/kg q12h. Ketoconazole (Nizoral) 5 to 10 mg/kg q12-24h is given when otitis media occurs with *Malassezia* infection. Otoscopic examination is also required.

Although not approved for this use, ivermectin is an extremely effective systemic therapy for *Otodectes* infection. When given subcutaneously at 250 μg/kg and repeated three times at 10-day intervals, it eradicates the ear mites. This form of therapy treats the whole pet and will eliminate a carrier state; it therefore can be used to rule out *Otodectes* from the differential. In some recurrent cases related to ear mites the use of ivermectin in all the household pets has been very rewarding. **Collies and Collie crosses should not be treated with ivermectin!**

Systemic glucocorticoid therapy is indicated in markedly inflamed endematous otitis and when chronic pathologic changes cause marked stenosis of the canal lumen. Some cases of allergic otitis can be treated with systemic glucocorticoids, allowing the initial topical therapy to be a low-potency glucocorticoid product. Injectable dexamethasone is useful if only 2 to 3 days' action is required. For the uncommon case with stenosis primarily of the vertical canal, intralesional triamcinolone acetonide may be helpful. Triamcinolone is particularly effective for inhibiting fibroblasts and reducing collagen. When long-term treatment is expected, alternate-day, short-acting glucocorticoid therapy is indicated. In some dogs, especially Cocker Spaniels with markedly proliferative ear canals, intralesional triamcinolone may be more effective at reducing the fribrosis and swelling. Vetalog Injectable is deposited through a spinal needle in a ring pattern around the canal, approximately 0.2 ml in each of three or four locations for a total of up to 1 ml. This will generally be better than systemic or topical therapy for reducing fibrosis.

Isotretinoin (Accutane) and etretinate (Tegison) have been helpful in a limited number of cases of otitis externa. Isotretinoin was used in a few dogs and cats that had histologic evidence of sebaceous hyperplasia. Although it appeared to be helpful, it was stopped because of side effects or expense. Etretinate may be helpful in some cases with hyperproliferative forms of primary keratinization disorders. One study of etretinate in Cocker Spaniels with primary keratinization disorders (Power, 1989) showed no benefit in the dogs' ear disease. However, in these cases other perpetuating factors were not adequately treated. When the ears are repetitively cleaned and concurrent infections are treated, the drug may have some benefit. Further work and more studies with both these drugs are needed.

Surgery

Surgery is indicated when there is stenosis of the canal, when a tumor or polyps need to be removed, or when the animal has a medically resistant otitis media. It is imperative, for best results, that the primary diagnosis be determined prior to surgery. Many dogs have undergone a surgical procedure and then continued to suffer from otitis externa. In some cases that have undergone a modified Lacroix Zepp the otitis has persisted. This procedure should be restricted to cases with stenosis of the vertical canal only. Although some cases may be easier to treat following a Lacroix Zepp, clients not properly educated regarding what to expect from it may be dissatisfied with its results. Even cases that have been successfully ablated have had persistent pruritus and inflammation of the pinnae.

Surgical intervention is indicated when otitis media does not respond to a combination of flushing and aspiration of the bulla along with systemic and topical therapy. Although bulla osteotomy and various drainage procedures are sometimes sufficient, other more severe cases may require a total ear ablation. In my experience, ear ablations have been the only completely effective solution in animals with calcified external ear canals and otitis media.

REFERENCES

August JR: Diseases of the ear canal. In Solvay Veterinary Inc: The complete manual of ear care, Trenton NJ, 1986, Veterinary Learning Systems USA, p 37.

Frost RC: Canine otoacariasis, J Small Anim Pract 2:253, 1961.

Galle HG, Venker-van Haagen AJ: Ototoxicity of the antiseptic combination chlorhexidine/cetrimide (Savlon): effects on equilibrium and hearing, Vet Q 8:56, 1986.

Igarashi Y, Oka Y: Vestibular ototoxicity following intratympanic applications of chlorhexidine gluconate in the cat, Arch Otorhinolaryngol 245:210, 1988.

Little CJL, Lane JG: An evaluation of tympanometry, otoscopy and palpation for assessment of the canine tympanic membrane, Vet Rec 124:5, 1989.

Little CJL, et al: Inflammatory middle ear disease of the dog: the pathology of otitis media, Vet Rec 128:293, 1991a.

Little CJL, et al: Inflammatory middle ear disease of the dog: the clinical and pathological features of cholesteatoma—a complication of otitis media, Vet Rec 128:319, 1991b.

Macy DW: Diseases of the ear. In Ettinger SJ (ed): Textbook of veterinary internal medicine, ed 3, Philadelphia, 1989, WB Saunders, p 246.

Mansfield PD: Ototoxicity in dogs and cats, Compend Contin Educ Pract Vet 12:331, 1990.

Mansfield PD, et al: Infectivity of *Malassezia pachydermatis* in the external ear canal of dogs, J Am Anim Hosp Assoc, 26:97, 1990.

Merchant S: Quantitative and qualitative analysis of bacteria and yeast from normal canine ears. In Proceedings, Annual members' meeting AAVD & ACVD, Washington DC, 1988, p 12.

Moriello KA, et al: Adrenocortical suppression associated with topical otic administration of glucocorticoids in dogs, J Am Vet Med Assoc 193:329, 1988.

Powell MB, et al: Reaginic hypersensitivity in *Otodectes cynotis* infestation of cats and mode of mite feeding, Am J Vet Res 41:877, 1980

Power HT: The efficacy of etretinate (Tegison) in the treatment of keratinization disorders in dogs. In Proceedings, Annual members' meeting AAVD & ACVD, St Louis, 1989, p 17.

Rosser EJ. In Bigler B, Merchant SR: Otitis externa (Workshop report 8). In von Tscharner C, Halliwell REW (eds): Advances in veterinary dermatology, vol 1, London, 1990, Ballière Tindall, p 414.

Stout-Graham M, et al: Morphologic measurements of the external horizontal ear canal of dogs, Am J Vet Res 51:990, 1990.

Thomas ML: Development of a bacterial model for canine otitis externa. In Proceedings, Annual members' meeting AAVD & ACVD, San Francisco, 1990, p 28.

Trettien AL: The role of *Malassezia pachydermatis* in the external ear canal of normal dogs. In Proceedings, Annual members' meeting AAVD & ACVD, Phoenix, 1987, p 26.

Weisbroth SH, et al: Immunopathology of naturally occurring otodectic otoacariasis in the domestic cat, Am J Vet Res 165:1088, 1974.

Cutaneous Manifestations of Internal Disease

25

Canine Hypothyroidism

Robert J. Kemppainen   John M. MacDonald

Diagnostic Criteria for Canine Hypothyroidism

SUGGESTIVE
History and clinical findings

COMPATIBLE
Suggestive plus a borderline low T_4/T_3, a nonregenerative anemia, and a compatible dermatohistopathology

TENTATIVE
Supportive history and clinical findings with a low T_4

DEFINITIVE
Abnormal TSH response test or thyroid biopsy *or* a low T_4 and a sustained response to thyroid hormone supplementation

Importance

Hypothyroidism has long been recognized as a common problem causing skin disease in dogs (although, based on samples submitted to the Auburn University Endocrine Diagnostic Laboratory, hyperadrenocorticism is actually more common). The thyroid is undoubtedly the most frequently evaluated endocrine tissue in canine species, in which measurement of serum thyroxine is often an automatic component of a laboratory data base. The relatively low cost and commercial availability of tests measuring thyroxine (T_4) and triiodothyronine (T_3) permit the routine acquisition of these hormone assays. However, misdiagnosis of hypothyroidism occurs commonly by the erroneous interpretation of borderline-low thyroid hormone levels (T_4/T_3). These values usually result from coexisting nonthyroidal diseases or the effect of medication.

Therapeutic trials with thyroid hormones are often conducted to determine clinical response and aid in the diagnosis of thyroid dysfunction. Many times the trials are performed despite normal test values. Misinterpretation of treatment response may also occur since some transient changes of skin and hair are seen in euthyroid dogs placed on supplementation. Hypothyroidism is one of the most overdiagnosed diseases in veterinary dermatology. Bilaterally symmetric alopecia with hyperpigmentation and lichenification is often assumed to be associated with thyroid dysfunction when actually it is the result of an allergic dermatopathy or some other primary disease. Dogs with the disease may have a secondary suppression of thyroid activity. Glucocorticoid therapy may further depress the thyroid hormone levels. Anxiousness to find new explanations for the problem often leads to over interpretation of the thyroid test results. Many disease symptoms overlap with the expected lesions of hypothyroidism. Primary keratinization defects (Chapters 16 and 17) or other causes of scaling are often attributed to hypothyroidism without thorough evaluation. Differentiation by clinical presentation is not possible. Evaluating the patient for coexisting diseases is usually necessary.

Although thyroid function is easily evaluated in dogs using the measurement of basal T_4 (and T_3), it is often best to consider more extensive (and expensive) diagnostic tests for accurate confirmation. Unfortunately, the array of clinically useful, definitive tests of thyroid function for the canine is quite limited. Several tests currently promoted have not been validated.

Pathogenesis

Receptors for thyroid hormones are present in virtually all tissues of the body. Thyroid hormones are critical regulatory substances at the cellular level, controlling enzymes and other proteins involved in metabolic regulation. Thyroid hormones are important in the skin for maintaining normal keratinization, sebum production, hair growth cycle activity (telogen, anagen shifting) and bacterial flora. Since thyroid hormones are necessary for hair growth, reductions in T_4 and T_3 lead to increased numbers of inactive (telogen) hair follicles.

By far, the most common form of thyroid disease in dogs is primary hypothyroidism as a result of either lymphocytic thyroiditis or idiopathic atrophy of the gland. It is not clear whether idiopathic atrophy simply represents an end stage of lymphocytic thyroiditis or occurs as a spontaneous condition. Autoimmune mechanisms are thought to be involved in the initial attack upon the thyroid (at least in lymphocytic thyroiditis). Thyroid biopsies taken during acute stages of lymphocytic thyroiditis show a tissue infiltrate consisting of lymphocytes and plasma cells. Secondary hypothyroidism caused by deficient secretion of pituitary thyrotropin (TSH) has been documented, albeit rarely.

Clinically it is important to note that loss of thyroidal function is a slow, progressive process. The amount of T_4 and T_3 secreted by the gland declines as loss of thyroid tissue occurs. However, the remaining functional tissue attempts to compensate by secreting thyroid hormones at proportionately higher rates. This latter response is a direct consequence of an increase in circulating TSH concentrations, the pituitary hormone responsible

for T_4 and T_3 synthesis and secretion. Thus clinical signs of thyroid failure are not apparent until the majority of thyroidal tissue is lost. During this stage the thyroid is **incapable** of responding normally to an injection of exogenous TSH since it is already functioning at near maximal capacity due to high endogenous TSH in circulation.

CLINICAL DISEASE
History

Hypothyroidism is most commonly diagnosed in middle aged dogs of either sex and appears to be more common in mid to large breeds. Breeds often demonstrating antithyroglobulin antibodies include Doberman Pinschers, Great Danes, Irish Setters, and Old English Sheepdogs (Haines et al. 1984). Familial lymphocytic thyroiditis has been reported in Borzois (Conaway et al. 1985). Spontaneous occurring hypothyroidism has not been convincingly documented in the cat although it has been incriminated as the cause of skin conditions.

Disease features develop gradually and may not have been apparent to the pet owner at the onset, thereby influencing the history of the problem. Recognition of clinical signs by the owner may become apparent only when they have reached more dramatic proportions. Hypothyroidism may result in the following:

Lethargy
Mental dullness
Reproductive failure
Heat seeking
Dry, brittle, lusterless hair coat
Bilaterally symetric alopecia
Hyperpigmentation
Recurrent pyoderma

Early signs of lethargy, weakness, decreased appetite, or weight gain can sometimes distract one's attention from cutaneous changes. Decreased pet function may be the primary complaint, particularly in sporting dogs or breeding animals. Prolonged anestrus and/or loss of libido are related to reduced or deficient cellular metabolic activity. Secondary cardiac changes (bradycardia and first degree heart block) may be a cause of exercise intolerance. The classic historical features (including thermophilia) may not be present.

Pruritus is not a direct consequence of hypothyroidism, but can occur subsequent to bacterial infections. Hypothyroidism may be the primary cause of chronic recurrent superficial or deep pyodermas and should be considered in any case with this background. Coexisting pruritic dermatopathies (canine atopy, flea allergy, food allergy, bacterial pyoderma) may obscure the historical and physical examination features.

Historical questions should include a review of constitutional features, including activity level, mental acuity, performance, sexual characteristics of intact animals, heat-seeking tendencies, recurrent skin infections (bacterial pyoderma or dermatophytosis), water consumption, and urination. Differentiation from or association with pruritic diseases should be pursued by questions related to itching habits observed in the pet.

Physical Examination

Although the loss of general metabolic activity may be the first indication of thyroid hormone deficiency, clients often present their hypothyroid

dogs for veterinary evaluation when dermatologic abnormalities become evident. The first dermatologic signs of hypothyroidism usually include development of a dry, scaly coat and constant shedding (Fig. 25-1). Failure of hair regrowth is also apparent early in the course of the disease and existing hairs lack luster, are dry and brittle, and epilate easily (Fig. 25-2). Hair loss in the classic case is bilateral and symmetric and most evident at frictional surfaces, especially the axillae, ventrocervical and thoracic areas, and the tail (Fig. 25-3).

The skin is occasionally thickened in hypothyroidism due to the dermal deposition of mucopolysaccharides. If profound, this deposition may lead to myxedema, which is noted classically as a "tragic" facial expression (Fig. 25-4). Hyperpigmentation often occurs in chronic cases (Fig. 25-5) but should not be strictly associated with thyroid dysfunction since the most common cause is a cutaneous response to inflammation. (See Chapter 23.)

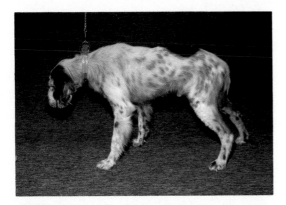

Figure 25-1. Primary hypothyroidism in an adult English Setter. Note the truncal distribution of the hair loss and the depressed attitude of the dog. An electroencephalogram revealed minimal electrical activity.

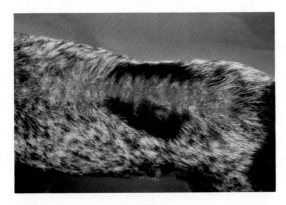

Figure 25-2. A localized area of alopecia with scales and crust on a hypothyroid dog with a history of failure to regrow hair. The existing hair was dry, brittle, and easily epilated.

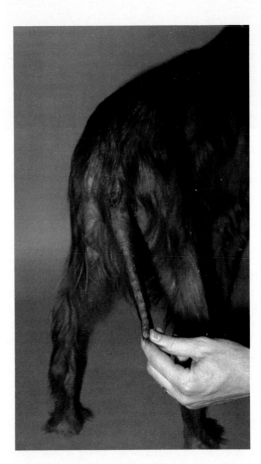

Figure 25-3. The tail of this hypothyroid dog shows the typical ratlike appearance. Hair loss was also noticeable over the trunk.

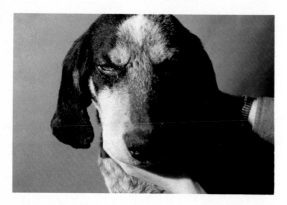

Figure 25-4. Facial features of the hypothyroid dog in Fig. 25-2, showing signs of myxedema and a "tragic expression." The dog was presented for depression and lethargy.

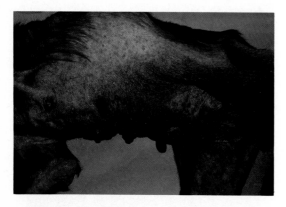

Figure 25-5. The caudal abdomen of this hypothyroid Irish Setter demonstrates intense secondary hyperpigmentation. Note also the papular eruption on the trunk caused by a secondary staphylococcal pyoderma.

Hypothyroidism has a variety of clinical appearances. Although the majority of dogs with end stage primary hypothyroidism will present with lethargy and bilateral nonpruritic alopecia, one should not rule out the disease in the absence of these signs. Since thyroid hormones influence virtually all tissues of the body, hypothyroidism should be considered when any clinical sign explainable by a reduction in cellular metabolic activity is observed.

DIAGNOSIS

Once the presenting clinical signs and history suggest the possibility of hypothyroidism, confirmation or exclusion of the diagnosis is usually based on supporting laboratory findings and sub-

sequent direct measurement of deficient thyroid hormone secretion. Laboratory findings commonly associated with canine hypothyroidism include hypercholesterolemia (mainly due to reduced cholesterol clearance) and a normocytic, normochromic anemia (probably secondary to reduced oxygen utilization and erythropoietin production). Although these findings are commonly observed in documented cases of hypothyroidism (occurring in 50% to 70% of cases), they are not specific but occur in association with a variety of other disorders. Confirmation of hypothyroidism requires documentation of reduced or absent thyroid function, based upon direct evaluation of this endocrine system.

Routine Endocrine Tests Used to Diagnose Canine Hypothyroidism

Basal Measurements of T_4 and T_3 Concentrations

Measurement of serum or plasma concentrations of T_4 and T_3 in dogs under nonstimulated or basal conditions is the most common method of evaluation. Generally these measurements should be viewed as a screening procedure—i.e., measurement of T_4 and T_3 concentrations that are well within the normal range established for a particular diagnostic laboratory rules out hypothyroidism. For example, in the Auburn University Endocrine Diagnostic Laboratory, a T_4 concentration greater than 20 nmol/L (1.5 μg/100 ml) is interpreted as consistent with normal thyroid function (Table 25-1). It is unlikely that a dog would develop clinical signs of thyroid hormone deficiency if circulating T_4 concentrations were at this level or higher. One should attempt to utilize diagnostic laboratories that have validated their assays for samples from dogs and that can provide normal ranges established using those procedures.

A more difficult situation arises when the T_4 or T_3 concentration is below this "cutoff" level. In dogs with a failing thyroid one would expect to measure borderline concentrations of both hormones for a time as clinical signs of deficiency developed. Nonthyroidal factors, however, can profoundly influence (lower) circulating concentrations of T_4, and especially T_3. Such factors include therapy with drugs (glucocorticoids, anticonvulsants, phenylbutazone) and a variety of illnesses (renal failure, liver disease, diabetes mellitus, hyperadrenocorticism, systemic infection, pyoderma, demodicosis, blastomycosis). The magnitude of suppression likely varies directly with the

Table 25-1. Flow chart for endocrine evaluation of canine hypothyroidism

	MEASURE BASAL T_4 AND T_3			
T_4 CONCENTRATION* T_3 CONCENTRATION	>20 >0.7	<10 <0.7	<10 <0.7	>10 but <20 VARIABLE
Nonthyroid illness or drugs (from history)?	Yes or no	No	Yes	Yes or no
Diagnosis	Normal	Hypothyroid	Not sure	Not sure
Next step	Consider another diagnosis	Treat with T_4	TSH stimulation	TSH stimulation

*All concentrations in nmol/L.
Normal values (Auburn University Endocrine Diagnostic Laboratory): T_4 = 20 to 55 nmol/L; T_3 = 0.7 to 2.3 nmol/L.

severity of the illness, the dose of medication, and the form of drug administered. Much individual variation is observed. Reductions in circulating thyroid hormone concentration are believed to be normal metabolic adaptations to either the medication or disease, and are not thought to reflect thyroidal failure. However, such influences have direct impact upon evaluation of thyroid hormone concentrations determined under basal conditions. Generally most animals with borderline-low thyroid hormones will demonstrate an adequate response when the TSH response test is performed. Repeating basal levels is a method of monitoring thyroid status. Further depression of basal levels from specimens collected 6 to 8 weeks later may indicate a failing thyroid, or a return to normal following elimination of the illness may suggest normal thyroid function.

In the absence of concurrent therapy with these drugs or evidence of other relatively severe illness, measurement of very low serum T_4 and T_3 concentrations in a dog with clinical hypothyroidism should be sufficient evidence to make a clinical diagnosis. However, quite commonly concentrations of these hormones will be in the "borderline" range in dogs who also have been treated with glucocorticoids for skin problems. Thyroid function should be further evaluated in these patients with more definitive tests of thyroid function (which currently involve TSH stimulation testing).

For two main reasons basal T_4 levels are a more accurate measure of thyroid function than T_3 levels. First, T_4 is the major hormone secreted by the thyroid. Second, the majority of T_3 in the body resides inside cells and is not in circulation. Levels of T_3 may be more sensitive to alteration by nonthyroidal influences. Comparing T_3 with T_4 does assist in the confirmation of hypothyroidism, since concentrations of both should be low. This is one way to check for laboratory errors. Measurement of T_3 may also permit the identification of dogs with T_3 autoantibodies, which may have prognostic significance.

TSH Stimulation Test

The TSH stimulation test is currently recommended for practitioners to use in definitively diagnosing canine hypothyroidism. It assesses the ability of the thyroid to respond to exogenous (bovine) TSH by determining the increase in serum T_4 after TSH injection (Table 25-2). It is necessary only to determine T_4 (not T_3) concentrations after TSH. The normal thyroid is not under maximal stimulation by endogenous TSH, so a marked increase in serum T_4 concentrations from the pre-TSH to the post-TSH sample is to be expected in normal dogs. The test is performed by acquiring a serum specimen followed by an intravenous or intramuscular injection of TSH (Dermathycin) at 0.1 to 0.25 IU/kg with a maximum dosage of 5.0 IU. The post-TSH specimen is collected in 6 to 8 hours if administered IV or 8 to 12 hours if administered IM. TSH may be reconstituted and stored at 4° C in smaller volumes for as long as 6 months without affecting activity (Rosychuck, 1992). This will avoid waste when less than 5 IU is required for a given case. In advanced primary hypothyroidism little or no functional thyroidal tissue is present, so the low serum T_4 concentrations show little or no increase in response to TSH. In early compensating hypothyroidism, circulating T_4 concentrations may be near normal; however, the **endogenous** TSH levels cause the remaining tissue to secrete at near maximal capacity and, conse-

Table 25-2. TSH stimulation test

T_4 CONCENTRATION AFTER TSH	>45	<15	>15 BUT <45
Interpretation	Normal thyroid	Hypothyroid	Not sure
Next step	Consider another diagnosis	Treat with T_4	Evaluate T_4 increase due to TSH (see below)
T_4 Increase from pre-TSH to post-TSH sample			Increase <15 nmol/L → Hypothyroid Increase >15 nmol/L → Reevaluate later

T_4 concentrations in nmol/L.

Method for TSH stimulation test: Draw pre-TSH serum and inject TSH at 0.1 to 0.25 unit/kg to a maximum of 5 units. If TSH given IV, collect post-TSH serum at 6 to 8 hours. If TSH given IM, collect post-TSH serum at 8 to 12 hours. Measure T_4 concentration in both samples.

Normal TSH stimulation test results (Auburn University Endocrine Diagnostic Laboratory): pre-TSH T_4 = 20 to 55 nmol/L; post-TSH T_4 = >45 nmol/L.

quently, dogs in the early stages of hypothyroidism may have borderline-low basal T_4 concentrations that show little increase after TSH injection.

Although the results of TSH stimulation testing in normal (euthyroid) and advanced hypothyroid dogs are relatively easy to evaluate, intermediate values often present a dilemma. The TSH response test in dogs with nonthyroidal illnesses or receiving drugs that suppress basal T_4 and T_3 will have values parallel to normal, except lower pre- and post-TSH T_4 concentrations. Differentiating borderline TSH stimulation test results between those due to non-thyroidal factors and those to early primary thyroid failure is difficult, if not impossible. One option is to repeat the TSH stimulation later, following recognition and/or treatment of a nonthyroidal illness or after withholding drugs that possibly interfere with thyroid function. Progressive failure of thyroid gland function (leading to end stage hypothyroidism) would result in a continued decline in the concentrations of T_4 before and after TSH. Although TSH stimulation is the best test for definitively evaluating the thyroid, the problems noted above illustrate that a single TSH stimulation may not provide a conclusive answer. The rather high cost of bovine TSH (Dermathycin), the frequent unavailability of the material, and the time required to perform the test add to its disadvantages.

Other Diagnostic Tests of Thyroid Function

Measurement of Endogenous TSH

Since pituitary TSH forms a negative feedback loop with thyroid hormones, measurement of endogenous TSH would likely provide an excellent tool for evaluating this gland. One would expect endogenous TSH concentrations to be above nor-

mal in dogs with primary hypothyroidism, as is the case in humans with this disease. However, at the present time, no satisfactory, clinically available procedure is available to measure canine TSH. Since TSH structure varies between species, procedures already validated for human or nonhuman TSH do not work with dog serum. It is hoped that a valid assay for canine TSH will be developed in the near future.

Thyrotropin-Releasing Hormone (TRH) Stimulation Test

The TRH stimulation test is used in human medicine for thyroid evaluation. Injection of TRH normally causes an increase in TSH, which is accentuated in primary hypothyroidism but severely diminished in hyperthyroidism. Since canine TSH cannot be routinely measured, the increase in serum T_4 and T_3 concentrations following TRH administration have been used instead of TSH measurement in dogs to assess pituitary and thyroid function. Two major problems affect the usefulness of this test in dogs. First, the increase in serum T_4 and T_3 concentrations in normal dogs after TRH is quite small and somewhat variable. Second, the influence of nonthyroidal factors on this response have not been determined. Consequently the TRH stimulation test using measurement of the increase in serum T_4 and T_3 concentrations in dogs appears to be of little diagnostic value and is not recommended by the authors at the present time.

Determination of Free T_4 and Free T_3 Concentrations

Theoretically measurement of the amounts of T_4 and T_3 free or not bound to carrier proteins provides an accurate test for the amount of active thyroid hormone present for cellular uptake. The levels of free T_4 and T_3 are quite low, less than 1% of the total circulating concentration of either hormone. Kit procedures for measurement of free thyroid hormones have been developed for use with human samples, and are now being used and evaluated for use by veterinary laboratories for assay in the dog. Unfortunately, it appears that because of species differences in binding proteins and other factors, these kits may not be valid for use in dog sera. Problems with values from the kits become especially profound in conditions involving nonthyroid illnesses or during treatment with drugs that alter thyroid hormone concentrations. Additionally, dilution of sera as recommended in many of the kit procedures results in artifactually low estimates of free hormones in dog sera. Finally, the results of some studies using the kit procedures to measure free T_4 and T_3 in dog sera have found that the tests are no better than measuring total T_4 and T_3 in the diagnosis of hypothyroidism. Until more reliable and clinically applicable procedures for the measurement of free T_4 and T_3 are developed for dogs, there seems to be no advantage to using them over the more routine measurements of total T_4 and T_3.

Formulas Combining Several Criteria

Some groups have suggested that several indices of thyroid function, indirect and direct, can be combined arithmetically to generate a value that would be more diagnostic for thyroid status than any single measurement. An example of this utilizes free T_4 and serum cholesterol concentrations to generate a k value (Larsson, 1988). Although one would expect that use of multiple discriminatory information would be better than using single measurements, few controlled studies have been performed to convincingly demonstrate this fact. In essence, the k value does not improve the diagnostic accuracy.

Other Issues in Canine Hypothyroidism

T_3 Autoantibodies

Autoantibodies to T_3 occur in less than 1% of samples submitted to Auburn University Endocrine Diagnostic Laboratory. Typically, the presence of such autoantibodies is suspected when the reported T_3 concentration is elevated above normal, or when the T_3 is in the high-normal range with a concurrently low T_4. Depending on the radioimmunoassay (RIA) method used to measure T_3, results may be high or low with regard to the T_3 autoantibody. Most diagnostic laboratories today use solid phase separation methods in their RIAs, which produce high T_3 values in the presence of autoantibody. This

elevation is an artifact. It is not a true representation of thyroid function. Practitioners may think that a dog has hyperthyroidism when the report of a high serum T_3 concentration is received because the apparent T_3 concentration can be extremely elevated (up to 100 times normal). However, actual T_3 concentrations in dogs with this condition are either slightly above normal or low. The autoantibody artifactually elevates (or lowers) the RIA estimate for total T_3 because it competes with the antibody used in the RIA.

Currently, the exact clinical significance of the T_3 autoantibody phenomenon is not known. In our experience this phenomenon occurs in association with hypothyroidism (docmented with the TSH stimulation test) in slightly over half the cases. However, some dogs with the autoantibody have absolutely normal T_4 responses to TSH and appear clinically normal. Whether these dogs are in the early stages of autoimmne thyroid attack is not known. It is our recommendation not to institute therapy in dogs with T_3 autoantibodies and otherwise normal thyroid function but instead to continue to monitor thyroid function at 6-month intervals. We recommend that dogs with hypothyroidism and the T_3 autoantibody receive treatment with synthetic T_4 in exactly the same regimen as other dogs with hypothyroidism. It appears that the autoantibody does not interfere with the response to thyroid hormone replacement therapy.

Poor Converters: Deficiency of T_4 to T_3 Conversion

It has been proposed that some dogs have a defect in the enzyme that converts T_4 to T_3. This claim was based on the finding of normal serum T_4 concentrations but subnormal T_3 levels in samples either obtained to evaluate thyroid status or collected for a "post-pill" evaluation. This type of enzymatic deficiency has never been documented, and it appears more likely that the pattern is due to nonthyroidal factors that are selectively lowering T_3 or that these dogs have T_3 autoantibodies that manifest in artifactually low levels of T_3. Consequently, there is no evidence to suggest that dogs whose serum thyroid hormone profile shows such a pattern require thyroid hormone replacement, in the form of T_4 or T_3.

Therapeutic Trials Using Synthetic T_4

In some instances definitive proof of hypothyroidism cannot be obtained using TSH stimulation, because of diagnostic restrictions or lack of TSH availability or because of borderline T_4 responses to TSH. An alternative to retesting at a later date is a therapeutic trial with synthetic T_4. A 12-week period will allow sufficient time for resolution of all signs, including hair regrowth, if hypothyroidism is present. When using such a trial, one must remember that primary hypothyroidism is a nonreversible disease that will require thyroid hormone replacement for the life of the dog. Consequently, it is usually worth the effort and expense to make the definitive diagnosis during the initial evaluation. It is certainly advisable to at least **measure** basal T_4 and probably T_3 concentrations prior to initiating a trial dose with T_4, which may demonstrate circulating levels of thyroid hormones in the low to borderline-low range. Evaluation of thyroid function after dogs have received treatment is complicated by the fact that T_4 replacement therapy feeds back negatively upon the hypothalamus, pituitary, and thyroid, suppressing the entire axis while the dog becomes "dependent" on exogenous T_4. In such cases it is best to stop T_4 treatment for at least 4 weeks before evaluating thyroid function with basal T_4 and T_3 measurements or TSH stimulation testing.

TREATMENT

Because T_4 is the major product of the thyroid and the body can regulate the conversion of T_4 to T_3 in different tissues, synthetic thyroxine is the only recommended therapy for canine hypothyroidism. Therapy with T_3, combinations of T_3 and T_4, or crude or desiccated thyroid is not recommended; either the treatments bypass this regulatory conversion step, providing thyroid hormones in nonphysiologic ratios, or their content of thyroid hormones varies.

The recommended starting dose for synthetic T_4 is 20 to 40 μg/kg q24h (i.e., 0.02 to 0.04 mg/kg q24h or 0.01 to 0.02 mg/lb q24h). Initially it is recommended that the dose start at 20 μg/kg q12h PO for 6 weeks after which time it can be reduced to 20 μg/kg q24h. Many, but not all, dogs with hypothyroidism can be successfully maintained on once-a-day therapy with T_4. Since it is quite common for obese dogs to lose considerable weight during the first few months after initiating thyroid hormone replacement, it is necessary to monitor body weight frequently during this time and adjust the dose accordingly.

Clinical signs should begin to resolve within a few weeks after initiating thyroid hormone replacement. The hair coat should be dramatically improved within 6 weeks, although a total 12 weeks of treatment will be necessary for complete eval-

uation of a therapeutic trial. A post-pill T_4 measurement is recommended after 6 weeks of treatment. The post-pill sample is collected 4 to 8 hours after a dose of T_4 is administered. Concentrations of T_4 should be near the top of the normal range (T_4 = 45 to 60 nmol/L) when sampled at this time. The dosage can be adjusted by using these values together with the clinical evaluation. Causes for low post-pill thyroid hormone levels include bioavailability problems and difficulties with pill administration. If post-pill values are low and problems with pill administration can be ruled out, the dosage should be increased and post-pill values reevaluated at 6 week intervals until the T_4 value is within the ideal range given above. Occasionally, changing to a different brand of T_4 is recommended when the thyroid hormone levels are continually low. Changing the source of T_4 has been successful in some cases. For initial treatment any brand of synthetic T_4 can be used (Synthroid, Soloxine, Thyro-Tabs). Once the thyroid hormone levels are stabilized, it is best to perform post-pill tests every 6 to 12 months for the remainder of the dog's life and adjust the dosage accordingly.

REFERENCES

Conaway DH, et al: Clinical and histological features of primary, progressive, familial thyroiditis in a colony of Borzoi dogs, Vet Pathol 22:439, 1985.

Haines DM, et al: The detection of canine autoantibodies to thyroid antigens by enzyme-linked immunosorbent assay, hemagglutination, and indirect immunofluorescence, Can J Comp Med 48:262, 1984.

Larsson MG: Determination of free thyroxine and cholesterol as a new screening test for canine hypothyroidism, J Am Anim Hosp Assoc 24:209, 1988.

Rosychuck RAW: Personal communication, 1992.

SUPPLEMENTAL READING

Beale KM: Techniques for evaluating thyroid function in the dog. In DeBoer DJ (ed): Advances in clinical dermatology, Vet Clin North Am 20:1429, 1990.

Belshaw BE: Thyroid diseases. In Ettinger SJ (ed): Textbook of veterinary internal medicine: diseases of the dog and cat, ed 2, Philadelphia, 1983, WB Saunders.

Ferguson DC: Thyroid hormone replacement therapy. In Kirk RW (ed): Current veterinary therapy IX, Philadelphia, 1986, WB Saunders.

Nelson RW: Treatment of canine hypothyroidism. In Kirk RW (ed): Current veterinary therapy X, Philadelphia, 1989, WB Saunders.

Peterson ME, Ferguson DC: Thyroid diseases. In Ettinger SJ (ed): Textbook of veterinary internal medicine: diseases of the dog and cat, ed 3, Philadelphia, 1989, WB Saunders.

26

Canine and Feline Cushing's Syndrome

Carole A. Zerbe   John M. MacDonald

Diagnostic Criteria for Spontaneous Hyperadrenocorticism

SUGGESTIVE
History and cutaneous features of endocrinopathy

COMPATIBLE
Suggestive plus clinical findings of polyuria-polydipsia, lack of hair regrowth, muscle wasting, excessive panting, bullous impetigo, poor wound healing, hepatomegaly
Laboratory findings of increased serum alkaline phosphatase, diabetes mellitus, skin biopsy suggestive of endocrinopathy

TENTATIVE
Compatible plus skin biopsy revealing epidermal atrophy and/or calcinosis cutis, specialized testing: radiographic adrenal calcification, ultrasonographic adrenomegaly

DEFINITIVE
Tentative plus abnormal ACTH stimulation test, abnormal low-dose dexamethasone suppression test, and abnormal urine corticoid/creatinine ratio

CANINE HYPERADRENOCORTICISM
Importance

Cushing's syndrome has been recognized for many years in dogs as a result of excessive glucocorticoids. When hyperglucocorticoidism results from exogenous sources, it may be referred to as iatrogenic Cushing's or the misnomer "iatrogenic hyperadrenocorticism." Endogenous hypercortisolemia results from excessive adrenocortical activity and may be referred to as Cushing's syndrome, or naturally occurring or spontaneous hyperadrenocorticism. "Cushing's disease" refers specifically to Cushing's syndrome of pituitary tumor origin. Glucocorticoid administration is by far the most common cause of Cushing's syndrome. Naturally occurring hyperadrenocorticism was often considered an uncommon disease. Only recently has it been recognized as the most common endocrinopathy of dogs, surpassing in frequency hypothyroidism. Although the condition is extremely uncommon in cats, it (likewise) is being recognized more frequently.

Classical physical or clinicopathologic abnormalities are not observed in many cases, making the suggestive diagnostic signs more obscure and requiring a broader base of suspicion than previously considered. Prominent dermatologic features may actually represent secondary complications such as chronic pyoderma or dermatophytosis, thereby overlooking the diagnosis of hyperadrenocorticism. The relevancy of hyperadrenocorticism often goes well beyond the external features and may include pathology of many organ systems.

Left untreated, the hyperadrenocortical patient

risks several sequelae of sustained hyperglucocorticoidism. These include diabetes mellitus, hepatopathy, infection, alteration of cardiac and skeletal muscle, and overall catabolic changes as well as dermatopathies. Early recognition and treatment can lead to satisfactory control of the problem. Unfortunately, there is no single laboratory test that provides all the diagnostic or rule-out criteria for this syndrome. Often several tests are required to determine the etiopathology. The availability of these tests and the therapeutic options make canine and feline Cushing's syndrome a treatable disease.

Pathogenesis

The underlying cause in more than 85% of spontaneous hyperadrenocorticism in dogs is an excessive secretion of adrenocorticotrophic hormone (ACTH) by the pituitary (box). This may be due to either a functional tumor or a defect in the hypothalamic-pituitary axis. Both conditions are categorized as pituitary-dependent disease. The result of pituitary-dependent disease from either cause is hyperplastic adrenal cortices with excess production of cortisol. Pituitary tumors are the most common cause of pituitary-dependent Cushing's and usually arise from the pars distalis but may also develop in the pars intermedia of the pituitary lobe. They generally occur in brachiocephalic breeds and may become quite large, resulting in neurologic signs. Functional adrenal tumors are a less common cause of spontaneous hyperadrenocorticism. Glucocorticoid treatment is the cause of iatrogenic Cushing's in dogs, representing more than half the cases.

Clinical Disease

History

The history of hyperglucocorticoidism usually, but not necessarily, includes cutaneous changes.

Etiologic Classification of Cushing's Syndrome

Iatrogenic
Naturally occurring (spontaneous)
  Pituitary-dependent hyperadrenocorticism (85% to 90%)
    Hypothalamic-pituitary axis defect
    Pituitary tumor (Cushing's disease)
  Adrenocortical tumor (10% to 15%)

These often occur gradually over a period of several months. Historical questions concerning glucocorticoid therapy must be pursued in any case with suspicious clinical features or abnormal laboratory data suggesting Cushing's syndrome. Owners should be questioned with regard to pruritic dermatopathies and associated treatment. Documentation of both systemic (parenteral and oral) and topical treatments should be made. Otic preparations often contain glucocorticoids and are routinely used to treat allergic otitis associated with canine atopy or food allergy. Ophthalmic medications, likewise, may contain glucocorticoids and, either by themselves or in combination with systemic drugs, be responsible for the development of Cushing's syndrome. Topical medications containing glucocorticoids prescribed for focal dermatopathies are sometimes used to excess. Owners may not be aware of the glucocorticoid content of a therapy. "Itch pills" or "itch shots" are often used to describe glucocorticoid products. There is no glucocorticoid treatment that does not cause iatrogenic Cushing's syndrome. Single injections of triamcinolone have resulted in generalized hair loss, calcinosis cutis, and biochemical abnormalities of glucocorticoid excess.

Spontaneous hyperadrenocorticism is a disease of middle-aged to older dogs. Dachshunds, Boston Terriers, Poodles, and Boxers are the breeds most commonly predisposed to pituitary-dependent hyperadrenocorticism; large-breed dogs more commonly develop adrenal tumors. Historical questions should include reference to systemic signs, particularly increased water consumption, increased urination, decreased activity, increased appetite, and weight gain. It may be desirable to monitor water consumption to quantify the history of polydipsia. Normal dogs should not consume more than 100 ml of water per kilogram per day. Questions regarding the animal's reproductive status should be included, both to obtain relevant information about possible Cushing's and to provide historical background for primary sex hormone endocrinopathies. A history of chronic or recurrent infections from either bacterial or fungal agents should arouse suspicion of hyperglucocorticoidism. Recognition of liver disease through previous laboratory data may indicate hyperadrenocorticism.

The response to previous therapy should be documented, with particular reference to specific drugs, dosages, and duration of therapeutic trials. Hypothyroidism is often misdiagnosed in dogs with Cushing's syndrome because of practitioner conditioning and possible borderline thyroid hormone levels. Thyroxine levels with hyperglucocorticoidism may be low or borderline low due to excess glucocorticoid. This often leads to a wrong diagnosis and treatment with a thyroid hormone. The thyroid axis of hyperadrenocortical dogs can be evaluated accurately only by a TSH response test or by reevaluating the thyroid axis after treatment of the Cushing's. Failure of a therapeutic trial of thyroxine is expected in dogs with Cushing's syndrome and normal thyroid status. The results of other hormone therapy trials should be documented, as well as the response to neutering if this has been performed.

Chronic superficial pyoderma or folliculitis may be the most striking feature of a hyperadrenocortical case. The response to antibiotic therapy should be determined in cases with recurrent pyoderma. Adult-onset demodicosis with poor response to demodicidal therapy should signal concern for hyperadrenocorticism. A combination of demodicosis and superficial or deep pyoderma may be observed concurrently. Coexistent diabetes mellitus may also be associated with hyperadrenocorticism, and the combination may affect the pyoderma and demodicosis components.

Combinations of cutaneous problems are often observed. Further complication occurs when the atopic dog also develops spontaneous hyperadrenocorticism, which can be overshadowed both historically and diagnostically by treatment with systemic glucocorticoids. The ACTH stimulation test should be used to distinguish spontaneous hyperadrenocorticism from iatrogenic Cushing's syndrome in these dogs. If ACTH stimulation testing produces normal values in the presence of clinical and laboratory findings highly suggestive of Cushing's, then glucocorticoid therapy should be withheld for 2 weeks and a repeat ACTH stimulation test performed. If there is an exaggerated response after ACTH testing, a diagnosis of spontaneous, not iatrogenic, Cushing's syndrome is made.

Physical Examination

Clinical features of Cushing's syndrome vary but usually are insidious and slowly progressive. Some of the classical features include the "five P's": polydipsia, polyuria, polyphagia, pendulous abdomen, and panting. Polydipsia and polyuria may be the first signs observed and usually precede cutaneous changes. Behavioral changes include lethargy and reluctance to exercise. Less common behavioral changes may include aggressiveness or psychotic behavior. Self-mutilation has been observed. Obesity results from the excess food consumption, which further influences the animal's inactivity. Muscle weakness, caused by the catabolic effect of the hyperglucocorticoidism, also intensifies the sedentary life-style. Atrophy of muscle groups may be profound. The masseters are classically involved and should serve as a signal of suspicion for hyperadrenocorticism when atrophy is observed in association with cutaneous changes. Most females have prolonged anestrus or irregular estral cycles whereas males lack libido and have testicular atrophy.

Classical cutaneous changes include hair loss, usually in a bilateral and symmetric pattern without evidence of inflammation unless secondary complications are present or dystrophic mineralization has taken place (Fig. 26-1). Hyperpigmentation is variable. The skin is thin and has decreased elasticity with a wrinkled appearance (Fig. 26-2). Fragility of blood vessels results in easy bruising, particularly where venipunctures have been performed. Phlebectasias are infrequently observed as red macules or papules, usually on the ventral abdomen, that fail to blanch with diascopy. These have sometimes been referred to as "cherry hemangiomas." Calcinosis cutis is observed in 35% to 40% of Cushing's cases and may be confused with mycotic dermatoses or neoplastic disease. It is more commonly observed with iatrogenic disease (Fig. 26-3). Scaling disorders are less common with hyperglucocorticoidism than with other endocrine dermatoses but may be seen as light desquamating scale.

Large comedones are generally seen on the ventral abdomen (Fig. 26-4). Milia-type lesions are also observed, as small, single, white, superficial,

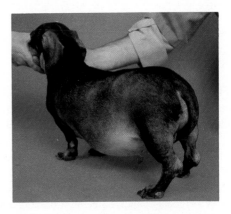

Figure 26-1. Pituitary-dependent hyperadrenocorticism in a Dachshund, demonstrating sparsity of hair on the trunk with a pendulous abdomen. The hair loss was bilateral and the skin was thin.

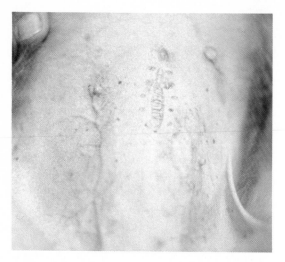

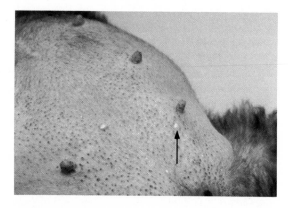

Figure 26-2. Abdomen of a dog with pituitary-dependent hyperadrenocorticism, showing distension, extremely thin skin, and prominent vasculature. Note the scar associated with the skin incision from an ovariohysterectomy.

Figure 26-3. Abdomen of a Poodle with pituitary-dependent hyperadrenocorticism, showing thin skin, comedones, and miliary lesions. Note the rotund appearance of the body.

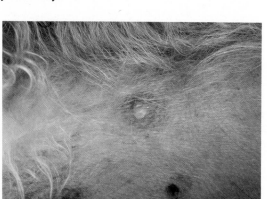

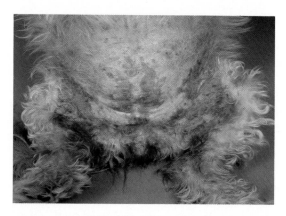

Figure 26-4. A large flaccid pustule (bullous impetigo) caused by *Staphylococcal* spp organisms on the abdomen of a dog with Cushing's syndrome. The erythemic border noted here is absent in many cases of pyoderma with Cushing's syndrome.

Figure 26-5. Dystrophic mineralization (calcinosis cutis) observed bilaterally in the inguinal region of a dog with Cushing's syndrome. This lesion is most often seen in iatrogenic Cushing's syndrome.

dome-shaped structures. Scars from surgical incisions (neutering) may be more prominent, showing evidence of stretching. Areas shaved have typically not regrown hair for a prolonged time. Alternatively, when hair regrowth has been observed, it was considerably slower and usually of poorer quality. A change in hair coloration has been observed; originally black hairs may have taken on an auburn hue. The hair quality is typically poor, with dry, lusterless, brittle hairs.

Adult dogs that suddenly develop pyodermas should be suspected of having hyperglucocorticoidism. Pustules found in these cases are usually large (bullous) and may lack surrounding erythema

(Fig. 26-5). The distribution of pyodermatous lesions may be atypical, affecting the head, face, or pinnas. Poor antibiotic response or sudden relapse after termination of therapy is common. Dogs with adult-onset demodicosis should, likewise, be suspected of having hyperadrenocorticism. A coexisting pyoderma may be present.

The physical evaluation for Cushing's syndrome should include close inspection of the skin. Evaluating skin thickness and elasticity is important but often overlooked. Inspecting for subtle changes, including comedones, may produce supportive diagnostic information. Abdominal palpation should be performed to detect hepatomegaly. Auscultation of the lung field and heart should be done routinely, since respiratory signs (e.g., panting) are a consistent finding. Neurologic signs may be observed in cases with large pituitary tumors. A neurologic examination should be performed if historical facts or clinical features on the general physical suggest a neuropathy.

Diagnosis

A tentative diagnosis of Cushing's syndrome in dogs can be made based on the animal's gross appearance, clinical signs, historical abnormalities, and discrepancies in the CBC, biochemical tests, and urinalysis. Other important tests include radiographic and sonographic evaluation of the adrenals. For example, if calcification is noted on abdominal radiographs of the dog, an adrenal tumor is likely. However, caution must be used in cats since calcification can occur in older individuals without an adrenal tumor. In addition, more specialized tests such as computed tomography (CT) and magnetic resonance imaging (MRI) may be used to identify adrenal and pituitary tumors.

Specifically with regard to the skin, a minimal database for cutaneous evaluation should include skin scrapings and a dermatophyte test medium (DTM) culture for dermatophytosis. If pustules are present, their contents require cytologic examination. Skin biopsies are often helpful but may reveal changes not diagnostic of Cushing's. The following dermatohistopathologic changes, observed collectively, are highly suggestive of hyperadrenocorticism: atrophy of the epidermis and follicular epithelium, follicular dilation and hyperkeratosis; thin dermis, atrophy or absence of arrector pili muscles, and dystrophic mineralization. Changes observed that are compatible with a number of endocrinopathies include orthokeratotic hyperkeratosis, epidermal atrophy, epidermal melanosis, follicular hyperkeratosis, and sebaceous gland atrophy. Diagnostic assessment of the adrenal axis should be performed when dystrophic mineralization is included in the histologic report.

A definitive diagnosis of hyperadrenocorticism can be made only by evaluating the hypothalamic-pituitary-adrenal (HPA) axis. Two questions should be addressed in approaching the diagnosis of hyperadrenocorticism, First, does the patient have hyperadrenocorticism? This can be determined by specific screening tests. Second, what form of hyperadrenocorticism does the dog have? In other words, does it have pituitary-dependent hyperadrenocorticism or an adrenal tumor? Differentiating or discriminating tests are used to answer this question.

Screening Tests for Hyperadrenocorticism

Basal plasma cortisol concentration (not recommended)
Urinary corticoid/creatinine ratio
ACTH stimulation test
Low-dose dexamethasone suppression test (0.01 mg/kg)
Combined dexamethasone suppression–ACTH stimulation test

Screening Tests of the Hypothalamic-Pituitary-Adrenal Axis

Examples of screening tests for the HPA axis include basal plasma cortisol concentrations, urinary corticoid/creatinine ratios, the ACTH stimulation test, the low-dose dexamethasone suppression test (0.01 mg/kg), and the combined dexamethasone suppression–ACTH stimulation test (box). It should be emphasized that normal ranges from different endocrine diagnostic laboratories vary and the practitioner should contact the laboratory with regard to specific values used for interpretation. Representative values from Auburn University Endocrine Diagnostic Laboratory are provided in Table 26-1.

Basal or resting plasma or serum cortisol. A basal or resting plasma or serum cortisol test is not generally recommended for Cushing's syndrome. Single basal cortisol levels in animals with HPA disease overlap with cortisol levels in normal dogs. For example, stress associated with sample collection or with the visit to a veterinary clinic, or normal episodic secretion of cortisol in individual animals, may cause values higher than normal in samples taken from animals with normal HPA function. Furthermore, recent administration of glucocorticoids such as hydrocortisone, prednisolone, or prednisone may falsely elevate values as a result of cross-reactivity in many cortisol radioimmunoassays.

Urinary corticoid/creatinine ratio determinations. Urinary corticoid/creatinine ratios may be used to screen for canine hyperadrenocorticism and to monitor response to Lysodren therapy (Rijnberk and van Wees, 1988; Jones et al., 1990; Smiley and Peterson, 1990). This test involves having the owner collect a urine sample from the dog at home and bring it in, and then assessing the cortisol and creatinine for a corticoid/creatinine

Table 26-1. Laboratory test values* for hyperadrenocorticism screening

CORTISOL (nmol/L)	DOGS	CATS
Baseline cortisol (pre-ACTH or pre-dexamethasone)	10-160	10-110
Post-dexamethasone (low dose)	<30	<30
Post-ACTH	220-560	110-280

*Auburn University Endocrine Diagnostic Service.

ratio. Two consecutive morning urine samples should be evaluated when used as a screening test for hyperadrenocorticism. However, caution should be used when interpreting test results because false-positives may occur with nonadrenal illness (as with many tests of adrenal function).

Recently (Jones et al., 1990) measurement of the urinary corticoid/creatinine ratio was shown to be useful assessing adrenal suppression after Lysodren treatment. A morning urine sample should be collected by the owner at home before Lysodren therapy is begun and also at the completion of the loading-dose regimen.

ACTH stimulation test. The ACTH stimulation test is used to do the following:

1. Screen for hyperadrenocorticism
2. Distinguish spontaneous hyperadrenocorticism from iatrogenic Cushing's syndrome
3. Diagnose Addison's disease
4. Monitor the response to mitotane (Lysodren) (or to ketoconazole or metyrapone)

This is a test of adrenocortical reserve. With adrenal hyperplasia or an adrenal tumor, for example, there should be a greater reserve and, therefore, a hyperresponsiveness to exogenous ACTH stimulation. The test is easy to perform and requires from 1 to 2 hours depending on the ACTH preparation used and the animal species tested. In dogs a pre-ACTH blood sample is collected for plasma or serum cortisol determination. Then 2.2 IU/kg of ACTH gel (Acthar) is injected IM and a post-ACTH sample drawn 2 hours later. Alternatively, 0.25 mg of synthetic ACTH (Cosyntropin) is injected IV and a post-ACTH sample drawn 1 hour later. In cats a pre-ACTH blood sample for plasma or serum cortisol determination is collected and 2.2 IU/kg of ACTH gel injected. Then two post-ACTH samples are taken, one at 1 hour and another at 2 hours. Alternatively, 0.125 mg per cat of synthetic

ACTH may be injected IV and two post-ACTH samples taken, one at 30 minutes and another at 60 minutes. Two post-ACTH samples are recommended, because some cats will show peak cortisol concentration with the first or second sample.

A normal response to ACTH suggests functional integrity of the HPA axis; however, some 15% to 20% of dogs with hyperadrenocorticism will show a normal response to ACTH. A low-dose dexamethasone suppression test is recommended when this occurs in dogs suspected of having the disease. A reduced response is seen in Addison's disease, adrenocortical suppression resulting from glucocorticoid treatment, and during or after mitotane therapy.

Exaggerated responses to ACTH are seen in approximately 75% of dogs with pituitary-dependent hyperadrenocorticism, whereas about 50% of dogs with functional adrenocortical tumors show excessive response to ACTH. Exaggerated responses to ACTH have also been documented in dogs with chronic illness (e.g., chronic liver disease or diabetes mellitus) not directly involving the HPA axis (Chastain, 1986). It is worth noting that dogs with diabetes mellitus may have an exaggerated response to ACTH and not have Cushing's disease. For this reason it is generally recommended that the low-dose dexamethasone suppression test be used as the initial screening test for dogs with diabetes mellitus.

If the dog or cat has recently been treated with or is currently undergoing glucocorticoid therapy, the ACTH stimulation test is the recommended initial screening procedure. Other tests, such as dexamethasone suppression, may yield inappropriate results due to activation of the negative feedback pathway from exogenous glucocorticoid administration.

Low-dose dexamethasone suppression test. The low-dose dexamethasone suppression test is the most accurate screening device used for canine hyperadrenocorticism. It has the added advantage of being able to distinguish the pituitary-dependent form of hyperadrenocorticism from adrenal tumors in as many as 40% of dogs with Cushing's syndrome. Unlike the ACTH stimulation test, which reflects the capacity of the adrenal gland to secrete ACTH, the low-dose dexamethasone suppression test measures the integrity of the negative feedback pathway. The pituitary-adrenal axis is abnormally resistant to suppression by dexamethasone in animals with hyperadrenocorticism; by contrast, in normal animals dexamethasone inhibits pituitary ACTH release through negative feedback inhibition, and cortisol concentrations decrease.

In dogs and cats a pre-dexamethasone blood sample is collected for plasma or serum cortisol determination. Dexamethasone (0.01 or 0.015 mg/kg, IV) is injected, and two post-dexamethasone samples are collected, one at 4 hours and the next at 8 hours. It often is advantageous to dilute the dexamethasone (1:10 dilution with sterile saline) for more accurate dosing in smaller patients.

Some 90% to 95% of dogs with hyperadrenocorticism fail to show normal suppression of cortisol with the low-dose desamethasone suppression test. The 8-hour sample is the most critical for interpretation. Failure to suppress cortisol at 4 and/or 8 hours is consistent with a diagnosis of Cushing's syndrome and may represent either an adrenal tumor or pituitary-dependent disease (Table 26-1). However, suppression of cortisol concentrations at 4 hours with a rebound at 8 hours would be consistent with pituitary-dependent hyperadrenocorticism (PDH).

Although the low-dose dexamethasone suppression test is an excellent screening test in the dog, it appears that a certain percentage of normal cats have an escape of serum cortisol suppression at the 8-hour sample (Smith and Feldman, 1987; Peterson, 1988). Thus this test may not be as useful for diagnosis of hyperadrenocorticism in the cat.

Combined dexamethasone suppression–ACTH stimulation test. The combined dexamethasone suppression–ACTH stimulation test serves principally as a means of screening for hyperadrenocorticism. The addition of dexamethasone suppression permits (1) identification of a percentage of animals with hyperadrenocorticism that respond normally to ACTH but fail to show normal cortisol suppression in response to dexamethasone and (2) immediate diagnosis of PDH in some animals. This test examines both negative feedback (high-dose dexamethasone suppression) and adrenocortical secretory capacity (ACTH stimulation) in a relatively short time. Although its use has been controversial among endocrinologists (Eiler and Oliver, 1984; Feldman, 1985; Zerbe et al., 1987c), it nevertheless is a valid and useful test recommended by the Auburn University Endocrine Diagnostic Service. It will be discussed further in the next section.

Differentiating Tests of the Hypothalamic-Pituitary-Adrenal Axis

Once a definitive diagnosis of hyperadrenocorticism has been made by the use of screening tests, it is important to determine which form of hyper-

Differentiating Tests for Hyperadrenocorticism
Basal ACTH concentrations
High-dose dexamethasone suppression (0.1 or 1 mg/kg)
CRH stimulation

adrenocorticism the animal has. In other words, does it have pituitary-dependent hyperadrenocorticism or an adrenal tumor? Dogs with pituitary-dependent hyperadrenocorticism have bilateral adrenal hyperplasia, which is caused by excessive secretion of ACTH. Glucocorticoid negative feedback continues to operate, but at a greater threshold than normal. Adrenocortical tumors are either adenomas or carcinomas affecting one adrenal gland. Because glucocorticoid negative feedback is in operation, ACTH levels are low and atrophy of the normal adrenal cortex occurs. Most differentiating tests, therefore, are designed to take advantage of the fact that pituitary disease is associated with high ACTH and a raised glucocorticoid negative feedback whereas animals with an adrenal tumor have low levels of ACTH and a normal glucocorticoid negative feedback.

Examples of differentiating tests include basal ACTH concentrations, high-dose dexamethasone suppression (0.1 mg/kg is "high dose," 1 mg/kg "mega-dose"), and the CRH stimulation test (box). It is important to note that some screening tests (e.g., the low-dose dexamethasone suppression and the combined dexamethasone suppression–ACTH stimulation test) may have results consistent with a diagnosis of pituitary-dependent hyperadrenocorticism. Hence, in addition to accurately identifying Cushing's syndrome in 75% to 95% of dogs, these screening tests also differentiate pituitary-dependent disease from adrenal tumors in approximately 40% to 50% of dogs with hyperadrenocorticism (Eiler and Oliver, 1984; Zerbe et al., 1987c).

High-dose dexamethasone suppression test. The high-dose dexamethasone suppression test is used to differentiate pituitary-dependent hyperadrenocorticism from adrenal tumor. The principle of this test is that a high dose of dexamethasone is expected to suppress cortisol concentrations in animals with pituitary-dependent hyperadrenocorticism but not in those with an adrenal tumor.

In dogs and cats a pre-dexamethasone blood

sample is collected for plasma or serum cortisol determination. Then 0.1 or 1 mg/kg of dexamethasone is injected IV and two post-dexamethasone samples drawn, one at 4 hours and another at 8 hours. The 0.1 mg/kg dose of dexamethasone should be the initial dose used in dogs. The 1 mg/kg dose of dexamethasone is used only when cortisol concentrations are not suppressed in response to the 0.1 mg/kg dose of dexamethasone. The 1 mg/kg dose of dexamethasone should be used with caution in dogs with diabetes mellitus and in dogs with basal cortisol concentrations in excess of approximately 12 μg/dl (331 nmol/L). The high-dose dexamethasone suppression test is designed for use only in animals with confirmed hyperadrenocorticism. A cortisol concentration less than 50% of the pre-dexamethasone value at either 4 or 8 hours post-dexamethasone is consistent with pituitary-dependent hyperadrenocorticism (PDH). As many as 20% of dogs with PDH do not show suppression of cortisol to high doses of dexamethasone. Therefore, failure to suppress adequately with high doses of dexamethasone cannot be taken as confirmation of an adrenal tumor. Further diagnostic procedures (an ACTH assay or corticotropin stimulation) are required.

Unlike the situation in dogs, it appears that in cats the dexamethasone suppression test using a dose of 0.1 mg/kg is more reliable. It may, in fact, be preferred over the low-dose dexamethasone suppression test, whereas a dexamethasone suppression test using a dose of 1 mg/kg may be appropriate for distinguishing pituitary-dependent hyperadrenocorticism from adrenal tumors in cats.

Combined dexamethasone suppression–ACTH stimulation test. The combined dexamethasone suppression–ACTH stimulation test serves principally as a screening device for hyperadrenocorticism. (See p. 279) It is performed in dogs and cats by collecting a pre-dexamethasone blood sample for plasma or serum cortisol determination and then injecting 0.1 mg/kg of dexamethasone IV; 4 hours later a post-dexamethasone sample is drawn. Immediately after the post-dexamethasone sample has been collected, ACTH is administered in accordance with the ACTH stimulation test. A post-ACTH sample (two post-ACTH samples in cats) is then collected. In dogs, lack of suppression in response to dexamethasone, an exaggerated response to ACTH, or both would be consistent with hyperadrenocorticism; a post-dexamethasone cortisol value less than 50% of the pre-dexamethasone value, together with an exaggerated response to ACTH, would be consistent with PDH.

This response pattern occurs in approximately 40% to 50% of dogs with hyperadrenocorticism. Inadequate suppression of cortisol to dexamethasone, together with an exaggerated response to ACTH, is also consistent with hyperadrenocorticism; however, further tests are required to differentiate PDH from an adrenal tumor. Additional tests might include the ACTH assay or corticotropin stimulation test. Similarly, further evaluation is required in a dog that exhibits a lack of suppression in response to dexamethasone but has a normal response to ACTH. The lack of cortisol suppression by dexamethasone is highly suggestive of hyperadrenocorticism, provided the dog has not recently received glucocorticoids.

Normal results of the combined test do not absolutely rule out a diagnosis of hyperadrenocorticism. The low-dose dexamethasone suppression test is recommended if equivocal results are obtained with the combined test, or if normal results are observed in a dog strongly suspected of having hyperadrenocorticism. Conversely, as with other screening tests, abnormal results are possible in animals with chronic non–hypothalamic-pituitary-adrenal axis disease (e.g., renal failure, diabetes mellitus, or chronic liver dysfunction) or in animals treated with certain drugs (glucocorticoids or anticonvulsants) (Chastain, 1986; Zerbe, personal observation).

Endogenous plasma ACTH measurement. Endogenous plasma ACTH measurement is used to differentiate pituitary-dependent hyperadrenocorticism from an adrenal tumor. Plasma ACTH will be normal to high in patients with pituitary-dependent disease but low in dogs with an adrenal tumor because of the negative feedback of cortisol. ACTH is measured using radioimmunoassay (RIA) of a plasma sample. Blood should be collected from nondisturbed animals in tubes with EDTA or heparin and ideally should be centrifuged at 4° C immediately after collection. Plasma should be rapidly harvested and stored frozen in plastic tubes for shipment. Packing in dry ice and using an overnight mail service are usually necessary to keep the sample frozen until the time of assay in the laboratory.

As with other differentiating tests, plasma ACTH determination is of little diagnostic value for the initial evaluation of suspected hyperadrenocorticism. It is best used as a differentiating test once hyperadrenocorticism has been confirmed. Proper collection, storage, and shipment of samples are critical to obtain an accurate assay. Using a reference laboratory with a validated assay for dog or cat samples is also mandatory. The practitioner should contact the reference laboratory before drawing the sample to obtain recommendations on specific collection and handling. Since most Pomeranians have elevated values, this test must be interpreted cautiously. Determining plasma ACTH concentrations is the most accurate means of differentiating PDH from an adrenal tumor. A second ACTH measurement usually provides the answer when a single sample is not diagnostic for either form.

CRH stimulation test. The corticotropin-releasing hormone (CRH) stimulation test is a test of pituitary ACTH reserve used to distinguish dogs with PDH from dogs with an adrenal tumor. Plasma ACTH will be normal to high in patients with pituitary-dependent hyperadrenocorticism but low in dogs with an adrenal tumor because of the negative feedback of cortisol. CRH stimulates the release of ACTH from the anterior pituitary. The CRH stimulation test appears to be a good means of differentiating but is not generally available for private practitioners, and the cost may be high.

Treatment

The treatment and prognosis for pituitary-dependent hyperadrenocorticism (PDH) and adrenal tumors vary with age, concurrent illness, and specific etiology. In general, treatment modalities include medical, surgical and/or radiation therapy.

Treatment of Pituitary-Dependent Hyperadrenocorticism

The primary disease of PDH occurs at the level of the pituitary, either as hyperplastic pituitary tissue or as a pituitary tumor capable of secreting excessive ACTH. The increased ACTH, in turn, causes a bilateral adrenal hyperplasia, with resultant excessive secretion of cortisol. Treatment of PDH may be aimed specifically at the pituitary tumor or at the target organ (the adrenal cortex). Although the adrenal glands are only secondarily affected by PDH, they often are the target of therapy.

Medical management. Medical therapy aimed at decreasing cortisol production by the adrenal cortex is the most common treatment for pituitary-dependent hyperadrenocorticism. Four drugs may be used to decrease cortisol synthesis: Lysodren, aminoglutethimide, metyrapone, and ketoconazole.

The drug most commonly used to treat PDH is

Lysodren (also known as mitotane or o,p'-DDD). It effectively reduces cortisol secretion by causing a selective necrosis and atrophy of the adrenocortical zona fasciculata and zona reticularis. The zona glomerulosa, the zone of the adrenal cortex responsible for mineralocorticoid production, is relatively resistant. Because Lysodren therapy does not effect a cure, dogs require weekly to biweekly lifelong therapy.

Lysodren therapy is divided into two phases, loading and maintenance. The initial phase consists of "loading" Lysodren, with the objective of returning the dog to a eucortisolemic state. The general recommendation is 40 to 50 mg/kg q24h PO for 7 to 10 days. It may be best to start with lower dosages of Lysodren, such as 25 to 40 mg/kg, for large dogs or dogs whose owners cannot provide more continuous observation. This can be supplemented with prednisolone or prednisone 0.2 to 0.4 mg/kg q24h at the same time to reduce the side effects of glucocorticoid withdrawal.

Complications of Lysodren therapy include lethargy, vomiting, diarrhea, weakness, anorexia, and ataxia. These occur in about 25% of dogs. Vomiting, which may be related to a direct effect of Lysodren, can be prevented by dividing the dose and giving it twice daily, if loading, or three times weekly if maintaining. Administering the drug with food may also help (Watson et al., 1987). Weakness, anorexia, diarrhea, and vomiting may be related to a decrease in cortisol, which drops rapidly into the normal range, causing a relative glucocorticoid deficiency. Lysodren therapy should be stopped if this happens, and prednisone or prednisolone administered at 0.2 to 0.4 mg/kg until the dog can be evaluated. Generally, the signs will resolve within 3 hours of glucocorticoid supplementation. ACTH stimulation testing should be done to document adrenal suppression and to monitor recovery of the hypothalamic-pituitary-adrenal axis (see below). Because Lysodren usually spares the zona glomerulosa, mineralocorticoid deficiency associated with the electrolyte changes of hyperkalemia and hyponatremia are uncommon. Alternatively, there may be a relapse of clinical signs of hyperadrenocorticism, in which case the dose of Lysodren may need to be increased.

Recall that Lysodren therapy will not affect a pituitary tumor itself and therefore an expanding macroadenoma may cause neurologic signs even though the excess cortisol level has been adequately controlled. It would be appropriate to consider cobalt irradiation of the pituitary tumor in such a case.

(See "Radiation.") The animal should be monitored for water consumption, appetite, and attitude while undergoing Lysodren therapy, particularly the loading dose. The best method to assess Lysodren therapy is the ACTH stimulation test, performed immediately after the loading dose of Lysodren. Both pre-cortisol and post-cortisol values should remain within the normal *resting* range (Table 26-1). Lysodren therapy should be continued if the cortisol values are not within the resting range at the conclusion of the loading dose. The animal should be evaluated at 5-to-10-day intervals until cortisol values remain in the normal resting range on an ACTH response test. Occasionally a dog may require months of daily treatment to reduce cortisol levels. In a recent study, dogs that required prolonged induction for more than 20 days were all small-breed dogs (Kintzer and Peterson, 1991). Lysodren therapy should be stopped if cortisol levels fall below normal resting range, and glucocorticoids should be administered if necessary. Cortisol usually increases within 2 to 3 weeks, but it may take months for some dogs to recover. The corticoid/creatinine ratio before and after Lysodren treatment may also be used to assess adrenal suppression and response to therapy (Jones et al., 1990). (See p. 277.)

A maintenance dosage of Lysodren may be started once eucortisolemia has been obtained. The objective of a maintenance dosage is to maintain the dog in the eucortisolemic state. This involves administering 50 mg/kg q7d in two to three divided doses. Lower dosages may result in an increased incidence of relapse. Glucocorticoid supplementation generally is not necessary. An ACTH stimulation test should be repeated after 3 and 6 months of maintenance therapy, and every 6 months thereafter. If cortisol levels rise above the normal range, Lysodren therapy should be given at 50 mg/kg q24h for 5 days, and the weekly maintenance dosage should be increased by about 50%. Approximately half the dogs treated with Lysodren relapse within 12 months. Occasionally dogs develop a resistance to Lysodren therapy and require very high dosages (100 to 300 mg/kg q7d).

Ketoconazole, an antifungal agent, also decreases cortisol levels. It interferes with adrenal steroid synthesis by blocking enzymes in the cortisol synthetic pathway. This is a safe and effective therapeutic agent for treatment of canine hyperadrenocorticism (Bruyette and Feldman, 1988). Ketoconazole has been used as an alternative to Lysodren therapy, particularly when Lysodren is unsuccessful because of drug resistance or severe side effects. However, it is expensive in the large-breed dog (up to six times more than Lysodren per month). The initial dosage is 10 mg/kg q24h, divided and given twice daily for 7 to 10 days. Treatment success is monitored with an ACTH stimulation test after 7 to 10 days. It is not necessary to discontinue ketoconazole before testing. The dosage may need to be increased to achieve successful treatment. Failure to respond to dosages as high as 30 mg/kg q24h occurs in up to 20% of cases, and reported side effects include anorexia, vomiting, and a lightening of the hair coat. Lifelong therapy twice daily must be used to be effective, because the drug blocks adrenal steroid synthesis without destroying adrenal tissue. This drug has shown promise in the treatment of feline hyperadrenocorticism. (See "Treatment of Feline Hyperadrenocorticism," p. 286, for more specific details.)

Aminogluthimide also decreases steroidogenesis by inhibiting conversion of cholesterol to cortisol. **Metyrapone** decreases steroidogenesis by inhibiting conversion of 11-deoxycortisol to cortisol. This drug also has shown promise in the treatment of feline hyperadrenocorticism.

Medical therapy directed toward the pituitary to decrease ACTH release includes cyproheptadine (Periactin), an antiserotonin drug, or bromocriptine (Parlodel), a dopamine agonist. These drugs are not usually used because of their frequent side effects and infrequent success in dogs.

Surgery. Surgical approaches to the treatment of pituitary-dependent hyperadrenocorticism include hypophysectomy and bilateral adrenalectomy. These procedures, which are not generally done in dogs, require a skilled surgeon, intensive monitoring, and lifelong hormone replacement therapy. Unlike the situation in dogs, bilateral adrenalectomy in cats appears to be the most successful treatment for pituitary-dependent hyperadrenocorticism. The reader is referred to Matthieson and Mullen (1990) for additional information about hypophysectomy and adrenalectomy. Adrenalectomy is discussed with treatment of adrenocortical tumors and in the section on feline hyperadrenocorticism.

Radiation. Radiation therapy has also been used to treat pituitary tumors. Pituitary tumors may be microadenomas or infrequently macroadenomas. Occasionally macroadenomas may be associated with neurologic signs such as blindness, stupor, and seizure activity because of their large size. Cobalt irradiation has been used successfully in these cases to reduce the size of the pituitary tumor (Dow and LeCouteur, 1989; Mauldin and Burk, 1990). Although cobalt therapy can reduce the size of the tumor and ameliorate neurologic complications, it does not appear to decrease pituitary ACTH secretion. Therefore Lysodren or ketoconazole therapy must be used concurrently to reduce serum cortisol concentrations.

Treatment of Adrenocortical Tumors

The treatment for adrenal tumors should be directed at destroying or removing the cancerous tissue. Surgical adrenalectomy is the treatment of choice for an adrenal tumor. Approximately 50% of the tumors are benign adenomas, and the dog should be cured with an adrenalectomy. The remaining 50% are metastatic adenocarcinomas, where surgical removal of all neoplastic tissue usually is impossible. Adrenalectomy may be associated with high morbidity and mortality, and should be done by a skilled surgeon. Great care must be taken to prevent acute adrenocortical insufficiency. Remember that the contralateral adrenal gland is atrophic so large doses of glucocorticoids should be given during and immediately after surgery. Generally dexamethasone (0.1 to 0.2 mg/kg IV) or prednisolone sodium succinate (1 to 2 mg/kg IV) is given at anesthetic induction (Matthieson and Mullen, 1990). The dosage of steroids is gradually tapered and can usually be discontinued within 2 months of surgery. If a metastatic adrenal carcinoma is found at the time of surgery and euthanasia is not desired by the owner, cortisol production can sometimes be temporarily reduced with large doses of Lysodren (50 to 150 mg/kg q24h) (Kintzer and Peterson, 1989). Medical therapy should be considered if the owner does not allow surgery, if a nonresectable tumor is present, or if the dog is not a suitable surgical patient. Some authorities advocate using Lysodren as the primary treatment for an adrenal tumor, since it has the potential to destroy the cancerous tissue. It would seem prudent to administer Lysodren at dosages large enough to effectively destroy all adrenocortical tumor as well as normal tissue. The dog could then be managed as an addisonian patient. The advantage of surgical cure in 50% of adrenal tumor patients is worth the risk in most animals. Ketoconazole, which blocks the cortisol synthetic pathway, can be used temporarily to achieve eucortisolemia. This treatment is used to stabilize the patient in preparation for later surgery or for the animal who has extremely high levels of cortisol or is unsuitable as a surgical candidate at the time of diagnosis.

Treatment for Iatrogenic Cushing's Syndrome

Treatment of iatrogenic Cushing's, also referred to as "secondary adrenocortical insufficiency,"

does not require surgery or Lysodren therapy. The adrenals are bilaterally atrophic in this condition despite the outward signs of hyperglucocortioidism. Depending on the degree of adrenocortical insufficiency, the dog should be started on a course of short-acting glucocorticoids (i.e., prednisone or prednisolone at 1 mg/kg q48h) and the dosage slowly reduced over 3 to 6 months. An alternative to prednisone or prednisolone therapy is treatment with oral hydrocortisone (Cortef) at 0.1 mg/5 kg q24h. The advantage of this approach is the replacement of maintenance glucocorticoid with more consistent blood levels from daily treatment while allowing restoration of adrenocortical function. The therapy can be monitored through ACTH stimulation tests, which should show recovery of the hypothalamic-pituitary-adrenal axis. Withdrawal of glucocorticoids from dogs with severe iatrogenic Cushing's syndrome can result in death.

Therapy for Dogs with Both Diabetes Mellitus and Hyperadrenocorticism

Diabetes mellitus and hyperadrenocorticism occur concurrently and require special therapeutic (and diagnostic) considerations. Cortisol excess causes an insulin resistance and glucose intolerance, by altering either receptor binding or receptor coupling. Thus dogs often require larger doses of insulin when they have concurrent hyperadrenocorticism. Lysodren therapy reduces cortisol concentration and daily insulin requirements in these patients and may lead to insulin overdosage, hypoglycemia, shock, and death. The standard Lysodren loading protocol (50 mg/kg q24h) is dangerous in these animals but is made safer by using a lower initial dosage of 25 mg/kg q24h and a higher daily dosage of prednisolone (0.4 mg/kg). Rapid reduction in daily insulin requirements is prevented, and the diabetes mellitus is easier to regulate.

Prognosis of Canine Hyperadrenocorticism

Adrenal adenocarcinoma may result in metastasis and death. Pituitary tumors may result in enlargement and secondary neurologic dysfunction. Chronic hypercortisolemia may include increased susceptibility to infection, glucose intolerance leading to diabetes mellitus, pulmonic thromboembolism, cardiovascular disease, and hypertension. Euthanasia may be elected if the dog has become unacceptable due to severe polyuria and polydipsia or chronic therapy for complicating problems. Most dogs do well with therapy for pituitary-dependent hyperadrenocorticism. Of 200 dogs who were treated with Lysodren for more than

3 months (Kintzer and Peterson, 1991) more than 80% were considered to have good to excellent response. Many dogs, because of their age, die or are euthanized for unrelated reasons within 2 years of diagnosis. Kintzer and Peterson (1991) reported that the mean survival time of 200 dogs was 2.2 years, with a range of 10 days to 8.2 years. Dogs with pituitary-dependent hyperadrenocorticism that do not have cortisol suppression after the 1 mg/kg of dexamethasone testing may have a more guarded long-term prognosis.

The prognosis for dogs with an adrenal tumor depends on whether the tumor is a benign adenoma or a malignant adenocarcinoma. Generally dogs with benign adenomas and adrenalectomy have an excellent prognosis. They are essentially cured. However, one must consider the morbidity and mortality associated with the surgical procedure. Alternatively, adrenal adenocarcinoma is associated with a guarded to grave prognosis, and death usually occurs shortly after diagnosis.

FELINE HYPERADRENOCORTICISM

Canine hyperadrenocorticism and feline hyperadrenocorticism are similar in many respects; however, there are some major differences, and these will be discussed in the following section. (The reader is referred to pp. 273 and 274 for a more general explanation of disease related to cortisol excess.) Unlike in dogs, which seem to have Cushing's as the most common endocrinopathy, in cats it is most uncommon (less than 20 cases having been described in the literature).*

Clinical Disease

Cats with hyperadrenocortcism are middle-aged or older. They are more frequently females (69%), and there is no apparent breed predilection. Polyuria, polydipsia, pendulous abdomen, and polyphagia are the most frequently observed signs of feline hyperadrenocorticism (Table 26-2). Cutaneous abnormalities such as truncal and abdominal alopecia, unkempt hair coat, thin skin, bruising and abscesses are also common. Some cats have exremely fragile skin, which is easily torn with normal manipulation or handling (Fig. 26-6). These cats are best managed with occlusive dressings and body bandages to promote healing and

*These have been reviewed by Zerbe (1989) and more recently by Nelson and Feldman (1991).

Table 26-2. Incidence of historical and clinical signs of spontaneous feline hyperadrenocorticism

SIGN	NUMBER OF CATS (%)
Polyuria-polydipsia	15/16 (94)
Pendulous abdomen	15/16 (94)
Polyphagia	14/16 (88)
Hair loss	11/16 (69)
Muscle wasting	10/16 (63)
Weight gain	9/16 (56)
Hepatomegaly	9/16 (56)
Thin skin	7/16 (44)
Infections	6/16 (38)
Depression	4/16 (25)
Weight loss	3/16 (19)
Easy bruising	3/16 (19)

From Zerbe CA. In Kirk RW (ed): Current veterinary therapy X. Philadelphia, 1989, WB Saunders, p 1038.

help prevent further damage, as well as therapy to promote eucortisolemia.

Although polyuria and polydipsia are common in both canine and feline hyperadrenocorticism, the cause and time of onset of the polyuria and polydipsia differ. In dogs they occur early in the syndrome and are secondary to glucocorticoid inhibition of the secretion or action of antidiuretic hormone. In cats they result from a glucocorticoid-induced hyperglycemia with subsequent glucosuria and osmotic diuresis. Of reported cats with hyperadrenocorticism, 81% had concurrent overt diabetes mellitus (only 10% to 15% of dogs with hyperadrenocorticism developed diabetes mellitus). In addition, the onset of polyuria and polydipsia in cats appears to be delayed. Therefore it is possible that hyperglycemia, and thus poluria and polydipsia, may not be detected in the early states of hyperadrenocorticism.

Recurrent infections may be life-threatening and can include facial abscesses, bacterial and fungal cystitis, pyothorax, bronchitis, rhinitis, pancreatitis, and enteritis. One cat had demodicosis.

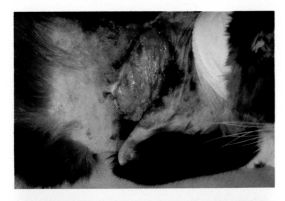

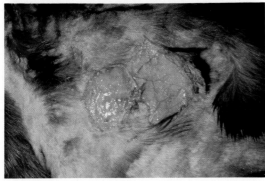

Figure 26-6. A, Large full-thickness tears in the skin of a cat with hyperadrenocorticism and diabetes mellitus. Note the associated hair loss and very thin skin. **B,** Additional tears occurred during hospitalization with routine handling of the cat.

(Courtesy Dr. Catherine Daley, Auburn, Ala.)

Laboratory Findings

Serum Biochemistries

The most common biochemical abnormalities in cats with hyperadrenocorticism are hyperglycemia and hypercholesterolemia (Table 26-3). Hyperglycemia tends to develop more frequently in cats, and cats tend to have higher glucose concentrations than dogs with Cushing's syndrome. The hypercholesterolemia is probably related to the poorly controlled diabetic state rather than to the glucocorticoid excess per se. Mild to moderate increases in alanine aminotransferase (ALT) and serum alkaline phosphatase (SAP) develop in 50% and 40% of cats respectively. This is in contrast to dogs, in which SAP is frequently (more than 90% of cases), very high.

Selecting the Appropriate Test for Adrenocortical Evaluation in Cats

Because feline hyperadrenocorticism is an uncommon disease, it will probably be some time

Table 26-3. Incidence of laboratory abnormalities in spontaneous feline hyperadrenocorticism

FINDING	NUMBER OF CATS (%)*
Hyperglycemia	14/15 (93)
Glucosuria	13/15 (87)
Hypercholesterolemia	10/13 (77)
Lymphopenia	10/14 (71)
Eosinopenia	9/14 (64)
Neutrophilia	9/14 (64)
Increased alanine aminotransferase	7/14 (50)
Increased serum alkaline phosphatase	5/15 (40)
Mature leukocytosis	3/14 (21)
Decreased blood urea nitrogen (BUN)	3/15 (20)

*Not all cats received all tests.
From Zerbe CA. In Kirk RW (ed): Current veterinary therapy X. Philadelphia, 1989, WB Saunders, p 1038.

before firm recommendations can be made as to the best endocrine test to use when screening for and differentiating among its etiologies in cats. However, it would currently seem that the ACTH stimulation test, the combined dexamethasone suppression–ACTH stimulation test, and the high-dose dexamethasone suppression test (0.1 mg/kg IV) are the most useful. Nonetheless, it is important to realize the limitations of these tests; the veterinarian should carefully consider clinical signs and laboratory abnormalities, as well as results of adrenal function studies, before making a diagnosis of hyperadrenocorticism. For example, if a cat has a normal response to one of the screening tests but hyperadrenocorticism is still suspected, a different screening test should be used or the test repeated in 3 to 4 weeks. Likewise, caution must be used before diagnosing hyperadrenocorticism in a cat with equivocal test results since some normal cats and cats with nonadrenal illness may have exaggerated cortisol response to ACTH stimulation (Zerbe et al., 1987b).

Once a diagnosis of hyperadrenocorticism has been made, differentiating tests can be used to determine whether the cat has pituitary-dependent hyperadrenocorticism (PDH) or an adrenal tumor. The ACTH assay and possibly the 1 mg/kg dexamethasone suppression test appear to be useful for this. However, it could be argued that it is not necessary to distinguish PDH from an adrenal tumor in cats since the current recommended treatment of feline hyperadrenocorticism is unilateral adrenalectomy for adrenal tumor and bilateral adrenalectomy for PDH.

Treatment of Feline Hyperadrenocorticism

Treatment of hyperadrenocorticism includes surgical, medical, and radiation modalities and has been attempted in 7 of 13 cats with pituitary-dependent hyperadrenocorticism and in 2 of 3 cats with an adrenal tumor. These therapies have met with varying degrees of success. Lysodren therapy, cobalt irradiation, metyrapone therapy, and bilateral adrenalectomy have been used for the treatment of pituitary-dependent hyperadrenocorticism (Zerbe et al., 1987c). Lysodren, tried in one cat, was ineffective in controlling clinical signs but did not induce any side effects or adrenocortical suppression. Furthermore, only 2 of 4 normal cats experienced adrenocortical suppression after Lysodren therapy with dosages typically used in dogs. Cobalt irradiation of the pituitary tumor was then unsuccessfully attempted in that same cat. Metyrapone, a drug that decreases cortisol synthesis by inhibiting an enzyme in the cortisol synthetic pathway, has been used with mixed results to treat feline hyperadrenocorticism. Clinical improvement was noted in one cat treated with metyrapone at a dosage of 65 mg PO q8h for 6 months; however, the cat was lost to follow-up. Peterson (1988) reported using metyrapone at dosages of 200 to 250 mg q24h in two cats; one showed slight clinical improvement with some regrowth of hair and resolution of polyuria and polydipsia after 6 months of therapy; the other died after 1 month of therapy without clinical improvement. Another case, previously unpublished, was successfully treated with metyrapone; a dose of 65 mg orally q8h was used initially and then reduced to 65 mg PO q12h when an ACTH response test showed adrenocortical suppression. This cat, which had extremely fragile skin with several large tears, had remarkable wound healing (Fig. 26-7) and decreased insulin requirements within 1 month of initiating metyrapone therapy, after which she underwent uneventful adrenalectomy. Ketoconazole has also been used with mixed success in cats. Of four that were

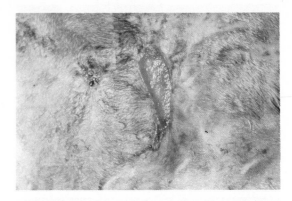

Figure 26-7. Same cat as in Fig. 26-6 following 2 weeks of metyrapone therapy and return to eucortisolemia. Note the dramatic improvement in wound healing.

(Courtesy Dr. Catherine Daley, Auburn, Ala.)

treated, one had no clinical improvement after more than 2 months, another developed severe thrombocytopenia after 7 days of therapy, and two others showed clinical improvement after receiving ketoconazole at an initial dosage of 5 mg/kg q12h for 7 days and then 10 mg/kg q12h indefinitely (Nelson and Feldman, 1991).

The following is a recently published protocol for treatment with adrenalectomy in the cat (Nelson and Feldman, 1991): dexamethasone (0.05 mg/kg body weight) is placed in the fluid infusion bottle and given over 6 hours, beginning at the time of adrenal removal. This is repeated every 12 hours until the cat is eating and drinking. Glucocorticoids are then supplemented with prednisone or prednisolone at 1 mg/kg PO q12h for 2 to 4 days, after which the dosage can be gradually reduced. If a bilateral adrenalectomy was performed, daily prednisone (2.5 mg/day) and mineralocorticoid supplementation (Florinef, 0.05 mg q12h) are necessary. At the time of bilateral adrenalectomy, hydrocortisone hemisuccinate or hydrocortisone sodium succinate can be used at 2 mg/kg q6h, then 1 mg/kg q6h the second day, and then 1 mg/kg q12h thereafter until the cat can be switched to oral medication.

Bilateral adrenalectomy, followed by mineralocorticoid and glucocorticoid replacement therapy, appears to be the most successful treatment for feline pituitary-dependent hyperadrenocorticism. As with dogs, this surgery should be performed by a skilled surgeon. This surgery was performed in six cats, all of which showed clinical improvement with resolution of polyuria and polydipsia and regrowth of hair. Five of these hyperadrenocorticoid cats had concurrent diabetes mellitus. After surgery four cats no longer required insulin therapy, and one remained a diabetic but was controlled on approximately 1 unit of protamine zinc insulin per day. Two cats underwent unilateral adrenalectomy, and at a 6-week recheck clinical signs of hyperadrenocorticism were resolving in one; the remaining cat progressively improved, lost its insulin dependency, and survived 14 months before being killed by a car. Thus four of the five diabetic cats that were successfully treated for their hyperadrenocorticism no longer required insulin therapy.

It is worth noting that all cats that were treated with adrenalectomy for either PDH or an adrenal tumor survived the surgery and experienced no reported complications. Dogs that undergo this type of operation have significantly higher morbidity and mortality. If the cat exhibits extremely fragile skin that tears easily with handling, we recommend the animal be treated initially with metyrapone until cortisol levels are normal and the cutaneous lesions are healing. Ketoconazole may be used if the response to metyrapone is not adequate. At that time the adrenalectomy should be performed.

Prognosis for Feline Hyperadrenocorticism

Untreated or unsuccessfully treated spontaneous feline hyperadrenocorticism appears to be a progressive disorder with a grave prognosis. Cats died of severe infection, uncontrolled diabetes mellitus, or euthanasia in all reported cases that were not treated. Cats with adrenal adenomas or pituitary-dependent hyperadrenocorticism appear to have a good to excellent prognosis with proper treatment. One cat, however, did develop neurologic abnormalities, presumably related to an expanding pituitary tumor. Since this is a disease of middle-aged to older cats, it is not unreasonable to expect that some will die or be euthanized because of problems unrelated to their hyperadrenocorticism. It is likely that cats with adrenal carcinoma will have a grave prognosis, as do dogs.

REFERENCES

Bruyette DS, Feldman EC: Ketoconazole and its use in the management of canine Cushing's disease, Compend Contin Educ Pract Vet 10:1379, 1988.

Chastain CB: Evaluation of the hypothalamic pituitary axis in clinically stressed dogs, J Am Anim Hosp Assoc 22:435, 1986.

Dow SW, LeCouteur RA: Radiation therapy for canine ACTH-secreting pituitary tumors. In Kirk RW (ed): Current veterinary therapy X, Philadelphia, 1989, WB Saunders, p 1031.

Eiler H, Oliver JN: Stages of hyperadrenocorticism: response of hyperadrenocorticoid dogs to the combined dexamethasone suppression/ACTH stimulation test, J Am Vet Med Assoc 185:289, 1984.

Feldman EC: Evaluation of a combined dexamethasone suppression/ACTH stimulation test in dogs with hyperadrenocorticism, J Am Vet Med Assoc 187:49, 1985.

Jones CA et al: Changes in adrenal cortisol secretion as reflected in the urinary cortisol/creatinine ratio in dogs, Domest Anim Endocrinol 7:559, 1990.

Kintzer PP, Peterson ME: Mitotane (O,P'DDD) treatment of cortisol-secreting adrenocortical neoplasia. In Kirk RW (ed) Current veterinary therapy X, Philadelphia, 1989, WB Saunders, p 1034.

Kintzer PP, Peterson ME: Mitotane (o,p'-DDD) treatment of 200 dogs with pituitary-dependent hyperadrenocorticism, J Vet Intern Med 5:182, 1991.

Matthieson DT, Mullen HS: Problems and complications associated with endocrine surgery in the dog and cat, Probl Vet Med Endocrinol 2(4):627, 1990.

Mauldin GN, Burk RL: The use of diagnostic computerized tomography and radiation therapy in canine and feline hyperadrenocorticism, Probl Vet Med Endocrinol 2:557, 1990.

Nelson RW, Feldman EC: Hyperadrenocorticism. In August JR (ed): Consultations in feline internal medicine, Philadelphia, 1991, WB Saunders, p 267.

Peterson ME: Endocrine disorders in cats: four emerging diseases, Compend Contin Educ Pract Vet 10:1353, 1988.

Peterson ME, Graves TK: Effects of low dosages of intravenous dexamethasone on serum cortisol concentrations in the normal cat, Res Vet Sci 44:38, 1988.

Rijnberk A, van Wees A: Assessment of two tests for the diagnosis of canine hyperadrenocorticism, Vet Rec 122:178, 1988.

Smiley LE, Peterson ME: Urinary corticosteroid/creatinine ratio at a screening test for canine hyperadrenocorticism. In Proceedings, Eighth ACVIM forum, Washington DC, 1990, p A31.

Smith MC, Feldman EC: Endogenous ACTH and plasma cortisol response to synthetic ACTH and dexamethasone sodium phosphate in normal cats, Am J Vet Res 48:1719, 1987.

Watson ADJ, et al: Systemic availability of o,p'-DDD in normal dogs, fasted and fed, and in dogs with HAC, Res Vet Sci 43:160, 1987.

Zerbe CA: Feline hyperadrenocorticism. In Kirk RW (ed): Current veterinary therapy X, Philadelphia, 1989, WB Saunders, p 1038.

Zerbe CA, et al: Adrenal function testing in dogs with hyperadrenocorticism. Abstract 8. In Proceedings, Fifth Annual Veterinary Medical Forum, 1987a, p 883.

Zerbe CA, et al: Effect of nonadrenal illness on adrenal function in the cat, Am J Vet Res 48:451, 1987b.

Zerbe CA, et al: Hyperadrenocorticism in a cat, J Am Vet Med Assoc 190:559, 1987c.

CHAPTER

27

Growth Hormone–Responsive Dermatosis

Edmund J. Rosser Jr.

Diagnostic Criteria for Growth Hormone–Responsive Dermatosis

SUGGESTIVE

Age, breed, sex, and distribution pattern of alopecia and hyperpigmentation; hair coat color changes (especially red, brown, or black streaks); no pruritus, secondary pyoderma, or keratinization abnormality

COMPATIBLE

Suggestive plus no response to thyroid supplementation; skin biopsies compatible with an endocrine dermatosis (non-scarring alopecia) with a prominent number of hair follicles showing hyper-eosinophilic tricholemmal keratinization ("flame follicles")

TENTATIVE

Suggestive plus normal basal thyroid hormone values and/or normal TSH response test; normal adrenal function tests (both cortisol and adrenal androgens); normal reproductive hormone values (estradiol, progesterone, testosterone); no response to castration; regrowth of a tuft of hair at skin biopsy sites.

DEFINITIVE

Tentative plus abnormal growth hormone stimulation test and response to growth hormone injection therapy

---

Importance

Growth hormone–responsive dermatosis is a rare endocrine dermatosis that initially appears as a nonpruritic skin disease with symmetric alopecia. It is often confused with other endocrine dermatoses (Chapters 25, 26, and 28) and is difficult to diagnose due to the unavailability of canine growth hormone assays.

Pathogenesis

The pathogenesis of growth hormone–responsive dermatosis is unknown. The primary defect was once believed to be a maturity-onset growth hormone deficiency (so-called maturity-onset hyposomatotropism) (Parker and Scott, 1980; Eigenmann and Patterson, 1984; Scott and Walton, 1986). This belief was based on the observation that affected dogs had either a low or a normal basal serum level of growth hormone and poor response to xylazine or clonidine (growth hormone stimulation test). However, responses to treatment utilizing growth hormone injections varied considerably. They included no regrowth of hair, partial regrowth of hair, regrowth of hair followed by a recurrence of the alopecia, and permanent regrowth of hair (Rosser, 1987). These observations resulted in further evaluation of this disease for other underlying causes.

Patients with abnormal growth hormone–response tests may have concurrent abnormalities related to gonadal sex hormone production (Rosser, 1990). (See Chapter 28.) Recent work in Pomeranians (Schmeitzel and Lothrop, 1990; Lothrop and

Schmeitzel, 1990) suggests the possibility of an adrenal gland sex hormone abnormality. The findings included various combinations of elevations in serum levels of progesterone, 17-hydroxyprogesterone, dehydroepiandrosterone sulfate (DHEAS), androstenedione, and endogenous ACTH. It was hypothesized that the sex hormone abnormalities were primarily of adrenal origin and that a partial deficiency of the adrenal enzyme 21-hydroxylase might be the cause. The study also revealed that Pomeranians that appear clinically normal have low basal serum levels of growth hormone and a poor response to xylazine. Hyperglucocorticoidism, hypothyroidism, and sex hormone abnormalities may also alter the results of a growth hormone stimulation test (Peterson and Altszuler, 1981; Jansson et al., 1982; Medleau et al., 1985). Therefore, simply finding abnormally low results on a growth hormone stimulation test is not sufficient evidence to establish that the pathophysiology is related to a primary growth hormone deficiency.

For these reasons primary growth hormone deficiency is considered a relatively rare cause of endocrine skin disease and should be diagnosed only after exclusion of the other, more common, endocrine dermatoses discussed.

CLINICAL DISEASE

Growth hormone–responsive dermatosis most commonly occurs in adult male dogs before 2 years of age. However, it has been reported in females and in dogs of various ages. The breeds most commonly affected include Pomeranians, Chow Chows, Poodles, Keeshonds, and Samoyeds. The initial chief complaint is a bilaterally symmetric alopecia, which is not associated with pruritus and affects the perineal region, genital region, and neck (often in a bandlike pattern). The posterior and medial thighs, ventral abdomen, tail, and ears may be affected as the disease progresses. Severe cases develop more generalized truncal alopecia. Marked hyperpigmentation frequently develops in the areas of alopecia, often simultaneously with the alopecia. The hair coat becomes dull and dry, may have a "fuzzy" appearance, and easily epilates. A change in hair coat color usually develops (may become lighter or darker) with red, brown, or black streaks within the hair coat. An interesting feature is that hair will regrow in a tuftlike manner at any site of full-thickness skin trauma (e.g., skin biopsy sites, lacerations). This occurs within 1 to 3 months in a previously alopecic area (Rosser and Sams, 1991).

There are no signs of systemic illness or other metabolic problems on clinical presentation. Patients have a normal activity level and are mentally alert; thus the owner's primary concern is the change in the appearance of the skin and hair coat. Secondary pyodermas and keratinization abnormalities (often observed in hypothyroidism and hyperglucocorticoidism) rarely develop.

DIAGNOSIS

The age, breed, sex, and physical findings may lead one to suspect growth hormone responsive dermatosis but only after ruling out other endocrine dermatoses. The diagnosis of a primary growth hormone deficiency, requiring growth hormone replacement therapy, is rare and other causes for the clinical appearance of these patients can usually be found. In attempting to establish this diagnosis, it is important to first rule out hypothyroidism (Chapter 25), hyperadrenocorticism (Chapter 26), and

---

ACTH Stimulation Test– Reproductive Hormone Panel

1. Collect baseline EDTA (2 ml blood) and clot (5 ml blood) tube samples.
2. Centrifuge and remove the plasma from the EDTA tube as quickly as possible (cortisol binds to RBCs).
3. Centrifuge and remove serum from clot tube as soon as the sample has clotted. Freeze the serum.
4. Administer ACTH (Cosyntropin) at a dose of 0.5 IU/kg IV.
   Alternatively, use ACTH gel at a dose of 0.22 USP unit/kg IM
5. Collect post-ACTH stimulation samples (2 ml EDTA tube and 5 ml clot tube) 1 hour after ACTH administration. If ACTH gel is used, collect 1- and 2-hour samples.
6. Freeze the plasma and serum samples; ship on dry ice by overnight express mail. (See Appendix for mailing addresses.)
7. Samples will be measured for cortisol, 11-deoxycortisol, DHEAS, androstenedione, 17-hydroxyprogesterone, progesterone, testosterone, and estradiol.

sex hormone abnormalities, especially castration-responsive dermatosis (Chapter 28). Having done this, one should next assess the dog for a possible adrenal sex hormone abnormality by performing an ACTH stimulation test–reproductive hormone panel (box on p. 289) (Schmeitzel and Lothrop, 1990). This protocol is based on the observation that many patients with "growth hormone–responsive dermatosis" may actually have a primary abnormality in adrenal sex hormone function. The test involves prestimulation and poststimulation measurements of serum cortisol, 11-deoxycortisol, DHEAS, androstenedione, 17-hydroxyprogesterone, progesterone, testosterone, and estradiol. A sample should also be submitted for the measurement of endogenous levels of serum ACTH. If there is an adrenal sex hormone abnormality, serum progesterone, 17-hydroxyprogesterone, DHEAS, androstenedione, and endogenous ACTH should be elevated (Schmeitzel and Lothrop, 1990; Lothrop and Schmeitzel, 1990).

The objective of this test is to determine whether the primary problem is an adrenal sex hormone disorder. If this is proved, one must question whether the condition should even be referred to as "growth hormone–responsive dermatosis." Finally, the growth hormone stimulation test can be performed. A baseline sample for measurement of serum growth hormone is taken, followed by the IV administration of 0.1 mg/kg of xylazine (Rompun). Serum samples are drawn 15 and 30 minutes after the injection for measurement of growth hormone. Unfortunately, a commercial assay for the measurement of serum levels of growth hormone in dogs is no longer available.

Skin biopsies may also be submitted for histopathologic examination. This will usually support a diagnosis of endocrine skin disease with additional changes suggestive of growth hormone–responsive dermatosis or castration-responsive dermatosis. Unfortunately, these two diseases cannot be differentiated by histologic changes. The histologic changes include surface and follicular hyperkeratosis, epidermal atrophy and melanosis, follicular dilation and atrophy, telogen hair follicles, atrophy of sebaceous glands, and a prominent number of hair follicles exhibiting hypereosinophilic tricholemmal keratinization (so-called "flame follicles").

TREATMENT

It is easy for the clinician or practitioner to become confused when selecting the best treatment for a patient with so-called growth hormone–responsive dermatosis. The patient should first be evaluated for any thyroid, glucocorticoid, or sex hormone abnormalities (especially castration-responsive dermatosis and adrenal sex hormone abnormality). If these diseases have been ruled out and the patient has an abnormally low growth hormone stimulation test, growth hormone injection therapy may be tried. The recommended treatment (Schmeitzel and Lothrop, 1990) is human growth hormone at a dosage of 0.15 IU/kg subcutaneously two times a week for 6 weeks. A complete response should occur within 3 months. It is important to note the diabetogenic effect of exogenous growth hormone therapy, so blood glucose must be measured before the treatment is started and on a weekly basis for the 6-week injection period. If hyperglycemia is noted, the injections should be stopped immediately and the diabetes is usually reversible. However, if the patient is not monitored closely and the growth hormone injections are not stopped early enough, permanent diabetes mellitus may result. For this reason I do not currently recommend using growth hormone injections to treat this disease. If the patient is left untreated, the only consequences are persistence of the skin and hair coat changes and the animal is not at risk for the development of any systemic illness or metabolic disease.

An alternative treatment is the use of o,p'-DDD (Lysodren) when an adrenal sex hormone dysfunction has been documented through the ACTH stimulation test–reproductive hormone panel and measurement of endogenous serum ACTH (Lothrop and Schmeitzel, 1988). As previously mentioned, one must question use of the term "growth hormone–responsive dermatosis" once this abnormality has been established. Information pertaining to o,p'-DDD therapy may be found in Chapter 26. The owner should be first advised that this disease appears to affect only the skin and hair coat (i.e., produces only aesthetically displeasing changes) and is not associated with the development of any systemic illness or metabolic disease. The owner should then be cautioned that therapy with o,p'-DDD is potentially toxic to the dog and the dog can become ill.

REFERENCES

Eigenmann JE, Patterson DF: Growth hormone deficiency in the mature dog, J Am Anim Hosp Assoc 20:741, 1984.

Jansson JO, et al: Effects of gonadectomy and testosterone replacement on growth hormone response to alpha-2 adrenergic stimulation in the male rat, Psychoneuroendocrinology 7:245, 1982.

Lothrop CD, Schmeitzel LP: Growth hormone-responsive alopecia in dogs, Vet Med Rep 2:81, 1990.

Medleau L, et al: Congenital hypothyroidism in a dog, J Am Anim Hosp Assoc 21:341, 1985.

Parker WM, Scott DW: Growth hormone-responsive alopecia in the mature dog: a discussion of 13 cases, J Am Anim Hosp Assoc 16:824, 1980.

Peterson ME, Altszuler N: Suppression of growth hormone secretion in spontaneous canine hyperadrenocorticism and its reversal after treatment, Am J Vet Res 42:1881, 1981.

Rosser EJ: Growth hormone-responsive dermatosis vs castration responsive dermatosis, Derm Dialogue, Fall, 1987.

Rosser EJ: Castration-responsive dermatosis in the dog. In von Tscharner C, Halliwell REW (eds): Advances in veterinary dermatology, London, 1990, Baillière Tindall.

Rosser EJ, Sams A: Alopecia. In Allen DG (ed): Small animal medicine, Philadelphia, 1991, JB Lippincott.

Schmeitzel LP, Lothrop CD: Hormonal abnormalities in Pomeranians with normal coat and in Pomeranians with growth hormone–responsive dermatosis, J Am Vet Med Assoc 197:1333, 1990.

Scott DW, Walton DK: Hyposomatotropism in the mature dog: a discussion of 22 cases, J Am Anim Hosp Assoc 22:467, 1986.

28

Sex Hormones

Edmund J. Rosser Jr.

Importance

The sex hormone–related dermatoses have traditionally been considered rare forms of endocrine skin diseases; and compared to hypothyroidism and hyperadrenocorticism, they certainly are. Since hypothyroidism and hyperadrenocorticism occur relatively more often, it is necessary to perform the appropriate diagnostic tests to rule them out first before considering a sex hormone–related dermatosis. The incidence with which sex hormone–related dermatoses are diagnosed has increased as our understanding of sex hormone production and the physiology of the gonads, adrenal glands, and peripheral target tissues (e.g., the dermis and epidermis) has improved. The recent availability of serum or plasma analysis of the various sex hormones at commercial and research laboratories has also aided our understanding of these diseases. In many instances the basal level of a given sex hormone may be sufficiently elevated or lowered to support the suspicion of a sex hormone abnormality. However, patients with sex hormone imbalances can also have basal levels within normal limits and these results alone may not be sufficient to rule out a suspected problem; thus it may become necessary to treat the patient according to the suspected diagnosis, with ultimately the response to therapy confirming or denying the diagnosis. In the future sex hormone stimulation and function tests should prove more helpful in establishing a definitive diagnosis. The normal values for these tests are currently being established, and the results of preliminary tests are not yet available.

OVARIAN IMBALANCE TYPE I

Ovarian imbalance type I is an abnormality involving the excess production of sex hormones from the ovaries. It may consist of elevations in estradiol (most common), progesterone, or testosterone (Muller et al., 1989; Rosser and Sams, 1991). Any one or a combination of these three hormones may be elevated. Cystic ovaries with endometrial hyperplasia or a functional ovarian tumor are most often observed in these patients. In rare instances the disease can present in an iatrogenic form due to the administration of estrogens in treating urinary incontinence, mismatings, and hypoestrogenism.

Clinical Disease

Ovarian imbalance type I is usually first noted in middle-aged and older intact female dogs. It is always important to take a thorough history, reviewing the estrous cycles and reproductive capabilities of an intact female presented for a dermatologic examination. The earliest suggestion of ovarian sex hormone excess is an abnormality in one of these areas.

The skin condition may be noted first in association with the estrous cycles, pregnancy, or pseudopregnancy and be present only during that time. This cyclic nature of the disease may continue for several years, or cease and the problem become continuous. In some instances it may be continuous with exacerbations noted only during changes in the estrous cycle. Abnormal findings include short

Diagnostic Criteria for Ovarian Imbalance Type I

SUGGESTIVE

Age, sex, and distribution patterns of alopecia and hyperpigmentation; may be pruritic; history of estrous cycle abnormalities; alopecia may initially coincide with estrous cycles; presence of a keratinization abnormality or ceruminous otitis externa

COMPATIBLE

Suggestive plus gynecomastia and enlarged vulva; skin biopsy compatible with an endocrine dermatosis (nonscarring alopecia)

TENTATIVE

Compatible plus normal basal thyroid hormone values and/or normal thyroid-stimulating hormone (TSH) response test, absence of clinical signs or clinicopathologic data suggesting hyperadrenocorticism; persistent elevations of serum estradiol, testosterone, or progesterone

DEFINITIVE

Tentative plus response to ovariohysterectomy

or long cycles, absent cycles, abnormal intervals between cycles, minimal or excess vaginal bleeding or discharge during the cycle, repeated and severe or prolonged pseudopregnancies, and inability of the bitch to be successfully bred.

The most common dermatologic abnormality is a bilaterally symmetric alopecia beginning in the perineal and perivulvar region that may progress anteriorly along the ventral trunk and neck. Hyperpigmentation of the skin in the alopecic areas usually occurs. In some instances the alopecia and hyperpigmentation are localized to the flank regions and may change in severity with the onset of estrus or changes in the seasons of the year (Miller, 1989; Muller et al., 1989; Rosser and Sams, 1991). A unique feature sometimes seen is early development of pruritus, long before any secondary complications are observed. Other findings on physical examination may include a keratinization abnormality (seborrheic changes), ceruminous otitis externa, and areas of lichenified skin. Gynecomastia and an enlarged vulva are often no-

ticed (especially with excess estradiol and/or progesterone) but may be absent (especially if the excess hormone is testosterone).

Diagnosis

The history and physical findings are the most important criteria for a suggestive diagnosis of ovarian imbalance type I. If the owner is not opposed to having an ovariohysterectomy performed on the dog, that should be the first recommendation. The ovaries should be submitted for histopathologic examination, in case of an ovarian tumor, which in some instances is malignant. If the diagnosis is correct, improvement will be noted within 3 to 6 months. If further support for the diagnosis is desired, before an ovariohysterectomy, the first step is to submit serum samples obtained during diestrus for measurement of estradiol, progesterone, and testosterone. If any one or a combination of these hormones is elevated, the ovariohysterectomy should be performed. An exception would be elevation of progesterone alone. If serum progesterone is elevated, measurements should be repeated on a monthly basis for 3 to 4 months to extend into the anestrus period. Sustained elevations suggest persistently functioning corpora lutea, and an ovariohysterectomy should be performed.

Several representative skin biopsies submitted for histopathologic examination will usually suggest the presence of an endocrine skin disease, but the changes noted are not specific for ovarian imbalance type I. The histologic changes include a surface and follicular hyperkeratosis, epidermal atrophy and melanosis, follicular dilation and atrophy, telogen hair follicles, and atrophy of sebaceous glands. When the patient is pruritic, additional histologic changes may include a superficial perivascular dermatitis reaction.

Treatment

Ovariohysterectomy is the treatment of choice, and a response occurs within 3 to 6 months. Secondary complications such as a keratinization abnormality (seborrheic changes) or ceruminous otitis externa should be treated with appropriate symptomatic therapy. (See Chapters 18 and 24.) If the patient is extremely pruritic or has lichenified areas of skin, a brief course of short-acting corticosteroid is recommended. Prednisone or prednisolone may be given orally at a dosage of 0.5 mg/kg q12h for 5 to 7 days, then 0.5 mg/kg q24h for 5 to 7 days, and then 0.5 mg/kg q48h for 1 week.

OVARIAN IMBALANCE TYPE II

Ovarian imbalance type II is a cutaneous abnormality occurring after ovariohysterectomy that is caused by a deficiency of sex hormones. It may consist of a deficiency in estradiol, progesterone, or testosterone. The ovaries are responsible for significant production of all three of these hormones during various stages of the estrous cycle (Pineda, 1989). Any one or a combination of these three hormones may be deficient, but deficiencies of estradiol are most common, with basal levels being essentially zero (Rosser and Sams, 1991). However, instances in which a spayed female has responded favorably to replacement therapy with testosterone have been reported (Miller, 1989). The exact pathogenesis as to how the disease develops in a given individual is not known at present. One possibility is that the body is responding to an absolute deficiency of these hormones simply due to removal of the ovaries. It is assumed that the adrenal glands are responsible for maintaining an adequate level of these hormones after an ovariohysterectomy. Therefore, it is also possible that the primary defect is an inadequate level of basal sex hormones produced by the adrenal glands. It is now known (Ebling and Hale, 1983) that a significant amount of sex hormone metabolism takes place peripherally within the skin. This occurs by means of various receptors within cells of the skin and the response of these receptors to the decrease in sex hormones; alternatively, a defect within the receptor system itself may be the cause.

Clinical Disease

Most female dogs that develop ovarian imbalance type II have had an ovariohysterectomy early in life. The first sign noted is a bilaterally symmetric alopecia of the perineal and perivulvar region. The alopecia may progress to the medial thighs and along the ventral trunk and neck region. As it progresses, hyperpigmentation of the skin is usually absent. Alopecia may also be noted around and on the pinnae. In some instances the alopecia is isolated to the flank regions and may change in severity with changes in the seasons of the year (Muller et al., 1989; Scott, 1990; Rosser and Sams, 1991). On physical examination the vulva and nipples have a juvenile appearance. Rarely the dog may also have a history of urinary incontinence, which may respond to estrogen replacement or phenylpropanolamine.

Diagnosis

An area of endocrinology in which a deficiency of knowledge seems apparent is our understanding of the normal sex hormone levels after neutering. At this writing none of the endocrinology laboratories have established a reference range for the major ovarian hormones (estradiol, progesterone, and testosterone) after ovariohysterectomy. For this reason ovarian imbalance type II disease is often treated according to history and physical examination findings alone, and a therapeutic response trial is recommended. The diagnosis of ovarian imbalance type II is made if the patient responds to treatment and the hair coat grows back to normal. However, it is often helpful to measure the basal levels of these hormones to guide selection of the replacement hormone. Estradiol, progesterone, and testosterone should be measured simultaneously. The diagnosis of ovarian imbalance type II can be suspected if the level of any of these hormones is found to be essentially zero. In my experience, estradiol is the sex hormone that most commonly has a value at or near zero, followed by testoster-

---

Diagnostic Criteria for Ovarian Imbalance Type II

SUGGESTIVE

Age, sex, and distribution patterns of alopecia; history of ovariohysterectomy early in life; hyperpigmentation usually absent; absence of pruritus, secondary pyoderma, or keratinization abnormality

COMPATIBLE

Suggestive plus juvenile vulva and nipples; concurrent urinary incontinence; skin biopsy compatible with an endocrine alopecia (nonscarring alopecia)

TENTATIVE

Compatible plus normal basal thyroid hormone values and/or normal TSH response test, absence of clinical signs or clinicopathologic data suggestive of hyperadrenocorticism; serum estradiol or testosterone levels of essentially zero

DEFINITIVE

Tentative plus response to treatment using estrogen or testosterone replacement therapy

one. At this writing, an abnormally low progesterone level has not been recognized. The hormone measurement closest to zero should then be selected as the one for replacement therapy.

Skin biopsies can be submitted to help suggest the presence of an endocrine skin disease, but the changes are not specific for ovarian imbalance type II. The histologic changes include surface and follicular hyperkeratosis, epidermal atrophy, follicular dilation and atrophy, telogen hair follicles, and atrophy of sebaceous glands.

Treatment

The treatment of ovarian imbalance type II is usually estrogen replacement, but testosterone replacement also may be effective. The decision as to which hormone to use should be based on the basal sex hormone levels, as discussed above. The recommended dosage of diethylstilbestrol (DES) is 0.1 to 1 mg q24h PO for 3 to 4 weeks and then once or twice weekly thereafter as needed to maintain a normal hair coat. Since exogenous estrogen treatment can cause bone marrow suppression, a CBC, including platelet numbers, should be obtained. Initial monitoring is performed every 2 weeks for the first month. Once maintenance therapy has begun, blood cell monitoring can be decreased to every 3 to 6 months. This treatment may rarely cause signs of estrus.

The recommended dosage of methyltestosterone is 1 mg/kg q48h PO, not to exceed a total dose of 30 mg. This dosage is given for 1 to 3 months (until some hair regrowth is noted) and then reduced to twice weekly. Since exogenous testosterone treatment is capable of causing hepatotoxicity, serum alanine aminotransferase (ALT), aspartate aminotransferase (AST), and alkaline phosphatase levels should be monitored. Initially this is done every 3 to 4 weeks for the first 1 to 3 months of treatment. Once maintenance therapy has begun, liver enzyme monitoring can be decreased to every 4 to 6 months. A behavioral change (increased aggression) is rarely observed. A complete response to hormone replacement therapy usually occurs within 3 months.

TESTICULAR TUMORS

Three types of primary tumors of the testis occur in dogs: Sertoli cell tumors, interstitial cell tumors, and seminomas. There may be a single tumor type, two tumor types, or all three tumor types present in the same patient (Feldman and Nelson, 1987;

Diagnostic Criteria for Testicular Tumors

SUGGESTIVE

Age, breed, sex, and distribution pattern of alopecia and hyperpigmentation; frizzy, dull, and dry hair coat; presence of secondary keratinization abnormality or ceruminous otitis externa; presence of cryptorchidism

COMPATIBLE

Signs of male feminization; cryptorchidism with a palpable abdominal mass; palpable testicular mass or hardening with atrophy of the opposite testicle; tail gland or perianal gland hyperplasia or neoplasia; skin biopsy compatible with an endocrine dermatosis (nonscarring alopecia)

TENTATIVE

Presence of linear preputial dermatoses or macular melanosis of the inguinal and perianal skin; decreased spermatogenesis, blood dyscrasias, bone marrow suppression, prostatomegaly, or prostatitis; elevation of basal serum estradiol or elevation or decrease in serum testosterone

DEFINITIVE

Response to castration; presence of testicular tumor on biopsy

---

Madewell and Theilen, 1987). The clinical manifestations often relate to the tumor type and location of the neoplastic testicle. In general, the Sertoli cell tumor is the type most commonly associated with male feminization, but this may occur with seminomas and interstitial cell tumors as well (Muller et al., 1989). Intraabdominal and inguinal testicular tumors are most frequently Sertoli cell tumors or seminomas and are often associated with changes of male feminization. Estrogen levels may or may not be elevated, and testosterone levels may be either normal or decreased. All three tumors occur with equal frequency when located within the scrotum. However, most reported interstitial cell tumors are located within the scrotum and this is the type with the greatest capability of producing excess androgens.

Clinical Disease

Testicular tumors usually occur in middle-aged to older dogs, with a breed predisposition for Boxers, Shetland Sheepdogs, Weimaraners, German Shepherd Dogs, Cairn Terriers, Pekingeses and Collies (Feldman and Nelson, 1987; Madewell and Theilen, 1987; Muller et al., 1989). The most common dermatologic sign associated with testicular tumors is the development of a bilaterally symmetric alopecia beginning in the perineal and genital region that may progress anteriorly along the ventral trunk and neck. The hair coat may take on a frizzy appearance and be dull and dry. Hyperpigmentation is variable but is usually present in patients with male feminization. Signs of male feminization include gynecomastia of all mammary glands, lactation, a pendulous prepuce, attraction of male dogs, decreased libido, and squatting in a female posture to urinate or simply failing to lift a leg while urinating (Fig. 28-1).

Other possible dermatologic changes include secondary keratinization abnormalities (seborrheic changes) and ceruminous otitis externa. A fairly unique lesion, referred to as "linear preputial dermatosis," may be observed (Griffin and Rosenkrantz, 1986). This is a linear, erythematous or melanotic, macule present along the ventral aspect of the prepuce extending to the scrotum. It has also been suggested (Miller, 1989) that a macular melanosis of the inguinal and perianal skin may be observed as a specific change in patients with testicular tumors.

The abdomen, inguinal region, and scrotum should be carefully palpated for testicular tumors. The nontumorous testicle is usually soft and atrophic due to the effects of excess estrogens and/or androgens from the tumorous testicle on regulatory centers in the hypothalamus and pituitary glands via negative feedback. Occasionally there is no palpable testicular abnormality. Other abnormalities associated with excess estrogens include decreased spermatogenesis, bone marrow suppression, and prostatitis or prostatomegaly from squamous metaplasia of the epithelial cells of the prostate gland. Abnormalities to consider from excess androgens include tail gland hyperplasia, perianal gland hyperplasia or neoplasia, and benign

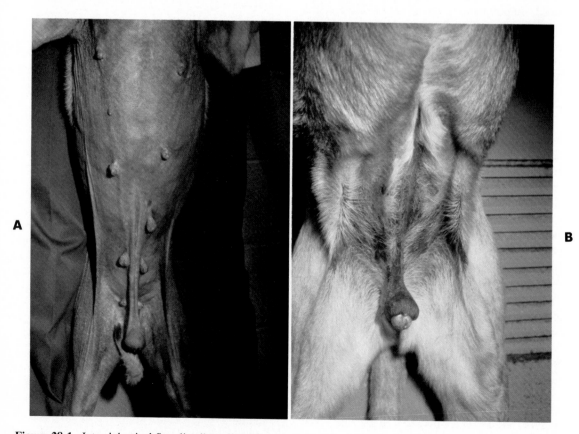

Figure 28-1. Intraabdominal Sertoli cell tumor with ventral alopecia, hyperpigmentation, gynecomastia, and a pendulous prepuce. **A,** Prior to castration. **B,** Following castration.

prostatic hypertrophy. One case has been reported (Fadok et al., 1986) of a patient with a Sertoli cell tumor producing excess progesterone that presented with a bilaterally symmetric alopecia over the flank regions.

Diagnosis

The suspicion that a testicular tumor is responsible for dermatologic changes found at physical examination is based exclusively on the historical development of the disease and physical findings. If the owner is not opposed to having the animal castrated, this should be the first recommendation. If the diagnosis is correct, histopathology of the testicles will determine the tumor type. A response to castration is observed within 3 months. If further support of the diagnosis is required before castration, serum samples should be submitted for the measurement of estradiol, progesterone, and testosterone. In most instances one of these three hormones will be abnormally elevated. However, the owner should be cautioned that some patients with a testicular tumor do not have a measurable abnormality in their sex hormone levels. A CBC should be performed to evaluate any blood dyscrasias, especially thrombocytopenia and anemia.

Although most testicular tumors are benign, they all have the potential of metastasizing to the regional lymph nodes, liver, lungs, spleen, kidneys, and pancreas. The Sertoli cell tumor is the most capable of metastasizing, especially if located intraabdominally, followed by the seminoma; the interstitial cell tumor is least likely to metastasize. Therefore, both abdominal and thoracic radiographs should be taken and examined for evidence of tumor metastasis.

Several representative skin biopsies can be submitted to further suggest the presence of an endocrine skin disease, but the changes are not specific for testicular tumors. The histologic changes include a surface and follicular hyperkeratosis, epidermal atrophy with or without melanosis, follicular dilation and atrophy, telogen hair follicles, and atrophy of sebaceous glands. The presence of linear preputial erythema or melanosis would suggest a Sertoli cell tumor.

Treatment

As discussed above, bilateral castration is the recommended treatment of choice after radiographic examination for tumor metastasis. The testicles should be submitted for histopathologic ex-amination. A complete response to castration is usually observed within 3 months. Tumor metastasis is suspected if there is no response to castration or if an initial response is followed by a recurrence of clinical signs. Should this occur, the prognosis is poor, although some limited success has been reported (Crow, 1980; Madewell and Theilen, 1987) when chemotherapy was attempted with various protocols using vinblastine, cyclophosphamide, and methotrexate.

If concurrent bone marrow suppression or prostatic gland disease is also present, these will require specific treatment as an adjunct to castration. In general, advanced bone marrow suppression carries a grave prognosis for complete recovery.

HYPOANDROGENISM OF MALE DOGS (testosterone-responsive dermatosis)

The development of hypoandrogenism may be due to a testosterone deficiency in dogs that have been castrated early in life (usually between 6 and 9 months of age). When the patient has responded

---

Diagnostic Criteria for Hypoandrogenism of Male Dogs

SUGGESTIVE

Age, sex, and distribution patterns of alopecia; hyperpigmentation usually absent; history of castration early in life or soft atrophied testicles in an intact older male dog

COMPATIBLE

Suggestive plus history of concurrent urinary incontinence; skin biopsy compatible with an endocrine dermatosis (nonscarring alopecia)

TENTATIVE

Suggestive plus normal basal thyroid hormone values and/or normal TSH response test, absence of clincial signs of clinical pathologic data suggesting hyperadrenocorticism; serum testosterone values of essentially zero

DEFINITIVE

Tentative plus response to treatment using testosterone replacement therapy

to testosterone replacement, initial basal levels of testosterone have been essentially zero (Rosser and Sams, 1991). A similar condition may be seen in older intact male dogs but is extremely rare. The exact pathogenesis of the cutaneous changes is not known. One possibility is that the body is responding to an absolute deficiency of androgens simply due to the removal of the testes, or as a function of the normal aging process in older intact male dogs. However, once the testes have been removed or become atrophied with age, it is assumed that the adrenal gland is then responsible for maintaining an adequate basal level of androgens. Therefore, it is also possible that the primary defect is an inadequate level of basal androgens from the adrenal gland. Finally, it is now known (Ebling and Hale, 1983) that a significant amount of androgen metabolism occurs peripherally within the skin. This occurs via receptors within various cells of the skin and the response of these receptors to the decrease in androgens, or perhaps because of a defect in the receptor system itself.

Clinical Disease

Most male dogs that develop hypoandrogenism have a history of being castrated early in life (usually between 6 and 9 months of age) but do not develop clinical signs until they are middle-aged or older dogs. The condition may develop in older intact male dogs with atrophied and soft testicles in rare instances. The most common clinical sign is bilaterally symmetric alopecia that initially affects the perineal and genital regions. The alopecia may progress to the medial thighs and along the ventral trunk and neck region. In rare cases the only presenting clinical sign is a bilaterally symmetric alopecia over the flank region. The hair coat may be dull and dry with secondary keratinization abnormalities (seborrheic changes). In rare cases a dog may have a history of urinary incontinence that responds to testosterone replacement.

Diagnosis

An area of endocrinology where a deficiency of knowledge seems apparent is our understanding of the normal androgen levels after neutering. At this writing, none of the endocrinology laboratories have established a reference range for androgens in normal castrated dogs versus intact or castrated dogs responsive to testosterone replacement. The serum testosterone levels measured have been essentially zero in patients that respond to replace-

ment therapy. It is important to note that older intact male dogs with atrophied, soft testicles and an endocrine-like alopecia should first be evaluated for possible hypothyroidism, hyperadrenocorticism, or the exogenous use of glucocorticoids. This process often proves to be quite rewarding, since these are common causes of secondary hypoandrogenism. Skin biopsies may be submitted from several representative areas to help support the diagnosis of an endocrine skin disease, but the changes are not specific for hypoandrogenism. The histologic changes include surface and follicular hyperkeratosis, epidermal atrophy, follicular dilation and atrophy, telogen hair follicles, and atrophy of sebaceous glands.

Treatment

The treatment of choice for hypoandrogenism in males dogs is methyltestosterone at a dosage of 1 mg/kg q48h PO, not to exceed an individual dose of 30 mg. This dosage is given for 1 to 3 months until some hair regrowth is noted and is then reduced to twice weekly. Occasionally male dogs may not respond to oral replacement but may respond to injectable testosterone. Repositol testosterone is given at a dosage of 2 mg/kg intramuscularly, not to exceed a total dose of 30 mg, and is given every 1 to 4 months as needed to maintain a normal hair coat. Since exogenous testosterone treatment may cause hepatotoxicity, the alanine aminotransferase (ALT), aspartate aminotransferase (AST), and alkaline phosphatase should be monitored. Initial monitoring should be performed every 3 to 4 weeks for the first 1 to 3 months of treatment. Once maintenance therapy has begun, liver enzyme monitoring can be decreased to every 4 to 6 months. A behavioral change of increased aggression is rarely observed.

CASTRATION-RESPONSIVE DERMATOSIS

Castration-responsive dermatosis is seen in male dogs that have palpably normal testes, that respond to castration as the only treatment, and that do not have a testicular tumor when biopsied. In most cases (Medleau, 1989; Muller et al., 1989; Rosser, 1990) a primary abnormality in gonadal sex hormones has been described, consisting of various combinations of altered basal levels of serum estradiol and testosterone. Abnormalities in basal levels of serum progesterone are less common and seem to be minimally affected by castration, since

Diagnostic Criteria for Castration-Responsive Dermatosis

SUGGESTIVE

Age, breed, sex, and distribution pattern of alopecia and hyperpigmentation; presence of hair coat color changes (especially red, brown, or black); absence of pruritus, secondary pyoderma, or keratinization abnormality; history of normal descent of testicles, which are normal on palpation

COMPATIBLE

Suggestive plus lack of response to thyroid supplementation; skin biopsies compatible with an endocrine dermatosis (nonscarring alopecia) with a prominent number of hair follicles showing hypereosinophilic tricholemmal keratinization ("flame follicles")

TENTATIVE

Compatible plus normal basal thyroid hormone values and/or normal TSH response test; absence of clinical signs or clinicopathologic data suggesting hyperadrenocorticism; elevation or decrease in basal serum estradiol and/or testosterone; abnormal GnRH-response test; regrowth of a tuft of hair at skin biopsy sites.

DEFINITIVE

Tentative plus response to castration

---

dog may be an effective treatment. Under these circumstances, one has to question whether the condition should even be referred to as "growth hormone–responsive dermatosis." Finally, it has been shown (Schmeitzel and Lothrop, 1990) that certain breeds of dogs (e.g., Pomeranians) that appear to be clinically normal may have low basal levels of growth hormone with poor responses on a growth hormone stimulation test. This suggests that a poor response to xylazine on a growth hormone stimulation test may be completely normal in certain breeds. Therefore the role of a growth hormone deficiency in these patients remains unclear at this time, but it does not appear to be the primary defect in patients with castration-responsive dermatosis. (See Chapter 27.) Hopefully, continued research that integrates observations about the gonadal sex hormones, adrenal sex hormones, and growth hormone and their responses to various hypothalamic and pituitary stimuli will further clarify the pathophysiology of this disease.

Clinical Disease

Castration-responsive dermatosis most frequently occurs in intact male, sexually mature, young adult dogs. There is a history of normal descent of the testicles, and the testicles are normal on palpation. The disease has been most commonly reported in Pomeranians, Chow Chows, Alaskan Malamutes, Siberian Huskies, Keeshonds, and Miniature Poodles. The initial chief complaint is a bilaterally symmetric alopecia affecting the perineal region, genital region, and neck (often in a bandlike pattern, Fig. 28-2). As the disease progresses, the posterior and medial thighs, ventral abdomen, and tail may be affected. Severe cases may develop a generalized truncal alopecia. Marked hyperpigmentation often develops in the areas of alopecia. The hair coat becomes dull and dry with excessive scaling and may have a "fuzzy" appearance. A change in hair coat color usually develops (may become lighter or darker), with red, brown, or black streaks (Fig. 28-3). An interesting feature is that hair is noted to regrow in a tuftlike manner at any site of full-thickness trauma to the skin (e.g., skin biopsy sites, lacerations) within 1 to 3 months in a previously alopecic area (Rosser and Sams, 1991).

Diagnosis

The age, breed, sex, and physical examination findings lead one to suspect the diagnosis of cas-

most of the basal progesterone is produced by the adrenal gland in the male dog.

An interesting finding in many of these patients is the concurrent abnormality of low basal levels of serum growth hormone and a poor response to xylazine when performing a growth hormone stimulation test. In one study (Rosser, 1990) it was demonstrated that dogs that responded completely to castration had low results on both precastration and postcastration growth hormone stimulation tests. They did not require growth hormone injection treatments for complete recovery, suggesting that the growth hormone abnormality was not the cause of the dermatosis. Articles describing growth hormone–responsive dermatosis (Lothrop, 1988) have mentioned that castration of an intact male

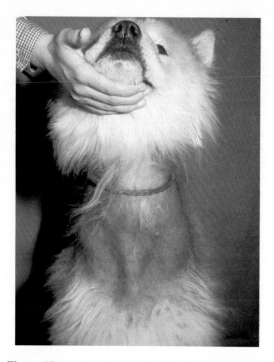

Figure 28-2. Castration-responsive dermatosis in a Chow Chow with a bandlike area of alopecia around the neck.

(From Rosser EJ, Sams AW: Small animal medicine, Philadelphia, 1991, JB Lippincott.)

tration-responsive dermatosis. Basal levels of serum estradiol, testosterone, and progesterone should be determined. The results will usually reveal various combinations of an increased or decreased serum estradiol and/or an increased or decreased serum testosterone. A gonadotropin-releasing hormone (GnRH) (Cystorelin) response test may be performed to demonstrate response of the gonads to stimulation. The test is performed by submitting baseline serum samples for measurement of estradiol, testosterone, and progesterone. GnRH is then administered IV at a dosage of 0.22 μg/kg and serum samples are collected at 1 and 2 hours after injection for measurement of all three hormones. This test is especially useful when the basal gonadal hormone levels are normal. The values expected will vary based on the established normals for each individual laboratory. The normal values for these tests are currently being established, and the results of preliminary tests are not yet available.

Several representative skin biopsies may be submitted for histopathologic examination and will usually support a diagnosis of endocrine skin disease with additional changes suggestive of castration-responsive or growth hormone–responsive dermatosis. Unfortunately, these two diseases cannot be differentiated on the basis of histologic changes. The histologic changes include surface and follicular hyperkeratosis, epidermal atrophy and melanosis, follicular dilation and atrophy, te-

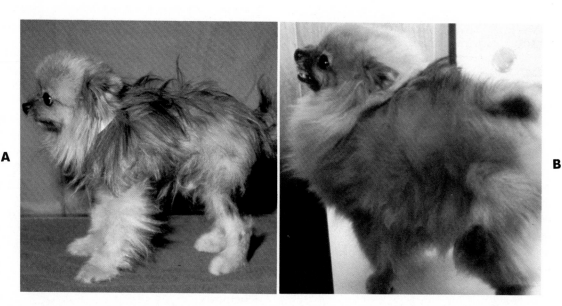

A **B**

Figure 28-3. A, Castration-responsive dermatosis in a Pomeranian with alopecia and hair-coat color changes. **B,** Three months following castration.

(From Rosser EJ, Sams AW: Small animal medicine, Philadelphia, 1991, JB Lippincott.)

logen hair follicles, atrophy of sebaceous glands, and a prominent number of hair follicles exhibiting hypereosinophilic tricholemmal keratinization (so-called flame follicles). Testicular biopsies submitted for histopathologic examination reveal normal testes.

Treatment

Castration is obviously the treatment of choice for this disease. However, certain criteria may be helpful in deciding when to recommend castration. These include the clinical disease (described earlier), abnormal basal levels of estradiol, testosterone, or progesterone; regrowth of tufts of hair at skin biopsy sites; and the histologic changes described earlier. If all of these criteria are met, the first treatment recommendation should be castration, and a complete response should be noticed within 3 months. It is important to note that some animals have fulfilled these criteria but have either not responded to castration or demonstrated an initial response to castration, only to redevelop the disease several months or years later. Interestingly, many of these patients have subsequently responded to testosterone replacement therapy. (See "Hypoandrogenism of Male Dogs," p. 297, for the treatment protocol. For further recommendations, should all these measures prove unrewarding, see Chapter 27.)

REFERENCES

Crow SE: Neoplasms of the reproductive organs and mammary glands of the dog. In Morrow, DA (ed): Current therapy in theriogenology, Philadelphia, 1980, WB Saunders.

Ebling FJ, Hale PA: Hormones and hair growth. In Goldsmith LA (ed): Biochemistry and physiology of the skin, New York, 1983, Oxford University Press.

Fadok VA, et al: Hyperprogesteronemia associated with Sertoli cell tumor and alopecia in a dog, J Am Vet Med Assoc 188:1058, 1986.

Feldman EC, Nelson RW: Disorders in the canine male reproductive tract. In Feldman EC, Nelson RW (eds): Canine and feline endocrinology and reproduction, Philadelphia, 1987, WB Saunders.

Griffin CE, Rosenkrantz W: Linear preputial erythema (abstr). In Proceedings, Annual members' meeting AAVD & ACVD, 1986.

Lothrop CD: Pathophysiology of canine growth hormone-responsive alopecia, Compend Contin Educ Pract Vet 10:1346, 1988.

Madewell BR, Theilen GH: Tumors of the genital system. In Theilen GH, Madewell BR (eds): Veterinary cancer medicine, Philadelphia, 1987, Lea & Febiger.

Medleau L: Sex hormone-associated endocrine alopecias in dogs, J Am Anim Hosp Assoc 25:689, 1989.

Miller WH: Sex hormone-related dermatoses in dogs. In Kirk RW (ed): Current veterinary therapy X, Philadelphia, 1989, WB Saunders.

Muller GH, et al: Cutaneous endocrinology. In Muller GH, et al (eds): Small animal dermatology, Philadelphia, 1989, WB Saunders.

Pineda MH: Reproductive patterns of female dogs. In McDonald LE, Pineda MH (eds): Veterinary endocrinology and reproduction, Philadelphia, 1989, Lea and Febiger.

Rosser EJ: Castration-responsive dermatosis in the dog. In von Tscharner C, Halliwell REW (eds): Advances in veterinary dermatology, London, 1990, Baillière Tindall.

Rosser EJ, Sams A: Alopecia. In Allen DG (ed): Small animal medicine, Philadelphia, 1991, JB Lippincott.

Schmeitzel LP, Lothrop CD: Hormonal abnormalities in Pomeranians with normal coat and in Pomeranians with growth hormone–responsive dermatosis, J Am Vet Med Assoc 197:1333, 1990.

Scott DW: Seasonal flank alopecia in ovariohysterectomized dogs, Cornell Vet 80:187, 1990.

29

Metabolic Epidermal Necrosis

Donna Walton Angarano

Diagnostic Criteria for Metabolic Epidermal Necrosis

SUGGESTIVE

Clinical features and history; crusting dermatopathy; lack of response to routine therapy, including glucocorticoids or zinc

COMPATIBLE

Crusting acral dermatopathy; hyperkeratosis and/or ulceration of foot pads; lack of acantholytic cells in impression smears

TENTATIVE

Compatible plus hepatopathy, diabetes mellitus, hyperadrenocorticism, or hypoaminoacidemia

DEFINITIVE

Tentative plus dermatohistopathology; hepatic cirrhosis or glucagonoma

Importance

Canine metabolic epidermal necrosis is a rare disease that in most cases is found to be a cutaneous marker for a specific metabolic disorder. It has some similar findings to necrolytic migratory erythema (NME) in humans. In humans NME is associated with a glucagon-secreting pancreatic tumor. Metabolic epidermal necrosis is most often associated with hepatic cirrhosis. A small number of cases in both humans and dogs have manifested a different metabolic disease.

Metabolic epidermal necrosis is a rare but significant syndrome. The cutaneous lesions mimic pemphigus foliaceus and systemic lupus erythematosus. In addition, the disorder is indicative of concurrent serious internal disease with a poor prognosis.

Necrolytic Migratory Erythema

Necrolytic migratory erythema (NME) was originally described (by Becker et al., 1942) as a unique cutaneous eruption in a woman later found to have a pancreatic tumor. Subsequently, the disease in humans has been referred to as "glucagonoma syndrome," since most affected humans have a glucagon-secreting, alpha-cell neoplasm of the pancreas. The pathomechanism of the cutaneous eruption is debatable; however, most researchers believe the cutaneous changes are the result of elevated circulating glucagon and decreased amino acid (specifically tryptophan and niacin) levels. Hypoaminoacidemia is thought to result in epidermal protein depletion and subsequent cutaneous necrosis. There have been human cases (Norton et al., 1979) in which total parenteral nutrition and correction of hypoaminoacidemia led to remission of cutaneous signs despite persistent hyperglucagonemia. The exact pathomechanism is unknown.

Pseudoglucagonoma was reported (Doyle et al., 1979) in a human patient with NME and hepatic cirrhosis who had no evidence of pancreatic neoplasia on postmortem examination.

Metabolic Epidermal Necrosis

Metabolic epidermal necrosis (MEN) (the hepatodermal syndrome) was first described (Ehrlein et al., 1968) in eight dogs with unusual cutaneous lesions and concurrent liver disease. Five of these dogs were shown to have hepatic cirrhosis. Four similar cases were reported later (Walton et al., 1986), and the association with necrolytic migratory erythema in humans was made. These cases were called canine diabetic dermatopathy, which may have been an oversight of other pathomechanisms.

The disease is often, but not always, associated with hepatic cirrhosis in dogs. Glucagon-secreting pancreatic neoplasms have been reported (Gross and O'Brien, 1989) in two canine cases.

The most commonly reported concurrent diseases are hepatic cirrhosis and diabetes mellitus (Walton et al, 1986). Other associated abnormalities include hypoalbuminemia, renal disease, and hyperadrenocorticism. Elevated glucagon levels have been associated with canine necrolytic erythema and hepatic cirrhosis (Miller et al., 1990).

CLINICAL DISEASE

Twenty-six cases of canine metabolic epidermal necrosis (under various names) have been described since the first report. There does not appear to be any breed predilection. Published reports include 13 mixed-breed dogs, 2 Bedlington Terriers, 2 West Highland White Terriers, and 2 Cocker Spaniels. There were single reports of an English Cocker Spaniel, Dachshund, Scottish Terrier, Fox Terrier, Beagle, Bichon Frise, and German Shepherd Dog. Either sex may be affected, but males have been reported to have the disease almost twice as often as females (17 versus 9). Older dogs are most likely to be affected. The age ranges from 1 to 14 years, with an average of 10 years. Only one of these dogs was under 5 years old.

Although metabolic epidermal necrosis is a metabolic disease, the cutaneous manifestations usu-

ally precede clinical evidence of internal disease. Cutaneous signs are striking and follow a waxing and waning course. Lesions are well-demarcated and typically consist of erythema, crusts, and erosions around the mouth and eyes and on the legs, feet, and external genitalia (Figs. 29-1 and 29-2). Foot pads are usually hyperkeratotic and may be

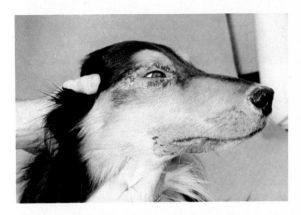

Figure 29-1. Periocular and perioral crusts on the face of a dog with metabolic epidermal necrosis.

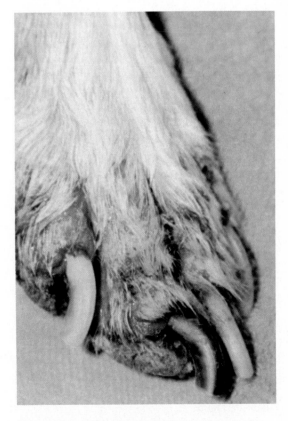

Figure 29-2. Crusts on the distal extremity of a dog with metabolic epidermal necrosis.

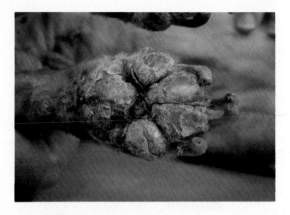

Figure 29-3. Hyperkeratosis of the foot pads of a dog with metabolic epidermal necrosis.

mildly to severely affected with fissures and ulceration (Fig. 29-3). The planum nasale is usually unaffected, which is not the case with most of the autoimmune dermatoses. Erythema is more pronounced on the distal extremities. In some cases superficial epidermal separation will lead to the formation of vesicles.

Lesions may be mildly pruritic or painful. A positive Nikolsky sign may be observed with some lesions.

The cutaneous signs of metabolic epidermal necrosis are generally not responsive to treatment; however, the erythema and severity of the lesions may lessen with glucocorticoid therapy. This can be of historical significance but is not a recommended form of therapy due to the metabolic disorders.

Differential Diagnosis

The differential diagnoses for this type of facial crusting in dogs include demodicosis, dermatophytosis, and bacterial folliculitis. The mucocutaneous distribution of lesions suggests pemphigus foliaceus, systemic lupus erythematosus, zinc-responsive dermatosis, toxic epidermal necrolysis, drug eruption, vasculitis, and mycosis fungoides.

The distal extremity erythema and foot pad hyperkeratosis observed in metabolic epidermal necrosis are unique. The differential diagnoses of the foot pad lesions include pemphigus foliaceus, systemic lupus erythematosus, zinc-responsive dermatosis, toxic epidermal necrolysis, and contact-irritant dermatitis.

Secondary bacterial or fungal infections may result from the ulceration. Dermatophyte infections

have been observed in the foot pads of several affected dogs (Walton et al., 1986).

Our understanding of this disease is incomplete at present, although at least two metabolic syndromes appear to be associated. Both hepatic cirrhosis and glucagon-secreting pancreatic tumors have been reported to occur individually with this disease.

Cutaneous signs may precede evidence of internal disease by weeks or months.

DIAGNOSIS

The diagnosis of metabolic epidermal necrosis is based on several test findings. The disease should be suspected on the basis of the history and physical examination. A typical case would be a middle-aged or older dog with a progressive, crusting dermatitis affecting the face, distal extremities, and external genitalia. Foot pad involvement is most consistent and suggestive of the diagnosis.

Skin scrapings and fungal cultures are negative. Impression smears reveal primarily neutrophils. Acantholytic cells (the hallmark of pemphigus) are absent.

Examination of skin biopsies reveals a unique combination of diffuse parakeratotic hyperkeratosis, epidermal necrosis, marked superficial epidermal edema, irregular epidermal hyperplasia, and mild superficial perivascular dermatitis. The epidermal edema consists of intercellular and intracellular edema localized to the upper half of the epidermis. Severe edema may result in intraepidermal clefts and vesicles. At low-power examination of the epidermis there is a striking microscopic appearance of a zone of pink, followed by white and then blue, representing respectively necrosis and parakeratosis, severe superficial edema, and epidermal hyperplasia. Epidermal edema may not be as pronounced in older lesions, requiring several skin biopsies for histologic examination.

Secondary bacterial and/or fungal infections often are present and frequently are found in foot pad lesions.

Clinicopathologic abnormalities vary, depending on the specific organ system involved (liver versus pancreas) and progression of the disease. Hemogram changes include anemia (either regenerative or nonregenerative), abnormalities in red cell morphology (polychromasia, anisocytosis, poikilocytosis, and target cells), neutrophilic leukocytosis, and toxic neutrophilic changes.

Frequent serum biochemical abnormalities include increased levels of liver enzymes (SAP, ALT, and AST), total bilirubin, bile acids, and BSP retention. Blood urea nitrogen is usually decreased, although cases with concurrent azotemia have been documented. Hypoalbuminemia is a common finding, and most dogs develop hyperglycemia during the course of the disease. This latter finding is interesting in that dogs with hepatic cirrhosis typically develop hypoglycemia as opposed to hyperglycemia and glucose intolerance.

Glucagon levels have been elevated in some cases when it was measured (Miller et al., 1990) but not in all (Turnwald et al., 1989). Concurrent pituitary-dependent hyperadrenocorticism has also been seen.

Immunofluorescence testing is generally negative, although a weakly positive ANA titer and positive staining at the basement membrane zone using direct immunofluorescence testing have been reported (Miller et al., 1990).

Postmortem examination may confirm hepatic cirrhosis or a glucagon-secreting tumor of the pancreatic alpha cells. The latter has been shown by Gross and O'Brien (1989) utilizing immunoperoxidase (PAP) staining of pacreatic tumors from two affected dogs. Chronic pancreatitis, renal pathology, and adrenohyperplasia may also be found.

TREATMENT

Specific treatment for metabolic epidermal necrosis is aimed at correcting the underlying metabolic disease, which is not usually accomplished. Although it may be possible in a dog with a glucagon-secreting tumor of the pancreatic alpha cells if the tumor can be surgically removed, this is rarely the case. Unfortunately, most cases of metabolic epidermal necrosis are associated with irreversible chronic liver disease and hepatic cirrhosis.

Therapy is primarily symptomatic. Antibiotic or antifungal agents are indicated for secondary infections. If the dog is diabetic, insulin therapy is indicated; however, in most cases, regulation is difficult. Hydrotherapy and shampoo therapy can help remove crusts and lessen the pruritus and pain that may be present.

Glucocorticoid therapy has been associated with an improvement in cutaneous signs. Since glucose intolerance is usually present, glucocorticoid therapy is contraindicated.

Correcting hypoaminoacidemia may be considered if a deficiency is determined to be present. Although there are no reports of this treatment in dogs, it has been helpful in humans (Norton et al., 1979).

Due to our lack of knowledge regarding the pathogenesis of metabolic epidermal necrosis, surgical or postmortem findings of hepatic cirrhosis or a glucagon-secreting pancreatic tumor are a great aid in establishing the definitive diagnosis. As our understanding of this unusual syndrome increases, the evidence needed for a suggestive, compatible, tentative, and definitive diagnosis will surely change. In order to better understand this syndrome, data on bile acid levels, the glucose tolerance test, liver biopsies, adrenal function tests, and glucagon assays need to be reported.

A decrease in serum amino acids (especially tryptophan and niacin) has been reported in humans. This abnormality needs to be evaluated in dogs.

REFERENCES

Becker SW, et al: Cutaneous manifestations of internal malignant tumors, Arch Dermatol Syphilol 45:1069, 1942.

Doyle JA, et al: Hyperglucagonemia and necrolytic migratory erythema in cirrhosis: possible pseudoglucagonoma syndrome, Br J Dermatol 101:581, 1979.

Ehrlein HJ, et al: Ekzem and Lebererkrankung beim Hund (Hepatodermales Syndrom), Kleint Prax 13:123, 1968.

Gross TL, O'Brien TD: Superficial necrolytic dermatitis (diabetic dermatopathy) in two dogs with glucagon-producing pancreatic endocrine tumors, Proc Am Acad Vet Dermatol, p 59, 1989.

Miller WH, et al: Necrolytic migratory erythema in dogs: a hepatocutaneous syndrome, J Am Anim Hosp Assoc 26:573, 1990.

Norton JA, et al: Amino acid deficiency and the skin rash associated with glucagonoma, Ann Intern Med 91:213, 1979.

Turnwald GH, et al: Failure to document hyperglucagonemia in a dog with diabetic dermatopathy resembling necrolytic migratory erythema, J Am Anim Hosp Assoc 25:363, 1989.

Walton DK, et al: Ulcerative dermatoses associated with diabetes mellitus in the dog: a report of four cases, J Am Anim Hosp Assoc 22:79, 1986.

SUGGESTED READINGS

Hashizume T, et al: Glucagonoma syndrome, J Am Acad Dermatol 19:377, 1988.

Muller GH, et al: Small animal dermatology, ed 4, Philadelphia, 1989, WB Saunders.

Swenson KH, et al: The glucagonoma syndrome: a distinctive cutaneous marker of systemic disease, Arch Dermatol 114:224, 1978.

Photodermatitis

30

Solar Dermatitis

Wayne S. Rosenkrantz

Diagnostic Criteria for Solar Dermatitis

SUGGESTIVE

History of sun exposure; physical signs of erythema in depigmented locations

COMPATIBLE

Suggestive plus normal adjacent pigmented sites with history of regression with reduced sun exposure or use of sunscreens

TENTATIVE

Compatible plus histopathology with epidermal hyperplasia and solar elastosis

DEFINITIVE

Tentative plus histopathology with squamous cell dysplasia, dyskeratosis, follicular hyperkeratosis—follicular cysts, furunculosis, scarring, and occasionally squamous cell carcinoma in situ

Importance

The cutaneous effects of sun exposure are directly related to wavelengths and the total dose of ultraviolet (UV) radiation. UVA (320 to 400 nm) is more abundant than UVB (290 to 320 nm) and is more frequently associated with photosensitivity reactions (Kocheuar et al., 1987; Parrish et al., 1987). "Photodermatitis" is a term often used to refer to an abnormal reaction of the skin to sun exposure. Photodermatitis can be divided into phototoxic, photosensitive, photoallergic, and miscellaneous disorders. Phototoxic reactions are dose-related responses seen in all animals that cause acute or chronic damage. The emphasis of the current discussion is on phototoxic reactions.

Phototoxic reactions as they occur in dogs and cats generally appear on areas of the body with white skin, depigmented skin, or lightly haired skin. Solar dermatitis and subsequent squamous cell carcinoma in white cats and nasal solar dermatitis in dogs are good examples of these phototoxic reactions. More recently, the recognition of solar dermatitis in white Bull Terriers with histories of chronic sun exposure also supports the importance of phototoxic reactions. In addition, phototoxic reactions are thought to play a role in the aggravation of other diseases. Lupus erythematosus and pemphigus erythematosus are autoimmune diseases thought to have a photoaggravated component.

Pathogenesis

The effects of ultraviolet radiation are attenuated by the hair coat, by absorption by melanin, and by reflection and refraction in the stratum corneum. The obvious photoprotector in animals is their hair coat. The amount of protection offered by the coat depends on its color, length, and density. Certain breeds, and individual animals of any breed, that are lightly colored or have a sparse hair coat have less protection. In general, areas with the least hair density (e.g., the ventrum, flanks, face, and ears) are more prone to a photodermatitis. Most cases of canine solar dermatitis in white Bull Terriers present with lesions on the flanks and abdomen, areas that are commonly sparsely covered by hair.

Melanin is considered a major defense of the skin against the effects of the sun. Dark hair coats also contain melanin and provide extra melanin protection over nonglabrous areas. Specifically, melanin absorbs radiation, which is utilized in the oxidation of melanin, causing the skin to darken. An example of the protective role melanin supplies can be seen in cases of nasal solar dermatitis. In dogs with mottled pigment over their planum nasale, pigmented sites are rarely or only mildly affected compared to nonpigmented areas.

The stratum corneum, with its variable content of melanin, is a major optically protective element. Loss of the stratum corneum will increase the potential for phototoxicity. Chronically affected solar dermatitis in white cats can be associated with erosions and ulcerations. Such sites are often where more invasive squamous cell carcinomas develop.

Other epidermal components (carotenoids and surface lipids) may act as photoprotective agents as well.

The mechanism and the subsequent pathology that occurs in a photodermatitis reaction are very complex and not completely understood. Cellular nucleic acids, membranes, and enzymes may be altered, causing functional and structural changes that lead to altered metabolism, mutation, or cell death. Partial or complete repair may occur, with subsequent changes in metabolic or mitotic kinetics in the surviving cells. Damaged cells release chemical mediators such as histamine, serotonin, kinins, prostaglandins, and leukotrienes.

Ultraviolet radiation can alter the immune system, possibly by decreasing the number of epidermal Langerhans cells by 20% to 50% (Thiers et al., 1984). Such changes in local immune function, cell kinetics, and cell damage could contribute to skin cancer. Extensive epidemiologic data support a causal role for sun exposure in most basal cell and squamous cell carcinomas and melanomas in humans. Certainly similar evidence exists to support the causal role of sun exposure in feline and canine solar dermatitis. Both of these entities can progress into squamous cell carcinomas.

CLINICAL DISEASE
Canine Nasal Solar Dermatitis

Canine nasal solar dermatitis occurs in dogs with a poorly pigmented planum nasale. Affected dogs may be born without pigment or may acquire a noninflammatory depigmentation (Ihrke, 1981).

The Australian Shepherd has this condition more commonly than any other breed. Cases in these dogs have been diagnosed as immune-mediated disorders (e.g., discoid lupus erythematosus or pemphigus erythematosus) (Rosenkrantz, 1990). Although definite proof is lacking, most appeared to be a form of nasal solar dermatitis. Previous breeds such as Collies with so-called "collie nose" and German Shepherd Dogs with ulcerated/crusted nasal lesions were also considered part of this entity. Over the years we have learned that many cases are autoimmune although sun exposure appears to be involved in the pathogenesis of some.

Cases may resolve or become quiescent during months of reduced UV radiation. The most intense sun exposure generally occurs in the summer months. However, dogs living in snow climates can have aggravated lesions as a result of UV reflection.

Lesions may begin initially either at the junction of the haired and nonhaired planum nasale or on the planum itself. Sites devoid of pigment initially appear erythematous. This early erythema most closely resembles a true sunburn as occurs in humans (Fig. 30-1). With more chronic sun exposure, affected areas can ulcerate and crust. Mild, limited, intermittent episodes of "sunburn" will generally not produce gross permanent alterations. However, with continued sun exposure the healed sites often appear scarred, with loss of their normal "cobblestone" architecture, hair, and glandular structures. It is rare for lesions to progress to squamous cell carcinoma. Severe chronic cases can end up with marked nasal ulceration and deformity of the nares and distal planum nasale. The underlying cartilage may also become eroded, which adds to the clinical deformity (Fig. 30-2). When severe ulceration is present, blood vessels are readily exposed and minor trauma can produce hemorrhage.

The major differential is autoimmune disease. Lupus erythematosus, particularly the discoid variety, can cause nasal depigmentation, ulceration, and crusting. Lupus erythematosus is a sun-aggravated disease. Systemic lupus usually will have more severe generalized skin lesions as well as a greater potential for systemic involvement. Pem-

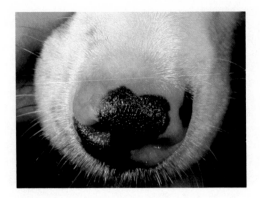

Figure 30-1. An Australian Shepherd with early sunburn. Note the erythema in depigmented areas.
(Courtesy Dr. Irv Ameti, Orange, Calif.)

phigus erythematosus and pemphigus foliaceus can also produce erosive vesicular or pustular nasal lesions, but these generally also affect the haired portion of the nasal area and (with pemphigus foliaceus) other body locations can be affected. Dermatomyositis, a disease seen primarily in Shetland Sheepdogs and Collies, can present with nasal lesions although it usually has facial and extremity lesions as well.

Infectious conditions, including bacterial and fungal nasal infections, occasionally resemble a nasal solar lesion. Tumors occurring in the nasal region can resemble a nasal solar-induced lesion. Such tumors include squamous cell carcinoma, basal cell carcinoma, epitheliotropic lymphoma, and fibrosarcoma. Other differential diagnoses include drug eruption, topical drug hypersensitivity, contact reaction, and trauma.

Canine Solar Dermatitis

Recently (Mason, 1987; Rosenkrantz, 1990) an increased recognition of solar-induced dermatitis has been noted in light-colored, sparsely haired breeds such as white Bull Terriers and American Staffordshire Terriers and their crosses, German Shorthaired Pointers, Dalmatians, white Boxers, Whippets, and Beagles. The most common history coinciding with the development of skin disease is that the dog likes to sunbathe. Often it will lie on one side more than the other, and the clinical disease will be more severe on areas with greater sun exposure. Some cases will be aggravated by additional environmental factors: dogs kept on white cement runs or patios, or dogs from climates with much snow.

The flanks and ventrolateral abdomen are most

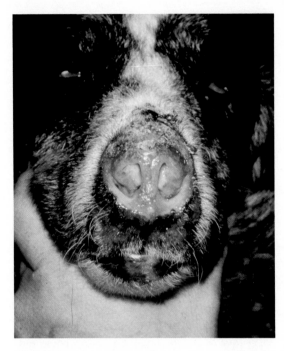

Figure 30-2. An Australian Shepherd with end-stage solar damage and ulceration with deformity of the planum nasale and nasal cartilage.

commonly involved. The bridge of the nose, pinnas, and lateral or medial hock areas can also be affected. The earliest lesions are erythema and scale (Fig. 30-3). Advanced lesions appear thicker and often have a roughened but glistening erythematous surface. Palpation of the affected areas allows recognition of how thickened these depigmented sites feel. The surrounding unaffected pigmented areas palpate normally. Closer visual inspection often reveals comedone formation, follicular cysts, hemorrhagic bullae, folliculitis, furunculosis, and scarring. In more chronic progressive cases squamous cell carcinoma can develop (Fig. 30-4).

The differential diagnosis of canine solar dermatitis includes infectious conditions, particularly chronic scarring staphylococcal pyoderma. Early cases may resemble lupus erythematosus, not only clinically (by the diffuse erythema) but also histopathologically and immunopathologically. An example (Rosenkrantz, 1990) was seen in an 8-year-old white Boxer that had been initially misdiagnosed with lupus erythematosus due to (1) hydropic vacuolar changes on routine histopathology and (2) IgG deposition at the basement membrane zone on immunofluoresence. Other possible differentials that can present with comedones and follicular plugging are keratinization disorders, de-

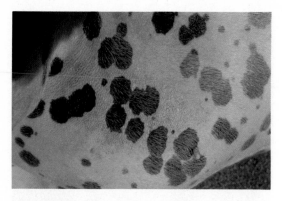

Figure 30-3. A white Boxer with early lesions of solar dermatitis. Note the diffuse erythema in a nonpigmented truncal location.

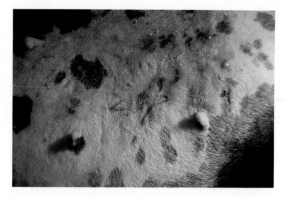

Figure 30-4. Progressive solar dermatitis in a dog with a lichenified glistening erythematous surface, follicular cysts, pyoderma, scarring, and early squamous cell carcinoma.

modicosis, and dermatophytosis. The diffuse erythematous phase may be confused clinically with epitheliotropic lymphoma. In advanced cases, when squamous cell carcinomas form, other nodular tumors (e.g., lymphosarcoma, mast cell tumors, hemangiosarcomas, and metastatic neoplasia) need to be considered. There also appears to be a higher incidence of primary hemangiosarcomas and hemangiomas developing on solar-damaged skin (Hargis, 1989), but these seem to metastasize at a lower rate than nonsolar hemangiosarcomas.

Feline Solar Dermatitis

Feline solar dermatitis is a chronic actinic dermatitis occurring in cats with white-colored areas. It can progress to squamous cell carcinoma. Most patients have a history of liking to sit in the sun on a regular basis. Affected sites include the ears, eyelids, planum nasale, lips, and face. The earliest lesions often appear on the margins of the pinnae. This area is normally sparsely covered by hair and stands erect, so it is the site most vulnerable to solar radiation (Fig. 30-5). The first sign of the solar damage is erythema (sunburn). This early change often persists for months or even years and slowly progresses to thickened, erythematous, peeling, erosive, and crusting lesions. As the progression occurs, there may be some discomfort, exhibited by pruritus or twitching of the pinnae. With further progression it is not uncommon for the sites to become heavily crusted and bleed when traumatized. Pinnal margins may also curl and take on a scalloped appearance. At this point the lesions most likely have progressed to squamous cell carcinoma.

Another site commonly affected is the dorsal aspect of the planum nasale, with progression to the alar folds and development into squamous cell carcinoma with severe erosion, ulceration, and necrosis (Fig. 30-6). The margins of the eyelids and lips are also often affected, starting with erythema and progressing to ulceration and crusting. Another common site of involvement on the face that can be overlooked is the preauricular region. This area, like the pinnae, is often sparsely haired, allowing for penetration of solar radiation. Lesions here are similar to those at other sites but many times will progress from persistent erythema to brown pigmented macules and papules that eventually crust and ulcerate. With time most progress to squamous cell carcinoma and can metastasize to regional nodes.

The differential diagnosis includes autoimmune diseases that can affect the pinnae and facial area, such as pemphigus and lupus erythematosus. Drug reactions and epitheliotropic lymphoma (mycosis fungoides) can have an affinity for the face and ears of cats. Pruritic dermatopathies such as notoedric mange, otodectic acariasis, and food and inhalation allergies must also be considered. Bacterial infections may be a complicating factor. In cold climates, cold agglutinin disease and frostbite are differentials.

DIAGNOSIS

A suggestive diagnosis of solar dermatitis is made on the history and physical examination. Chronic sun exposure is reported in most cases. The finding of erythematous lesions in depigmented or sparsely haired sites following sun exposure is suggestive of a solar dermatitis. Adjacent

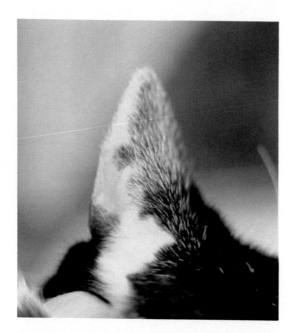

Figure 30-5. Feline solar dermatitis affecting the margin of the pinna. Often the earliest lesion is persistent erythema of the pinnal margin.

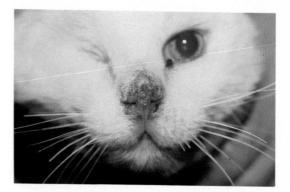

Figure 30-6. Squamous cell carcinoma developing at a site of solar dermatitis on the planum nasale of a cat.

pigmented areas appear normal and palpate normally compared to affected erythematous depigmented sites. A history of the regression of erythema and other lesions following sun avoidance or the use of sunscreens is also supportive. Many cases will have seasonal variation—more severe in the spring and summer, less severe in the fall and winter.

Both a tentative and a definitive diagnosis will require histopathology. In all three entities described—canine nasal solar dermatitis, canine solar dermatitis, and feline solar dermatitis—early features on routine histopathology include reduced numbers of melanocytes and pigment, mild intraepidermal edema, and vascular dilation. The intraepidermal edema can occur at the dermal/epidermal junction, making early solar lesions difficult to distinguish from lupus erythematosus. At this stage of the disease the histopathology is not definitive for solar dermatitis. As cases progress, epidermal hyperplasia with lymphocytic/mononuclear perivascular infiltrates can be seen. Solar elastosis (blue-staining elastic fibers) can occur in the superficial dermis. Elastic fibers may become curled or fragmented and eventually degenerate. The epidermis may ulcerate, with an overlying suppurative crust.

In more chronic cases the dermis and cartilage in areas such as the planum nasale or pinnae may be destroyed. As a case advances further, dyskeratotic, dysplastic, and occasionally atypical polyhedral squamous cells are visualized. Sometimes cords of atypical cells will invade the dermis, resulting in a squamous cell carcinoma. In canine solar dermatitis, additional features include dilated hyperkeratotic follicules with follicular cysts, folliculitis, furunculosis, and deep pyogranulomas. In all three entities, moderate scarring is common in chronic cases.

TREATMENT

The most obvious therapy in canine nasal solar dermatitis, canine solar dermatitis, and feline solar dermatitis is sun avoidance, and the most critical time for this is between 10 AM and 4 PM. Optimally, total sun avoidance is recommended, but this is often not practical.

When the pet cannot be kept out of the sun, alternatives must be considered. For outside dogs, providing shade with a patio or run cover is recommended. Sunscreens may also be utilized. Products with a high sun protection factor (SPF) and water resistance are recommended. SPF is defined by Taylor et al. (1990) as the ratio of the amount of UVB energy required to produce a minimal erythematous reaction through a sunscreen product film to the amount of energy required to produce the same erythema without any sunscreen application. Sunscreens with an SPF of 15 or higher filter more than 92% of the UVB responsible for erythema. The sunscreen should be applied q12h. In canine solar dermatitis, protective clothing such as T-shirts can help block sun exposure to truncal locations. Black felt-tipped marking pens may be used to color the depigmented planum nasale of dogs or cats with nasal solar lesions. Tattooing is a more permanent technique but currently is rarely used because allergic or irritant reactions to the injected ink can develop. Tattoo reactions may occur, more commonly in autoimmune diseases affecting the planum nasale. To rule out other differentials, skin biopsies should always be performed before tattooing. Antibiotics should also be used if any secondary infection is present.

In addition to sun avoidance, medical approaches to solar dermatitis may be tried. Early erythematous solar lesions on any part of the body can be treated with topical or systemic corticosteroids. Topical preparations need not be particularly potent. Products containing hydrocortisone in a cream (Pharmaderm 1% and 2.5%) or ointment (Pharmaderm 1%) base are mild enough to be used topically q12-24h for the first week and then as needed. If systemic therapy is necessary to reduce the erythema, a short course of oral prednisone at 1 mg/kg q24h for 3 to 5 days is usually sufficient. It can be continued on an alternate-day basis and slowly tapered to 0.5 mg/kg q48h and eventually discontinued.

Mild cases of solar dermatitis have also been treated with beta-carotene (Solatene) at a dosage of 30 mg twice a day (Mason, 1987). Carotenoids are vitamin A precursors, and beta-carotene is a free-radical scavenger that is thought to quench the triplet state of singlet oxygen and free radicals, forming a lipid-carotene complex that may absorb solar radiation. The benefits of carotenes are highly controversial, and most veterinarians believe they have minimal value in any of the solar dermatitis entities.

Other synthetic forms of vitamin A have also received attention. Isotretinoin (Accutane) and etretinate (Tegison) have been tried in canine solar dermatitis. Results have been variable, though more favorable with etretinate. In 10 dogs with solar-induced squamous cell carcinoma and preneoplastic lesions (Power, 1991), 3 showed complete resolution of the lesions following etretinate administration and 2 had partial responses at 90 days. The dosage was 1 mg/kg q12h PO. Isotretinoin (3 mg/kg q24h) has also been evaluated for solar-induced squamous cell carcinoma in cats (Evans et al., 1985). It was ineffective, but established synthetic retinoid drugs could have been used safely. Isotretinoin at a dosage of 2 mg/kg q12h has been ineffective in several cases of solar dermatitis in dogs (Rosenkrantz, 1990).

If response to the retinoids occurs, it should be seen within 4 to 6 weeks. Dosages can be reduced to a once-a-day or alternate-day basis. Initially the animal should be monitored monthly for keratoconjunctivitis sicca, musculoskeletal abnormali-

ties, triglyceride elevations, and hepatotoxicity. Monitoring can be reduced to quarterly if no complications are seen within the first 3 months.

More specialized therapeutic options include hyperthermia, cryosurgery, photochemotherapy, and radiation therapy.

Hyperthermia, or local current field radiofrequency at 50° C, for 30 to 60 seconds can adequately treat small focal solar lesions or early squamous cell carcinomas. Results are best in lesions of less than 5 mm diameter and 2 mm depth. However, this therapy should be avoided on the pinnae since it may cause necrosis and sloughing. In a feline study (Grier et al., 1980) results were favorable in 70% of the cases.

Cryosurgery, or the use of freezing temperatures, can be effective for solar dermatitis or early squamous cell carcinoma. Optimal results are seen in small focal lesions. Cell damage is more severe with rapid freezing and slow thawing with three freeze-thaw cycles. Ideally the final tissue temperature should be −20° C. Small lesions (less than 5 mm) can be treated by liquid nitrogen applications with an ordinary cotton stick. Larger lesions (greater than 5 mm) generally require more involved freezing techniques and are beyond the scope of this discussion. Additional information is available elsewhere (Withrow, 1980).

Photochemotherapy is a recent technique (Thoma, 1983) that utilizes selective wavelengths of light to increase the energy of a photosensitive drug that causes a selective cytotoxic effect on tumor cells. The drugs used currently are hematoporphyrin derivatives (photofrin-V, chloroaluminum sulfonated phthalocyanine), which have a greater affinity for neoplastic than for normal cells and subsequently accumulate in the atypical cells. The hematoporphyrin derivatives are injected IV at dosages of 1 mg/kg (for chloroaluminum sulfonated phthalocyanine) and 5 mg/kg (for photofrin-V). The affected sites are treated 48 to 72 hours after the hematoporphyrin is injected with an argon laser at wavelengths of 630 to 675 nm. The actual treatment takes 10 to 20 minutes per lesion and depends on the lesion's size and the joules and milliwatts used. Best results are seen in lesions smaller than 2.5 cm diameter and 5 mm depth.

In 10 cats with either squamous cell carcinoma (7) or solar dermatitis and early SCC in situ (3) that I treated with photofrin-V, results were poor in 6 with SCC lesions. However, this most likely reflected the density, severity, and progressive nature of the cases selected. The solar dermatitis cases (3) with early SCC in situ exhibited good responses. Some investigators (Berns, 1990) recommend surgical debulking or CO_2 laser therapy before utilizing the hematoporphyrin technique. In a recent study (Peavy et al., 1991) treatment of feline solar and squamous cell carcinoma lesions with phthalocyanine was more promising. Initially 19 of 23 treated sites (82.6%) were judged complete responses; at 12 months posttreatment, 10 of 14 (71.4%) were reevaluated and were still judged complete responses. Based on these results and the limited availability of equipment, this technique should be reserved for early solar lesions and for practitioners who have access to such equipment. Currently the equipment needed to perform photochemotherapy is limited. Three facilities that offer it are the Irvine Beckman Laser Institute at the University of California, Irvine; the University of California, Davis, School of Medicine; and the Town & Country Animal Hospital in Cheektowage, New York. The cost is reasonable, with average cases running $200 to $300.

Radiation therapy is expensive and has limited availability, but is highly effective. It is generally saved for more advanced lesions that progress to SCC. Most require a total dosage of 3000 to 4000 rads, and this may include three to ten treatments with multiple anesthesias.

Surgical excision of the affected tissue is one of the more drastic, but curative, forms of therapy for progressive solar lesions (and particularly squamous cell carcinoma). In cats with solar lesions that have progressed to SCC, partial pinnectomies are commonly performed. Nasal and eyelid lesions are less amenable to surgery, but occasionally surgery can result in an adequate cosmetic appearance. Many cases of canine solar dermatitis that progress to carcinoma with severe scarring and pyogranuloma formation are also amenable to surgical excision.

Optimal early therapy in all cases involves sun avoidance, the use of sunscreens, and the administration of antibiotics if a secondary pyoderma develops. Should this be ineffective, a short course of topical or systemic gluococorticoids can be evaluated. In cases that are refractory or that progress to early SCC in situ, treatment with one of the specialized procedures or drugs may be required: etretinate may be used in canine solar dermatitis; ink marking and tattooing should be considered for canine nasal solar dermatitis; and cryosurgery, hyperthermia, or phototherapy should be considered for feline or canine solar lesions that are small enough to be effectively treated. If a case continues to progress, radiation and surgery may become additional considerations.

REFERENCES

Berns MW: Personal communication, Beckman Laser Institute, 1990.

Evans AG, et al: A trial of 13-cis-retinoic acid for treatment of squamous cell carcinoma and preneoplastic lesions of the head in cats, Am J Vet Res 46:2553, 1985.

Grier RL, et al: Hyperthermic treatment of superficial tumors in cats, J Am Vet Med Assoc 177:227, 1980.

Hargis A: Cutaneous hemangiomas and hemangiosarcomas in dogs: a retrospective clinicopathological study of 212 dogs. In Proceedings, Annual member's meeting AAVD & ACVD, 1989.

Ihrke P: Nasal solar dermatitis. In Kirk RW (ed): Current veterinary therapy VIII, Philadelphia, 1983, WB Saunders, p 440.

Kocheuar IE, et al: Photophysics, photochemistry, and photobiology. In Fitzpatrick TB, et al (eds): Dermatology in general medicine, ed 3, New York, 1987, McGraw-Hill, p 1441.

Mason KV: The pathogenesis of solar-induced skin lesions in Bull Terriers. In Proceedings, Annual members' meeting AAVD & ACVD, 1987, p 12.

Parrish JA, et al.: Photomedicine. In Fitzpatrick TB, et al (eds): Dermatology in general medicine, ed 3, New York, 1987, McGraw-Hill, p 942.

Peavy GM, et al: The use of chloro-aluminum sulfonated phthalocyanine as a photosensitizer in the treatment of malignant tumors in dogs and cats. Proceedings, Society of Photo-optical Instrumentation Engineers, 1991, p 1424.

Power HT: Personal communication, 1991.

Rosenkrantz WS: Unpublished data, 1990.

Taylor CR, et al: Photoaging/photodamage and photoprotection, J Am Acad Dermatol 22:1, 1990.

Thiers BH, et al: The effect of aging and chronic sun exposure on human Langerhans cell populations, J Invest Dermatol 82:223, 1984.

Thoma RE: Phototherapy. In Kirk RW (ed): Current veterinary therapy VIII, Philadelphia, 1983, WB Saunders, p 438.

Withrow SJ (ed): Symposium on cryosurgery, Vet Clin North Am [Small Anim Pract] 10:753, 1980.

Dermatoses of Unknown Cause

31

Feline Eosinophilic Granuloma Complex

Wayne S. Rosenkrantz

Diagnostic Criteria for Idiopathic Feline Eosinophilic Granuloma Complex

SUGGESTIVE
History of clinical lesions

COMPATIBLE
Suggestive plus elimination of differentials through skin scrapings, cultures, cytology, food elimination, intradermal skin testing, and dermatohistopathology

TENTATIVE
Compatible plus dermatohistopathology consistent with one of the three reaction patterns: eosinophilic ulcer (variable eosinophilic collagenolysis), eosinophilic plaque (spongiotic dermatitis), or eosinophilic granuloma (eosinophilic collagenolysis)

DEFINITIVE
Tentative without identifying the underlying etiology

The eosinophilic granuloma complex (EGC) includes a group of lesions that affect the skin and oral cavity of cats. The term itself is often used as a final diagnosis when, in reality, there is another primary etiology. Three entities have traditionally been recognized: the eosinophilic ulcer, eosinophilic plaque, and linear granuloma.

These entities, considered common in practice, are seen more frequently in cats that have allergic and/or insect hypersensitivities (Reedy, 1982; Wilkinson and Bate, 1984; McDougal, 1986; Mason and Evans, 1991; Rosenkrantz, 1991ab). Bacterial involvement may be a factor, since antibiotic therapy occasionally resolves some lesions (Rosenkrantz, 1991ab). Because no single etiology or treatment is recognized as consistently effective, it is important that the practitioner stay current on thoughts regarding these reaction patterns. Understanding basic eosinophilic cellular function helps explain the association of eosinophils with proposed etiologies.

Eosinophils make up the major cell type found in the tissue, and in some cases the peripheral blood, of cats with EGC. Most inflammatory diseases in cats stimulate both mast cells and eosinophils. Mast cells contain numerous chemotactic mediators for eosinophils. Eosinophils are also attracted to parasites, microorganisms, and antigen-antibody complexes. The eosinophil granule proteins contain substances that downgrade inflammation and are active in the destruction of extracellular parasites. The most important of these are major basic protein (MBP) and eosinophilic cation protein (ECP). Both are involved with the collagenolysis seen in some forms of EGC.

Earlier thoughts on the etiology of this complex (Hess and MacEwen, 1977; Scott, 1980; Janik, 1983; Gelberg et al., 1985; Muller et al., 1989b) included genetic, viral, immune mediated, stress, and psychogenic factors as well as hypersensitivity reactions to normal anatomic structures. Two recent reports implicating genetics (Power, 1990, 1991) showed a heritable mode of transmission in a family of specific pathogen–free cats. The studies evaluated 25 related cats with EGC in which all the clinical manifestations of EGC were recognized. Food elimination testing and intradermal testing were conducted, and no detectable abnormalities occurred. However, hormonal evaluation in several of the intact female cats showed abnormally high testosterone values that had a cycling character corresponding somewhat to changes in estrogen levels. The studies documented a heritable form of the recognized eosinophilic skin diseases. Power (1991) concluded that in genetically predisposed cats these lesions can develop spontaneously, without allergic stimulus. Although hypersensitivities may cause them in many cats, when a hypersensitivity cannot be documented a heritable form of the diseases should be considered.

As just mentioned, the eosinophil contains granular proteins that can cause parasite destruction, specifically MBP and ECP. These products contribute to tissue injury. In humans, eosinophilic cellulitis (Wells' syndrome) is a disease presenting with recurrent edematous and infiltrative plaques characterized histologically by collagenolysis and foci of amorphous dermal eosinophilic material called "flame figures" (Wells and Smith, 1979). The most common documented etiology in humans is insect bites (Schorr et al., 1984). Many of these persons also have peripheral eosinophilia.

There are similarities between the eosinophilic cellulitis seen in humans and the eosinophilic/collagenolytic granuloma recognized in cats. A mosquito hypersensitivity reaction (Mason and Evans, 1991) has been reported on the bridge of the nose in cats with eosinophilic collagenolysis (Fig. 31-1). The investigators were able to experimentally reproduce both the clinical and the histologic features of these lesions. One investigator (Mason, 1990) was also able to identify insect–foreign body material on dermatopathology associated with an oral eosinophilic granuloma. In addition, I have had a case of mosquito and blackfly nasal EGC that was documented by positive intradermal skin testing and successfully hyposensitized; and other clinical cases of intradermal flea antigen–positive

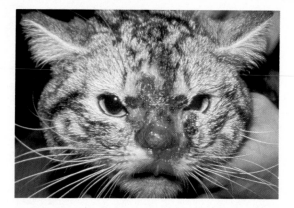

Figure 31-1. Nasal collagenolytic granuloma in a cat with mosquito hypersensitivity.

(Courtesy Dr. Kenneth Mason, Springwood, Queensland, Australia.)

cats have presented with multifocal papular eosinophilic/collagenolytic lesions over their lower abdomen with early eosinophilic collagenolysis.

Allergic etiologies gain support not only through the insect-induced collagenolytic granulomas but also with the pruritic eosinophilic plaques seen over the caudal abdomen and flanks. Many cases are flea antigen–positive. Food and inhaled allergies have also been associated with lesions of this complex. Cases responding to food-elimination diets (Muller et al., 1989b; Rosenkrantz, 1991ab), seasonal recurrent outbreaks (Wilkinson and Bate, 1984), and hyposensitization from positive skin testing (Reedy, 1982; McDougal, 1986) support food and inhaled allergies as etiologic factors in the complex.

Although no pathogenic bacteria have been isolated, there are unpublished cases in which upper lip ulcers and eosinophilic/collagenolytic granulomas have responded solely to antibiotics. In recurrent cases, different antibiotics may work equally well (Rosenkrantz, 1991ab). No controlled studies exist at present to determine whether this response is related to the antimicrobial property or to some other antiinflammatory effect of the antibiotic.

CLINICAL DISEASE

Depending on the type of lesion and body location, the disease can have a variable presenting history and physical examination.

Upper lip ulcerative lesions (also called eosinophilic ulcers, lip ulcers, or rodent ulcers) have been reported in a wide range of ages and are seen more frequently in females. No breed predilection has been noted (Hess and MacEwen, 1977). Lesions are often present for days or weeks prior to examination. Clinically they may appear as acute, firm swellings or fresh, moist ulcers; more chronic ones are brown-yellow depressed craters with raised edges (Fig. 31-2). Most lip ulcers appear on the midline of the upper lip. Less common and more controversial locations include other sites in the oral cavity and on the feet and neck. Once in the chronic stage, the ulcers tend to progress slowly. They are usually painless and nonpruritic. Scott (1980) has reported malignant transformation to squamous cell carcinoma and fibrosarcoma, but this is rare.

The pruritic eosinophilic plaques are generally seen in younger cats. No sex or breed predilections have been recognized. The lesions are intensely pruritic, and a history of pruritus precedes development of the lesion. The abdomen and flank are most commonly affected. Lesions appear as moist, erythematous papules and plaques. Often papules coalesce into plaques. The plaques are sharply demarcated and may have a cobblestone appearance (Fig. 31-3). Most occur in allergic cases, often as a result of a flea allergy.

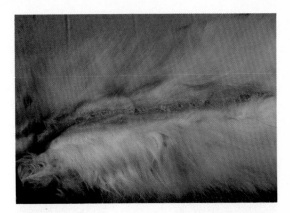

Figure 31-4. Linear collagenolytic granuloma along the lateral truncal aspect of a cat with flea allergy.

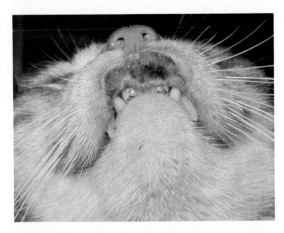

Figure 31-2. Idiopathic upper lip ulcerative lesion in a cat.

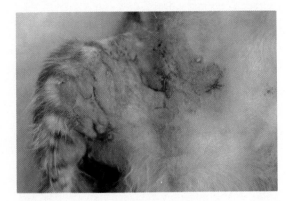

Figure 31-3. Pruritic eosinophilic plaque-type lesion associated with a flea allergy.

Eosinophilic/collagenolytic granuloma, also called "linear granuloma" or true granuloma, is seen primarily in young cats, with females more commonly affected. No breed predilections occur. The lesions can vary considerably in appearance. The classical location (Scott, 1980) is over the caudal aspect of the hind legs—a raised, linear, yellow to erythematous band 2 to 4 mm wide and 5 to 10 mm long—but variations may be seen. Some cats will present with symmetric bands on the trunk or irregular bands anywhere on the body (Fig. 31-4). Well-circumscribed papular, nodular, or plaque lesions may occur in the oral cavity, on the bridge of the nose, on the pinna, perirectally, and on the foot pads and paws (Wilkinson and Bate, 1984; Rosenkrantz, 1991ab) (Fig. 31-5). The granulomas can vary in color and hue but generally are shades of yellow to pink.

Occasionally all three types of lesions—eosinophilic ulcer, plaque, and granuloma—will be seen in the same case. Some lesions may even have histologic features consistent with those of two or more of the recognized clinical entities.

The differential for EGC includes ulcerative and granulomatous infections (bacterial, fungal, and foreign body), trauma, and neoplasms (squamous cell carcinoma, mast cell tumor, and lymphosarcoma). Rarely, in cases with ulcerative lesions, underlying feline leukemia virus or feline T-lymphotrophic virus may be involved as an immunosuppressive factor.

DIAGNOSIS

The history and physical findings are important in EGC, and correlating them with other diagnostic tests is essential to making a final diagnosis.

Skin scrapings and cytology are quick and easy

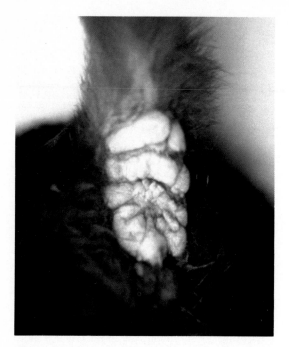

Figure 31-5. Idiopathic collagenolytic perirectal granuloma in a cat.

tests that will help eliminate parasitic diseases and provide information on bacterial involvement and cellular infiltrate. Many patients will have high numbers of eosinophils on cytologic examination; and if intracellular bacteria are present, antibiotics should be given as the primary therapy. If rods are seen on cytology, or to further document the bacterial component, a culture and sensitivity can be performed. Since many lesions are ulcerated, cytologic tests are best performed by impression smears or by lightly scraping the surface with a scalpel blade and smearing the material on a slide. For nodular lesons, needle aspiration works best.

Cultures are optimally taken by punch biopsy techniques after surface preparation. The laboratory should be instructed to tissue grind the sample prior to culturing. Most samples can be transferred to the laboratory in routine transport media. Aerobic bacterial cultures are usually performed, but occasionally with nodular or deeper ulcerative lesions anaerobic cultures will be indicated.

Complete blood counts are of value since some lesions may be associated with peripheral eosinophilia. The eosinophilic plaque and granuloma are more commonly associated with peripheral eosinophilia.

A skin biopsy is the most valuable test for eliminating differentials, defining the type of reaction pattern present, and finding clues to the underlying etiology. The best sites depend on the type of lesion present. Ulcerative lesions should be sampled by a junctional biopsy (normal/abnormal margin) us-ing either an elliptical incision or a few large (6 to 8 mm) punch biopsies. Nodular or plaque lesions should be sampled by means of punch biopsies directly through the lesion or, if small enough, by total excision.

The histopathologic features are variable. A spongiotic microvesicular epidermitis with massive dermal eosinophilia is typical of plaque lesions whereas the eosinophilic granuloma is the only one of the three lesions characterized by true granuloma formation, collagenolysis, and palisading granulomatous inflammation. As mentioned, the last lesion has histologically similar collagenolysis and flame figures as are seen in human patients with Wells' syndrome. The ulcerative lip lesion has been reported (Rosenkrantz, 1991ab) to contain little or no eosinophils or in some cases to look identical to an eosinophilic/collagenolytic granuloma. Since all entities have been associated with atopic disease, atopy and food and insect allergies must be pursued as possible underlying diseases. Food-elimination diets are best performed by utilizing a protein source not routinely fed. The diet is given for 4 to 6 weeks. If there is improvement at the end of the food trial, the cat is rechallenged with its regular food to document the allergy. Lamb or ham baby food has worked in many cases. Hill's Feline d/d may also be used but is less accurate; diarrhea and low palatability have been problems with this product (though less so than with Canine d/d). Inhaled and insect allergies can be determined by intradermal skin testing as in dogs. This procedure is more difficult to perform and interpret in cats because of their thinner skin and more subtle skin test reactions.

TREATMENT

A variety of therapeutic approaches can be taken in these eosinophilic disorders. Some cases will spontaneously resolve; others may be chronic and refractory to many drugs.

With allergic and parasitic hypersensitivities emphasized as etiologies, therapy needs to be directed toward these disorders. Dietary management based on positive responses to elimination diets has been reported to benefit all clinical entities of the complex. As mentioned under "Diagnosis," lamb or ham baby food (assuming that it is not routinely fed) makes an adequate elimination diet in cats. Long-term management can be accomplished by adding a commercial vitamin and mineral supplement. Also Hill's Feline d/d (canned) is now available and is completely balanced for cats. The previously mentioned problems with the Canine d/d (canned)—vomiting, diarrhea, lack of palatability—are far less with the feline product. Its low palatability may be overcome by heating the food. The taurine content of lamb muscle is considered adequate, and using clam juice, which is actually low in taurine, is no longer advocated. Furthermore, many of the commercial vitamin and mineral supplements contain extra taurine, which should protect against such a deficiency. Other alternatives for long-term management of food hypersensitivities include commercial canned cat foods with just one ingredient. (See Table 11-2, p. 131.)

There are two reports of successful hyposensitization for this complex. In the first (McDougal, 1986) three cases of eosinophilic granuloma complex (type unknown) had the following results: one of three cats had good responses, and two had moderate responses. The second report (Reedy, 1982) included a case of eosinophilic ulcer that was successfully hyposensitized.

Hyposensitization protocols are similar to those used in dogs. Based on the recently reported insect-induced hypersensitivity reactions (Wilkinson and Bate, 1984; Mason, 1990; Mason and Evans, 1991; Rosenkrantz, 1991ab), strict insect control for cats and the environment is required. (Environmental treatment and topical therapy are covered in Chapter 6.) Topical insect repellents (e.g., Avon Skin So Soft or Duocide LA) have proved effective and relatively safe for cats. Pyrethroids with and without diethyltoluamide (Deet) are also effective but have potential toxicity. (See Chapter 6 for details on pyrethroid-pyrethrin toxicity in cats.)

Oral antibiotics have produced reduction, and in some cases complete remission, of eosinophilic ulcers and collagenolytic granulomas. No controlled studies have presently been performed; however, other practitioners (Kunkle, 1988; MacDonald, 1988) report favorable results. The antibiotics used include trimethoprim-sulfadiazine (30 mg/kg q12h), cefadroxil (22 mg/kg q12h), and amoxicillin trihydrate–clavulanate potassium (12.5 mg/kg q12h). It is not known whether the responses are related to the antimicrobial or some other nonspecific antiinflammatory effect.

Glucocorticoids have been used extensively for all three clinical entities. Results are generally best with injectable methylprednisolone acetate (Depomedrol). Effective dosages are 4 mg/kg, with a minimum of 20 mg per cat. Initial therapy requires injections at 2-week intervals, and the average case receives two or three injections. Once resolution occurs, the injections should not be repeated any more often than every 2 months. The initial every-2-week schedule should be followed for more complete and longer remissions. Oral prednisone or methylprednisolone at high dosages (4 to 5 mg/kg

q24h) can also be tried initially to put the lesions into remission and then tapered to a lower, every-other-day dosage for chronic management (2 mg/kg q48h). Oral triamcinolone (Vetalog) at 0.5 to 0.75 mg/kg q24h PO can be used at an induction dosage for 7 to 10 days and then tapered to q48-72h. This has been effective in some cases (Rosenkrantz, 1991b). Topical glucocorticoids have limited value in this complex, since the product is often licked off.

Megestrol acetate (Ovaban, Megace) has been advocated for treating this complex. The dosages for induction therapy are 2.5 to 5 mg per cat q48h. Maintenance dosages are 2.5 to 5 mg q7-14d. These products are rarely used or recommended due to their potential side effects, the effectiveness of other forms of therapy, and the fact that they have not been approved for use in cats. Some of the severe side effects reported are reduced spermatogenesis, development of pyometra, postponed estrus, increased growth hormone levels, and potential acromegaly. Mammary gland fibroadenomatous hyperplasia may be seen in both intact and altered cats and in some animals will not resolve with drug withdrawal. Occasional cases develop mammary neoplasia. Diabetes mellitus, either transient or permanent, has resulted from progestogen therapy. Behavioral abnormalities are common: some cats become more affectionate, others more aggressive. Weight gain, polydipsia, and lethargy are also common. One of the most serious side effects is adrenocortical suppression, which occurs at even low doses and persists for weeks (Muller et al., 1989a).

Immunomodulating drugs, such as levamisole (2.2 mg/kg q48h PO) and thiabendazole (5 mg/kg q48h PO), have induced partial to complete remission in some cases (MacEwen and Hess, 1987; Rosenkrantz, 1991b); and in one case I had complete remission of a refractory perirectal collagenolytic granuloma with levamisole at the above dosage. However, a major complication in this case was marked bone marrow suppression, resulting in pancytopenia and near death, with an 8-week recovery from the time the drug was discontinued.

Other methods of treatment occasionally effective include surgery, cryosurgery, radiation therapy, and laser therapy:

1. Surgical excision of lip ulcers and focal collagenolytic granulomas has been successful but can leave deformities in and about the lip.
2. Cryosurgery has had variable and generally poor results (Willemse, 1980).
3. Radiation therapy has been advocated for solitary lesions that do not respond to med-

ical therapy (Biery, 1977). Four to eight weekly treatments with 300 to 400 rads per session are the recommended protocol. However, the technique is expensive, requires special equipment and general anesthesia, and is not practical in clinical situations.

4. Carbon dioxide laser therapy was used in three cats with refractory eosinophilic ulcers (Manning et al., 1987), and successful results were seen in two of the three cases.

Depending on the chronicity and refractoriness of a case, therapeutic and diagnostic approaches will vary. A first-time presentation may initially be treated with just a course of antibiotics and re-evaluated in 2 weeks. If the response is poor, a decision regarding more diagnostics (in the form of cytology, cultures, CBCs, and biopsies) may be indicated. If the client is reluctant to sanction such an extensive workup, a course of oral or parenteral glucocorticoids may be tried. If response is poor, the workup is mandatory. In cases that present with a long, recurrent, or chronic refractory nature, more aggressive diagnostics in the form of biopsies, food elimination diet, and intradermal allergy testing are recommended. If a primary disease (e.g., insect hypersensitivity or a food or inhaled allergy) cannot be determined or controlled, then systemic long-term glucocorticoid therapy will be called for. Injectable methylprednisolone should not be used more often than every 2 months in a maintenance program. Oral glucocorticoids need to be administered on an every-other-day or every-third-day basis. Depending on the glucocorticoid maintenance program, semiannual to yearly monitoring in the form of complete blood counts, chemistry, and urinalysis should be performed to screen for long-term steroid side effects. If a case is nonresponsive to glucocorticoids, more aggressive measures can be taken—in the form of laser therapy, surgery, immunomodulating drugs, and (as a last resort) megestrol acetate. Refractory cases should have consultation with a specialist.

REFERENCES

Biery DM: Radiation therapy in dermatology. In Kirk RW (ed): Current veterinary therapy VI, Philadelphia, 1977, WB Saunders, p 527.

Gelberg HB et al: Antiepithelial autoantibodies associated with the feline eosinophilic granuloma complex, Am J Vet Res 46:263, 1985.

Hess PW, MacEwen EG: Feline eosinophilic granuloma. In Kirk RW (ed): Current veterinary therapy VI, Philadelphia, 1977, WB Saunders, p 534.

Janik TA: An outbreak of eosinophilic plaques in a large group of felines, Vet Allergist, p 2, Summer 1983.

Kunkle G: Personal communication, 1988.

MacDonald JM: Personal communication, 1988.

MacEwen EG, Hess PW: Evaluation of effect of immunomodulation on the feline eosinophilic granuloma complex, J Am Anim Hosp Assoc 23:519, 1987.

Manning TO, et al: Three cases of feline eosinophilic granuloma complex (eosinophilic ulcer) and observations on laser therapy, Semin Vet Med Surg (Small Anim) 2:206, 1987.

Mason KV: Personal Communication, 1990.

Mason KV, Evans A: Feline eosinophilic granuloma complex: a further clinical manifestation and etiology. In Proceedings, Annual members' meeting AAVD & ACVD, Washington DC, 1988.

Mason KV, Evans AG: Mosquito bite–caused eosinophilic dermatitis in cats, J Am Vet Med Assoc 198:2086, 1991.

McDougal BJ: Allergy testing and hyposensitization for the three common feline dermatoses, Mod Vet Pract 67:629, 1986.

Muller GH, et al: Small animal dermatology, ed 4, Philadelphia, 1989a, WB Saunders, p 210.

Muller GH, et al: Small animal dermatology, ed 4, Philadelphia, 1989b, WB Saunders, p 561.

Power HT: Eosinophilic granuloma in a family of specific pathogen–free cats. In Proceedings, Annual members' meeting AAVD & ACVD, 1990.

Power HT: Personal communication, 1991.

Reedy LM: Results of allergy testing and hyposensitization in selected feline skin disease, J Am Anim Hosp Assoc 18:618, 1982.

Rosenkrantz WS: Eosinophilic granuloma confusion. In August JR (ed): Consultations in feline internal medicine, Philadelphia 1991a, WB Saunders, p 121.

Rosenkrantz WS: Unpublished data, 1991b.

Schorr WF, et al: Eosinophilic cellulitis (Wells' syndrome): histologic and clinical features in arthropod bite reactions, J Am Acad Dermatol 11:1043, 1984.

Scott DW: Feline dermatology 1900-1978: a monograph, J Am Anim Hosp Assoc 16:406, 1980.

Wells GC, Smith EP: Eosinophilic cellulitis, Br J Dermatol 100:101, 1979.

Wilkinson GT, Bate MJ: A possible further clinical manifestation of the feline eosinophilic granuloma complex, J Am Anim Hosp Assoc 20:325, 1984.

Willemse TA: Cryotherapy in small animal dermatology. In Kirk RW (ed): Current veterinary therapy VII, Philadelphia, 1980, WB Saunders, p 495.

32

Feline Stomatitis

Wayne S. Rosenkrantz

Importance

Feline stomatitis is a common inflammatory disease of the oral mucosa. Lesions can occur in confined areas such as the gums (gingivitis) or the tongue (glossitis). Many chronic cases produce plasmacytic inflammatory infiltrates and are often diagnosed as plasmacytic stomatitis. Some have underlying or coexistent disease, although diagnostic confirmation can be difficult, and idiopathic cases exist. The search for an underlying disease is often prematurely abandoned with a biopsy finding of plasmacytic stomatitis. Plasmacytic stomatitis is merely a cutaneous reaction pattern with multiple etiologies, and a diagnosis of idiopathic stomatitis should be made only after ruling out other causes.

Pathogenesis

Plasma cells may be present in a variety of disorders, particularly when a chronic antigenic stimulus exists in local tissue or in autoimmune diseases. Chronic viral diseases (e.g., herpesvirus and calicivirus), bacterial infections, or foreign body reactions should be considered a source for plasmacytic infiltrates. The significance of isolating normal oral flora from affected periodontal tissue has not been established; they may possibly be pathogenic in some cases. A common cause of tissue plasmacytic infiltrates in humans is spirochete infections. These organisms have not been documented in cases of feline stomatitis but are not readily isolated on routine cultures.

Periodontal disease is another source of chronic antigenic stimulus and subsequent plasmacytic stomatitis. It is thought to be caused by plaque, a layer of bacteria that adheres to the surface of the teeth. Plaque is controlled by a normal immune system and appropriate diet. Plaque flora may change from a gram-positive coccal population to a gram-negative anaerobic rod population in stressed or immune compromised cats. The affected teeth tend to develop "neck lesions," which are cavities that form in the root cementum at the junction of the crown and root. Although similar to caries, neck lesions have a histologic appearance that supports external odontoblastic resorption rather than chemical decalcification as the cause of periodontal disease (Reichart et al., 1984).

The cell type and corticosteroid responsiveness of plasmacytic stomatitis have led many to consider it an immune mediated disease. However, response to corticosteroids is a poor criterion for diagnosing immune mediated diseases, and it is inappropriate to add this disorder to that list of diseases.

CLINICAL DISEASES

The clinical presentation of feline stomatitis in cats is variable. No age or sex predilection occurs. The Abyssinian breed is overrepresented. Patients may have a history of halitosis, salivation, anorexia, and pain associated with eating, or a combination of these, or they may be totally asymptomatic. Most owners do not routinely examine their cat's mouth and may not detect early or milder

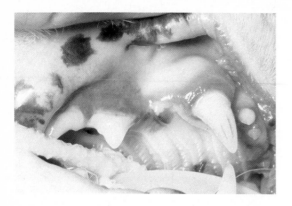

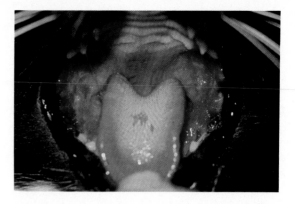

Figure 32-1. Early feline stomatitis (red line at the junction of the tooth crown and gingiva).

(Courtesy Dr. Karen Helton-Rhodes, New York, N.Y.)

Figure 32-2. Progressive feline stomatitis. Note the proliferative, vegetative, fleshy, ulcerated lesions at the tooth gum margins.

(Courtesy Dr. Karen Helton-Rhodes, New York, N.Y.)

chronic lesions (which are commonly asymptomatic).

Early lesions with a mild marginal gingivitis appear clinically as a red line at the junction of the tooth crown and gingiva (Fig. 32-1). Many cases will progress no further. Others will also have physical findings of halitosis, salivation, and pain upon oral examination. Some will develop proliferative, vegetative, fleshy, ulcerated lesions at the tooth-gum margins, glossopalatine arch, and pharyngeal walls (Fig. 32-2). Buccal, lingual, and palatel contact ulcers may be seen in more advanced cases. These are painful upon examination, and the patients are often underweight. Some cases with idiopathic plasmacytic stomatitis will develop concurrent plasma cell pododermatitis, which typically starts as a swelling of the central or metatarsal pads and may be associated with ulceration and pain or lameness.

The differentials for feline stomatitis are extensive (Table 32-1). Viral infections such as herpes, calici, and panleukopenia can cause lingual, palatal, and pharyngeal ulcerations. Thompson et al. (1984) have isolated virus from affected cats with gingival lesions.

Periodontal disease, which starts with marginal gingivitis, can produce soft tissue proliferative to ulcerative lesions that spread to the glossopalatine area and pharyngeal walls.

Immunocompromising viruses such as feline leukemia virus (FeLV) and feline T-lymphotropic virus (FTLV) have been associated with chronic stomatitis. However, it should be noted that cats that have primarily oral lesions are rarely FeLV-positive (Johnessee and Hurvitz, 1983). Chronic gingivitis is a more common finding in cats with FTLV (Pedersen et al., 1987).

Autoimmune disease is another cause of stomatitis (Scott, 1984). Pemphigus vulgaris and systemic lupus erythematosus would be the likely considerations for autoimmune-induced stomatitis. These are serious diseases that generally cause severe, widespread oral ulcerative lesions and often affect other mucocutaneous junctions. Ulcerative stomatitides that can mimic autoimmune diseases include drug reactions, erythema multiforme, and toxic epidermal necrolysis.

Oral hyperplastic and neoplastic diseases can resemble gingival hyperplasia associated with stomatitis. Eosinophilic/collagenolytic granulomas usually present with focal plaques or nodules and occasionally with ulceration. The most common oral tumor of cats is squamous cell carcinoma. The gingiva, tongue, and lingual frenulum are the most common sites. Lymphosarcoma is another tumor to consider, but it usually has lesions in other body locations.

Infectious agents to consider as differentials or as complicating an ongoing stomatitis are bacterial and mycotic infections. The significance of isolating bacteria in stomatitis cases is difficult to determine, since recovered organisms are often part of the normal flora. *Pasteurella multocida,* beta-hemolytic streptococci, *Corynebacterium* spp, *Actinomyces* spp, fusiform bacilli, and *Bacteroides* spp are part of the normal flora in cats. However, antibiotic therapy based on sensitivity results has produced positive responses in some cases. Mycotic infections are a rare cause of feline stomatitis. Oral candidiasis is rare but may be seen in debilitated or immune suppressed cases.

Systemic or metabolic disorders can also produce oral lesions. Uremia may be associated with

Table 32-1. Feline stomatitis differential diagnosis

CAUSE	DIAGNOSTIC TEST
Viral Herpes Calici Panleukopenia	Viral cultures Dermatohistopathology
Bacterial Secondary component	Cultures and sensitivities Dermatohistopathology
Mycotic Candidiasis	Fungal culture Dermatohistopathology
Periodontal disease	Response to dental hygiene, radiographs, and tooth extractions
Immunocompromising virus FeLV FTLV	Specific antigen-antibody testing
Autoimmune disease Pemphigus vulgaris Systemic lupus erythematosus	Dermatohistopathology Direct immunofluorescence ANA
Drug reactions	History of compatible drug exposure
Erythema multiforme	Dermatohistopathology
Toxic epidermal necrolysis	
Insect, inhaled, and food hypersensitivities and idiopathic oral collagenolytic lesions	Allergy testing and food-elimination diets Dermatohistopathology
Neoplasia Squamous cell carcinoma Lymphosarcoma	Dermatohistopathology
Systemic-metabolic diseases Uremia Diabetes mellitus Cushing's disease	CBC Chemistry screens Urinalysis Endocrine screening tests
Protein-calorie malnutrition	History Physical
Toxicities Heavy metals Plant toxins	History of exposure Urine or blood levels for heavy metals
Physical injuries Chemical burns Thermal burns Electrical burns Foreign bodies	History Physical Dermatohistopathology
Idiopathic plasmacytic stomatitis	Elimination of other differentials

oral ulcerations. The irritation due to ammonia produced by the bacterial action on urea and a dry oral mucosa due to dehydration and clotting deficiencies may both contribute to oral ulcerations in chronic severe renal disease. Diabetes mellitus and Cushing's disease may be associated with progressive periodontitis and oral abscesses.

Malnutrition with a protein-calorie deficiency can lead to oral ulceration as a result of decreased epithelial cell turnover. In addition, such cases have obvious generalized malnutritional symptoms.

Toxicities in the form of heavy metal compounds like thallium or plant substances (e.g., *Dieffenbachia*) can cause oral ulcerations in cats.

Chemical, thermal, and electrical burns or foreign bodies can also produce oral lesions, which are generally localized to the site of contact of the offending agent. Foreign body reactions are often solitary but may be multifocal if the agent is diffusely infiltrated into the oral mucosa.

DIAGNOSIS

Although physical findings alone may be suggestive of feline stomatitis, it is important to approach these cases in a systematic fashion. This is a cutaneous reaction pattern, and the goal is to identify the underlying disease (Table 32-1).

Unfortunately, diagnostic tests may not always reveal a cause and a diagnosis of idiopathic stomatitis is settled upon. A detailed history, including dietary information and complete physical examination, should be performed. Depending on the degree of the cat's pain and its temperament, a complete examination of the oral cavity may need to be performed under sedation or anesthesia. The appearance, pattern, symmetry, and severity of lesions should be observed. As previously described, this can help rank differentials and, if cost is a factor, can indicate what tests to perform initially.

Laboratory testing should include cytology, a CBC count, chemistry screen, FeLV and FTLV testing, and biopsy of the affected sites. Bacterial, fungal, or viral cultures may also be helpful.

Cytology is a quick and easy test that can give immediate clues to the underlying etiology. When taking samples for cytology from the oral cavity, a light scraping of the gum tissue with a no. 10 scalpel blade works best. The material is smeared on a glass slide, heat-fixed, and stained with Wright's or Diff-Quik stain. The presence of intracellular bacteria may be an indication for antibiotic therapy; large numbers of eosinophils would raise suspicions about eosinophilic granuloma;

acantholytic cells would suggest pemphigus vulgaris; identifying specific cell lines with highly mitotic/bizarre cells would raise suspicions of neoplasms.

Bacterial, fungal, and viral cultures should be taken from the tissue, not from the mucosal surface. Tissue cultures should be performed by removing a small piece of tissue with a 4 mm punch biopsy and placing in an appropriate transport medium. Once at the laboratory, the sample should be tissue ground prior to plating on the medium. Before submitting samples for viral cultures, it is recommended that the practitioner check with the laboratory for availability and sample handling. The closest veterinary university may be the only facility with viral isolation capability.

Bacterial cultures should be interpreted carefully, since many resident bacteria are commonly isolated from normal cats. However, the results may be considered significant if bacteria are isolated from tissue samples that do not include surface epithelium. Positive culture results and identification of intracellular organisms on cytologic tests are significant.

Histologic evaluation of biopsies may reveal a specific diagnosis, such as pemphigus vulgaris or lupus erythematosus. In other cases histology helps select therapy or further diagnostic testing. If the biopsy supports a suppurative process and bacterial or fungal elements are seen, cultures and subsequent antimicrobial therapy should be performed. Many of these cases will also respond to a dental prophylaxis and extractions. If viral inclusions or "ballooning degeneration and edema" are histopathologic features, viral cultures may help identify the specific virus involved. The biopsy will demonstrate a tissue reaction pattern, such as plasmacytic stomatitis or eosinophilic/collagenolytic granuloma, and this can narrow the differential to causes of those patterns or their respective idiopathic diagnoses.

A complete blood count and chemistry screen may show only the changes of chronic inflammation (e.g., elevated WBC and protein levels, anemia). Metabolic disorders may be detected from the chemistry screen and will direct medical management. FeLV- or FTLV-positive cats have a poor prognosis, for these viruses often affect other organ systems and can result in chronic debilitation or death.

TREATMENT

If a primary underlying disease is identified, specific therapy is indicated. A diagnosis of chronic idiopathic plasmacytic stomatitis is appropriate when no underlying disease can be detected and a biopsy is compatible. Treatment options for idiopathic plasmacytic stomatitis are numerous.

Managing periodontal disease may eliminate gingivitis and some cases of idiopathic plasmacytic stomatitis. Aggressive dental prophylaxis, subgingival scaling, and resection of proliferative gingival tissue to eliminate pockets may produce positive results (Emily, 1991). Neck lesions should be cleaned and resected, and the tooth surface should be restored with an appropriate composite. Severely involved teeth must be extracted.

Radical therapy with extraction of all premolar and molar teeth in severely affected cats can yield good results. This will eliminate root lesions and pockets for accumulation of plaque. In a report of nine severely affected cats (Harvey, 1986) results were very good, with minimal signs of oral disease 7 months after extractions in six cases (67%). One of the six needed intermittent corticosteroids to control cyclic recurrences. Antibiotic therapy is often used in conjunction with aggressive prophylaxis, filling, and extraction procedures.

After the initial aggressive interventions, long-term management should combine daily brushing or rubbing of the teeth and gingivae to eliminate plaque. A specially designed toothbrush and commercial toothpaste are available for cats (under the trade name CET*). Topical application of zinc ascorbate, potassium permanganate, or vitamin E to promote healing after cleaning and help prevent recurrent lesions has also been recommended (Emily, 1991). These products can be brushed on or applied with cotton-tipped applicators. Proper diet, in the form of dry food rather than canned or moist foods, is preferred to help maintain chronically affected cats.

Antibiotic therapy is a more conservative approach to periodontal disease or when bacteria are thought to be a contributing cause of the stomatitis. In older or more debilitated cats, antibiotics can reduce inflammation and make the animal feel well enough to eat and drink. Antibiotics that have efficacy against gram-negative bacteria are recommended. Empirical selection of antibiotics includes trimethoprim-sulfadiazine (30 mg/kg q12h), potentiated amoxicillin–clavulanic acid (13.75 mg/kg q12h), enrofloxacin (2.5 mg/kg q12h), cefadroxil (22 mg/kg q12h), lincomycin (22 mg/kg q12h), tetracycline (20 to 30 mg/kg q12h), and metronidazole (10 to 20 mg/kg q12h). The cat's

painful mouth may make these antibiotics difficult to administer, and parenteral antibiotics may be given initially until the pain subsides. The duration of therapy varies, with a normal range of 3 to 6 weeks. Some cases can be managed chronically with long-term antibiotic therapy. Antibiotics may be given at one third to one half the daily dose. However, it is best to use pulse therapy (recommended dosages at set intervals). An example would be giving the antibiotic the first 3 days of the week and then holding off the remaining days. The practitioner should be aware that pulse and low-dose therapy can cause the development of resistant bacterial strains. When dental hygiene and antibiotics are ineffective, the practitioner is forced to suppress the chronic antigenic stimulus. This is generally achieved with antiinflammatory therapy. It should be emphasized that a thorough dental prophylaxis should be done prior to corticosteroid therapy.

Methylprednisolone acetate (4 mg/kg, 20 mg minimum, IM) is the recommended corticosteroid to start therapy. This is followed by oral prednisone (1 mg/kg q48h) for maintenance if the animal is in remission at a 2-week recheck. A repeat injection of methylprednisolone at the 2-week recheck is occasionally needed to induce remission prior to starting maintenance oral prednisone. Depending on the lesion's severity and rate of recurrence, injectable methylprednisolone acetate can be repeated every 2 to 4 months. The cat should be monitored for iatrogenic Cushing's disease and diabetes mellitus while on high-dose corticosteroids. This can be done by performing routine urinalysis, chemistry screens, and ACTH stimulation tests. Monitoring should be performed every 6 to 12 months.

Chrysotherapy (treatment with oral or parenteral gold salts) has produced favorable results in some cases of plasmacytic stomatitis and autoimmune skin disease. The most common protocol is to use aurothioglucose at a dosage of 1 to 2 mg/kg q7d IM. To rule out idiosyncratic reactions, a test dose of 1 to 2 mg should be administered the first week, followed by a second dose of 2 to 5 mg. There is a long lag period, and clinical response is not expected for 6 to 12 weeks. During the induction phase it is common to use corticosteroids concurrently. Once a response is seen, the injections should be tapered to every 2 weeks and eventually to every 1 or 2 months and then as needed. Side effects include hepatic necrosis, thrombocytopenia, toxic epidermal necrolysis, stomatitis, and proteinuria. Minor side effects are sterile abscesses at the injection sites and eosinophilia. Platelet

*VRX Products, Div. of St Jon Laboratories, Harbor City, Calif. 90710.

counts, complete blood counts, and urinalysis should be performed every 2 weeks during the first 16 weeks. Once maintenance therapy has been started, the monitoring can be decreased to monthly. When the blood test results have stabilized, monitoring can be reduced to quarterly.

Other immunosuppressive drugs to consider are chlorambucil and azathioprine. Chlorambucil (Leukeran) is an alkylating agent that can be used in conjunction with corticosteroids or as sole therapy. The dosage is 0.1 mg/kg q24-48h. Azathioprine (Imuran) is an antimetabolic that can also be used in conjunction with corticosteroids or as sole therapy. The dosage in cats is 1.1 mg/kg q48h. Both drugs work by myelosuppression and therefore can cause bone marrow toxicity. Of the two, azathioprine appears to be more dangerous in cats and chlorambucil is recommended initially. Because marked leukopenia has resulted in mortality in some cats, strict monitoring is required before and during treatment. Complete blood counts every 1 to 2 weeks are required the first 12 to 16 weeks. Maintenance monitoring should be performed every 4 to 8 weeks. A rare hepatotoxic reaction can occur with azathioprine. A periodic chemistry screen should also be performed to check for hepatic reactions.

The course of idiopathic plasmacytic stomatitis is often chronic and frustrating. Rarely do pets die from the stomatitis, but untreated cases may develop secondary infections and malnutrition that could result in death.

If an underlying etiology cannot be determined, the initial approach should be an aggressive dental prophylaxis. Then topical maintenance with regular brushing and applications of vitamin E, zinc ascorbate, or potassium permanganate can be tried. If the dental cleanings and subsequent topical maintenance are ineffective, empirical antibiotic therapy should be attempted. If this is helpful, a pulse therapy program can be instituted. If dental hygiene and antibiotics are ineffective, antiinflammatory therapy may be needed. Corticosteroids should be tried initially and then followed by golds salts, chlorambucil, and azathioprine.

REFERENCES

Emily P: Personal communication, 1991.

Harvey CE: Results following extraction of cheek teeth as treatment of severe periodontal disease in cats (abstr), Vet Dent 3(3):2, 1986.

Johnssee JS, Hurvitz AI: Feline plasma cell gingivitis, J Am Anim Hosp Assoc 19:179, 1983.

Pederson NC, et al: Isolation of a T-lymphotropic virus from cats with an immunodeficiency-like syndrome, Science 235:790, 1987.

Reichart PA, et al: Periodontal disease in the domestic cat: a histopathologic study, J Periodont Res 19:67, 1984.

Scott DW: Feline dermatology 1979-1982: introspective retrospections, J Am Anim Hosp Assoc 20:537, 1984.

Thompson RR, et al: Association of calicivirus infection with chronic gingivitis and pharyngitis in cats, J Small Anim Pract 25:207, 1984.

Appendix A
Formulary

DRUGS (generic and trade)	MANUFACTURER	DOSAGE & ROUTE OF ADMINISTRATION (Topical, PO, SQ, IM, IV)	DISEASE	MAJOR SIDE EFFECTS
Acetic acid 2.5% to 5%	Various	Topical (especially yeast)	Infectious otitis	Irritation
Adams Flea Off Mist		Topical (see label restrictions)	Flea control	Clinical signs of pyrethrin intoxication
Adams Pan-Otic	SmithKline-Beecham	Topical, 15 min prior to bathing	Local areas of severe greasy scale	Irritancy
Adams Pyrethrin Dip		Topical (see label restrictions)	Flea control	Clinical signs of pyrethrin intoxication
Allergroom Shampoo	Allerderm/ Virbac	Topical	Primary keratinization disorders (dry scale), secondary dry scale, allergic skin disease	Contact irritancy (rare)
Alpha-Sesame Oil Dry Skin Rinse	Veterinary Prescription	Topical	Primary keratinization disorders (dry scale), secondary dry scale	
Aluminum acetate *Domeboro*	Miles	Topical	Localized pruritus, acute moist dermatitis	
Amcinonide cream 0.1% *Cyclocort*	Lederle	Apply q12-24h for 10 days, then taper to q48-72h	DLE, PF, PE, inflammation	Cutaneous atrophy, cushingoid changes

DLE, Discoid lupus erythematosus; PF, pemphigus foliaceus; PE, pemphigus erythematosus.

Continued.

DRUGS (generic and trade)	MANUFACTURER	DOSAGE & ROUTE OF ADMINISTRATION (Topical, PO, SQ, IM, IV)	DISEASE	MAJOR SIDE EFFECTS
Amikacin *Amiglyde-V*	Aveco Fort Dodge	10 mg/kg q12h SQ or IM Topical, several drops per ear q12h	Gram-negative pyoderma, *Pseudomonas* otitis	Nephrotoxicity, ototoxicity, neurotoxicity, cutaneous drug reactions
Amitraz *Mitaban*	Upjohn	Topical (0.025% rinse) q1-2wk	Generalized demodicosis, canine scabies	Transient pruritus, sedation (especially in toy breeds)
Taktic	Nor-Am	Topical (0.125% rinse) applied to half the body q24h	Generalized demodicosis (resistant cases)	Transient pruritus, sedation (especially in toy breeds)
Amitriptyline *Elavil*	Stuart	1 to 2 mg q12h PO	Atopic disease	Drowsiness
Amoxicillin trihydrate with clavulanate potassium *Clavamox*	SmithKline-Beecham	12.5 mg/kg q12h PO (Kwochka, 22 mg/kg q12h PO)	Pyoderma, plasmacytic stomatitis	Vomiting, diarrhea, anorexia
Aquamist	Miles	Topical (see label restrictions)	Flea control	Clinical signs of pyrethrin intoxication
Astemizole *Hismanal*	Janssen	0.25 mg/kg q12h PO	Atopy	Drowsiness, hyperactivity
Auranofin *Ridaura*	SmithKline-Beecham	0.2 to 0.3 mg/kg q12h PO	DLE, PE, PF, eosinophilic feline dermatoses	Blood dyscrasias
Aurothiomalate *Myochrysine*	Merck	Test dose: initially 1 mg Cats: 1 mg/kg q7d IM	DLE, PF, PE, plasmacytic stomatitis	Hepatic necrosis, thrombocytopenia, stomatitis, proteinuria
Aurothioglucose *Solganal*	Schering	Test dose: initially 1 mg, then Dogs: 1 mg/kg q7d IM Cats: 1 to 2 mg/kg q7d IM	Plasmacytic stomatitis, PF (feline)	Hepatic necrosis, thrombocytopenia, stomatitis, proteinuria

DLE, Discoid lupus erythematosus; PF, pemphigus foliaceus; PE, pemphigus erythematosus.

DRUGS (generic and trade)	MANUFACTURER	DOSAGE & ROUTE OF ADMINISTRATION (Topical, PO, SQ, IM, IV)	DISEASE	MAJOR SIDE EFFECTS
Aveeno Colloidal Oatmeal	Rydelle	Topical rinse (1 Tbsp/gal H$_2$O)	Pruritus	Excessive greasiness
Aveeno Colloidal Oatmeal—oilated		Topical (½ to 1 Tbsp/gal H$_2$O)	Pruritus with dry skin	
Avon Skin So Soft	Avon	Topical moisturizer and insect repellent (1 oz/gal H$_2$O)	Eosinophilic feline dermatoses, flea allergic dermatoses, insect hypersensitivities	Excessive greasiness, contact irritancy (rare)
Azathioprine *Imuran*	Burroughs-Wellcome	Dogs: 1.1 to 2.2 mg/kg q24-48h PO Cats: 1.1 mg/kg q48h PO	DLE, PF, plasmacytic stomatitis	Bone marrow suppression, hepatotoxicity, demodicosis, dermatophytosis, pyoderma; especially toxic in cats, **use with caution**
Benzoyl peroxide gel *OxyDex Gel*	DVM	Topical	Chin acne of dogs and cats, localized pyoderma	Excessive drying, irritancy (rare), bleaching of fabrics
Pyoben Gel	Allerderm/ Virbac			
Benzoyl peroxide shampoo *OxyDex Shampoo*	DVM	Topical	Pyoderma, keratinization disorders with greasy scale, follicular keratinization disorders, *Malassezia* dermatosis	Excessive drying, irritancy (rare), bleaching of fabrics
Pyoben Shampoo	Allerderm/ Virbac	Topical		
Benzoyl peroxide/sulfur shampoo				

Continued.

DRUGS (generic and trade)	MANUFACTURER	DOSAGE & ROUTE OF ADMINISTRATION (Topical, PO, SQ, IM, IV)	DISEASE	MAJOR SIDE EFFECTS
Sulf-OxyDex Shampoo	DVM	Topical	Keratinization disorders with greasy scale, follicular keratinization disorders, *Malassezia* dermatosis, pyoderma	Excessive drying, irritancy (rare), bleaching of fabrics
Beta-carotene *Solatene*	Roche Generics	Capsules (30 mg, q12h PO)	Provitamin A; for reducing severity of photosensitivity reactions; not a sunscreen; requires fat in diet	Diarrhea (mild), joint soreness (rare)
Betamethasone dipropionate *Betasone* (0.5%)	Schering	Topical	Localized allergic reaction	Cutaneous atrophy, iatrogenic Cushing's
Diprolene	Schering	Topical q12-24h, then taper	Pruritus	Cutaneous atrophy, iatrogenic Cushing's
Betamethasone valerate 0.1% cream/ointment *Valisone*	Schering	Topical	Localized allergic reactions, immune-mediated PF, eosinophilic lesions	Cutaneous atrophy, iatrogenic Cushing's
Burow's H solution	*see* HB101 solution			
Captan Antifungal Shampoo	Burns	Bathe q5d	Dermatophytosis	Contact sensitivity; caution: carcinogenic in people
Captan powder, spray *Orthocide*	Ortho	Dilution 2% (2 Tbsp/gal), spray or rinse	Dermatophytosis	Contact sensitivity; caution: carcinogenic in people
Cefadroxil *Cefa Tabs, Cefa Drops*	Fort Dodge	22 mg/kg q12h PO	Pyoderma, plasmacytic stomatitis, eosinophilic feline dermatoses	Vomiting (rare), diarrhea, systemic hypersensitivity

DRUGS (generic and trade)	MANUFACTURER	DOSAGE & ROUTE OF ADMINISTRATION (Topical, PO, SQ, IM, IV)	DISEASE	MAJOR SIDE EFFECTS
Cephalexin *Keflex*	Eli Lilly Generics	20 to 30 mg/kg q12h PO	Pyoderma	Gastrointestinal disturbances, cutaneous drug reactions
Cephradine	Various	22 mg/kg q12h PO	Pyoderma	Vomiting (rare), diarrhea, systemic hypersensitivity
Chlorambucil *Leukeran*	Burroughs Wellcome	0.1 mg/kg q24-48h PO	Plasmacytic stomatitis, PF, DLE	Myelosuppression, gastrointestinal side effects, severe tissue necrosis
Chloramphenicol	Various	50 mg/kg q8h PO	Pyoderma	Vomiting, diarrhea; major concern is for serious and fatal blood dyscrasias in humans with accidental absorption
Chlorhexidine *Nolvasan Solution*	Fort Dodge	Topical	Dermatophytosis	Irritant reactions, eye irritation
Chlorhexidine shampoo *ChlorhexiDerm* *Nolvasan*	DVM Fort Dodge	Topical Topical	Pyoderma, *Malassezia* dermatitis, dermatophytosis	Irritant reactions, eye irritation
Chloroaluminum sulfonated phthalocyanine		1 mg/kg IV q48-72h prior to argon laser treatment	Feline solar dermatitis, preneoplastic squamous cell carcinoma	Severe tissue necrosis, swelling, anaphylaxis
Chlorpheniramine maleate	Generic	Canine: 2 to 8 mg q8-12h PO Feline: 2 mg q12h PO	Pruritus, atopy	Excessive sedation, hyperexcitability (rare)
Chlorpyrifos *Dursban*	3M	Topical	Flea control	Organophosphate toxicity

DLE, Discoid lupus erythematosus; PF, pemphigus foliaceus; PE, pemphigus erythematosus.

Continued.

DRUGS (generic and trade)	MANUFACTURER	DOSAGE & ROUTE OF ADMINISTRATION (Topical, PO, SQ, IM, IV)	DISEASE	MAJOR SIDE EFFECTS
Cimetidine *Tagamet*	Smith-Kline-French	3 to 4 mg/kg q12h PO	Chronic recurrent pyoderma (immune stimulant)	
Clear-X Ear Cleansing Solution	DVM	Topical, 15 min prior to bathing	Local areas of severe greasy scale	Irritancy
Clemastine *Tavist*	Sandoz	0.05 mg/kg q12h PO	Atopy	Drowsiness, hyperactivity
Clindamycin hydrochloride *Antirobe*	Upjohn	5.5 to 11 mg/kg q12h PO	Pyoderma	Vomiting, diarrhea, colitis
Clobetasol propionate *Temovate*	Glaxo	Topical q12-24h, then taper	Pruritus, localized allergy	Cutaneous atrophy, iatrogenic Cushing's
Clotrimazole *Lotrimin*	Schering	Topical	Focal dermatophytosis	Contact irritancy
Clotrimazole/ betamethasone dipropionate *Lotrisone Cream*	Schering	Topical	Focal dermatophytosis	Contact irritancy, steroid atrophy, iatrogenic Cushing's
Cyclophos-phamide *Cytoxan*	Bristol Myers	50 mg/m^2 PO (in AM) on first 4 days each treatment week for 8 wk	Lymphosarcoma	Myelosuppression, hemorrhagic cystitis, bladder fibrosis, teratogenesis, infertility
Cyclosporine *Sandimmune*	Sandoz	5 mg/kg q12h PO	Sebaceous adenitis, PF, PE	Vomiting, diarrhea, gingival hyperplasia, B-lymphocyte hyperplasia, hirsutism, papillomatous skin lesions, increased incidence of infections, nephrotoxicity, hepatotoxicity

DLE, Discoid lupus erythematosus; PF, pemphigus foliaceus; PE, pemphigus erythematosus.

DRUGS (generic and trade)	MANUFACTURER	DOSAGE & ROUTE OF ADMINISTRATION (Topical, PO, SQ, IM, IV)	DISEASE	MAJOR SIDE EFFECTS
Cytosine arabinoside *Cytosar*	Upjohn	100 mg/m² IV or SQ on first 4 days of first treatment week only	Lymphosarcoma	Leukopenia
Dapsone *Avlosulfon*	Wyeth-Ayerst	1 mg/kg q12-24h PO	Vasculitis	Thrombocytopenia, anemia, granulocytopenia
Desoximetasone *Topicort*	Hoechst-Roussel	Topical q12-24h, then taper	Pruritus, localized allergy	Cutaneous atrophy, iatrogenic Cushing's
Dexamethasone	Generics	Pulse therapy, one to two treatments: 0.1 to 0.2 mg/kg q12h IV Maintenance: 0.05 to 0.1 mg q48-72h PO	Vasculitis, PF Inflammatory diseases	Gastrointestinal disturbances
Diazepam	Generics	1 to 2 mg added to calculated ketamine dose IV, IM	Sedative with ketamine for intradermal testing and ear flushes	Seizure with overdose
Diethylstilbestrol	Eli Lilly	0.1 to 1 mg q24h for 3 to 4 wk, then q3-4d PO	Ovarian imbalance type II	Bone marrow suppression, stimulation of estrus signs
Diflorasone diacetate *Psorcon*	Dermik	Topical q12-24h, then taper	Pruritus	Cutaneous atrophy iatrogenic Cushing's
Diphenhydramine hydrochloride *Benadryl*	Parke-Davis Generics	2.2 mg/kg q8h PO	Atopy	Drowsiness, hyperactivity
Domeboro	Miles	Topical	Pruritus, allergic dermatitis	
Doxepin HCl *Sinequan*	Roerig Generics	1 mg/kg q12h PO	Atopy	Drowsiness, hyperactivity, vomiting, diarrhea

Continued.

DRUGS (generic and trade)	MANUFACTURER	DOSAGE & ROUTE OF ADMINISTRATION (Topical, PO, SQ, IM, IV)	DISEASE	MAJOR SIDE EFFECTS
Doxorubicin *Adriamycin*	Adria	30 mg/m^2 IV q14d	Lymphosarcoma	Mast cell degranulation, myelosuppression, and cardiotoxicity
Duocide LA Flea Spray	Allerderm/ Virbac	Topical (see label restrictions)	Flea control	Clinical signs of pyrethrin or permethrin intoxication
DuraKyl Flea Dip	DVM	Topical (see label restrictions)	Flea control	Clinical signs of pyrethrin or rotenone intoxication
Duratrol (pet and premise)	3M	Topical and premise treatment (see label restrictions)	Flea control	Clinical signs of organophosphate intoxication
DVM Derm Caps	DVM	Regular: 1 cap/20 kg PO ES: 1 cap/40-60 kg PO	Atopy, dry skin, sebaceous adenitis	Diarrhea, weight gain
Efa Vet	Efamol	1 cap/9 kg q24h PO	Atopy, dry skin, sebaceous adenitis	Diarrhea, weight gain
Emollient/ emulsifier rinse *Alpha-Sesame Oil Dry Skin Rinse*	Veterinary Prescription	Topical emollient rinse and spray	Primary keratinization disorders (dry scale), secondary dry scale; also used to counteract drying effects of degreasing shampoos and flea-control products	Greasiness
Emollient rinse and spray *Sesame Oil Spray*	Veterinary Prescription	Topical emollient rinse and spray	Primary keratinization disorders (dry scale), secondary dry scaling, control drying associated with degreasing shampoos and flea-control products	Greasiness

DLE, Discoid lupus erythematosus; PF, pemphigus foliaceus; PE, pemphigus erythematosus.

DRUGS (generic and trade)	MANUFACTURER	DOSAGE & ROUTE OF ADMINISTRATION (Topical, PO, SQ, IM, IV)	DISEASE	MAJOR SIDE EFFECTS
Enilconazol *Imaveraol*	Janssen	Apply topically as 1:50 dilution rinse q3-4d	*Malassezia* dermatitis, dermatophytosis	Slight odor, irritation
Enrofloxacin *Baytril*	Haver	2.5 to 5 mg/kg q12h PO	Plasmacytic stomatitis, gram-negative otitis, *Pseudomonas* pyoderma	Vomiting, diarrhea, anorexia, polyarteritis in young dogs (<1 to 1½ yr)
Erythromycin stearate	Various	10 to 15 mg/kg q8h PO	Pyoderma	Vomiting (up to 50% incidence)
Erythromycin estolate	Various	10 to 15 mg/kg q8h PO	Pyoderma	
Etretinate *Tegison*	Hoffman-LaRoche	1 to 2 mg/kg q24h PO	See p. 206	Keratoconjunctivitis sicca, triglyceride elevation, musculoskeletal abnormalities, heptatoxicity, teratogenicity
Evening primrose oil (EPO)	Efamol	500 mg q12h PO	Allergies, sebaceous adenitis, keratinization disorders	Vomiting, diarrhea, flatulence
Ex Spot	Pitman-Moore	Topical (see label restrictions)	Flea control	Clinical signs of permethrin intoxication
Fluocinolone acetonide 0.01% *Synotic*	Syntex Animal Health	Topical	Otitis/allergy/localized immune-mediated disease	Cutaneous atrophy, iatrogenic Cushing's
Fluoxetine *Prozac*	Dista	1 mg/kg q24h PO	Atopy, acral pruritic nodules	Lethargy, wheals, polydipsia-polyuria
Gentamicin *Gentocin*	Schering	2 mg/kg q8-12h SQ, IM	Gram-negative pyoderma	Nephrotoxicity, ototoxicity, neurotoxicity

Continued.

DRUGS (generic and trade)	MANUFACTURER	DOSAGE & ROUTE OF ADMINISTRATION (Topical, PO, SQ, IM, IV)	DISEASE	MAJOR SIDE EFFECTS
Griseofulvin microsize				
Fulvicin U/F	Schering	25 to 60 mg/kg q12h PO	Dermatophytosis	
Grifulvin V	Ortho			Anorexia, vomiting, blood dyscrasias, thrombocytopenia, ataxia
Grisactin	Wyeth-Ayerst			
Griseofulvin ultramicrosize				
Gris-PEG	Herbert	2.5 to 5 mg/kg q12-24h PO	Dermatophytosis	
HB101 (Burow's solution)	Burns	Topical	Allergic otitis, localized allergic reactions	Irritancy (rare)
Hematoporphyrin derivatives (photofrin V)		5 mg/kg IV 48 to 72 hr prior to argon laser	Canine and feline squamous cell carcinoma	Urticaria, photoactivated reaction; avoid direct sunlight 30 days posttreatment
Human growth hormone		0.15 IU/kg q3-4d for 6 wk SQ	Growth hormone–responsive dermatosis	Diabetogenic
Humectant rinse and spray				
Micro Pearls Humectant Spray	EVSCO			
Humilac Dry Skin Spray and Rinse	Allerderm/ Virbac	Topical	Dry skin, primary keratinization disorders (dry skin), control drying associated with amitraz dips, degreasing shampoos, flea-control products	Greasiness
Humectant/ emollient rinse and spray				
*HyLyt*efa Bath Oil Coat Conditioner*	DVM			

DLE, Discoid lupus erythematosus; PF, pemphigus foliaceus; PE, pemphigus erythematosus.

DRUGS (generic and trade)	MANUFACTURER	DOSAGE & ROUTE OF ADMINISTRATION (Topical, PO, SQ, IM, IV)	DISEASE	MAJOR SIDE EFFECTS
Hydrocortisone, 0.5% to 2.5%	Generics			
Cortispray	DVM	Apply q12-24h for 10 days, then taper to q48-72h	Allergic otitis, localized allergic reaction (antipruritic)	Contact irritancy (rare)
Dermacool	Allerderm/ Virbac			
PTD-HC	Veterinary Prescription			
Hydroxyzine *Atarax*	Generics Roerig	2.2 mg/kg q8h PO	Atopy and insect allergy	Drowsiness, hyperactivity
*HyLyt*efa Shampoo*	DVM	Topical	Allergic skin diseases, primary keratinization disorders (dry scale), secondary dry scale	Contact irritancy (rare)
Hypoallergenic diets				See pp. 126, 131
Hyposensitization allergens	Greer, Center	Variable dose and frequency, SQ	Atopic disease, insect allergy	Pruritus, wheals, angioedema, anaphylaxis
Insect allergenic testing and hyposensitization	Greer	Various doses and frequencies	Insect allergy	Pruritus, allergic reactions
Iodide (super-saturated solution, KI)		Dogs: 40 mg/kg q8h PO	Sporotrichosis	Ocular and nasal discharge, dry coat with excess scales, vomiting, depression
		Cats: 20 mg/kg q12h PO	Sporotrichosis	Anorexia, vomiting, depression, twitching, hypothermia, cardiovascular failure
Iodine complex shampoo *Weladol*	Pitman-Moore	Topical	Pyoderma	Contact irritancy, staining of light-colored hair coats
Iodine solution (povidone-I)	Generics	Topical antiseptic	Pyoderma, dermatophytoses	Contact irritancy, staining of light-colored hair coats

Continued.

DRUGS (generic and trade)	MANUFACTURER	DOSAGE & ROUTE OF ADMINISTRATION (Topical, PO, SQ, IM, IV)	DISEASE	MAJOR SIDE EFFECTS
Isotretinoin *Accutane*	Hoffman-LaRoche	2 mg/kg q12h PO	Canine solar dermatitis	Keratoconjunctivitis sicca, triglyceride elevation, musculoskeletal abnormalities, heptatoxicity, teratogenicity
		1 to 2 mg/kg q24h PO	Schnauzer comedo syndrome, sebaceous adenitis, ichthyosis	
Ivermectin *Ivomec 1% injection*	MSD AgVet	0.25 mg/kg q14d SQ 2 or 3 times	Canine scabies, *Otodectes, Notoedres, Cheyletiella,*	**Not in collies;** mydriasis, depression, tremors, ataxia, coma, death
		0.25 mg/kg q7-14d SQ	*Demodex*	
Ketamine *Ketaset*	Fort Dodge	10 to 15 mg/kg IV, IM	Sedative with diazepam for intradermal testing and ear flushes	Seizure with overdose
Ketoconazole *Nizoral Cream*	Janssen	Topical, q12h	Sporotrichosis, dermatophytosis, *Malassezia* otitis, *Malassezia* dermatitis	
Nizoral Shampoo	Janssen	Topical (refer to label restrictions)		
Nizoral Tablets	Janssen	10 mg/kg q12h PO (Mason); q12-24h (Rosser)		Anorexia, pruritus, alopecia, lightening of coat color
Lactated Ringer's	Abbott	80 ml/kg (initial dose) IV	Replacing and maintaining fluid and electrolyte balance for severe drug reactions	Overhydration

DLE, Discoid lupus erythematosus; PF, pemphigus foliaceus; PE, pemphigus erythematosus.

DRUGS (generic and trade)	MANUFACTURER	DOSAGE & ROUTE OF ADMINISTRATION (Topical, PO, SQ, IM, IV)	DISEASE	MAJOR SIDE EFFECTS
Lactic acid lotion *LactiCare*	Stiefel	Topical	Idiopathic nasal hyperkeratosis, calluses, ear margin dermatosis	
Levamisole hydrochloride *Levasole*	Pitman-Moore	2.2 mg/kg q48h PO	Chronic recurrent pyoderma, eosinophilic feline dermatoses	Vomiting, diarrhea, neurotoxicity, granulocytopenia, drug reactions
Lime Sulfur *LymDyp*	DVM	Topical, 2% to 5% rinse q7d	Feline generalized demodicosis, canine scabies, dermatophytosis, *Cheyletiella*	Rare contact irritancy, will stain light hair coats yellow
Lincomycin hydrochloride *Lincocin*	Upjohn	22 mg/kg q12h PO	Pyoderma, plasmacytic stomatitis	Vomiting, diarrhea, colitis
Lysodren (*o,p'*-DDD)	Bristol Myers	Loading: 40 to 50 mg/kg q24h PO for 7 to 10 days or longer (see text for duration) (lower dose for large or diabetic dogs) Maintenance: 50 mg/kg weekly	Spontaneous hyperadrenocorticism	Vomiting, diarrhea, weakness, anorexia, hypoadrenocorticism
Malathion *Adams Flea & Tick Dip*	SmithKline-Beecham	Topical: dilute 0.25 oz per gallon H$_2$O q7d	Feline generalized demodicosis (resistant cases)	Organophosphate toxicity; not approved for use in cats
Megestrol acetate *Megace* *Ovaban*	Bristol Myers Schering	Induction: 2.5 to 5 mg q48h PO for 7 to 14 days Maintenance: 2.5 to 5 mg q7-14d PO	Eosinophilic feline dermatoses	Pyometra, diabetes mellitus, behavioral lethargy, weight gain, polydipsia, polyphagia, adrenocortical suppression, mammary gland hyperplasia, mammary gland neoplasia

Continued.

DRUGS (generic and trade)	MANUFACTURER	DOSAGE & ROUTE OF ADMINISTRATION (Topical, PO, SQ, IM, IV)	DISEASE	MAJOR SIDE EFFECTS
Melatonin	Rickards	2 mg q48h SQ for four injections, then q14d	Idiopathic acanthosis nigricans	Antigenic sensitization
Methylprednisolone *Medrol*	Upjohn	Induction: 0.8 to 1.5 mg/kg q12h PO Maintenance: taper to q48h	Eosinophilic feline dermatoses, plasmacytic stomatitis, PF, DLE, atopy, flea allergy dermatitis	Iatrogenic Cushing's
Methylprednisolone acetate *DepoMedrol*	Upjohn	Feline only: 4 mg/kg IM (with maximum of 20 mg)	Eosinophilic granuloma, feline flea-allergy dermatitis, plasmacytic stomatitis	Iatrogenic Cushing's
Methylprednisolone succinate *Solu-Delta Cortef*	Upjohn	Pulse therapy: 1 mg/kg IV, give one to two times	PF	Iatrogenic Cushing's
Methyltestosterone Oral	Generics	1 mg/kg q48h PO, not to exceed 30 mg, for 1 to 3 mo, then q3-4d	Hypoandrogenism of male dogs	Hepatotoxicity, aggression
Repositol	Generics	2 mg/kg q1-4m IM, not to exceed 30 mg		
Metronidazole *Flagyl*	Searle	10 to 20 mg/kg q12h PO	Plasmacytic stomatitis	Vomiting, diarrhea, anorexia
Metyrapone *Metopirone*	Ciba	Cats: 65 mg q8h PO	Spontaneous hyperadrenocorticism	Anorexia, hypoadrenocorticism

DLE, Discoid lupus erythematosus; PF, pemphigus foliaceus; PE, pemphigus erythematosus.

DRUGS (generic and trade)	MANUFACTURER	DOSAGE & ROUTE OF ADMINISTRATION (Topical, PO, SQ, IM, IV)	DISEASE	MAJOR SIDE EFFECTS
Miconazole cream, lotion *Conofite*	Pitman-Moore	Apply q12-24h	*Malassezia* dermatitis, *Malassezia* otitis externa	Potential for irritancy, ototoxicity
Miconazole, chlorhexidine, selenium shampoo *Sebolyse Foam*	Dermcare	Shampoo q3-4d initially, then q7d; 10 min soak	*Malassezia* dermatitis	Irritancy, dry skin
Milbemycin oxime *Interceptor*	Ciba	0.5 to 1 mg/kg q24h PO	Generalized demodicosis	Potential for neurologic abnormalities at high doses
Mupirocin *Bactoderm*	SmithKline-Beecham	Topical antibiotic ointment, q12h	Localized pyoderma	
Mycodex Aqua Spray	SmithKline-Beecham	Topical (see label restrictions)	Flea control	Clinical signs of pyrethrin intoxication
Mycodex 14 Day				Clinical signs of pyrethrin or permethrin intoxication
Naftifine cream *Naftin*	Herbert	Apply q12-24h	Dermatophytosis	
Ophthaine Solution	Solvay	0.5% proparacaine	Topical otic anesthesia	Ototoxicity, irritancy
Ormetoprim/ sulfadimethoxine *Primor*	Roche	55 mg/kg q24h PO day 1, then 27.5 mg/kg q24h PO	Pyoderma	Sulfonamide-induced systemic hypersensitivity

Continued.

DRUGS (generic and trade)	MANUFACTURER	USE	MAJOR SIDE EFFECTS
Otic ceruminolytics			
Cerumenex (triethanolamine polypeptide oleate condensate)	Purdue-Frederick	Otitis externa	Irritancy, ototoxicity
Cerusol (dioctyl calcium sulfosuccinate)	Burns	Otitis externa	Irritancy, ototoxicity
Clear-X Cleanser (dioctyl sodium sulfosuccinate, carbamide peroxide)	DVM	Otitis externa	Irritancy, ototoxicity
Murine Ear Wax Remover (carbamide peroxide)	Ross	Otitis externa	Irritancy, ototoxicity
Surfac (dioctyl sodium sulfosuccinate)	Upjohn	Otitis externa	Irritancy, ototoxicity
Otic cleansers (mild)			
Cerumene	EVSCO	Otitis externa	Irritancy, ototoxicity
Epi Otic	Allerderm/ Virbac	Otitis externa	Irritancy, ototoxicity
Gent-L-Clens	Schering	Otitis externa	Irritancy, ototoxicity
Oticare A	ARC	Otitis externa	Irritancy, ototoxicity
Oti-Clens	SmithKline-Beecham	Otitis externa	Irritancy, ototoxicity
Oti Fresh	Pan America	Otitis externa	Irritancy, ototoxicity
Otic disinfectants			
Acetic acid			
Clear-X Treatment Dryer	DVM	Bacterial otitis	Irritancy, ototoxicity
Otic Domeboro Solution	Miles	Bacterial otitis	Irritancy, ototoxicity
White vinegar and water	Generics	Bacterial otitis	Irritancy, ototoxicity
Chlorhexidine			
ChlorhexiDerm Otic	DVM	Bacterial otitis	Irritancy, ototoxicity
Nolvasan Otic	Fort Dodge	Bacterial otitis	Irritancy, ototoxicity
Solvaprep	Solvay	Bacterial otitis	Irritancy, ototoxicity
Otic drying agents			
Clear-X Treatment Dryer	DVM	Bacterial otitis	Irritancy, ototoxicity
Oticare B	ARC	Bacterial otitis	Irritancy, ototoxicity
Otic-Clear	Butler	Bacterial otitis	Irritancy, ototoxicity
Panodry	Solvay	Bacterial otitis	Irritancy, ototoxicity

DLE, Discoid lupus erythematosus; PF, pemphigus foliaceus; PE, pemphigus erythematosus.

DRUGS (generic and trade)	MANUFACTURER	USE	MAJOR SIDE EFFECTS
Otic therapeutic topicals			
Aurimite (pyrethrin, piperonyl butoxide)	Schering	Ear mites	Irritancy, ototoxicity
Canex (rotenone)		Ear mites	Irritancy, ototoxicity
Cerumite (pyrethrin)	EVSCO	Ear mites	Irritancy, ototoxicity
Clear-X Treatment Dryer (acetic acid, sulfur, hydrocortisone)	DVM	Otitis externa	Irritancy, ototoxicity
Conofite Lotion (miconazole)	Pitman-Moore	*Malassezia* otitis	Irritancy, ototoxicity
Forte Topical (penicillin procaine, neomycin, polymyxin oil suspension with hydrocortisone)	Upjohn	Bacterial otitis	Irritancy, ototoxicity
Fungizone Lotion (amphotericin B)	Squibb	*Candida* otitis	Irritancy, ototoxicity
Gentocin Otic (gentamicin sulfate, betamethasone valerate)	Schering	Combination treatment	Irritancy, ototoxicity
HB101 (1% hydrocortisone, Burow's solution)	Burns	Allergic otitis	Irritancy, ototoxicity
Liquichlor (chloramphenicol)	EVSCO	Combination treatment	Irritancy, ototoxicity
Mitox (carbaryl)	SmithKline-Beecham	Ear mites	Irritancy, ototoxicity
Oticare (pyrethrin)	ARC	Ear mites	Irritancy, ototoxicity
Panolog (triamcinolone acetonide, nystatin, neomycin, thiostrepton)	Solvay	Combination treatment	Irritancy, ototoxicity
Silvadene Cream (silver sulfadiazine)	Marion Merrell Dow	*Pseudomonas* otitis	Irritancy, ototoxicity
Synotic (dimethyl sulfoxide, fluocinolone acetonide)	Syntex	Allergic otitis	Irritancy, ototoxicity
Tresaderm (thiabendazole, neomycin, dexamethasone)	MSD-AgVet	Combination treatment	Irritancy, ototoxicity
Unitop (cuprimyxin)	Hoffman-LaRoche	Fungal/yeast otitis	Irritancy, ototoxicity

Continued.

DRUGS (generic and trade)	MANUFACTURER	DOSAGE & ROUTE OF ADMINISTRATION (Topical, PO, SQ, IM, IV)	DISEASE	MAJOR SIDE EFFECTS
Ovitrol Plus Pet Spray	VetKem	Topical (see label restrictions)	Flea control	Clinical signs of synergized pyrethrins or methoprene intoxication
Oxacillin *Oxacillin Capsules Rx*	Biocraft	22 mg/kg q8h PO	Pyoderma	Vomiting (rare), diarrhea, systemic hypersensitivity
Prostaphlin	Squibb			
Paramite Dip	VetKem	Topical (see label restrictions)	Flea control, canine scabies	Clinical signs of organophosphate intoxication
Permectrin Dip	Bio-Ceutic	Topical (see label restrictions)	Flea control	Clinical signs of permethrin (pyrethroid) intoxication
Permethrin insecticide	Generics	Topical	Flea control	See p. 65
Potassium permanganate	Generics	Dilution with H_2O 1:10,000 to 1:30,000 solution; swab topically with cotton-tipped applicator	Plasmacytic stomatitis	Painful, staining
Prednisolone or prednisone	Generics	Cats: Induction 4 to 5 mg/kg q24h PO Maintenance: 2 mg/kg q48h PO	Eosinophilic feline dermatoses	Iatrogenic Cushing's
		Dogs: Induction 0.5 to 1 mg/kg q24h PO Maintenance: lowest possible dose q48h PO	Atopy, allergic skin diseases, solar dermatitis	Iatrogenic Cushing's
		Dogs: Induction 2 mg/kg q24h PO Maintenance: taper thereafter q48h PO	Drug reactions	Iatrogenic Cushing's
		Dogs: Induction 1.1 to 3.3 mg/kg q12h PO for 14 days Maintenance: 0.5 to 2 mg/kg q48h PO	Autoimmune dermatoses (DLE, PF, etc.)	Iatrogenic Cushing's

DLE, Discoid lupus erythematosus; PF, pemphigus foliaceus; PE, pemphigus erythematosus.

DRUGS (generic and trade)	MANUFACTURER	DOSAGE & ROUTE OF ADMINISTRATION (Topical, PO, SQ, IM, IV)	DISEASE	MAJOR SIDE EFFECTS
ProBan	Miles	Tablet: 30 mg/10 kg q3-4d PO Liquid: 1 ml/5 kg q3-4d PO	Flea control	Clinical signs of organophosphate intoxication
ProSpot	Miles	Topical, 4 to 8 mg/kg q14d	Flea control	Clinical signs of organophosphate intoxication
Retinol	Various	625 to 800 IU/kg q24h PO	Vitamin A–responsive dermatosis	
Rifampin *Rifadin*	Marion Merrell Dow	5 to 10 mg/kg q24h PO	Chronic recurrent pyoderma with scarring	Hepatotoxicity, hemagglutination, gastrointestinal disorders
Rimactane	Ciba			
Rotenone *Goodwinol Ointment*	Goodwinol	Topical, 1% ointment, q24h	Localized demodicosis	Contact irritancy
Salicylic acid/urea/sodium lactate gel *KeraSolv*	DVM	Topical	Idiopathic nasal hyperkeratosis, calluses, ear margin dermatosis, chin acne of dogs and cats	Contact irritancy (rare)
Salicylic acid/alcohol *Stridex Pads*	Glenbrook	Regular (0.5%) and maximum strength (2%) for topical use	Chin acne of dogs and cats	Contact irritancy (due to alcohol content)
Science Diet w/d	Hill's	Low-fiber; use with fatty acid supplement	Atopy	
Science Diet Feline d/d	Hill's		Maintenance for feline food allergy	
Sectrol Two Way Pet Spray or Mousse	3M	Topical (see label restrictions)	Flea control	Clinical signs of pyrethrin intoxication

DRUGS (generic and trade)	MANUFACTURER	DOSAGE & ROUTE OF ADMINISTRATION (Topical, PO, SQ, IM, IV)	DISEASE	MAJOR SIDE EFFECTS
Sectrol Premise Spray	3M	Premise application (see label restrictions)	Flea control	Clinical signs of pyrethrin intoxication
Selenium sulfide shampoo *Seleen* *Selsun Blue*	Ceva Ross	Shampoo q3-7d	*Malassezia* dermatitis, primary keratinization disorders (greasy scale), secondary greasy scaling	Drying of coat, contact irritancy (rare); **not for use in cats**
Sodium hypochlorite (0.5%)	Clorox	Dilute 1:20 rinse q5-7d	Dermatophytosis	Discoloration of black animals, mucous membrane irritation when used in unventilated area
Staphage Lysate	Delmont	0.5 ml q3-4d or 1 ml q7d SQ	Chronic recurrent pyoderma	Vomiting, diarrhea, possible systemic hypersensitivity
Sulfasalazine *Azulfidine*	Pharmacia	22 to 44 mg/kg q48h PO	Vasculitis	Keratoconjunctivitis sicca
Sulfur/salicylic acid *SebaLyt* *Sebolux*	DVM Allerderm/ Virbac	Topical shampoo	Skin infections, keratinization defects (dry or waxy scale)	Contact irritancy (rare), excess drying (rare)
Sulfur/sodium salicylate *Sebbafon*	Upjohn	Topical shampoo		
Sunscreens (high SPF [15 +], water resistant)		Creams, ointments	Solar dermatitis, DLE, PE	If licked off, causes drooling
Bullfrog *Sundowner*	Chattem Pitman-Moore	Creams, ointments	Solar dermatitis, DLE, PE	If licked off, causes drooling
SynerKyl (Spray & Shampoo)	DVM	Topical (see label restrictions)	Flea control	Clinical signs of pyrethrin or permethrin intoxication

DLE, Discoid lupus erythematosus; PF, pemphigus foliaceus; PE, pemphigus erythematosus.

DRUGS (generic and trade)	MANUFACTURER	DOSAGE & ROUTE OF ADMINISTRATION (Topical, PO, SQ, IM, IV)	DISEASE	MAJOR SIDE EFFECTS
Tar shampoo *Clear Tar*	Veterinary Prescription	Topical	Primary keratinization disorders (greasy scale), secondary greasy scaling	Contact irritancy (rare), excessive drying (rare); **not for use in cats**
Pentrax	GenDerm	Topical	Primary keratinization disorders (greasy scale), secondary greasy scaling	Strong tar odor, contact irritancy (especially of hair follicles), excessive drying, potential to stain light-colored coats; **not for use in cats**
Tar/essential fatty acid *LyTar*efa Therapeutic Bath Oil Spray Conditioner*	DVM	Topical spray	Primary keratinization disorders (waxy or greasy scale), secondary waxy or greasy scaling	Contact irritancy (rare), excess drying (rare); **not for use in cats**
Tar/lactic acid *Micro Pearls Coal Tar Medicated Spray*	EVSCO	Topical spray	Primary keratinization disorders (waxy or greasy scale), secondary waxy or greasy scaling	Contact irritancy (rare), excess drying (rare); **not for use in cats**
Tar/salycylic acid/menthol *NuSal-T*	DVM	Topical shampoo	Primary keratinization disorders (waxy or greasy scale), secondary waxy or greasy scaling	Contact irritancy (rare), excess drying (rare); **not for use in cats**
Tar/sulfur/salicylic acid *Allerseb T* *LyTar* *Mycodex High Potency*	Allerderm/Virbac DVM SmithKline-Beecham	Topical shampoo	Primary keratinization disorders (greasy scale), secondary greasy scale	Strong tar odor, contact irritancy (especially hair follicles), shampoo causes excessive drying, potential to stain light-colored coats; **not for use in cats**

Continued.

DRUGS (generic and trade)	MANUFACTURER	DOSAGE & ROUTE OF ADMINISTRATION (Topical, PO, SQ, IM, IV)	DISEASE	MAJOR SIDE EFFECTS
Tar/sulfur/ sodium salicylate *T-Lux*	Allerderm/ Virbac	Topical shampoo	Primary keratinization disorders (waxy or greasy scale), secondary waxy or greasy scaling	Contact irritancy (rare), excess drying (rare); **not for use in cats**
Tetracycline	Generics	20 to 30 mg/kg q12h PO	Plasmacytic stomatitis	Vomiting, diarrhea
Tetracycline and niacinamide	Generics	Less than 10 kg: 250 mg q12h PO Greater than 10 kg: 500 mg q12h PO	DLE, PE	Vomiting, diarrhea, anorexia, hepatitis
Thiabendazole	MSD AgVet	5 mg/kg q48h PO	Eosinophilic feline dermatoses	Vomiting, diarrhea, neurotoxicity, granulocytopenia
Thiabendazole/ dexamethasone/ neomycin sulfate solution *Tresaderm*	MSD AgVet	Topical use only	Otitis externa, focal dermatophytosis	Systemic absorption of dexamethasone, contact drug reaction
L-Thyroxine *Synthroid* *Soloxine* *Thyro-Tab*	Boots Daniels Vet-A-Mix	Induction: 0.02 to 0.04 mg/kg q12h PO Maintenance: 0.04 mg/kg q24h PO	Hypothyroidism	Weight loss, hyperexcitability, gastritis
Toothpaste *CET Animal Toothpaste*	Veterinary Prescription	Topical, toothbrush	Plasmacytic stomatitis	Drooling
Tretinoin *Retin-A*	Ortho	Topical q12-24h 0.05% cream, 0.025% gel, 0.01% gel	Chin acne, idiopathic nasal hyperkeratosis, idiopathic ear margin dermatosis, acanthosis nigricans	Irritancy
Triamcinolone *Vetalog*	Squibb	Induction: 0.5 to 0.75 mg/kg q24h PO Maintenance: 0.1 to 0.2 mg/kg q48-72h PO	Eosinophilic feline dermatoses, allergic diseases, DLE, PE, PF	Iatrogenic Cushing's, diabetes mellitus

DLE, Discoid lupus erythematosus; PF, pemphigus foliaceus; PE, pemphigus erythematosus.

DRUGS (generic and trade)	MANUFACTURER	DOSAGE & ROUTE OF ADMINISTRATION (Topical, PO, SQ, IM, IV)	DISEASE	MAJOR SIDE EFFECTS
Trichlorfon *Neguvon Pour-On*	Haver	Topical: dilute to 3% aqueous, rinse entire body, q4d	Generalized demodicosis (resistant cases)	Organophosphate toxicity
Trimethoprim/ sulfadiazine *Ditrim*	Syntex	22 to 30 mg/kg q12h PO	Pyoderma, eosinophilic feline dermatoses, plasmacytic stomatitis	Polysystemic drug reaction, keratoconjunctivitis sicca, drooling, salivation, anorexia; vomiting and blood dyscrasia in cats
Tribrissen	Coopers			
Trimethoprim/ sulfamethoxazole	Generics	*see* Trimethoprim/ sulfadiazine		
Vincristine *Oncovin*	Eli Lilly	0.5 mg/m² IV q7d for 8 wk	Lymphosarcoma	Perivascular sloughing, constipation, diarrhea, peripheral neuropathy
Vitamin E (D,L alpha-tocopherol) *Aquasol E*	Generics	Oral: 400 to 800 IU q12h PO	DLE, PE	Gastrointestinal disturbances, rare coat color changes
		Oral: 200 mg q5h PO	Generalized demodicosis (resistant cases)	
		Topical: open capsule and apply to gums	Plasmacytic stomatitis	Drooling
Witch hazel *PTD lotion* *Dermacool*	Veterinary Prescription Allerderm/ Virbac	Topical	Allergic dermatitis	
Xylazine	Haver	0.3 to 0.6 mg/kg IV	Sedative for intradermal testing and ear flushes	Vomiting, arrhythmia, bradycardia
Zinc ascorbate	Generics	Topical, toothbrush or cotton-tipped applicator	Plasmacytic stomatitis	Drooling

Appendix B
Diagnostic Tests and Supplies

PART I

TEST	WHERE TO SEND	WHY PERFORMED
ACTH stimulation/ reproductive hormone panel	University of Tennessee College of Veterinary Medicine Dept. of Environmental Practice Clinical Endocrinology Lab VTH A105 Neyland Dr. Knoxville, TN 37916	Further evaluation of patients suspected of having growth hormone–responsive dermatosis; also of patients with castration-responsive dermatosis that relapses after castration
Cytology	Local laboratory, or learn to do in house	Determining whether bacteria or yeast are present, characterizing cellular makeup of pustular contents or surface exudates, establishing nature of otic exudates to identify perpetuating factors
Dermatopathology	Conroy, James D., D.V.M., Ph.D. Professor of Veterinary Pathology College of Veterinary Medicine Mississippi State University P.O. Box 5204 Mississippi State, MS 39762 (601) 325-3432 Dunstan, Robert W., D.V.M. Department of Pathology Michigan State University East Lansing, MI 48824 (517) 355-6504 (517) 355-1750 Goldschmidt, Michael H., V.M.D. School of Veterinary Medicine University of Pennsylvania 3850 Spruce Street Philadelphia, PA 19104 (215) 898-8861 Laboratory of Pathology 3800 Spruce Street Philadelphia, PA 19104 (215) 898-8857 (215) 898-7871 Gross, Thelma Lee, D.V.M. Dermatopathology Service 3911 W. Capital Ave. West Sacramento, CA 95691 (916) 372-4200	Histologic examination and evaluation of tissue samples

TEST	WHERE TO SEND	WHY PERFORMED
Dermatopathology—cont'd	Hargis, Ann Mae, D.V.M., M.S. 2244 Mukilteo Speedway Mukilteo, WA 98275 (206) 348-6781 Johnson, Gary R., D.V.M. Procter & Gamble 790 Compton Road Cincinnati, OH 45231 (513) 522-1883 Stannard, Anthony, D.V.M., Ph.D. Department of Medicine School of Veterinary Medicine University of California Davis, CA 95616 (916) 752-1363 Walder, Emily J., V.M.D. A & E Clinical Veterinary Lab. 11518 Pico Blvd. Los Angeles, CA 90064 (213) 477-9725	Histologic examination and evaluation of tissue samples
Direct immunofluorescence	University of California Davis, CA 95616 Cornell University Ithaca, NY 14853 Other veterinary universities	Detection of tissue immunoglobulins and complement
Fluorescent antibody for sporotrichosis	Centers for Disease Control 1600 Clifton Rd. N.W. Atlanta, GA 30333	Establishing diagnosis of sporotrichosis in dogs when cytologic examination of exudates, fungal cultures, and histopathologic examination of affected tissues all have been negative for *Sporothrix schenckii* and one is still suspicious of the disease
GnRH response	Serum samples for estradiol, progesterone, and testosterone to appropriately equipped lab	Further evaluation of a patient suspected of having castration-responsive dermatosis that has normal basal levels of estradiol, progesterone, and testosterone
Growth hormone stimulation/xylazine response	Currently unavailable	Aid in diagnosis of growth hormone–responsive dermatosis
Immunoperoxidase	Colorado State University Fort Collins, CO 80521 (other veterinary universities)	Detection of tissue immunoglobulins and complement
In vitro allergy RAST (K-9 RAST test)	Spectrum Laboratories Mesa, AZ 85202	Diagnosing atopic disease

Continued.

TEST	WHERE TO SEND	WHY PERFORMED
EIA (liquid phase)	Veterinary Allergy Reference Laboratories Pasadena, CA 91114	Diagnosing atopic disease and insect hypersensitivity
ELISA		
AREST test	Bioproducts DVM, Inc. Tempe, AZ 85282	Diagnosing atopic disease
Pet ELISA	Bio Medical Services, Inc. Austin, TX 78759	Diagnosing atopic disease
Serum testing	Greer Laboratories Lenoir, NC 28645	Diagnosing atopic disease
Intradermal allergy	Local or regional veterinary dermatologist/allergist or develop technique in house	Diagnosing atopic disease or insect hypersensitivity

PART II

INSTRUMENT/PRODUCT	SOURCE (Manufacturer, city, state)	HOW USED
ACTH		
Acthar Gel	Rhone-Poulenc Rorer Collegeville, PA 19426	ACTH stimulation test
Cortrosyn	Organon, Inc. West Orange, NJ 07052	
Cosyntropin	Organon, Inc. West Orange, NJ 07052	ACTH stimulation test–reproductive hormone panel (see p. 289)
Acuderm biopsy punch *Acu-Punch*	Acuderm, Inc. Ft. Lauderdale, FL 33309	Collection of skin biopsy samples
Bacterial transport medium (modified Amies)	Various	Transportation of specimens (exudate and tissue) for aerobic bacterial culture
Baker biopsy punch	Baker Cummins Dermatologicals, Inc. Miami, FL 33178	Collection of skin biopsy samples
Buck ear curettes	Edward Weck & Co. Weck Drive, P.O. Box 12600 Research Triangle Park, NC 27709	Ear canal cleansing
Dermatophyte test medium	Baker Cummins Dermatologicals, Inc. Miami, FL 33178	Identification of dermatophytes
Derm-Duet	Bactilab P.O. Box 1179 Mountain View, CA 94042	Fungal culture medium

INSTRUMENT/PRODUCT	SOURCE (Manufacturer, city, state)	HOW USED
Dexamethasone	Various	Dexamethasone suppression test
Diff-Quik stain set (*Wright's Dip Stat*)	American Scientific Products McGaw Park, IL 60085 Medi-Chem, Inc. P.O. Box 445 Santa Monica, CA 90404	Rapid differential stain for examination of hematology cells, inflammatory cells from tissue and exudate, and microbial organisms
Dextrose–Saboraud agar with chloraphenicol and gentamicin	Various	*Malassezia* growth medium
Feeding tubes (no. 6, 8, 12 French)	Various	Ear flushing
Feline food elimination diet		Test/elimination diet
Feline d/d	Hill's Pet Products Division, Colgate-Palmolive Co. Topeka, KS 66601	Maintenance diet for food-allergic cats
Lamb or ham baby food	Local grocery	Test or elimination diet; 1 to 2 jars/day Gerber baby food; no other food source; rechallenge 4 to 6 wk
Flea antigen test kit	Greer Laboratories Lenoir, NC 28645	Flea allergy test
Frazier suction tip	Edward Weck & Co. Weck Drive, P.O. Box 12600 Research Triangle Park, NC 27709	Deep ear canal and middle ear cleansing with suction apparatus
Fungal culture plates (*Sub-Duet*)	Bacti-Lab P.O. Box 1179 Mountain View, CA 94042	Growth and identification of dermatophytes
Gomori methenamine stain	Local histopathology laboratory	Identification of yeasts and fungi on histopathology
Gonadotropin releasing hormone (GnRH) *Cystorelin*	Abbott Laboratories North Chicago, IL 60064	GnRH response test: collect baseline serum samples for estradiol, progesterone, and testosterone; give 0.045 µg/kg; collect serum samples at 1 and 2 hr postinjection
Gram stain	Local microbiology laboratory	Bacterial identification
Halogen otoscope	Welch Allyn State Street Rd. Skaneateles Falls, NY 13153-0220	Ear cleansing
Intradermal skin testing	Greer Laboratories Lenoir, NC 28645	Intradermal injections to check for immediate hypersensitivities

Continued.

INSTRUMENT/PRODUCT	SOURCE (Manufacturer, city, state)	HOW USED
Lactophenol cotton blue stain	Medi-Chem, Inc. P.O. Box 445 Santa Monica, CA 90404	Stain dermatophytes macroconidia
Michel's solution (medium)	WAMPO Cranberry, NJ 08512 Zeus Scientific, Inc. Raritan, NJ 08869	Tissue sample fixation for direct immunofluorescence: can be held for several months
MacKenzie brush technique (toothbrush)		Identification of affected cats
Otic bulb syringe	Davol, Inc. 100 Sockanossett Crossroad Cranston, RI 02920	Ear flushing (identify yeasts, fungal elements)
Otoscope cone	Welch Allyn State Street Rd. Skaneateles Falls, NY 13153-0220	Ear examination
Periodic acid–Schiff (PAS)	Local histopathology laboratory	Identification of fungal yeast elements
Potassium hydroxide 10%	Medi-Chem, Inc. P.O. Box 445 Santa Monica, CA 90404	Direct examination of fungal elements
Suction apparatus	Schuco Co. Division of American Caduceus Toledo, OH 43608	Ear cleansing, especially middle ears
Surgical otoscope head	Welch Allyn State Street Rd. Skaneateles Falls, NY 13153-0220	Otic examination, also visualization during cleansing procedures
Thyroid stimulating hormone *Dermathycin* *TSH*	Pitman-Moore Mundelein, IL 60060 Sigma Chemical Co. St. Louis, MO 63178	TSH response test
Water flow diffuser		Ear cleansing
Water Pic	Teledyne 1730 E. Prospect Rd. Ft. Collins, CO 80553	Ear cleansing
Wood's lamp	Burton Medical Products, Inc. Van Nyes, CA 91406	Rapid screening for *Microsporum canis*
Xylazine *Rompun*	Haver/Miles Agriculture Division Animal Health Products Shawnee, KS 66201	Growth hormone stimulation test or xylazine response test

Appendix C
Drug Company Addresses

MANUFACTURER	LOCATION	CITY, STATE, ZIP CODE
Acuderm, Inc.	5370 NW 35 Terrace	Ft. Lauderdale, Fl 33309
Adria Laboratories	7001 Post Rd.	Dublin, OH 43017
Allerderm/Virbac	P.O. Drawer 277	Hurst, TX 76053
Anthony Products	5600 Peck Rd.	Arcadia, CA 91006
ARC Laboratories	P.O. Box 18884	Irvine, CA 92713
Avco Company	800 5th St. N.W.	Fort Dodge, IA 66201
Baxter Healthcare Corporation Scientific Products Division	1210 Waukegan Rd.	McGaw Park, IL 60085-6787
Bio-Ceutic (Boehringer Ingelheim Animal Health, Inc.)	2621 N. Belt Hwy.	St. Joseph, MO 64506
Biocraft Laboratories	92 Route 46	Elmwood Park, NJ 07407
Bio Medical Services, Inc.	3921 Steck Ave., Suite A101	Austin, TX 78759
Bioproducts DVM, Inc.	2405 S. Industrial Park Dr.	Tempe, AZ 85282-1804
Boots Pharmaceuticals, Inc.	300 Tri-State International Center, Suite 200	Lincolnshire, IL 60069
Bristol Myers Oncology Division of Bristol Myers Squibb Co.	2400 W. Lloyd Expwy.	Evansville, IN 47721
Burns Veterinary Supply	2019 McKenzie Dr., Suite 109	Carrollton, TX 75006
Burroughs Wellcome Co.	3030 Cornwallis Rd.	Research Triangle Park, NC 27709
Center Laboratories Division of EM Industries, Inc.	35 Channel Dr.	Port Washington, NY 11050
Ceva Laboratories	10551 Barkley, Suite 500	Overland Park, KS 66212
Clorox Company		Oakland, CA 94612
Ciba-Geigy Animal Health	P.O. Box 18300	Greensboro, NC 27419

Continued.

MANUFACTURER	LOCATION	CITY, STATE, ZIP CODE
Ciba Pharmaceutical Co. Division Ciba-Geigy Corporation	556 Morris Ave.	Summit, NJ 07901
Coopers Animal Health	421 E. Hawley St.	Mundelein, IL 60060
Daniels Pharmaceuticals, Inc.	2517 25th Ave. N.	St. Petersburg, FL 33713
Delmont Laboratories	P.O. Box 269	Swarthmore, PA 19081-0269
Dermcare Veterinary Scientifics Proprietary, Ltd.	3331 Pacific Hwy.	Springwood 4127 Australia
Dermik	920A Harvest Dr.	Blue Bell, PA 19422
DVM Pharmaceuticals	8785 N.W. 13th Terrace	Miami, FL 33172-3013
Eli Lilly & Co.	Lilly Corporate Center	Indianapolis, IN 46206
EVSCO Pharmaceutical Corporation	P.O. Box 209, Harding Hwy.	Buena, NJ 08310
Fort Dodge Laboratories, Inc.	800 Fifth St.	Ft. Dodge, IA 50501
GenDerm Corporation	425 Huehl Rd.	Northbrook, IL 60062
Glenbrook Laboratories	90 Park Ave.	New York, NY 10016
Goodwinol Products Corporation		Pierce, CO 80650
Greer Laboratories	P.O. Box 800	Lenoir, NC 28645
Haver/Miles Agriculture Division, Animal Health Products	P.O. Box 390	Shawnee, KS 66201
Herbert Laboratories, Dermatology Division of Allergan, Inc.	2525 Dupont Dr.	Irvine, CA 92715
Hill's Pet Products Division Colgate-Palmolive Co.	P.O. Box 148	Topeka, KS 66601
Hoechst-Roussel	Route 202-206, P.O. Box 2500	Somerville, NJ 00876-1258
The Iams Company	P.O. Box 862	Lewiston, OH 45338
ImmunoVet	5910-G Breckenridge Pkwy.	Tampa, FL 33610
Janssen Pharmaceutica, Inc.	40 Kingsbridge Rd.	Piscataway, NJ 08854
Lick Your Chops	50 Water St.	South Norwalk, CT 06854
Marion Merrell Dow	9300 Ward Pkwy., P.O. Box 8480	Kansas City, MO 64114-0480
Merck, Sharp & Dohme Division of Merck & Co., Inc.		Westpoint, PA 19486

MANUFACTURER	LOCATION	CITY, STATE, ZIP CODE
Miles, Inc. Pharmaceutical Division	400 Morgan Lane	West Haven, CT 06516
MSD AgVet Division of Merck & Co., Inc.	P.O. Box 2000	Rahway, NJ 07065-0912
Natural Life Pet Products, Inc.	12975 16th Ave. North, Suite 100-B	Minneapolis, MN 55441
Nature's Recipe		Corona, CA 91720
Nor-Am Chemical Co.	3509 Silverside Rd.	Wilmington, DE 19810
Nutro Products, Inc.	445 Wilson Way	City of Industry, CA 91744
Organon, Inc.	375 Mt. Pleasant Ave.	West Orange, NJ 07052
Ortho Consumer Products Division Chevron Chemical Co.	P.O. Box 5047	San Ramon, CA 94583-0947
Ortho Pharmaceutical Corporation Dermatological Division	Route 202, P.O. Box 300	Raritan, NJ 08869-0602
Parke Davis Division of Warner-Lambert Co.	201 Taboy Rd.	Morris Plains, NY 07950
Pharmacia, Inc.	P.O. Box 1327	Piscataway, NJ 08855-1327
Pitman-Moore	421 E. Hawley St.	Mundelein, IL 60060
The Protocol Group	P.O. Box 430	Siloam Springs, AR 72761
The Purdue-Frederick Company	100 Connecticut Ave.	Norwalk, CT 06856
Rhone-Poulenc Rorer	500 Arcola Rd.	Collegeville, PA 19426
Rickards Research Foundation	18235 Euclid Ave.	Cleveland, OH 44112
Roerig Division Pfizer, Inc.	235 E. 42nd St.	New York, NY 10017
Roche Animal Health & Nutrition Hoffman–La Roche	340 Kingsland St.	Nutley, NJ 07110
Ross Laboratories Division of Abbott Laboratories	625 Cleveland Ave.	Columbus, OH 43216
Royal Canin USA, Inc.	1600 Heritage Landing, Suite 112	St. Charles, MO 63303
Rydell Laboratories		Racine, WI 53403
Sandoz Pharmaceuticals Corporation Dorsey Division	59 Route 10	East Hanover, NJ 07936

Continued.

MANUFACTURER	LOCATION	CITY, STATE, ZIP CODE
Schering-Plough Animal Health Division	27 Commerce Dr.	Cranford, NJ 07016
Sigma Chemical Co.	P.O. Box 14508	St. Louis, MO 63178
SmithKline-Beecham Animal Health	812 Springdale Dr.	Exton, PA 19341
Smith Kline & French	1500 Spring Garden St., P.O. Box 7929	Philadelphia, PA 19101
Solvay Animal Health	1201 Northland Dr.	Mendota Heights, MN 55120
Spectrum Laboratories, Inc.	1833 W. Main St., Suite 139	Mesa, AZ 85202
E.R. Squibb & Sons	P.O. Box 4000	Princeton, NJ 08543-4000
Stiefel Laboratories, Inc.	2801 Ponce De Leon Blvd.	Coral Gables, FL 33134
Syntex Animal Health	4800 Westown Pkwy., Suite 200	West Des Moines, IA 50265
3M Animal Care Products	Building 225-1N-07, 3M Center	St. Paul, MN 55144
Upjohn Company Animal Health Division	7000 Portage Rd.	Kalamazoo, MI 49001
Vet-A-Mix, Inc.	604 W. Thomas Ave.	Shenandoah, IA 51601
Veterinary Allergy Reference Laboratories	P.O. Box 41059	Pasadena, CA 91114-9982
Veterinary Prescription Division of St Jon Laboratories	1656 W. 240th St.	Harbor City, CA 90710
VetKem Division of Zoecon Corporation	12200 Denton Dr.	Dallas, TX 75234
Wyeth-Ayerst Laboratories	P.O. Box 8299	Philadelphia, PA 19101
Wysong Medical Corporation	1880 North Eastman	Midland, MI 48640

Index

Italicized page number denotes boxed summary; *t*, table.

Italicized page number denotes boxed summary; *t*, table.

Italicized page number denotes boxed summary; *t*, table.

Italicized page number denotes boxed summary; *t*, table.

Italicized page number denotes boxed summary; *t*, table.

Italicized page number denotes boxed summary; *t*, table.

Italicized page number denotes boxed summary; *t*, table.

Italicized page number denotes boxed summary; *t*, table.

Italicized page number denotes boxed summary; *t*, table.

Italicized page number denotes boxed summary; *t*, table.

Italicized page number denotes boxed summary; *t*, table.

Italicized page number denotes boxed summary; *t*, table.

Italicized page number denotes boxed summary; *t*, table.

Italicized page number denotes boxed summary; *t*, table.

Italicized page number denotes boxed summary; *t*, table.